Thoracic Oncology

Thoracic Oncology

Editor: Neil Thomas

AMERICAN
MEDICAL PUBLISHERS
www.americanmedicalpublishers.com

AMERICAN
MEDICAL PUBLISHERS
www.americanmedicalpublishers.com

Cataloging-in-Publication Data

Thoracic oncology / edited by Neil Thomas.
p. cm.
Includes bibliographical references and index.
ISBN 979-8-88740-571-1
1. Chest--Cancer. 2. Chest--Tumors. 3. Lungs--Cancer. I. Thomas, Neil.
RC280.C5 T46 2023
616.994 94--dc23

American Medical Publishers,
41 Flatbush Avenue,
1st Floor, New York,
NY 11217, USA

ISBN 979-8-88740-571-1 (Hardback)

Contents

Preface ... IX

Chapter 1 **Immune Checkpoint Blockade Therapy may be a Feasible Option for Primary Pulmonary Lymphoepithelioma-Like Carcinoma** ... 1
Zuohong Wu, Xinghong Xian, Ke Wang, Deyun Cheng, Weimin Li and Bojiang Chen

Chapter 2 **First-Line Treatment Options for PD-L1–Negative Non-Small Cell Lung Cancer: A Bayesian Network Meta-Analysis** ... 8
Ling Peng, Wen-Hua Liang, De-Guang Mu, Song Xu, Shao-Dong Hong, Justin Stebbing, Fei Liang and Yang Xia

Chapter 3 **KRAS-Mutant Non-Small Cell Lung Cancer: An Emerging Promisingly Treatable Subgroup** ... 17
Mingying Xie, Xiaoling Xu and Yun Fan

Chapter 4 **Peripheral Lung Squamous Carcinoma with ROS1 Rearrangement Sensitive to Crizotinib** ... 28
Guangdie Yang, Jie Wang, Yinan Yao, Jun Zhao, Zheyan Yu, Qiqi Gao, Jiani Ye and Wenjiang Ma

Chapter 5 **The Efficacy and Safety of Anlotinib Combined with PD-1 Antibody for Third-Line or Further-Line Treatment of Patients with Advanced Non-Small-Cell Lung Cancer** ... 32
Chongya Zhai, Xiaoling Zhang, Lulu Ren, Liangkun You, Qin Pan, Hongming Pan and Weidong Han

Chapter 6 **Peripheral Blood Autoantibodies Against to Tumor-Associated Antigen Predict Clinical Outcome to Immune Checkpoint Inhibitor-Based Treatment in Advanced Non-Small Cell Lung Cancer** ... 40
Juan Zhou, Jing Zhao, Qingzhu Jia, Qian Chu, Fei Zhou, Xiangling Chu, Wencheng Zhao, Shengxiang Ren, Caicun Zhou and Chunxia Su

Chapter 7 **Molecular Characteristics of Genes and the Immune Microenvironment of a Rare Chest Malignant Tumor (Pulmonary Clear Cell Sarcoma)** ... 48
Xiaoling Xu, Ding Wang, Wei Wu and Hongyang Lu

Chapter 8 **Clinical Relevance of PD-L1 Expression and CD8+ T Cells' Infiltration in Patients with Lung Invasive Mucinous Adenocarcinoma** ... 53
Xiaoling Xu, Na Li, Ding Wang, Wei Chen and Yun Fan

Chapter 9 **The Effect of Asymptomatic and/or Treated Brain Metastases on Efficacy of Immune Checkpoint Inhibitors in Metastatic Non–Small Cell Lung Cancer** ... 61
Sihan Li, Hongwei Zhang, Tingting Liu, Jun Chen and Jun Dang

Chapter 10 **PD-L1 Test-Based Strategy with Nivolumab as the Second-Line Treatment in Advanced NSCLC: A Cost-Effectiveness Analysis in China** 72
Qiao Liu, Xia Luo, Zhen Zhou, Liubao Peng, Lidan Yi, Xiaomin Wan, Chongqing Tan and Xiaohui Zeng

Chapter 11 **Pre-Treatment Tumor Growth Rate Predicts Clinical Outcomes of Patients with Advanced Non-Small Cell Lung Cancer Undergoing Anti-PD-1/PD-L1 Therapy** 82
Li-na He, Xuanye Zhang, Haifeng Li, Tao Chen, Chen Chen, Yixin Zhou, Zuan Lin, Wei Du, Wenfeng Fang, Yunpeng Yang, Yan Huang, Hongyun Zhao, Shaodong Hong and Li Zhang

Chapter 12 **Efficacy of Combination Chemo-Immunotherapy as a First-Line Treatment for Advanced Non-Small-Cell Lung Cancer Patients with HER2 Alterations** 92
Shuang Zhao, Xinghong Xian, Panwen Tian, Weimin Li, Ke Wang and Yalun Li

Chapter 13 **Development and Validation of a Nomogram for Predicting Prognosis to Immune Checkpoint Inhibitors Plus Chemotherapy in Patients with Non-Small Cell Lung Cancer** 98
Hao Zeng, Wei-wei Huang, Yu-jie Liu, Qin Huang, Sheng-min Zhao, Ya-lun Li, Pan-wen Tian and Wei-min Li

Chapter 14 **Combination of Immune Checkpoint Inhibitors and Anti-Angiogenic Agents in Brain Metastases from Non-Small Cell Lung Cancer** 110
Likui Fang, Wuchen Zhao, Bo Ye and Da Chen

Chapter 15 **A Computed Tomography-Derived Radiomics Approach for Predicting Uncommon EGFR Mutation in Patients with NSCLC** 119
Wufei Chen, Yanqing Hua, Dingbiao Mao, Hao Wu, Mingyu Tan, Weiling Ma, Xuemei Huang, Jinjuan Lu, Cheng Li and Ming Li

Chapter 16 **Age-Associated Changes in Adverse Events Arising from Anti-PD-(L)1 Therapy** 127
Xinyi Huang, Tiantian Tian, Yan Zhang, Shengjian Zhou, Pingping Hu and Jiandong Zhang

Chapter 17 **Blood Tumor Mutational Burden as a Predictive Biomarker in Patients with Advanced Non-Small Cell Lung Cancer (NSCLC)** 135
Yuhui Ma, Quan Li, Yaxi Du, Jingjing Cai, Wanlin Chen, Guangqiang Zhao, Xing Liu, Hongsheng Li, Luyao Ma, Yunchao Huang and Yongchun Zhou

Chapter 18 **Pembrolizumab Alone or Combined with Chemotherapy in Advanced NSCLC with PD-L1 ≥50%: Results of a Retrospective Study** 143
Ya Chen, Yanan Wang, Zhengyu Yang, Minjuan Hu, Yanwei Zhang, Fangfei Qian, Wei Zhang, Bo Zhang and Baohui Han

Chapter 19 **Efficacy and Safety of Anlotinib in the Treatment of Small Cell Lung Cancer** 151
Jing Yuan, Feng Cheng, Guodong Xiao, Xiaofeng Wang and Huijie Fan

Chapter 20 **Pembrolizumab Plus Chemotherapy or Anlotinib *vs.* Pembrolizumab Alone in Patients with Previously Treated EGFR-Mutant NSCLC** 159
Ya Chen, Zhengyu Yang, Yanan Wang, Minjuan Hu, Bo Zhang, Yanwei Zhang, Fangfei Qian, Wei Zhang and Baohui Han

Chapter 21 **Efficacy and Safety of Anti-PD-1 Plus Anlotinib in Patients with Advanced Non–Small-Cell Lung Cancer after Previous Systemic Treatment Failure....168**
Peiliang Wang, Xiaozhuang Fang, Tianwen Yin, Hairong Tian, Jinming Yu and Feifei Teng

Chapter 22 **A Combination of Cytokine-Induced Killer Cells with PD-1 Blockade and ALK Inhibitor Showed Substantial Intrinsic Variability Across Non-Small Cell Lung Cancer Cell Lines....176**
Yutao Li, Amit Sharma, Xiaolong Wu, Hans Weiher, Dirk Skowasch, Markus Essler and Ingo G. H. Schmidt-Wolf

Chapter 23 **Immunotherapy in Non-Small Cell Lung Cancer with Actionable Mutations other than *EGFR*....189**
Karan Seegobin, Umair Majeed, Nathaniel Wiest, Rami Manochakian, Yanyan Lou and Yujie Zhao

Chapter 24 **Considerations for the Surgical Management of Thoracic Cancers during the COVID-19 Pandemic: Rational Strategies for Thoracic Surgeons....202**
Jiahao Zhang, Yichao Han, Yajie Zhang, Dong Dong, Yuqin Cao, Xiang Chen and Hecheng Li

Chapter 25 **Homozygous Co-Deletion of Type I Interferons and *CDKN2A* Genes in Thoracic Cancers: Potential Consequences for Therapy....209**
Marion Grard, Camille Chatelain, Tiphaine Delaunay, Elvire Pons-Tostivint, Jaafar Bennouna and Jean-François Fonteneau

Chapter 26 **How to Better Understand the Influence of Host Genetics on Developing an Effective Immune Response to Thoracic Cancers....216**
Kiarash Behrouzfar, Kimberley Burton, Steve E. Mutsaers, Grant Morahan, Richard A. Lake and Scott A. Fisher

Chapter 27 **A Panel of Five-lncRNA Signature as a Potential Biomarker for Predicting Survival in Gastric and Thoracic Cancers....227**
Jiayue Shao, Wei Lyu, Jiehao Zhou, Wenhui Xu, Dandan Wang, Shanshan Liang, Jiayin Zhao and Yujing Qin

Permissions

List of Contributors

Indexe

Preface

In my initial years as a student, I used to run to the library at every possible instance to grab a book and learn something new. Books were my primary source of knowledge and I would not have come such a long way without all that I learnt from them. Thus, when I was approached to edit this book; I became understandably nostalgic. It was an absolute honor to be considered worthy of guiding the current generation as well as those to come. I put all my knowledge and hard work into making this book most beneficial for its readers.

Oncology is a branch of medicine that deals with the study, diagnosis, treatment and prevention of cancer. Thoracic oncology is a sub-specialty of oncology that focuses on cancers of the lung, mediastinum, esophagus and pleura. It deals with malignancies like mesothelioma, esophageal cancer, small cell lung cancer and non-small lung cancer. Thoracic cancer refers to any cancer located in the organs, glands, or structures of thoracic cavity, or chest. Its major types are lung cancer and esophageal cancer, while thymus cancer and pleural cancer are among its less common forms. The field of thoracic oncology is extensively involved in the research aimed at the development of more effective treatments for thoracic cancer. Some current therapies and treatment in thoracic oncology are chemotherapy, radiation therapy and surgical procedures. This book contains some path-breaking studies in the field of thoracic oncology. A number of latest researches have been included to keep the readers up-to-date with the global concepts in this area of study. Researchers and students actively engaged in this field will find this book full of crucial and unexplored concepts.

I wish to thank my publisher for supporting me at every step. I would also like to thank all the authors who have contributed their researches in this book. I hope this book will be a valuable contribution to the progress of the field.

Editor

1

Immune Checkpoint Blockade Therapy may be a Feasible Option for Primary Pulmonary Lymphoepithelioma-Like Carcinoma

Zuohong Wu[1†], *Xinghong Xian*[2†], *Ke Wang*[1], *Deyun Cheng*[1], *Weimin Li*[1] *and Bojiang Chen*[1*]

[1] *Department of Respiratory and Critical Care Medicine, West China Hospital of Sichuan University, Chengdu, China,*
[2] *West China School of Medicine, Sichuan University, Chengdu, China*

Correspondence:
Bojiang Chen
cjhcbj@gmail.com

[†]*These authors have contributed equally to this work*

Primary pulmonary lymphoepithelioma-like carcinoma (PPLELC) is a rare subtype of non-small cell lung cancer (NSCLC) for which there is currently no recognized treatment. Recently, favorable immune checkpoint blockade responses have been observed in PPLELC. This study aimed to review the effects of this regimen in patients with advanced PPLELC. PPLELC patients treated with immune checkpoint inhibitors at West China Hospital between January 2008 and December 2019 were retrospectively identified. Demographic parameters and antitumor treatment details were retrieved and reviewed. Among 128 patients diagnosed with PPLELC, 5 who received immune checkpoint inhibitors at advanced stages were included in the analysis. All of these patients were female nonsmokers with a median age of 55.6 (range 53-58) years at diagnosis. Their median PD-L1 expression was 40% (range, 30-80%). Although the patients underwent surgeries, chemotherapy and radiotherapy, all the treatments failed. Immune checkpoint inhibitors were administered palliatively, and three patients responded favorably, with the best overall response being partial remission (PR). Thus, immune checkpoint inhibitors may be a promising treatment for advanced PPLELC, and large clinical trials are warranted to obtain more evidence regarding this regimen.

Keywords: lung cancer, primary pulmonary lymphoepithelioma-like carcinoma, treatment, immune checkpoint inhibitors, immunotherapy

INTRODUCTION

Primary pulmonary lymphoepithelioma-like carcinoma (PPLELC) is a rare subtype of non-small cell lung cancer (NSCLC) that was first described by Begin et al. in 1987 (1). In the latest 2015 World Health Organization classification, PPLELC is categorized under "other and unclassified carcinomas" (2). Due to its rarity, the reported cases of PPLELC mainly occur in Southeast Asia and are believed to be associated with Epstein-Barr virus (EBV) infection (3).

Programmed cell death-1 (PD-1) is a member of the B7 family that is expressed by activated T cells along with its ligand, i.e., programmed death-ligand 1 (PD-L1), to mediate immunoregulation (4). PD-L1 is another immune checkpoint cell-surface protein that is expressed by tumor cells and host cells (5). The interaction between PD-1 in T cells and PD-L1 in tumor cells leads to inhibition of the proliferation of activated T cells (6). Thus, the inhibition of this interaction *in vivo* contributes to the enhancement of T-cell responses and can have antitumor activity (7).

Prior studies have shown higher than average expression of PD-L1 in PPLELC, which is also high compared with that in conventional NSCLCs (8, 9). Therefore, the high expression of PD-L1 in PPLELC suggests the potential benefit of using immunotherapy in this subtype of lung cancer. Currently, there has been no recognized treatment for PPLELC. Most patients diagnosed with PPLELC often present in early stages, and complete resection is performed (10). However, for advanced cases, multimodal therapy, including systematic chemotherapy and radiotherapy, is often needed (11). Recently, immune checkpoint inhibitors have emerged as treatment targets for NSCLCs, and favorable treatment responses against PPLELC have been reported (12–14).

In the present study, we enrolled patients with advanced PPLELC who underwent immune checkpoint blockade therapy with the aim of reviewing our preliminary experience with the use of this regimen in patients with advanced PPLELC.

MATERIALS AND METHODS

This retrospective study included patients with histologically confirmed PPLELC at West China Hospital between January 2008 and December 2019. The patients were identified through hospital pathological and medical electronic databases, and records regarding demographic parameters, clinical manifestations, laboratory test results, chest computed tomography (CT) features, diagnostic methods, antitumor treatment and treatment reactions were simultaneously retrieved. All eligible patients received immunotherapy as the treatment for PPLELC and were followed up until June 30, 2020.

The pathological diagnosis of PPLELC was based on a combination of hematoxylin-eosin (HE) and immunohistochemical (IHC) staining and Epstein-Barr encoding region (EBER) positivity of lung tissue resections, and all patients underwent CT, magnetic resonance imaging (MRI), or positron emission tomography (PET)/CT to rule out nasopharyngeal cancer or lymphoepithelioma-like carcinoma (LELCs) of other origins. The tumor staging classification was based on the tumor-node-metastasis staging system (15). The expression level of PD-L1 was detected by immunohistochemistry using anti-PD-L1 antibody (clone 28-8, ab205921, Abcam). The results are expressed as a tumor proportion score (TPS), indicating the percentage of viable tumor cells showing partial or complete membrane staining at some intensity in the tissue specimens, i.e., TPS of 0–1% was regarded as negative, 1%–49% as low and ≥ 50% as high expression (16). We adopted the Response Evaluation Criteria in Solid Tumors (RECIST) version 1.1 to assess changes in the tumor burden (17).

RESULTS

Patient Characteristics

In total, we screened 128 patients diagnosed with PPLELC, including 5 who received immunotherapy. The demographic characteristics of these 5 patients are displayed in **Table 1**. All of these 5 patients were female nonsmokers with a median age of 55.6 (range 53-58) years at diagnosis. Furthermore, almost all of them had a tumor size greater than 3 (median 5.1, range 4.7-6.4) cm. In two patients, the tumors were located in the right middle lobe; in the other 3, the tumors were in the right lower lobe, left upper lobe and left lower lobe. The stage distribution at initial diagnosis was IA in one patient, IIIA in one patient and IV in three patients. Moreover, three patients had a PD-L1 TPS of less than 50% (case 1, 40%; case two, 30%; case 5, 5%), and two patients had a PD-L1 TPS of more than 50% (case 3, 90%; case 4, 80%). Two patients showed evidence of EBV infection, and the overall TPS of PD-L1 was 40% (range, 30-80%), including two patients with high expression (≥50%) and three with low expression (5-49%). Notably, one patient (case 3) was misdiagnosed with pulmonary squamous cell carcinoma before her biopsy samples were sent to the Pathology Department of our hospital for consultation. Representative images of the HE and IHC staining of PD-L1 expression are shown in **Figure 1**.

Treatment Before Immune Checkpoint Blockade Therapy

The treatment details before application of immune checkpoint inhibitors are shown in **Table 2**. Only two patients underwent radical tumor resection, and adjuvant chemotherapy and gemcitabine plus cisplatin (GP regimen) were administered to Patient 1. Progression-free survival (PFS) in the first two patients was 19.4 months and 8.3 months, respectively. Palliative chemotherapies, including paclitaxel plus carboplatin (TC regimen), pemetrexed (Alimta) plus carboplatin (AC regimen), docetaxel plus cisplatin (DP regimen) and paclitaxel plus fluorouracil (TF regimen), were administered to all patients at advanced stages, and the median number of chemotherapy cycles given to them was 1. The first four patients received the TC regimen only and achieved stable disease (SD). The fifth regimen was administered sequentially to the AC, DP, and TF regimen patients and resulted in partial remission (PR). Additionally, three patients received thoracic radiotherapy. However, all patients ultimately had progressive disease (PD), and the median time to first tumor progression was 7.4 (range, 5.2-9.6) months.

Abbreviations: AC, pemetrexed plus carboplatin; AP, pemetrexed plus platinum; CT, computed tomography; DP, docetaxel plus cisplatin; EBER, Epstein-Barr encoding region; GP, gemcitabine plus cisplatin; HE, hematoxylin-eosin; IHC, immunohistochemical; MRI, magnetic resonance imaging; NSCLC, non-small cell lung cancer; OS, overall survival; PD, progressive disease; PD-1, programmed cell death-1; PD-L1, programmed death-ligand 1; PET, positron emission tomography; PFS, progression-free survival; PPLELC, primary pulmonary lymphoepithelioma-like carcinoma; PR, partial remission; RECIST, Response Evaluation Criteria in Solid Tumors; SD, stable disease; TC, paclitaxel plus carboplatin; TF, paclitaxel plus fluorouracil; TP, taxanes plus platinum; TPS, tumor proportion score.

TABLE 1 | Demographic characteristics of the patients with PPLELC.

Patient	Sex	Age (y)	Smoking status	Method of diagnosis	Site of tumor	Tumor size (cm)	TNM staging	Overall staging	Serum EBV examination	PD-L1 expression	*EGFR*	*ALK*	*ROS-1*
1	Female	58	N	Operation	RLL	5.1	T3N2M0	IIIA	unknown	40%	Negative	Negative	Negative
2	Female	53	N	Operation	LUL	2.3	T1bN0M0	IA2	unknown	30%	Negative	Negative	Negative
3	Female	48	N	EBUS bronchoscopy	RML	4.7	T2bN2M1	IV	unknown	90%	Negative	Negative	Negative
4	Female	56	N	CT-guided percutaneous needle lung biopsy	LLL	6.4	T4N2M1b	IV	EBV-EA-IgG positive	80%	Negative	Negative	Negative
5	Female	63	N	Bronchoscope biopsy	RML	7.0	T4N3M1	IV	EB-DNA 9.10E +03 copies/mL	5%	Negative	Negative	Negative

EBUS, endobronchial ultrasound; RLL, right lower lobe; LUL, left upper lobe; RML, right middle lobe; LLL, left lower lobe; EBV, Epstein-Barr virus; PD-L1, programmed cell death-1.

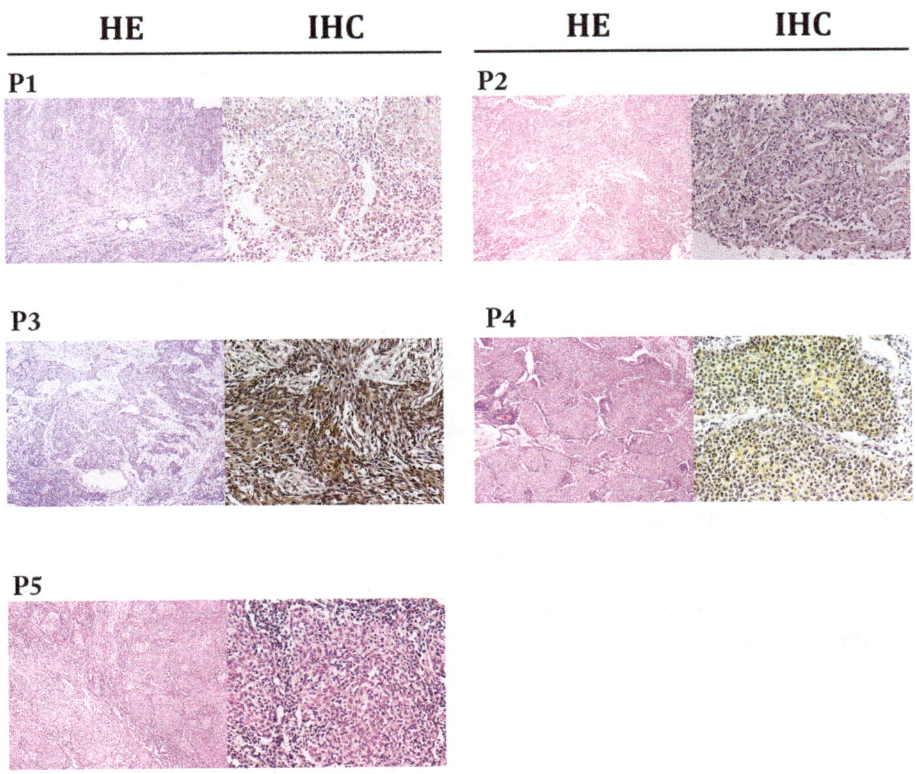

FIGURE 1 | Representative images for HE (×40) and IHC staining for PD-L1 expressions (×200). The expressions of PD-L1 in patients 1 to 5 were 40%, 30%, 90%, 80% and 5%, respectively.

Immune Checkpoint Blockade Therapy

Table 3 presents details on the immunotherapy regimen. In total, three types of immune inhibitors were used in our patients, including sintilimab, pembrolizumab and nivolumab. These five patients underwent a median of 8.8 (range, 5.5-14.7) months of palliative chemotherapy and/or radiation before immunotherapy was adopted. The median number of immunotherapy cycles administered to our patients was 8 (range, 6-19), and the best treatment response achieved was PR in two patients and SD in three patients. At the end of the final month, two of our patients had developed PD. Our second patient developed PD in the initial four cycles of pembrolizumab alone, but SD was subsequently achieved once she received pembrolizumab combined with nab-paclitaxel. We were unable to contact Patient 3 to obtain more information regarding her treatment details and subsequent status. Briefly, Patient 4 showed PD in the second follow-up after partial remission with a PFS following ICBT of 7.5 months. Unfortunately, she died 7.8 months after progression. Compared with the PFS of 4.2 months following chemotherapy, survival for 15.3 months following ICBT may be considered an improvement. Patient 5 also experienced PD in the final month (in May 2020), with SD for 24.5 months. A stable period of 24.5 months

TABLE 2 | Treatment details before immune checkpoint blockade therapy.

Patient	Surgery	Adjuvant chemotherapy	PFS since surgery (m)	No. of chemotherapy regimens	Chemotherapy regimens	PFS since following palliative chemotherapy (m)
1	Yes	Yes (GP)	19.4+	1	TC	15.7+
2	Yes	No	8.3	1	TC	10.6
3	No	No	NA	1	TC	5.6
4	No	No	NA	1	TC	4.2
5	No	No	NA	3	AC, DP, TF	9.3*, 9.7**

GP, gemcitabine plus cisplatin; PFS, progression-free survival, NA, not applicable; TC, paclitaxel plus carboplatin; AC, pemetrexed (Alimta) plus carboplatin; DP, docetaxel plus cisplatin; TF, paclitaxel plus fluorouracil; SD, stable disease; PR, partial remission.
**PFS1 with AC regimen; **PFS2 with DP regimen.*

TABLE 3 | Treatment details of immune checkpoint blockade therapy.

Patient	Time gap between ICBT and chemotherapy (m)	PD-L1 expression	ICBT	Cycles of ICBT received	Best overall response	PD to ICBT	PFS with ICBT	Duration of following the start of ICBT (m)	Living status	Survival from the start of ICBT (m)	Survival from the start of chemotherapy (m)
1	17.5+	40%	Sintilimab +Anlotinib	8 (ongoing)	PR	No	NA	8.3	Alive	8.3	25.8
2	11.6	30%	Pembrolizumab +nab-paclitaxel	6 (ongoing)	SD	No	NA	10.9	Alive	10.9	22.5
3	6	90%	Pembrolizumab	1	SD	UN	UN	4.2+	UN	4.2+	10.2+
4	4.1	80%	Nivolumab	19	PR	Yes	7.5	15.3	Dead	15.3	19.4
5	24.2	5%	Nivolumab +Anlotinib	21 (ongoing)	SD	Yes	24.5*	26.0	Alive	26.0	50.2

ICBT, immune checkpoint blockade therapy; PD-L1, programmed cell death-1; PD, progressive disease; PR, partial remission; SD, stable disease; UN, unknown.
**This patient had PD during the final month, with a PFS of 24.5 months, during which she suspended ICBT for more than 9 months due to hypothyroidism and financial reasons.*

following ICBT was a significant improvement over that resulting from the previous chemotherapy, especially because she suspended ICBT for more than 9 months due to financial reasons. Fortunately, both Patient 1 and Patient 2 continued to benefit from ICBT without progression. A summary of the overall treatment reaction is presented in **Figure 2**.

Images of the changes observed throughout treatment are displayed in **Supplementary Figures 1–5**, and additional information for the excluded 123 patients is presented in **Supplementary Table 1**.

DISCUSSION

We reviewed the efficacy of immune checkpoint inhibitors in patients with PPLELC, and based on our preliminary experience, most patients responded favorably to the PD1/PD-L1 blockade therapy. To the best of our knowledge, this study is the first to thoroughly summarize the treatment response of PPLELC patients to different checkpoint inhibitors.

Our patients had a median age of 55.6 years (range 53-58) and were predominantly female. The patients were all nonsmokers, which is quite a distinctive demographic characteristic of PPLELC, as it generally affects younger Asian nonsmoking females (18). The features of PPLELC that distinguish it from other subtypes of NSCLC indicate that PPLELC is a unique subtype of lung cancer. In addition, epidemiological differences in PPLELC exist across different regions worldwide (18, 19). As reported by other studies (13, 20, 21), PPLELC in our study mainly originated in the right lower lobe and rarely in the right upper lobe, with a median diameter of 5.1 cm. All of the patients had EBER positivity, and two showed evidence of EBV infection; although it is widely believed that a connection exists between EBV infection and the development of PPLELC (3), conflicting findings have been reported in Western populations (22). *In vitro* studies of nasopharyngeal carcinoma have shown that EBV has the ability to upregulate PD-L1 expression through IFN-γ and latent membrane protein 1 (18). The results of our study revealed a median PD-L1 TPS of 40%, and 60% of the patients had low PD-L1 expression, which is similar to the findings reported in the study by Zhanhong Xie et al. (23).

Patient 1 and Patient 2 first underwent radical tumor resection during early stages of the disease. In resectable cases, complete removal is the preferred approach to PPLELC. A study by Liang et al. suggested that a high survival rate can be achieved through radical resection (24). In their study, among 40 patients who underwent complete tumor resection, recurrence occurred in 6 patients, ranging from 10.6 to 41.1 months after the surgery. At the end of the final month of follow-up, these two patients were alive, with tumor progression times following surgery of 19.4 and 8.3 months. Notably, adjunct chemotherapy was administered to Patient 1, so whether longer progression-free survival could be achieved by adjuvant chemotherapy and/or radiation is unknown. Additionally, in Liang's study, the authors concluded that in PPLELC patients with stage IIIA disease who

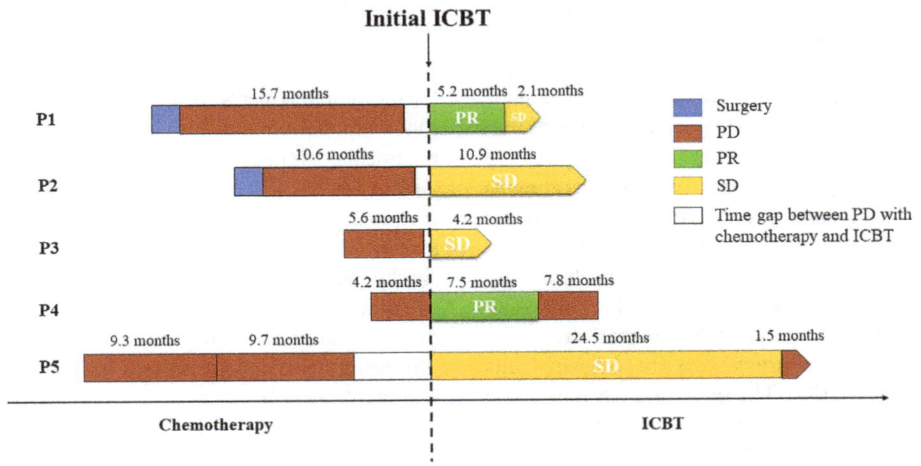

FIGURE 2 | Summary of treatment reactions to chemotherapy and immune checkpoint blockade therapy. All of the patients underwent PD before immunotherapy, and three of them responded favorably to ICBT. The bars on the left and right side of the dotted line denote the treatment details before and after the administration of immune checkpoint inhibitors, respectively.

underwent radical resection, a better prognosis could be achieved when adjuvant chemotherapy was administered (24). The results of a meta-analysis showed that NSCLC patients in stage IIIA benefited the most from adjuvant chemotherapy (25, 26). Therefore, postoperative adjuvant chemotherapy should be used for cases at locally advanced tumor stages. In addition, palliative chemotherapy and/or radiation are often used for patients in advanced or metastatic stages. In our study, the most commonly used chemotherapy was the TC regimen, and the corresponding patients achieved the best overall SD, regardless of the inclusion of radiotherapy in the treatment regimen. Currently, the optimal chemotherapy for PPLELC remains unclear. A study conducted in Macau compared the efficacy of taxane-based and non-taxane-based combinations, and the results did not show a significant difference in terms of response or survival (13). A retrospective study on Chinese Taiwan patients revealed that platinum-based doublet chemotherapy could be considered the first-line treatment for advanced PPLELC (27). Another study by Zuan Lin et al. assessed three first-line chemotherapy regimens, i.e., GP, taxanes plus platinum (TP) and pemetrexed plus platinum (AP); of these regimens, GP achieved the highest response rate and longest PFS (28). Furthermore, due to the uncertainty of adding thoracic radiotherapy to first-line chemotherapy, Zuan Lin et al. evaluated the value of radiotherapy and concluded that palliative thoracic radiotherapy was beneficial for prolonging the survival of PPLELC patients with advanced-stage disease (28). Consistent with our study, PFS was longer in Patients 1, 2, and 5, all of whom received thoracic radiotherapy.

Since our patients were all positive for PD-L1 expression, they received immunotherapy after systematic chemotherapy and radiotherapy either with or without concurrent treatments. The immune inhibitor administered to our first patient was sintilimab, and she achieved a response of PR. Initially approved for the treatment of classical Hodgkin's lymphoma, sintilimab is a fully humanized IgG4 monoclonal antibody that binds PD-1 to block the interaction between PD-1 and its ligands (29). To date, our patient is the first worldwide to receive sintilimab as a palliative treatment for PPLELC, and we confirmed its efficacy. The latest clinical trial conducted in mainland China evaluated the safety and outcome of sintilimab as a neoadjuvant treatment in patients with resectable NSCLC (stage IA-IIIB). The results showed that sintilimab was well tolerated, and a 40.5% major pathological response was obtained (30). Our results suggest that the use of the PD-1 inhibitor sintilimab in advanced PPLELC patients may be feasible. Pembrolizumab and nivolumab are other PD-1 antibodies approved for the treatment of unresectable NSCLC. Although patient 2 developed PD on pembrolizumab alone in the initial four cycles, she still had SD when it was subsequently combined with nab-paclitaxel. Patient 3 was treated with 1 cycle of pembrolizumab and was able to achieve SD. A study by Na Zhou et al. described a female patient from Macau treated with pembrolizumab after a three-line platinum-combined chemotherapy regimen, and SD was achieved (13), representing the first report of a favorable response to pembrolizumab in patients with advanced LELC. In patients with advanced NSCLC and a PD-L1 TPS of 50% or more, the first-line treatment has been pembrolizumab monotherapy instead of platinum doublet chemotherapy (31).

Moreover, a multicenter retrospective study recently conducted by Aguilar EJ showed that the treatment effect of the first-line treatment pembrolizumab was significantly better in NSCLC patients with PD-L1 expression ≥ 50% than in those with PD-L1 expression ≥ 90% (32). Their findings suggest that higher PD-L1 expression in NSCLC patients may lead to better clinical outcomes for patients receiving pembrolizumab. This finding may account for the effect difference of pembrolizumab in our patients. Unfortunately, we were unable to maintain contact with Patient 3, who only received one cycle of pembrolizumab, which may have affected the evaluation. Nevertheless, as mentioned above, our results still add evidence to the literature on the effectiveness of pembrolizumab for the treatment of unresectable PPLELC.

Regarding Patients 4 and 5, who received nivolumab, the former achieved PR, and the latter achieved SD. Evidence of nivolumab for the treatment of advanced PPLELC is limited to case reports (12, 33, 34). One case report in our study was for Patient 4, who was the first patient worldwide to respond favorably (PR) to nivolumab. However, she unfortunately developed PD during the final month of the evaluation. Patient 5 still achieved SD.

Additionally, three patients were given concurrent treatments during the course of immunotherapy, two with anlotinib and one with nab-paclitaxel. To date, reports regarding the effectiveness of anlotinib in PPLELC remain lacking due to its rarity. Subgroup analysis from the ALTER0303 trial suggested that anlotinib could improve PFS and overall survival (OS) in patients with adenocarcinoma, and prolonged survival was shown in patients with squamous cell carcinoma (35). The same findings may apply to PPLELC, but more evidence is needed to determine whether the addition of anlotinib leads to better outcomes. For nab-paclitaxel, there is no evidence indicating its efficacy in PPLELC. The KEYNOTE-407 study reported the immune-chemotherapy combination in the treatment of untreated metastatic squamous NSCLC and concluded that longer OS and PFS could be achieved when pembrolizumab was added to chemotherapy (carboplatin plus paclitaxel or nab-paclitaxel) compared with chemotherapy alone (36). According to our results, it is likely that the combination of pembrolizumab and nab-paclitaxel may be feasible in the treatment of advanced PPLELC, but more clinical trials are needed.

This study has several limitations that should be noted. The most obvious weakness is the small sample size. Due to the rare incidence of PPLELC, only 128 patients were diagnosed with PPLELC at our center over the last decade, which is among the top hospitals nationwide, with more than 5000 newly diagnosed lung cancer cases each year. Second, immunotherapy is a relatively new treatment method. Among the 128 PPLELC patients, 5 received immune checkpoint inhibitors with different treatment regimens. Whether heterogeneity exists between the different treatments requires further exploration. Additionally, the follow-up period was restricted due to the emergence of new treatments. Multicenter studies with sufficiently long observation periods will be carried out by our team in the future to provide more convincing evidence. Finally, this study represents a descriptive investigation. Research concerning the mechanism of immune checkpoint inhibitors in PPLELC is required.

In summary, we evaluated a small number of patients and demonstrated that immune checkpoint inhibitors may be promising beneficial treatments for advanced PPLELC. Optimal treatments for this type of disease remain lacking, and large clinical trials are warranted.

AUTHOR CONTRIBUTIONS

ZW and XX contributed to the collection and analysis of the data. ZW drafted the manuscript. DC, KW, and WL participated in interpreting the data and revising the manuscript. BC designed the study and reviewed the drafts. All authors contributed to the article and approved the submitted version.

ACKNOWLEDGMENTS

We thank all patients for participating in the study with patience and cooperation.

REFERENCES

1. Bégin LR, Eskandari J, Joncas J, Panasci L. Epstein-Barr virus related lymphoepithelioma-like carcinoma of lung. *J Surgical Oncol* (1987) 36 (4);280–3. doi: 10.1002/jso.2930360413
2. Travis WD, Brambilla E, Burke AP, Marx A, Nicholson AG. Introduction to The 2015 World Health Organization Classification of Tumors of the Lung, Pleura, Thymus, and Heart. *J Thorac Oncol* (2015) 10(9):1240–2. doi: 10.1097/JTO.0000000000000663
3. Han A-J, Xiong M, Zong Y-S. Association of Epstein-Barr virus with lymphoepithelioma-like carcinoma of the lung in southern China. *Am J Clin Pathol* (2000) 114(2):220–6. doi: 10.1309/148K-ND54-6NJX-NA61
4. Keir ME, Butte MJ, Freeman GJ, Sharpe AH. PD-1 and its ligands in tolerance and immunity. *Annual Rev Immunol* (2008) 26:677–704. doi: 10.1146/annurev.immunol.26.021607.090331
5. Gurung S, Khan F, Gunassekaran GR, Do Yoo J, Vadevoo SMP, Permpoon U, et al. Phage display-identified PD-L1-binding peptides reinvigorate T-cell activity and inhibit tumor progression. *Biomaterials* (2020) 274:119984. doi: 10.1016/j.biomaterials.2020.119984
6. Freeman GJ, Long AJ, Iwai Y, Bourque K, Chernova T, Nishimura H, et al. Engagement of the PD-1 immunoinhibitory receptor by a novel B7 family member leads to negative regulation of lymphocyte activation. *J Exp Med* (2000) 192(7):1027–34. doi: 10.1084/jem.192.7.1027
7. Topalian SL, Hodi FS, Brahmer JR, Gettinger SN, Smith DC, McDermott DF, et al. Safety, activity, and immune correlates of anti–PD-1 antibody in cancer. *New Engl J Med* (2012) 366(26):2443–54. doi: 10.1056/NEJMoa1200690
8. Jiang L, Wang L, Li P-F, Zhang X-K, Chen J-W, Qiu H-J, et al. Positive expression of programmed death ligand-1 correlates with superior outcomes and might be a therapeutic target in primary pulmonary lymphoepithelioma-like carcinoma. *OncoTargets Ther* (2015) 8:1451–7. doi: 10.2147/OTT.S84234
9. Chang Y-L, Yang C-Y, Lin M-W, Wu C-T, Yang P-C. PD-L1 is highly expressed in lung lymphoepithelioma-like carcinoma: A potential rationale for immunotherapy. *Lung Cancer (Amsterdam Netherlands)* (2015) 88 (3):254–9. doi: 10.1016/j.lungcan.2015.03.017
10. Sathirareuangchai S, Hirata K. Pulmonary Lymphoepithelioma-like Carcinoma. *Arch Pathol Lab Med* (2019) 143(8):1027–30. doi: 10.5858/arpa.2018-0149-RS
11. Chan AT, Teo PM, Lam KC, Chan WY, Chow JH, Yim AP, et al. Multimodality treatment of primary lymphoepithelioma-like carcinoma of the lung. *Cancer* (1998) 83(5):925–9. doi: 10.1002/(SICI)1097-0142(19980901)83:5<925::AID-CNCR18>3.0.CO;2-X
12. Qiu ZX, Zhou P, Wang K. Primary Pulmonary Lymphoepithelioma-Like Carcinoma Response Favorably To Nivolumab: A Case Report. *Onco Targets Ther* (2019) 12:8595–600. doi: 10.2147/OTT.S219512
13. Zhou N, Lin Y, Peng X, Wang Y, Wang Y. Thorough survey and analysis of pulmonary lymphoepithelioma-like carcinoma in Macau and multimodality treatment for advanced disease. *Lung Cancer* (2019) 138:116–23. doi: 10.1016/j.lungcan.2019.10.004
14. Narayanan A, Knollmann FD, Walby JAS, Lim S, Gandara DR, Riess JW. EBV-positive Primary Pulmonary Lymphoepithelioma-like Carcinoma Response to PD-L1 Blockade. *Clin Lung Cancer* (2019) 20(3):e238–e41. doi: 10.1016/j.cllc.2018.12.015
15. Goldstraw P, Crowley J, Chansky K, Giroux DJ, Groome PA, Rami-Porta R, et al. The IASLC Lung Cancer Staging Project: proposals for the revision of the

TNM stage groupings in the forthcoming (seventh) edition of the TNM Classification of malignant tumours. *J Thorac Oncol* (2007) 2(8):706–14. doi: 10.1097/JTO.0b013e31812f3c1a
16. Wang H, Agulnik J, Kasymjanova G, Wang A, Jiménez P, Cohen V, et al. Cytology cell blocks are suitable for immunohistochemical testing for PD-L1 in lung cancer. *Ann Oncol* (2018) 29(6):1417–22. doi: 10.1093/annonc/mdy126
17. Eisenhauer EA, Therasse P, Bogaerts J, Schwartz LH, Sargent D, Ford R, et al. New response evaluation criteria in solid tumours: revised RECIST guideline (version 1.1). *Eur J Cancer* (2009) 45(2):228–47. doi: 10.1016/j.ejca.2008.10.026
18. Fan Y, Li C, Qin J, Lu H. Primary pulmonary lymphoepithelioma-like carcinoma. *Med Oncol (Northwood London England)* (2020) 37(3):20. doi: 10.1007/s12032-020-1344-3
19. He J, Shen J, Pan H, Huang J, Liang W, He J. Pulmonary lymphoepithelioma-like carcinoma: a surveillance, epidemiology, and end results database analysis. *J Thoracic Dis* (2015) 7(12):2330–8. doi: 10.3978/j.issn.2072-1439.2015.12.62
20. Yu X, Wen Y, Qin R, Lin Y, Zhang X, Wang W, et al. Prognosis and distribution of lymph nodes metastases in resectable primary pulmonary lymphoepithelioma-like carcinoma: A large cohort from a single center. *Thorac Cancer* (2018) 9(3):360–7. doi: 10.1111/1759-7714.12586
21. Ma H, Wu Y, Lin Y, Cai Q, Ma G, Liang Y. Computed tomography characteristics of primary pulmonary lymphoepithelioma-like carcinoma in 41 patients. *Eur J Radiol* (2013) 82(8):1343–6. doi: 10.1016/j.ejrad.2013.02.006
22. Castro CY, Ostrowski ML, Barrios R, Green LK, Popper HH, Powell S, et al. Relationship between Epstein-Barr virus and lymphoepithelioma-like carcinoma of the lung: a clinicopathologic study of 6 cases and review of the literature. *Hum Pathol* (2001) 32(8):863–72. doi: 10.1053/hupa.2001.26457
23. Xie Z, Liu L, Lin X, Xie X, Gu Y, Liu M, et al. A multicenter analysis of genomic profiles and PD-L1 expression of primary lymphoepithelioma-like carcinoma of the lung. *Modern Pathol an Off J U States Can Acad Pathology Inc* (2020) 33(4):626–38. doi: 10.1038/s41379-019-0391-9
24. Liang Y, Wang L, Zhu Y, Lin Y, Liu H, Rao H, et al. Primary pulmonary lymphoepithelioma-like carcinoma: fifty-two patients with long-term follow-up. *Cancer* (2012) 118(19):4748–58. doi: 10.1002/cncr.27452
25. Dunant A, Pignon J-P. Adjuvant chemotherapy for non–small cell lung cancer: contribution of the International Adjuvant Lung Trial. *Clin Cancer Res* (2005) 11(13):5017s–21s. doi: 10.1158/1078-0432.CCR-05-9006
26. Pignon J-P, Tribodet H, Scagliotti GV, Douillard J-Y, Shepherd FA, Stephens RJ, et al. Lung adjuvant cisplatin evaluation: a pooled analysis by the LACE Collaborative Group. *J Clin Oncol* (2008) 26(21):3552–9. doi: 10.1200/JCO.2007.13.9030
27. Huang CJ, Feng AC, Fang YF, Ku WH, Chu NM, Yu CT, et al. Multimodality treatment and long-term follow-up of the primary pulmonary lymphoepithelioma-like carcinoma. *Clin Lung Cancer* (2012) 13(5):359–62. doi: 10.1016/j.cllc.2012.01.002
28. Lin Z, Fu S, Zhou Y, Zhang X, Chen C, He LN, et al. First-line platinum-based chemotherapy and survival outcomes in locally advanced or metastatic pulmonary lymphoepithelioma-like carcinoma. *Lung Cancer* (2019) 137:100–7. doi: 10.1016/j.lungcan.2019.09.007
29. Hoy SM. Sintilimab: First Global Approval. *Drugs* (2019) 79(3):341–6. doi: 10.1007/s40265-019-1066-z
30. Gao S, Li N, Gao S, Xue Q, Ying J, Wang S, et al. Neoadjuvant PD-1 inhibitor (Sintilimab) in NSCLC. *J Thorac Oncol* (2020) 15(5):816–26. doi: 10.1016/j.jtho.2020.01.017
31. Reck M, Rodriguez-Abreu D, Robinson AG, Hui R, Csoszi T, Fulop A, et al. Pembrolizumab versus Chemotherapy for PD-L1-Positive Non-Small-Cell Lung Cancer. *New Engl J Med* (2016) 375(19):1823–33. doi: 10.1056/NEJMoa1606774
32. Aguilar EJ, Ricciuti B, Gainor JF, Kehl KL, Kravets S, Dahlberg S, et al. Outcomes to first-line pembrolizumab in patients with non-small-cell lung cancer and very high PD-L1 expression. *Ann Oncol Off J Eur Soc Med Oncol* (2019) 30(10):1653–9. doi: 10.1093/annonc/mdz288
33. Kumar V, Dave V, Harris J, Huang Y. Response of advanced stage recurrent lymphoepithelioma-like carcinoma to nivolumab. *Immunotherapy* (2017) 9 (12):955–61. doi: 10.2217/imt-2017-0067
34. Kim C, Rajan A, DeBrito PA, Giaccone G. Metastatic lymphoepithelioma-like carcinoma of the lung treated with nivolumab: a case report and focused review of literature. *Trans Lung Cancer Res* (2016) 5(6):720–6. doi: 10.21037/tlcr.2016.11.06
35. Cheng Y, Han B, Li K, Wang Q, Zhang L, Shi J, et al. Effect of anlotinib as a third-or further-line therapy in advanced non-small cell lung cancer patients with different histologic types: Subgroup analysis in the ALTER0303 trial. *Cancer Med* (2020) 9(8):2621–30. doi: 10.1002/cam4.2913
36. Paz-Ares L, Luft A, Vicente D, Tafreshi A, Gümüş M, Mazières J, et al. Pembrolizumab plus Chemotherapy for Squamous Non-Small-Cell Lung Cancer. *N Engl J Med* (2018) 379(21):2040 51. doi: 10.1056/NEJMoa1810865

2

First-Line Treatment Options for PD-L1–Negative Non-Small Cell Lung Cancer: A Bayesian Network Meta-Analysis

Ling Peng[1†], Wen-Hua Liang[2†], De-Guang Mu[1], Song Xu[3], Shao-Dong Hong[4], Justin Stebbing[5], Fei Liang[6] and Yang Xia[7*]*

[1] Department of Respiratory Disease, Zhejiang Provincial People's Hospital, Hangzhou, China, [2] National Clinical Research Center for Respiratory Disease, The First Affiliated Hospital of Guangzhou Medical University, Guangzhou, China, [3] Department of Lung Cancer Surgery, Lung Cancer Institute, Tianjin Medical University General Hospital, Tianjin, China, [4] Department of Medical Oncology, Sun Yat-sen University Cancer Center, Guangzhou, China, [5] Division of Cancer, Department of Surgery and Cancer, Imperial College London, London, United Kingdom, [6] Department of Biostatistics, Zhongshan Hospital, Fudan University, Shanghai, China, [7] Department of Respiratory and Critical Care Medicine, The Second Affiliated Hospital, School of Medicine, Zhejiang University, Key Laboratory of Respiratory Disease of Zhejiang Province, Hangzhou, China

***Correspondence:**
Yang Xia
yxia@zju.edu.cn
Fei Liang
liangfei0726@163.com*

[†]These authors have contributed equally to this work

Background: First-line treatment strategies for programmed death-ligand 1 (PD-L1) negative non-small cell lung cancer (NSCLC) patients include chemotherapy and combination with anti-angiogenesis drugs and/or immune checkpoint inhibitor. We conducted a Bayesian network meta-analysis to evaluate the efficacy of these therapeutic options.

Methods: We included phase III randomized controlled trials comparing two or more treatments in the first-line setting for NSCLC, including data in PD-L1–negative patients. First-line strategies were compared and ranked based on the effectiveness in terms of overall survival (OS) and progression-free survival (PFS). A rank was assigned to each treatment after Markov Chain Monte Carlo analyses.

Results: Fourteen trials involving 14 regimens matched our eligibility criteria. For OS, none of the treatment were significantly more effective than chemotherapy. Nivolumab plus ipilimumab plus chemotherapy was probably the best option based on analysis of the treatment ranking (probability = 30.1%). For PFS, nivolumab plus chemotherapy plus bevacizumab, atezolizumab plus chemotherapy plus bevacizumab, and atezolizumab plus chemotherapy were statistically superior to chemotherapy in pairwise comparison. Nivolumab plus chemotherapy plus bevacizumab was likely to be the preferred option based on the analysis of the treatment ranking (probability = 72.9%).

Conclusions: Nivolumab plus chemotherapy, in combination with angiogenesis inhibition or anti-cytotoxic T-lymphocyte–associated antigen 4 (CTLA-4), had maximal benefits for NSCLC patient of PD-L1–negative expression. These findings may facilitate individualized treatment strategies. Safety at an individual patient level should be considered in decision making. Further validation is warranted.

Keywords: programmed death-ligand 1, non-small cell lung cancer, immune checkpoint inhibitor, network meta-analysis, immunotherapy

INTRODUCTION

Non-small cell lung cancer (NSCLC) accounts for ~85% of all lung cancer cases, and the prognosis for patients with advanced/metastatic NSCLC remains limited (1). Platinum-based chemotherapy has long been the first-line treatment of choice for advanced NSCLC patients who do not harbor activating driver mutations. Checkpoint blockade has led to a paradigm shift in the treatment landscape of NSCLC, making long-term survival possible (2).

Thus far, several effective first-line systemic treatment options have been shown to be effective in advanced NSCLC. Programmed death-ligand (PD-L1) expression on tumor or immune cells emerged as the first potential predictive biomarker for the sensitivity to immune checkpoint blockade and patient stratification (3). For NSCLC patients with PD-L1 expression in ≥50% of tumor cells, pembrolizumab confers a superior progression-free survival (PFS) and overall survival (OS) compared with platinum-doublet chemotherapy in the first-line setting (4). For PD-L1 expression of 1% to 49%, programmed death-1 (PD-1) or PD-L1 inhibition has been shown to be comparable to chemotherapy (5, 6). In contrast, for patients with negative PD-L1 expression, no definite optimal therapeutic strategy has been defined. Most importantly, this group accounts for about half of the whole NSCLC patient population (7). A lack of head-to-head randomized controlled trials (RCTs) comparing chemotherapy, anti-angiogenesis drugs, and immunotherapies leaves uncertainty regarding optimal first-line treatment for advanced NSCLC patients with negative PD-L1 expression.

Network meta-analysis offers the unique opportunity to perform indirect comparisons between treatments never directly compared in RCTs but compared to a common treatment, as well as to rank multiple treatments (8). The present study aims to probe optimal therapeutic management with advanced NSCLC with negative PD-L1 expression.

MATERIALS AND METHODS

Search Strategy

A literature search was performed using databases including PubMed, Embase, and Cochrane databases. The upper date limit of October 30, 2020, was applied, with no lower date limit. Our search strategy included the following Medical Subject Headings (MeSH) terms and keywords: "NSCLC", "(advanced) or (metastatic) or (stage IV)", "(first-line) or (untreated) or (front-line)". Searches were performed using the filter "clinical trial" or "study" or "investigation" or "phase 3". We also reviewed abstracts and presentations from conference proceedings, including American Society of Clinical Oncology (ASCO), World Conference on Lung Cancer (WCLC), European Society for Medical Oncology (ESMO), European Lung Cancer Conference (ELCC), and American Association for Cancer Research (AACR). To ensure that no RCTs were missing, reference lists of published reviews, meta-analyses, and included RCTs were manually checked, and www.clinicaltrials.gov was searched.

Study Selection

Eligibility criteria for inclusion in this meta-analysis were as follows: (1) prospective phase III RCTs in patients with advanced NSCLC who had received no previous treatment for metastatic disease; (2) English language; (3) data available regarding PD-L1 expression negative population; and (4) in cases of duplicate

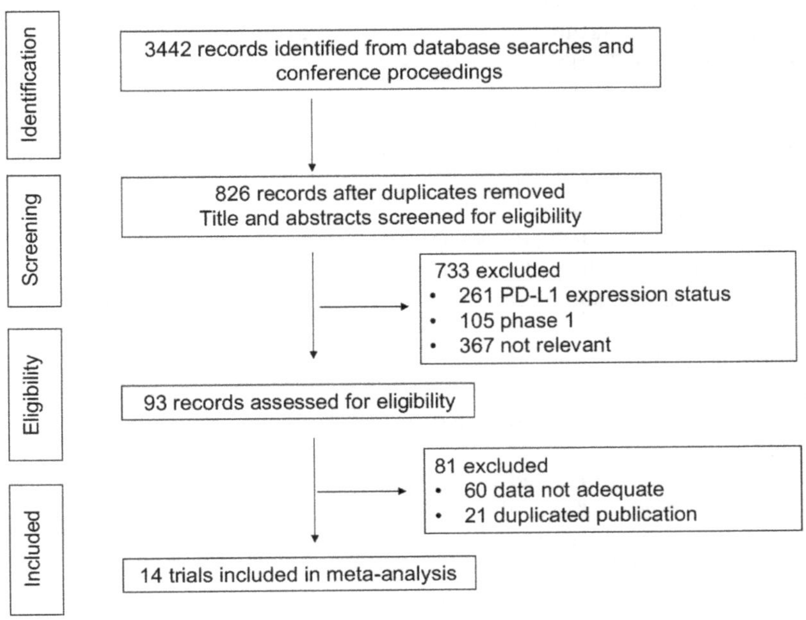

FIGURE 1 | Selection process for the trials included in the meta-analysis. PRISMA diagram. NSCLC, non-small cell lung cancer; RCT, randomized-controlled trial.

publications, only the most recent and updated report of the clinical trial were also included. Review articles, non-randomized trials, and observational studies, non-English studies were excluded from the analysis. The selection process is shown in **Figure 1**.

Articles that could not be categorized based on title and abstract alone were retrieved for full-text review. Disagreements were resolved by consensus between the authors. To determine the issue of multiple publications from the same data sets, we confirmed clinical trial information, such as the trial number and the period of patient recruitment of the articles. We also assessed the eligibility of the articles and abstracts identified by the search, and discrepancies were resolved by consensus. Study quality was assessed using the Jadad five-item scale, which takes into account randomization, double blinding, and withdrawals. The final score ranged from 0 to 5 (9).

Data Extraction

The meta-analysis was performed based on outcomes coming from the included studies. Data were extracted from eligible studies, which include the following items: study name, year of publication, source of publication, histology, number of patients, treatment arm and control arm, hazard ratio (HR), and 95% confidence intervals (CIs) of PFS and OS. In the case of trials that did not report PD-L1 expression subgroup, we reviewed each published trial's supplementary material. If data from any of the above categories were not reported in the study, items were treated as NR (not reported). The primary variables of interest were HRs with 95% CIs for OS or PFS.

Statistical Analysis

All calculations were performed using R (version 4.0.2) and STATA (version 14.0, Stata Corp LP, College Station, TX). OS and PFS were treated as time-to-event variables; therefore, these parameters were expressed as HR and 95% CI for each study. The primary endpoints of this network meta-analysis were the HRs for OS and PFS in PD-L1–negative patients. The Bayesian network meta-analysis (NMA) used a non-informative uniform prior to distribution to the parameters. For each outcome, three Markov chains with different starting values, generated using the method described by Gelman and Rubin were run in parallel for 100,000 iterations to obtain the posterior distribution. We used 10,000 burn-ins and a thinning interval of 10 for each chain. The model fit of each analysis was assessed by deviance information criterion (DIC) (10). Result heterogeneity across studies was evaluated with Cochrane's Q statistic and quantified with the inconsistency statistic (I^2). Statistical significance was considered at p less than 0.05, and heterogeneity was considered low, moderate, or high for I^2 values under 25%, between 25% and 50%, and over 50%, respectively (11). Effect sizes for the Bayesian network meta-analysis were described with 95% credible interval (CrL), the Bayesian equivalent of 95% CIs. Relative ranking of OS and PFS was presented as the probabilities. The probability of each regimen being the best among all regimens was computed by ranking the relative efficacies of all regimens in each iteration and then calculating the proportion of each regimen being ranked first across all iterations, which equals to 1 when a treatment is certain to be the best and 0 when a treatment is certain to be the worst.

TABLE 1 | Main characteristics and results of the eligible studies.

No	Year	Author	Source	Study	Histology	Phase	Sample size	Treatment	Control	OS (95% CI)	PFS (95% CI)
1	2019	West	Lancet Oncol	IMpower130 (12)	NSQ	3	356	Atezo+CT	CT	0.81 (0.61–1.08)	0.72 (0.56–0.91)
2	2020	Jotte	JTO	IMpower131 (13)	SQ	3	331	Atezo+CT	CT	0.87 (0.67–1.13)	0.81 (0.64–1.03)
3	2021	Papadimitrakopoulou	JTO	IMpower132 (14)	NSQ	3	143	Atezo+CT	CT	NR	0.45 (0.31–0.64)
4	2020	Socinski	AACR	IMpower150 (15)	NSQ+SQ	3	575	Atezo+CT	CT+Bev	0.96 (0.76–1.22)	1.10 (0.89–1.36)
								Atezo+CT+Bev	CT+Bev	0.90 (0.71–1.14)	0.77 (0.61–0.99)
5	2020	Zhou	Lancet Respir Med	CAMEL (16)	NSQ+SQ	3	118	Camre+CT	CT	NR	0.74 (0.44–1.23)
6	2020	Rizvi	JAMA Oncol	MYSTIC (17)	NSQ+SQ	3	254	Durva	CT	1.18 (0.86–1.62)	NR
								Durva+Treme	CT	0.73 (0.51–1.04)	NR
7	2020	Ramalingam	ASCO	CheckMate 227 Part 1b (18)	NSQ+SQ	3	550	Nivo+Ipi	CT	0.64 (0.51–0.81)	0.75 (0.59–0.95)
								Nivo+CT	CT	0.82 (0.66–1.03)	0.73 (0.58–0.92)
8	2021	Paz-Ares	Lancet Oncol	CheckMate 9LA (19)	NSQ+SQ	3	264	Nivo+Ipi+CT	CT	0.62 (0.45–0.85)	NR
9	2020	Lee	ESMO	ONO-4538-52/TASUKI-52 (20)	NSQ	3	550	Nivo+CT+Bev	CT+Bev	NR	0.55 (0.38–0.78)
10	2018	Gandhi	NEJM	KEYNOTE-189 (21)	NSQ	3	190	Pembro+CT	CT	0.59 (0.38–0.92)	0.75 (0.53–1.05)
11	2018	Paz-Ares	NEJM	KEYNOTE-407 (22)	SQ	3	104	Pembro+CT	CT	0.61 (0.38–0.98)	0.68 (0.47–0.98)
12	2020	Yang	JTO	ORIENT-11 (23)	NSQ	3	397	Sinti+CT	CT	NR	0.66 (0.41–1.09)
13	2021	Wang	JAMA Oncol	RATIONALE-307 (24)	SQ	3	91	Tisle+CT	CT	NR	0.64 (0.37–1.10)
										NR	0.69 (0.41–1.18)
14	2020	Lu	ESMO	RATIONALE-304 (25)	NSQ	3	334	Tisle+CT	CT	NR	0.76 (0.47–1.22)

Summary table of studies included in the meta-analysis.

OS, overall survival; PFS, progression-free survival; CI, confidence interval; CT, chemotherapy; Atezo, atezolizumab; Bev, bevacizumab; Nivo, nivolumab; Ipi, ipilimumab; Pembro, pembrolizumab; Carem, caremlizumab; Durva, durvalumab; Treme, tremelimumab; Tisle, tislezumab; Sinti, sintilimab; NR, not reported.

RESULTS

Study Selection and Characteristics

We found 4,125 potentially relevant articles. After initial exclusion of irrelevant, duplicate, and non-randomized studies, 14 original studies were considered eligible for the meta-analysis (**Figure 1**). The major baseline characteristics of the 14 eligible studies were represented in **Table 1**. Ten studies were double-arm design, whereas the remaining four referring three-arms. Overall, there were 14 different treatment strategies: chemotherapy, chemotherapy plus bevacizumab, atezolizumab plus chemotherapy, atezolizumab plus chemotherapy plus bevacizumab, nivolumab plus chemotherapy, nivolumab plus ipilimumab, nivolumab plus ipilimumab plus chemotherapy, nivolumab plus chemotherapy plus bevacizumab, pembrolizumab plus chemotherapy, caremlizumab plus chemotherapy, durvalumab, durvalumab plus tremelimumab, tislezumab plus chemotherapy, and sintilimab plus chemotherapy.

Studies were chosen and systemically reviewed in accordance with the Preferred Reporting Items for Systematic Reviews and Meta-Analyses (PRISMA) statement (26). Similarity was evaluated by reviewing characteristics of the trials with respect to any of those characteristics that are potential treatment effect modifiers, assuring validity of making indirect comparisons. It was impossible to calculate the Jadad's score for 2 of the studies (RATIONALE-304 and ONO-4538-52), which have not yet been published at the time of the analysis. The Jadad's score was evaluated for the rest 12 studies with scores ranging from 3 to 5.

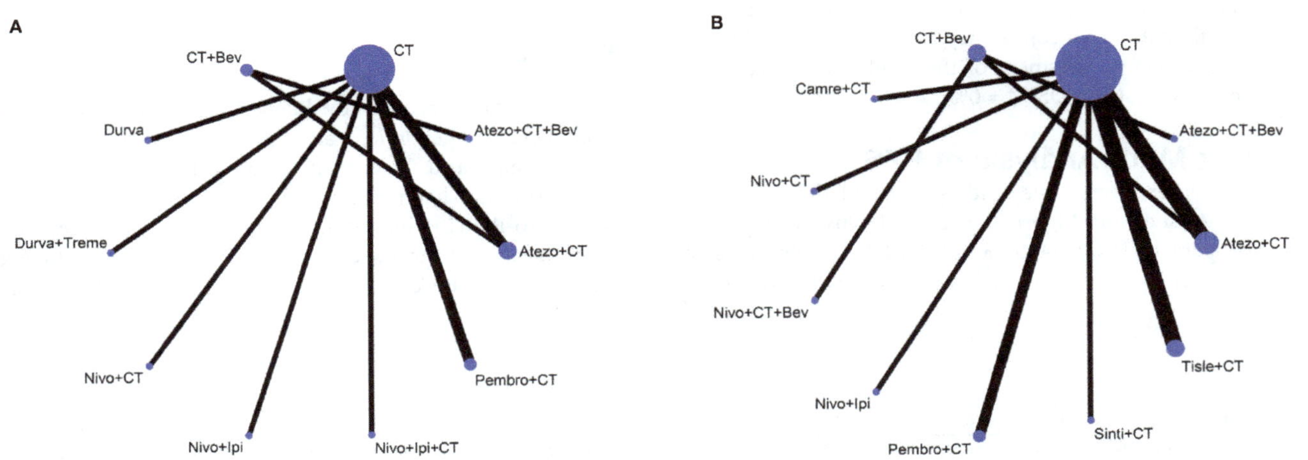

FIGURE 2 | Network plot for effectiveness of 10 and 9 different treatment modalities for patients with PD-L1–negative expression for OS **(A)** and PFS **(B)**, respectively. Circles represent the intervention as a node in the network and their size is proportional to the number of included studies; lines represent direct comparisons within the frame of randomized clinical trials (RCTs); the line thickness indicates the number of RCTs included in each comparison. CT, chemotherapy; Atezo, atezolizumab; Bev, bevacizumab; Nivo, nivolumab; Ipi, ipilimumab, Pembro, pembrolizumab; Carem, caremlizumab; Durva, durvalumab; Treme, tremelimumab; Tisle, tislezumab; Sinti, sintilimab; NR, not reported.

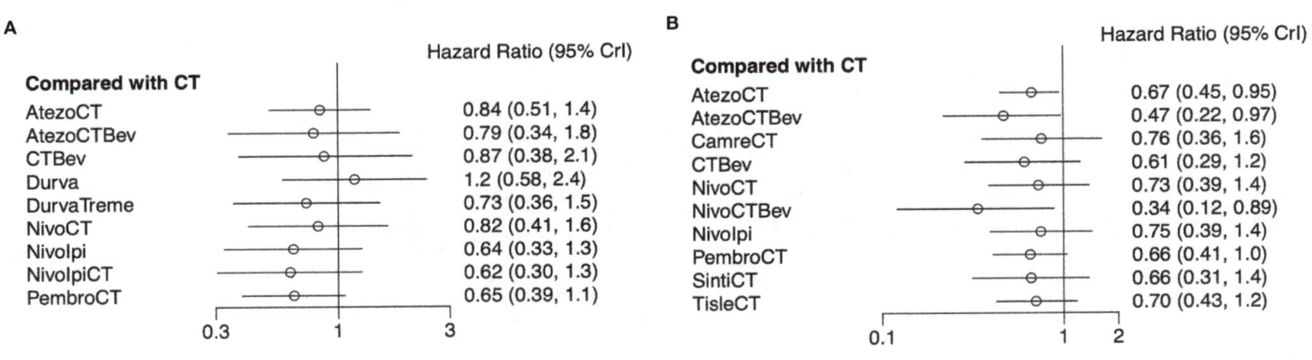

FIGURE 3 | Forest plots showing OS **(A)** and PFS **(B)** hazard ratio analyses. Efficacy of 10 and 11 treatment modalities for OS and PFS, respectively. Outcome measure: hazard ratio (HR). PrI, predictive interval; CT, chemotherapy; Atezo, atezolizumab; Bev, bevacizumab; Nivo, nivolumab; Ipi, ipilimumab; Pembro, pembrolizumab; Carem, caremlizumab; Durva, durvalumab; Treme, tremelimumab; Tisle, tislezumab; Sinti, sintilimab; NR, not reported.

Network Meta-Analysis of OS

Eight studies provided HR values for OS. The comparisons between treatments were shown by network plot (**Figure 2**). The forest plot of OS for pairwise comparison results were presented in **Figure 3**. In pairwise comparison, compared with chemotherapy, none of the treatments had a significant lower hazard risk of OS. The results providing indirect comparisons between treatments are presented in **Figure 4**, with none of the treatments performing significantly better than other treatment regimen in terms of OS. Comparative efficacy of treatments for OS based on treatment ranking was shown in **Figure 5** and **Table 2**, among which, combination of nivolumab and ipilimumab and chemotherapy was the most possible therapy to be ranked as first for OS (probability = 30.1%), nivolumab plus ipilimumab ranked the second (probability = 22.4%), and pembrolizumab plus chemotherapy ranked the third (probability = 18.8%). Comparing the DIC between the consistency and inconsistency models suggests that the consistency model has a similar fit to the data with inconsistency model (21.35 *vs.* 21.39). The overall heterogeneity assessment of the results showed that the heterogeneity was low for OS (I^2 = 0%).

Network Meta-Analysis of PFS

As for PFS, there were nine studies reported the HR values (**Figure 2**). As shown in **Figure 3**, nivolumab plus chemotherapy plus bevacizumab (HR, 0.34; 95% CrI, 0.12–0.89), atezolizumab plus chemotherapy plus bevacizumab (HR, 0.47; 95% CrI, 0.22–0.97), and atezolizumab plus chemotherapy (HR, 0.67; 95% CrI, 0.45–0.95) were statistically superior to chemotherapy in pairwise comparison. Indirect comparison results were illustrated in **Figure 4**, with nivolumab plus chemotherapy plus bevacizumab, atezolizumab plus chemotherapy plus bevacizumab, and atezolizumab plus chemotherapy have better PFS than chemotherapy. The probabilities of rank plot (**Figure 5** and **Table 2**) were as follows: combination of nivolumab, chemotherapy, and bevacizumab was most likely to be the best regimen (probability = 72.9%), atezolizumab plus chemotherapy plus bevacizumab ranked the second (probability = 11.9%). The DIC between the consistency and inconsistency models suggests that the consistency model has a similar fit to the data inconsistency model (27.05 *vs.* 27.06). The overall heterogeneity assessment of the results showed that the heterogeneity was low for PFS (I^2 = 22.1%).

DISCUSSION

The PD-L1 axis is regulated by different stimuli through multiple levels, including genomic, transcriptional, post-transcriptional, translational, and post-translational levels (27). PD-L1 expression has been proposed as distinct biomarker of response to PD-(L)1 inhibitor. In NSCLC, PD-L1 expression is highly variable and is associated with distinct clinicopathologic and genomic features (28). Clinical studies in NSCLC have

A

Atezo+CT	0.94 (0.47, 1.88)	1.19 (0.72, 1.96)	1.04 (0.53, 2.08)	1.40 (0.58, 3.35)	0.87 (0.37, 2.12)	0.98 (0.42, 2.26)	0.76 (0.33, 1.75)	0.74 (0.32, 1.76)	0.77 (0.38, 1.55)
1.06 (0.53, 2.13)	Atezo+CT+Bev	1.27 (0.55, 2.93)	1.11 (0.55, 2.22)	1.50 (0.49, 4.57)	0.93 (0.30, 2.84)	1.04 (0.35, 3.09)	0.81 (0.27, 2.44)	0.79 (0.26, 2.39)	0.82 (0.31, 2.19)
0.84 (0.51, 1.38)	0.79 (0.34, 1.83)	CT	0.87 (0.38, 2.07)	1.18 (0.58, 2.39)	0.73 (0.36, 1.51)	0.82 (0.41, 1.63)	0.64 (0.33, 1.26)	0.62 (0.30, 1.26)	0.65 (0.39, 1.07)
0.96 (0.48, 1.89)	0.90 (0.45, 1.82)	1.15 (0.48, 2.65)	CT+Bev	1.35 (0.44, 4.13)	0.84 (0.27, 2.53)	0.94 (0.31, 2.76)	0.73 (0.25, 2.19)	0.71 (0.24, 2.18)	0.74 (0.27, 1.95)
0.71 (0.30, 1.71)	0.67 (0.22, 2.03)	0.85 (0.42, 1.73)	0.74 (0.24, 2.25)	Durva	0.62 (0.29, 1.32)	0.70 (0.26, 1.92)	0.54 (0.20, 1.46)	0.53 (0.19, 1.46)	0.55 (0.23, 1.30)
1.15 (0.47, 2.73)	1.08 (0.35, 3.30)	1.37 (0.66, 2.80)	1.20 (0.40, 3.66)	1.61 (0.76, 3.44)	Durva+Treme	1.12 (0.42, 3.05)	0.87 (0.32, 2.34)	0.85 (0.31, 2.36)	0.88 (0.36, 2.11)
1.02 (0.44, 2.38)	0.96 (0.32, 2.89)	1.22 (0.62, 2.43)	1.07 (0.36, 3.18)	1.44 (0.52, 3.87)	0.89 (0.33, 2.39)	Nivo+CT	0.78 (0.40, 1.57)	0.76 (0.29, 2.03)	0.79 (0.33, 1.83)
1.31 (0.57, 3.03)	1.23 (0.41, 3.71)	1.56 (0.79, 3.07)	1.37 (0.46, 4.03)	1.84 (0.68, 4.98)	1.14 (0.43, 3.09)	1.28 (0.64, 2.53)	Nivo+Ipi	0.97 (0.36, 2.56)	1.01 (0.43, 2.32)
1.35 (0.57, 3.17)	1.27 (0.42, 3.83)	1.61 (0.79, 3.29)	1.40 (0.46, 4.24)	1.89 (0.68, 5.21)	1.18 (0.42, 3.27)	1.32 (0.49, 3.49)	1.03 (0.39, 2.75)	Nivo+Ipi+CT	1.04 (0.43, 2.47)
1.30 (0.64, 2.65)	1.22 (0.46, 3.28)	1.55 (0.94, 2.57)	1.35 (0.51, 3.66)	1.83 (0.77, 4.35)	1.13 (0.47, 2.78)	1.27 (0.55, 2.99)	0.99 (0.43, 2.32)	0.96 (0.41, 2.30)	Pembro+CT

B

Atezo+CT	0.70 (0.37, 1.35)	1.13 (0.50, 2.71)	**1.49 (1.05, 2.23)**	0.91 (0.48, 1.71)	1.09 (0.53, 2.34)	0.50 (0.20, 1.28)	1.11 (0.54, 2.45)	0.97 (0.55, 1.84)	0.99 (0.44, 2.28)	1.05 (0.57, 2.06)
1.43 (0.74, 2.70)	Atezo+CT+Bev	1.61 (0.57, 4.79)	**2.12 (1.03, 4.58)**	1.30 (0.68, 2.45)	1.55 (0.59, 4.32)	0.71 (0.28, 1.82)	1.59 (0.61, 4.41)	1.39 (0.58, 3.47)	1.41 (0.50, 4.01)	1.50 (0.62, 3.86)
0.88 (0.37, 2.00)	0.62 (0.21, 1.74)	Camre+CT	1.32 (0.61, 2.81)	0.81 (0.27, 2.23)	0.96 (0.36, 2.58)	0.44 (0.12, 1.51)	0.99 (0.37, 2.67)	0.86 (0.35, 2.10)	0.87 (0.30, 2.52)	0.93 (0.37, 2.37)
0.67 (0.45, 0.95)	**0.47 (0.22, 0.97)**	0.76 (0.36, 1.63)	CT	0.61 (0.29, 1.24)	0.73 (0.39, 1.39)	**0.34 (0.12, 0.89)**	0.75 (0.39, 1.44)	0.66 (0.41, 1.04)	0.66 (0.31, 1.38)	0.70 (0.43, 1.18)
1.10 (0.58, 2.09)	0.77 (0.41, 1.47)	1.24 (0.45, 3.70)	1.64 (0.81, 3.49)	CT+Bev	1.20 (0.46, 3.22)	0.55 (0.28, 1.10)	1.23 (0.47, 3.38)	1.07 (0.46, 2.65)	1.09 (0.39, 3.10)	1.15 (0.49, 2.92)
0.92 (0.43, 1.87)	0.65 (0.23, 1.70)	1.04 (0.39, 2.81)	1.37 (0.72, 2.59)	0.84 (0.31, 2.16)	Nivo+CT	0.46 (0.14, 1.48)	1.03 (0.54, 1.96)	0.9 (0.40, 1.97)	0.91 (0.34, 2.39)	0.97 (0.42, 2.20)
2.00 (0.78, 5.08)	1.40 (0.55, 3.57)	2.27 (0.66, 8.10)	**2.97 (1.13, 8.26)**	1.82 (0.91, 3.57)	2.18 (0.68, 7.31)	Nivo+CT+Bev	2.23 (0.70, 7.42)	1.95 (0.66, 6.02)	1.98 (0.57, 6.86)	2.10 (0.71, 6.67)
0.90 (0.41, 1.84)	0.63 (0.23, 1.65)	1.01 (0.37, 2.71)	1.33 (0.70, 2.54)	0.81 (0.30, 2.11)	0.97 (0.51, 1.86)	0.45 (0.13, 1.43)	Nivo+Ipi	0.87 (0.39, 1.93)	0.88 (0.33, 2.35)	0.94 (0.42, 2.15)
1.03 (0.54, 1.83)	0.72 (0.29, 1.71)	1.16 (0.48, 2.82)	1.53 (0.96, 2.45)	0.93 (0.38, 2.18)	1.12 (0.51, 2.48)	0.51 (0.17, 1.51)	1.14 (0.52, 2.55)	Pembro+CT	1.01 (0.42, 2.39)	1.07 (0.54, 2.17)
1.01 (0.44, 2.27)	0.71 (0.25, 2.00)	1.15 (0.40, 3.36)	1.51 (0.72, 3.19)	0.92 (0.32, 2.56)	1.10 (0.42, 2.91)	0.50 (0.15, 1.74)	1.13 (0.43, 3.06)	0.99 (0.42, 2.38)	Sinti+CT	1.06 (0.43, 2.68)
0.95 (0.49, 1.76)	0.67 (0.26, 1.62)	1.08 (0.42, 2.72)	1.42 (0.85, 2.34)	0.87 (0.34, 2.05)	1.04 (0.46, 2.36)	0.48 (0.15, 1.41)	1.07 (0.47, 2.41)	0.93 (0.46, 1.85)	0.94 (0.37, 2.32)	Tisle+CT

FIGURE 4 | Comparative efficacy of treatments for OS **(A)** and PFS **(B)** in network meta-analysis. Comparisons should be read from left to right. HR (95% credible interval) for comparisons is in cells in common between column-defining and row-defining treatment. Bold cells are significant. HR >1 favors row-defining treatment, and HR <1 favors column-defining treatment. CT, chemotherapy; Atezo, atezolizumab; Bev, bevacizumab; Nivo, nivolumab; Ipi, ipilimumab; Pembro, pembrolizumab; Carem, caremlizumab; Durva, durvalumab; Treme, tremelimumab; Tisle, tislezumab; Sinti, sintilimab; NR, not reported.

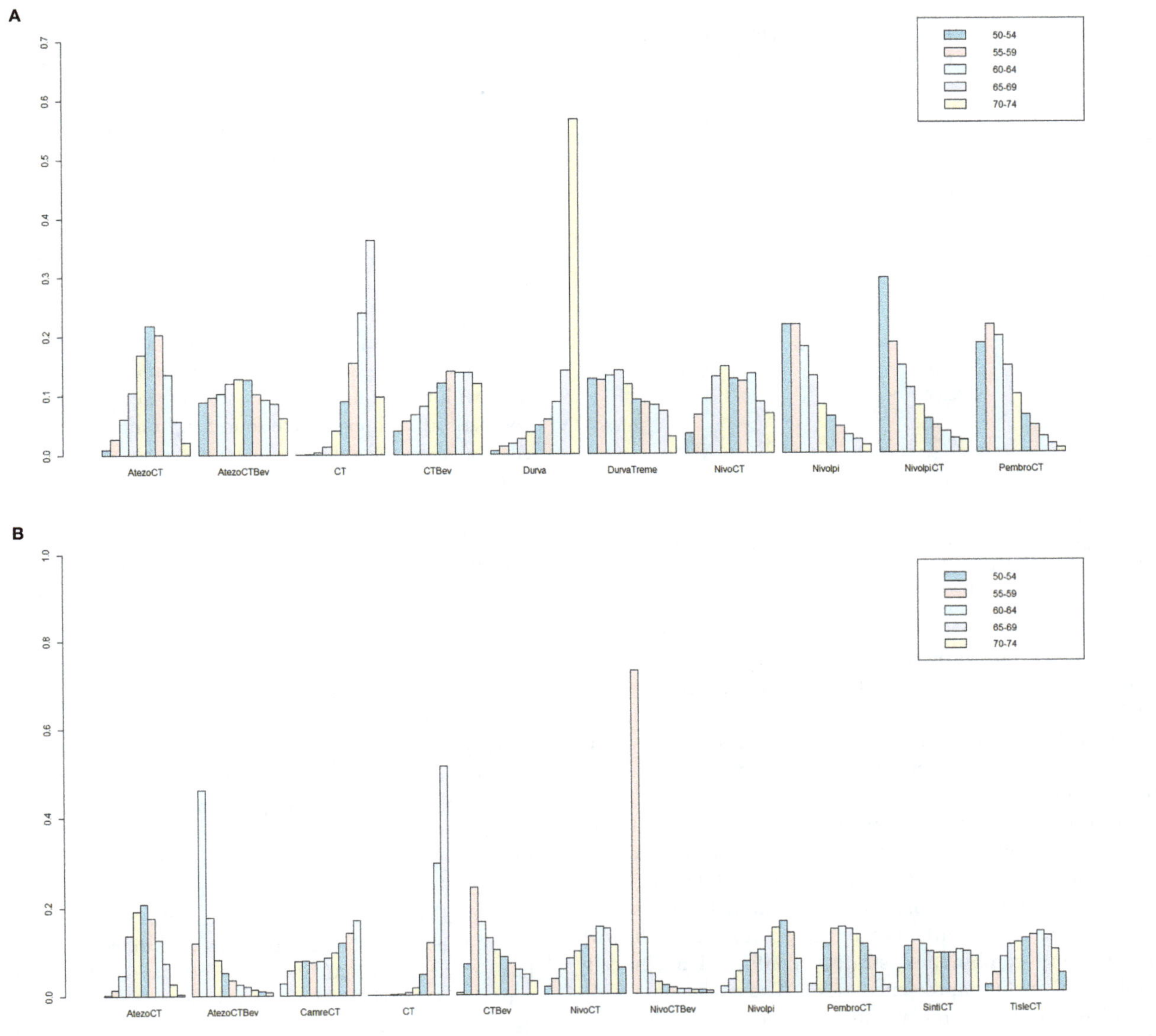

FIGURE 5 | Ranking probabilities based on the multiple comparisons on OS **(A)** and PFS **(B)** in NSCLC patients with PD-L1–negative expression. CT, chemotherapy; Atezo, atezolizumab; Bev, bevacizumab; Nivo, nivolumab; Ipi, ipilimumab; Pembro, pembrolizumab; Carem, caremlizumab; Durva, durvalumab; Treme, tremelimumab; Tisle, tislezumab; Sinti, sintilimab; NR, not reported.

demonstrated that PD-L1 expression on tumor and/or immune cells has a positive correlation with the efficacy of anti-PD-(L)1 therapy. A real-world EXPRESS study evaluated the PD-L1 expression profile in locally advanced or metastatic NSCLC, revealing that PD-L1–negative patients account for about 40% to 53% (7). Efficacies of PD-(L)1 blockade treatment in patients that are PD-L1 positive or negative are significantly different (29). Here, our analysis is designed to answer the open question of the optimal therapeutic management in advanced NSCLC with negative PD-L1 expression.

The expression of PD-L1 can be classified into constitutive and inducible expression depending on the extrinsic or intrinsic stimuli (30). Constitutive expression is dependent on cell genomics, while inducible PD-L1 expression is dependent on exposure of cells to cytokines, such as IFNγ, TNFα, IL-1α, and IL-1β *via* TLRs or IFN receptors (31). PD-L1–negative expression of a tumor is sometimes considered as the tumor being "cold" to use a somewhat colloquial term (32). The absence of PD-L1 expression on tumor cells might, for example, indicate impaired IFN-γsignaling (33). By turning "cold" tumors to "hot", combination strategies emerge, which involve different immune checkpoint inhibitors (ICIs) with chemotherapy, anti-angiogenesis, and other new classes drugs or, for example, oncolytic viruses (34).

The 14 treatment modalities in our meta-analysis for PD-L1–negative NSCLC can be categorized into seven types:

TABLE 2 | Ranking probabilities of different first-line treatment strategies for PD-L1–negative NSCLC patients.

	Ranking probability for the best (OS, %)	Ranking probability for the best (PFS, %)
Atezo + CT	0.71	0.20
Atezo + CT + Bev	8.46	11.93
Camre + CT	NR	2.71
CT	0.00	0.00
CT + Bev	3.46	0.46
Durva	0.48	NR
Durva + Treme	12.61	NR
Nivo + CT	2.97	1.77
Nivo + CT + Bev	NR	**72.92**
Nivo + Ipi	22.39	1.44
Nivo + Ipi + CT	**30.09**	NR
Pembro+CT	18.81	1.86
Sinti + CT	NR	5.26
Tisle + CT	NR	1.45

OS, overall survival; PFS, progression-free survival; CT, chemotherapy; Atezo, atezolizumab; Bev, bevacizumab; Nivo, nivolumab; Ipi, ipilimumab; Pembro, pembrolizumab; Carem, caremlizumab; Durva, durvalumab; Treme, tremelimumab; Tisle, tislezumab; Sinti, sintilimab; NR, not reported.
Bold means the the highest ranking probablity.

chemotherapy, chemotherapy plus angiogenesis inhibition, mono anti-PD-(L)1, anti-PD-(L)1 plus chemotherapy, anti-PD-(L)1 plus anti-cytotoxic T-lymphocyte–associated antigen 4 (CTLA-4), anti-PD-(L)1 plus anti-CTLA-4 plus angiogenesis inhibition, and anti-PD-(L)1 plus anti-CTLA-4 plus chemotherapy.

Chemotherapy was previously considered to be immunosuppressive, whereas cytotoxic drugs may also exert an immunomodulatory role in NSCLC and other solid tumors (35). A recent pooled analysis of three randomized trials assessing PD-L1–negative patients receiving pembrolizumab with chemotherapy combination strategy confirmed a clinically meaningful benefit improvement (36). The inclusion of HR from phase II studies might influence the results; therefore, only phase III trials were included in this analysis, leaving phase II KEYNOTE-021G trial (37) ineligible for our analysis.

The rationale for combining anti-angiogenesis drug with ICIs rests in aspects, including immuno-metabolism and tumor microenvironment (38), which leads to a synergistic effect. Therapeutic regimens of chemotherapy with anti-angiogenesis drugs, such as ECOG-4599 (39), BEYOND (40), were not included in the network meta-analysis because of lack of PD-L1 expression status. In the IMpower150 trial, ACP (atezolizumab plus chemotherapy) and BCP (bevacizumab plus chemotherapy) had similar outcomes for the PD-L1–negative population (15).

Another combination choice for PD-(L)1 inhibitor is the combination of a CTLA-4 inhibitor, as used by CheckMate 227. Anti-PD-1 and anti–CTLA-4 dual blockade offers a "chemo-free" choice for PD-L1–negative patients. Dual blockade of CTLA-4 and PD-1 therapy is sufficient to induce unique cellular responses compared with either monotherapy, which has been proven in preclinical studies (41). However, the toxicity of adding another ICI to a PD-(L)1 inhibitor leads to more toxicity (42). In our network meta-analysis, we have no data for toxicity regarding PD-L1–negative patients receiving different treatment strategies. However, based on a previous meta-analysis, combination with CTLA-4 inhibitor might lead to more toxicities (42).

For OS and PFS, based on treatment ranking probabilities, nivolumab plus chemotherapy plus ipilimumab/bevacizumab ranked first, respectively. However, nivolumab plus chemotherapy plus ipilimumab (CheckMate 9LA) did not report PFS subgroup data regarding PD-L1–negative patients, whereas nivolumab plus chemotherapy plus bevacizumab (ONO-4538-52) did not report OS data in PD-L1 negative patients. These subgroup data are missing and will thus impact the result of network meta-analysis comparison. Although these four-drug combinations prevailed in survival than the other regimens by ranking probability, more toxicities might also occur in four-drug combinations. In CheckMate 9LA trial, three times of treatment-related adverse events (TRAEs) of nivolumab plus ipilimumab plus two cycles of chemotherapy than control arm render a four-drug combination, an option for PD-L1 negative patients but may not be the standard of care.

Our meta-analysis has several limitations. First, there were no clinical trials investigating only PD-L1–negative NSCLC patients. Therefore, data were derived from subgroup analysis of each primary study, and none of these trials were powered to detect the difference in OS or PFS in the PD-L1–negative subgroup, which explained why none of the treatment were significantly more effective in OS than chemotherapy. Some of the trials did not report OS, making comparisons not identical between PFS and OS. Second, the antibodies using to detect PD-L1 expression varied in different trials. Spatial and temporal heterogeneity of PD-L1 expression and different test platforms have made PD-L1 an imperfect biomarker. However, PD-L1 expression especially in tumor cells is currently the most widely used biomarker in patient stratification. Third, we have no access to toxicity data for patients with PD-L1–negative expression, and such expression is often heterogenous (43). Balancing the benefit/risk to a specific patient population is always challenging (44).

In summary, our meta-analysis is the first study to systematically investigate the treatment options for PD-L1–negative patients of NSCLC. In the absence of an RCT directly comparing first-line treatment options for NSCLC of PD-L1–negative expression, our findings suggest that two combined therapies, nivolumab plus ipilimumab plus chemotherapy, and nivolumab plus chemotherapy plus bevacizumab, both appear the most effective therapeutic strategies for this patient population in terms of OS and PFS, respectively. Further research, particularly phase III RCTs comparing treatment options in PD-L1–negative patients are required.

AUTHOR CONTRIBUTIONS

YX and FL had full access to all the data in the study and takes responsibility for the integrity of the data and the accuracy of the data analysis. YX, WHL, and LP participated in the concept and design. All authors participated in the acquisition, analysis, or interpretation of data. All authors participated in the drafting of the manuscript. All authors participated in the critical revision of the manuscript. LP, FL, and YX participated as the administrative, technical, or material support. YX and FL participated in the supervision. All authors contributed to the article and approved the submitted version.

ACKNOWLEDGMENTS

We are grateful to the authors of the primary studies.

REFERENCES

1. Siegel RL, Miller KD, Fuchs HE, Jemal A. Cancer Statistics, 2021. *CA Cancer J Clin* (2021) 71(1):7–33. doi: 10.3322/caac.21654
2. Herbst RS, Morgensztern D, Boshoff C. The Biology and Management of Non-Small Cell Lung Cancer. *Nature* (2018) 553(7689):446–54. doi: 10.1038/nature25183
3. Brody R, Zhang Y, Ballas M, Siddiqui MK, Gupta P, Barker C, et al. PD-L1 Expression in Advanced NSCLC: Insights Into Risk Stratification and Treatment Selection From a Systematic Literature Review. *Lung Cancer* (2017) 112:200–15. doi: 10.1016/j.lungcan.2017.08.005
4. Reck M, Rodriguez-Abreu D, Robinson AG, Hui R, Csoszi T, Fulop A, et al. Pembrolizumab Versus Chemotherapy for PD-L1-Positive Non-Small-Cell Lung Cancer. *N Engl J Med* (2016) 375(19):1823–33. doi: 10.1056/NEJMoa1606774
5. Mok TSK, Wu YL, Kudaba I, Kowalski DM, Cho BC, Turna HZ, et al. Pembrolizumab Versus Chemotherapy for Previously Untreated, PD-L1-expressing, Locally Advanced or Metastatic Non-Small-Cell Lung Cancer (KEYNOTE-042): A Randomised, Open-Label, Controlled, Phase 3 Trial. *Lancet* (2019) 393(10183):1819–30. doi: 10.1016/S0140-6736(18)32409-7
6. Xu Y, Wan B, Chen X, Zhan P, Zhao Y, Zhang T, et al. The Association of PD-L1 Expression With the Efficacy of Anti-PD-1/PD-L1 Immunotherapy and Survival of Non-Small Cell Lung Cancer Patients: A Meta-Analysis of Randomized Controlled Trials. *Transl Lung Cancer Res* (2019) 8(4):413–28. doi: 10.21037/tlcr.2019.08.09
7. Dietel M, Savelov N, Salanova R, Micke P, Bigras G, Hida T, et al. Real-World Prevalence of Programmed Death Ligand 1 Expression in Locally Advanced or Metastatic Non-Small-Cell Lung Cancer: The Global, Multicenter EXPRESS Study. *Lung Cancer* (2019) 134:174–9. doi: 10.1016/j.lungcan.2019.06.012
8. Salanti G, Ades AE, Ioannidis JP. Graphical Methods and Numerical Summaries for Presenting Results From Multiple-Treatment Meta-Analysis: An Overview and Tutorial. *J Clin Epidemiol* (2011) 64(2):163–71. doi: 10.1016/j.jclinepi.2010.03.016
9. Jadad AR, Moore RA, Carroll D, Jenkinson C, Reynolds DJ, Gavaghan DJ, et al. Assessing the Quality of Reports of Randomized Clinical Trials: Is Blinding Necessary? *Control Clin Trials* (1996) 17(1):1–12. doi: 10.1016/0197-2456(95)00134-4
10. Higgins JP, Jackson D, Barrett JK, Lu G, Ades AE, White IR. Consistency and Inconsistency in Network Meta-Analysis: Concepts and Models for Multi-Arm Studies. *Res Synth Methods* (2012) 3(2):98–110. doi: 10.1002/jrsm.1044
11. Higgins JP, Thompson SG, Deeks JJ, Altman DG. Measuring Inconsistency in Meta-Analyses. *BMJ* (2003) 327(7414):557–60. doi: 10.1136/bmj.327.7414.557
12. West H, McCleod M, Hussein M, Morabito A, Rittmeyer A, Conter HJ, et al. Atezolizumab in Combination With Carboplatin Plus Nab-Paclitaxel Chemotherapy Compared With Chemotherapy Alone as First-Line Treatment for Metastatic Non-Squamous Non-Small-Cell Lung Cancer (Impower130): A Multicentre, Randomised, Open-Label, Phase 3 Trial. *Lancet Oncol* (2019) 20(7):924–37. doi: 10.1016/S1470-2045(19)30167-6
13. Jotte R, Cappuzzo F, Vynnychenko I, Stroyakovskiy D, Rodriguez-Abreu D, Hussein M, et al. Atezolizumab in Combination With Carboplatin and Nab-Paclitaxel in Advanced Squamous NSCLC (Impower131): Results From a Randomized Phase III Trial. *J Thorac Oncol* (2020) 15(8):1351–60. doi: 10.1016/j.jtho.2020.03.028
14. Nishio M, Barlesi F, West H, Ball S, Bordoni R, Cobo M, et al. Atezolizumab Plus Chemotherapy for First-Line Treatment of Nonsquamous NSCLC: Results From the Randomized Phase 3 IMpower132 Trial. *J Thorac Oncol* (2021) 16(4):653–64. doi: 10.1016/j.jtho.2020.11.025
15. Socinski M, Mok TSK, Nishio M, Jotte RM, Cappuzzo F, Orlandi F, et al. Impower150 Final Analysis: Efficacy of Atezolizumab (Atezo) + Bevacizumab (Bev) and Chemotherapy in First- Line (1L) Metastatic Nonsquamous (Nsq) Non-Small Cell Lung Cancer (NSCLC) Across Key Subgroups. *AACR* (2020) 80(16):CT216. doi: 10.1158/1538-7445.AM2020-CT216
16. Zhou C, Chen G, Huang Y, Zhou J, Lin L, Feng J, et al. Camrelizumab Plus Carboplatin and Pemetrexed Versus Chemotherapy Alone in Chemotherapy-Naive Patients With Advanced Non-Squamous Non-Small-Cell Lung Cancer (CameL): A Randomised, Open-Label, Multicentre, Phase 3 Trial. *Lancet Respir Med* (2021) 9(3):305–14. doi: 10.1016/S2213-2600(20)30365-9
17. Rizvi NA, Cho BC, Reinmuth N, Lee KH, Luft A, Ahn MJ, et al. Durvalumab With or Without Tremelimumab vs Standard Chemotherapy in First-line Treatment of Metastatic Non-Small Cell Lung Cancer: The MYSTIC Phase 3 Randomized Clinical Trial. *JAMA Oncol* (2020) 6(5):661–74. doi: 10.1001/jamaoncol.2020.0237
18. Ramalingam S, Ciuleanu TE, Płużański A, Lee JS, Schenker M, Caro RB, et al. Nivolumab + Ipilimumab Versus Platinum-Doublet Chemotherapy as First-Line Treatment for Advanced Non-Small Cell Lung Cancer: Three-Year Update From CheckMate 227 Part 1. *J Clin Oncol* (2020) 15:9500. doi: 10.1200/JCO.2020.38.15_suppl.9500
19. Paz-Ares L, Ciuleanu TE, Cobo M, Schenker M, Zurawski B, Menezes J, et al. First-Line Nivolumab Plus Ipilimumab Combined With Two Cycles of Chemotherapy in Patients With Non-Small-Cell Lung Cancer (CheckMate 9LA): An International, Randomised, Open-Label, Phase 3 Trial. *Lancet Oncol* (2021) 22(2):198–211. doi: 10.1016/S1470-2045(20)30641-0
20. Lee JS, Sugawara S, Kang JH, Kim HR, Inui N, Hida T. Randomized Phase III Trial of Nivolumab in Combination With Carboplatin, Paclitaxel, and Bevacizumab as First-Line Treatment for Patients With Advanced or Recurrent Non-Squamous NSCLC. *Ann Oncol* (2020) 31:S1184–5. doi: 10.1016/j.annonc.2020.08.2287
21. Gandhi L, Rodriguez-Abreu D, Gadgeel S, Esteban E, Felip E, De Angelis F, et al. Pembrolizumab Plus Chemotherapy in Metastatic Non-Small-Cell Lung Cancer. *N Engl J Med* (2018) 378(22):2078–92. doi: 10.1056/NEJMoa1801005
22. Paz-Ares L, Luft A, Vicente D, Tafreshi A, Gumus M, Mazieres J, et al. Pembrolizumab Plus Chemotherapy for Squamous Non-Small-Cell Lung Cancer. *N Engl J Med* (2018) 379(21):2040–51. doi: 10.1056/NEJMoa1810865
23. Yang Y, Wang Z, Fang J, Yu Q, Han B, Cang S, et al. Efficacy and Safety of Sintilimab Plus Pemetrexed and Platinum as First-Line Treatment for Locally Advanced or Metastatic Nonsquamous NSCLC: A Randomized, Double-Blind, Phase 3 Study (Oncology pRogram by InnovENT Anti-PD-1-11). *J Thorac Oncol* (2020) 15(10):1636–46. doi: 10.1016/j.jtho.2020.09.028
24. Wang J, Lu S, Yu X, Hu Y, Sun Y, Wang Z, et al. Tislelizumab Plus Chemotherapy vs Chemotherapy Alone as First-line Treatment for Advanced Squamous Non-Small-Cell Lung Cancer: A Phase 3 Randomized Clinical Trial. *JAMA Oncol* (2021) 7(5):709–17. doi: 10.1001/jamaoncol.2021.0366
25. Lu S, Yu Y, Yu X, Hu H-H, Ma Z, Li X, et al. Tislelizumab + Chemotherapy vs Chemotherapy Alone as First-Line Treatment for Locally Advanced/Metastatic Nonsquamous NSCLC. *Ann Oncol* (2020) 31:S816–7. doi: 10.1016/j.annonc.2020.08.1577
26. Moher D, Liberati A, Tetzlaff J, Altman DG. Preferred Reporting Items for Systematic Reviews and Meta-Analyses: The PRISMA Statement. *PloS Med* (2009) 6(7):e1000097. doi: 10.1371/journal.pmed.1000097

27. Zhang J, Dang F, Ren J, Wei W. Biochemical Aspects of PD-L1 Regulation in Cancer Immunotherapy. *Trends Biochem Sci* (2018) 43(12):1014–32. doi: 10.1016/j.tibs.2018.09.004
28. Lamberti G, Spurr LF, Li Y, Ricciuti B, Recondo G, Umeton R, et al. Clinicopathological and Genomic Correlates of Programmed Cell Death Ligand 1 (PD-L1) Expression in Nonsquamous Non-Small-Cell Lung Cancer. *Ann Oncol* (2020) 31(6):807–14. doi: 10.1016/j.annonc.2020.02.017
29. Shen X, Zhao B. Efficacy of PD-1 or PD-L1 Inhibitors and PD-L1 Expression Status in Cancer: Meta-Analysis. *BMJ* (2018) 362:k3529. doi: 10.1136/bmj.k3529
30. Topalian SL, Taube JM, Anders RA, Pardoll DM. Mechanism-Driven Biomarkers to Guide Immune Checkpoint Blockade in Cancer Therapy. *Nat Rev Cancer* (2016) 16(5):275–87. doi: 10.1038/nrc.2016.36
31. Chen DS, Irving BA, Hodi FS. Molecular Pathways: Next-Generation Immunotherapy–Inhibiting Programmed Death-Ligand 1 and Programmed Death-1. *Clin Cancer Res* (2012) 18(24):6580–7. doi: 10.1158/1078-0432.CCR-12-1362
32. Ribas A, Hu-Lieskovan S. What Does PD-L1 Positive or Negative Mean? *J Exp Med* (2016) 213(13):2835–40. doi: 10.1084/jem.20161462
33. Theelen W, Kuilman T, Schulze K, Zou W, Krijgsman O, Peters D, et al. Absence of PD-L1 Expression on Tumor Cells in the Context of an Activated Immune Infiltrate may Indicate Impaired IFNgamma Signaling in Non-Small Cell Lung Cancer. *PloS One* (2019) 14(5):e0216864. doi: 10.1371/journal.pone.0216864
34. Bonaventura P, Shekarian T, Alcazer V, Valladeau-Guilemond J, Valsesia-Wittmann S, Amigorena S, et al. Cold Tumors: A Therapeutic Challenge for Immunotherapy. *Front Immunol* (2019) 10:168. doi: 10.3389/fimmu.2019.00168
35. Heinhuis KM, Ros W, Kok M, Steeghs N, Beijnen JH, Schellens JHM. Enhancing Antitumor Response by Combining Immune Checkpoint Inhibitors With Chemotherapy in Solid Tumors. *Ann Oncol* (2019) 30 (2):219–35. doi: 10.1093/annonc/mdy551
36. Borghaei H, Langer CJ, Paz-Ares L, Rodriguez-Abreu D, Halmos B, Garassino MC, et al. Pembrolizumab Plus Chemotherapy Versus Chemotherapy Alone in Patients With Advanced Non-Small Cell Lung Cancer Without Tumor PD-L1 Expression: A Pooled Analysis of 3 Randomized Controlled Trials. *Cancer* (2020) 126(22):4867–77. doi: 10.1002/cncr.33142
37. Gadgeel S, Rodriguez-Abreu D, Speranza G, Esteban E, Felip E, Domine M, et al. Updated Analysis From KEYNOTE-189: Pembrolizumab or Placebo Plus Pemetrexed and Platinum for Previously Untreated Metastatic Nonsquamous Non-Small-Cell Lung Cancer. *J Clin Oncol* (2020) 38 (14):1505–17. doi: 10.1200/JCO.19.03136
38. Giannone G, Ghisoni E, Genta S, Scotto G, Tuninetti V, Turinetto M, et al. Immuno-Metabolism and Microenvironment in Cancer: Key Players for Immunotherapy. *Int J Mol Sci* (2020) 21(12):4414. doi: 10.3390/ijms21124414
39. Tyagi P. Bevacizumab, When Added to Paclitaxel/Carboplatin, Prolongs Survival in Previously Untreated Patients With Advanced Non-Small-Cell Lung Cancer: Preliminary Results From the ECOG 4599 Trial. *Clin Lung Cancer* (2005) 6(5):276–8. doi: 10.1016/S1525-7304(11)70220-0
40. Zhou C, Wu YL, Chen G, Liu X, Zhu Y, Lu S, et al. Beyond: A Randomized, Double-Blind, Placebo-Controlled, Multicenter, Phase III Study of First-Line Carboplatin/Paclitaxel Plus Bevacizumab or Placebo in Chinese Patients With Advanced or Recurrent Nonsquamous Non-Small-Cell Lung Cancer. *J Clin Oncol* (2015) 33(19):2197–204. doi: 10.1200/JCO.2014.59.4424
41. Wei SC, Anang NAS, Sharma R, Andrews MC, Reuben A, Levine JH, et al. Combination Anti-CTLA-4 Plus Anti-PD-1 Checkpoint Blockade Utilizes Cellular Mechanisms Partially Distinct From Monotherapies. *Proc Natl Acad Sci USA* (2019) 116(45):22699–709. doi: 10.1073/pnas.1821218116
42. Xu C, Chen YP, Du XJ, Liu JQ, Huang CL, Chen L, et al. Comparative Safety of Immune Checkpoint Inhibitors in Cancer: Systematic Review and Network Meta-Analysis. *BMJ* (2018) 363:k4226. doi: 10.1136/bmj.k4226
43. McLaughlin J, Han G, Schalper KA, Carvajal-Hausdorf D, Pelekanou V, Rehman J, et al. Quantitative Assessment of the Heterogeneity of PD-L1 Expression in Non-Small-Cell Lung Cancer. *JAMA Oncol* (2016) 2(1):46–54. doi: 10.1001/jamaoncol.2015.3638
44. Johnson DB, Jakubovic BD, Sibaud V, Sise ME. Balancing Cancer Immunotherapy Efficacy and Toxicity. *J Allergy Clin Immunol Pract* (2020) 8(9):2898–906. doi: 10.1016/j.jaip.2020.06.028

3

KRAS-Mutant Non-Small Cell Lung Cancer: An Emerging Promisingly Treatable Subgroup

Mingying Xie[1], *Xiaoling Xu*[2,3,4] *and Yun Fan*[2,3,4*]

[1] Department of Medical Oncology, The Second Clinical Medical College of Zhejiang Chinese Medical University, Hangzhou, China, [2] Department of Medical Oncology, The Cancer Hospital of the University of Chinese Academy of Sciences (Zhejiang Cancer Hospital), Hangzhou, China, [3] Institute of Basic Medicine and Cancer (IBMC), Chinese Academy of Sciences, Hangzhou, China, [4] Department of Thoracic Medical Oncology, Zhejiang Cancer Hospital, Hangzhou, China

***Correspondence:**
Yun Fan
fanyun@zjcc.org.cn

Lung cancer, the leading cause of cancer-related deaths worldwide, can be classified into small cell lung cancer and non-small cell lung cancer (NSCLC). NSCLC is the most common histological type, accounting for 85% of all lung cancers. Kirsten rat sarcoma viral oncogene (KRAS) mutations, common in NSCLC, are associated with poor prognosis, likely due to poor responses to most systemic therapies and lack of targeted drugs. The latest published clinical trial data on new small-molecule KRAS G12C inhibitors, AMG510 and MRTX849, indicate that these molecules may potentially help treat KRAS-mutant NSCLC. Simultaneously, within the immuno-therapeutic process, immune efficacy has been observed in those patients who have *KRAS* mutations. In this article, the pathogenesis, treatment status, progress of immunotherapy, and targeted therapy of KRAS-mutant NSCLC are reviewed.

Keywords: KRAS-mutant, NSCLC, targeted therapy, immunotherapy, AMG510, MRTX849

INTRODUCTION

Lung cancer ranks first worldwide for malignant tumour-related deaths. Non-small cell lung cancer (NSCLC) is the most common histological subtype, accounting for 85% of all lung cancers (1). Compared with other mutations, Kirsten rat sarcoma viral oncogene (KRAS) mutations are among the most common mutations in NSCLC. However, patients with NSCLC harbouring KRAS mutations respond poorly to chemotherapy and have a poor overall prognosis (2). The rapid development of immunotherapy has brought hope for patients, improving the clinical outcomes of patients with KRAS-mutant NSCLC (3, 4). Currently, there are no KRAS-mutant NSCLC targeted drugs; however, promising clinical trial data on new small-molecule *KRAS* G12C inhibitors (2), AMG510 (5) and MRTX849 (6), showing that they may potentially treat KRAS-mutant NSCLC have come to light. Moreover, many different targeted drugs are currently being developed. This article summarises the current treatment options for patients with KRAS-mutant NSCLC.

MOLECULAR BIOLOGICAL FUNCTIONS OF KRAS

The rat sarcoma viral oncogene (*RAS*) gene mainly encodes a low molecular weight G protein (21 kD), with guanosine triphosphatase activity that acts as a molecular signal transduction switch and participates in regulating cell growth and differentiation. RAS protein is activated upon binding to guanosine triphosphate (GTP) and/or upstream signalling factors, activating downstream molecules and different signalling pathways that regulate basic cellular processes. The main RAS-mediated signalling pathways include the mitogen-activated protein kinase (MAPK) pathway (7–9); RAS-rapidly accelerated fibrosarcoma (RAF)-MAPK extracellular signal-regulated kinase (ERK) kinase (MEK)-ERK pathway, which mainly regulates cell proliferation and survival; and the phosphatidylinositol 3-kinase (PI3K)-protein kinase B (AKT)-mechanistic target of rapamycin (mTOR) pathway, which primarily controls cell proliferation. The RAS-like proto-oncogene guanine nucleotide dissociation stimulator pathway primarily stimulates the transcription of genes that promote survival and cell cycle progression. However, RAS is inactivated by guanosine diphosphate (GDP) (7). This activation/deactivation process involves GTP hydrolysis and GDP/GTP exchange, and both steps involve other regulatory proteins, such as guanine nucleotide exchange factors (GEFs) and guanosine triphosphatase activating protein (GAP).

In summary, RAS proteins regulate signal transduction by activating different effectors, thereby controlling different cellular functions.

There are three genes related to human tumours in the *RAS* gene family, Harvey rat sarcoma viral oncogene (*HRAS*), *KRAS*, and Neuroblastoma rat sarcoma viral oncogene (*NRAS*), which are located on chromosomes 11, 12, and 1, respectively (10). Among them, *KRAS* most significantly impacts human cancer (**Figure 1**). The small G protein encoded by the mutated *KRAS*

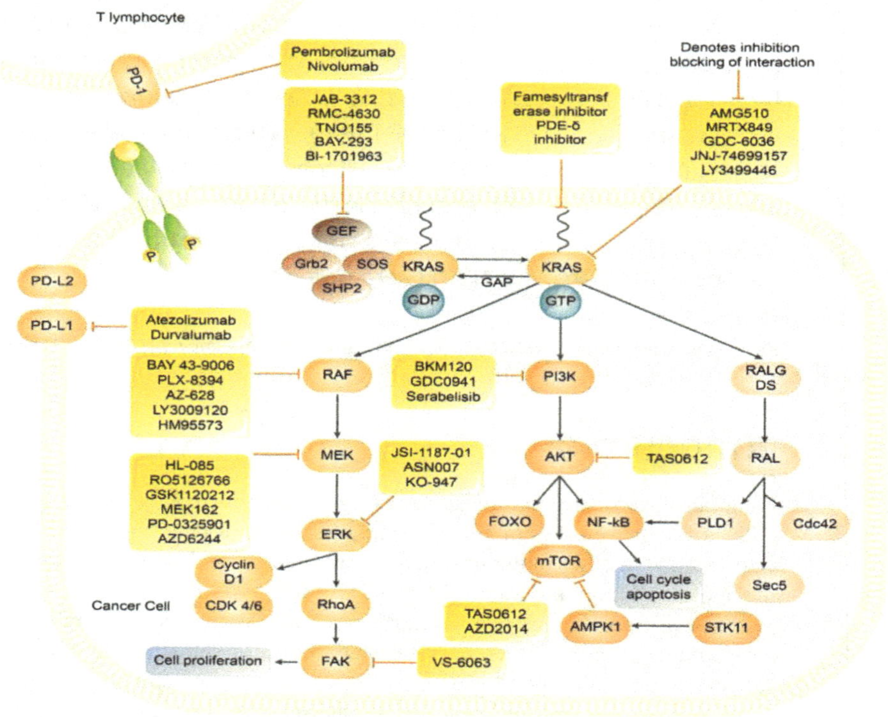

FIGURE 1 | Inhibitors of Kirsten rat sarcoma viral oncogene homolog (KRAS) effector signalling. RAS protein acts as a binary molecular switch in a variety of signal transduction pathways. It is active when combined with GTP, but doesn't have activity when combined with GDP. The GDP/GTP cycle is regulated by GEFs, which can promote the formation of active RAS - GTP and GAP stimulates GTP hydrolysis and forms inactive RAS - GDP. Normal RAS can be activated by upstream signalling factors, which in turn activates multiple downstream signalling pathways, including: MAPK, pathway; PI3k - AKT - mTOR, and pathway; RALGDS pathways. MAPK pathway, PI3K, pathway and JAK-STAT pathways promote the transcription of genes related to cell proliferation, metastasis, and drug resistance. PD -1 exists on the surface of activated T cells. When it is combined with PD-L1/2, it causes a series of immunosuppressive effects. Many Several methods have been developed to directly inhibit KRAS and inhibit KRAS downstream signalling pathways. Many new treatment strategies for KRAS inhibitors, KRAS downstream signalling pathway inhibitors, and ICIimmune checkpoint inhibitors are under investigation.

oncogene can still bind to GTP but prevents the GAP from increasing guanosine triphosphatase activity, inhibiting GTP hydrolysis to GDP and facilitating KRAS binding to GTP to maintain the active state. Without extracellular signals, an intracellular cascade reaction is initiated, resulting in unlimited cell growth and inducing tumourigenesis (7).

KRAS MUTATIONS AND THEIR ROLE IN NSCLC

KRAS mutations are some of the most common drivers of NSCLC and are almost only detected in lung adenocarcinoma and rarely found in squamous cell carcinoma. Over 80% of KRAS mutations occur in codon 12, and the most common mutations are *KRAS* G12C (mutation of glycine to cysteine; approximately 40%), *KRAS* G12V (mutation of glycine to valine; approximately 18–21%), and *KRAS* G12D (mutation of glycine to aspartic acid; approximately 17–18%), amongst others. Unlike other mutation types, *KRAS* mutations are mostly associated with smoking habits; approximately only 5% of *KRAS* mutations occur in light- or non-smokers. Notably, non-smokers are more likely to have *KRAS* G>A transformation mutations (mainly G12D) than smokers, while the most common mutation in smokers is a G>T translocation mutation (1, 7). Patients with KRAS-mutant NSCLC have a shorter median overall survival (OS) and a lower two-year survival rate (1).

PROGNOSIS OF KRAS-MUTANT NSCLC

At present, for NSCLC patients harbouring KRAS mutations, platinum-containing chemotherapy is central to a variety of treatments. However, the use of *KRAS* mutations as predictive markers for the onset of chemotherapy is disputable. A variety of studies have shown that *KRAS* mutations adversely affect OS and progression-free survival (PFS) and lower disease control rate (DCR) in patients with advanced NSCLC (11, 12). Furthermore, an earlier study showed that patients carrying KRAS mutations had high frequencies of liver (P = 0.01) and brain (P = 0.04) metastasis at baseline by radiological evaluation, suggesting that the presence of KRAS mutations may lead to more aggressive disease manifestations (11). As the epidermal growth factor receptor (*EGFR*) gene is located upstream of *KRAS*, a decrease in the tyrosine kinase activity of these receptors can reduce KRAS activation. However, *KRAS* mutations can counteract the therapeutic effects of EGFR tyrosine kinase inhibitors (TKIs), such as gefitinib and erlotinib, which are approved for the treatment of EGFR-mutant NSCLC but have poor efficacy in KRAS-mutant NSCLC (13).

In summary, currently available therapeutic options have little, if any, effect on NSCLC patients carrying KRAS mutations, whose prognoses remain poor.

PROGRESS IN IMMUNOTHERAPY OF KRAS-MUTANT NSCLC

In recent years, immunotherapy based on immune checkpoint inhibitors has been successful in treating NSCLC, especially in patients with a high tumour mutation burden (TMB), $CD8^+$ tumour cell infiltration, and programmed death-ligand 1 (PD-L1) expression (14). In a retrospective study, Valero et al. showed that neutrophil-to-lymphocyte ratio (NLR) is a suitable and promising biomarker for immunotherapy (15). They suggested that higher NLR is associated with poor prognosis after immune checkpoint inhibitors (ICI) therapy. In addition, lymphocyte-to-monocyte ratio (LMR) is also associated with immune responses (16). In contrast to the NLR, the higher the LMR, the better the immune effect (16). It was recently discovered that a normal expression of the human leukocyte antigen (HLA) class is a marker of favourable responses to immunosuppressive agents/ immunoinhibitors. Patients with complete loss respond poorly compared to patients with partial loss or normal expression of HLA class I (17). A recent study showed that in NSCLC, *KRAS* mutation status positively correlated with TMB, PD-L1 expression, and T cell infiltration (14). Since KRAS-mutant NSCLC is smoking-related lung cancer, high T cell infiltration and high TMB are usually observed in smokers with *KRAS* mutations (18, 19). The high T cell infiltration suggests that KRAS-mutant NSCLC may respond well to immunotherapy.

However, the influence of *KRAS* mutation status on the immune responses of NSCLC patients remains controversial. In a study of multi-line nivolumab treatment in those patients who have KRAS-mutant NSCLC (20), regardless of KRAS status, there were similar remission rates: overall response rate ([ORR] 20% vs. 17%; P = 0.39), DCR (47% vs. 41%; P = 0.23), median PFS (4 months vs. 3 months; P = 0.5), and OS (11.2 months vs. 10 months; P = 0.8). However, compared with the KRAS wild-type, the three-month PFS rate of patients with KRAS-mutant NSCLC was significantly increased (53% vs. 42%; P = 0.01). A subgroup analysis of randomised phase III study CheckMate057 indicated that during the second-line treatment for patients who carry *KRAS* mutations, nivolumab monotherapy had a higher OS benefit than docetaxel monotherapy (HR = 0.52; 95% CI: 0.29–0.95). Additionally, the subgroup with *KRAS* mutations had the highest OS benefit in nivolumab monotherapy, while the OS benefit of patients with wild-type KRAS was limited (HR = 0.98; 95% CI: 0.29–0.95) (4). According to the KRAS mutation status, the results of OS analysis in the OAK research, a randomised, double-blind III period clinical study, showed that patients with KRAS-mutant NSCLC could also benefit from atezolizumab treatment in terms of OS (HR = 0.71; 95% CI: 0.38–1.35) (3). First-line studies using immunosuppressants indicate some benefits for patients with KRAS-mutant NSCLC. The exploratory analysis of KEYNOTE-042 showed that the first-line pembrolizumab monotherapy in patients with KRAS-mutant NSCLC has higher PFS (12 months vs. 6 months; HR = 0.51; 95% CI: 0.29-0.87) and OS (28 months vs. 11 months; HR = 0.42; 95% CI: 0.22-0.81) than platinum-containing chemotherapy (21). The subgroup analysis of KEYNOTE-189 (21) showed that first-line pembrolizumab combined with platinum-containing chemotherapy has improved clinical efficacy compared with platinum-containing chemotherapy alone in patients with advanced NSCLC (PFS: 9 months vs. 5 months; HR = 0.47; 95% CI: 0.29-0.77; OS: 21 months vs. 14 months; HR = 0.79; 95% CI: 0.45-1.38). However, regardless of the *KRAS* mutation status, the PFS (9 months vs. 9 months), OS (21 months vs. 23 months), and ORR (40.7% vs. 47.6%) benefits are similar in pembrolizumab combined with platinum-containing chemotherapy. Furthermore, many studies have suggested that there may be a synergistic effect between KRAS G12C inhibitors and immunotherapy drugs. In preclinical studies, the use of AMG510 in immune-competent mice allowed T cells, especially $CD8^+$ T cells, to infiltrate a large number of tumours, resulting in a pro-inflammatory tumour microenvironment that produced durable responses alone or in combination with ICI (22). Another study also verified the immunomodulatory effect of KRAS G12C inhibitors, that is, the ability to reshape the immune microenvironment (23). Therefore, the combination therapy model using KRAS G12C inhibitors and anti-PD-1 therapy is expected to become a new treatment direction.

Interestingly, the different *KRAS* mutation subtypes may be related to the immune responses of patients with NSCLC. A retrospective study suggested that (24), among the common subtypes of *KRAS* mutations, the *KRAS* G12D mutation was related to poor OS (HR: 2.43; 95% CI: 1.15–5.16; P = 0.021), while the remaining *KRAS* mutation subtypes had no significant correlation with OS. This indicates that for patients with KRAS-mutant NSCLC, the *KRAS* G12D mutation is a negative prognostic factor compared to the negative expression of PD-L1 (<1%). Additionally, *KRAS* G12C mutation is related to weakly positive expression of PD-L1 (1%–49%) which suggests that it may predict immunotherapy benefits. Another retrospective study of patients with advanced KRAS-mutant NSCLC treated with immunosuppressive agents showed no significant differences in OS or PFS among the main *KRAS* mutation subtypes (G12A, G12C, G12D, G12V, and G13C) (25).

Furthermore, *KRAS* may have co-mutations with other master genes, which may affect immunity. In one Lung Cancer Mutation Consortium (LCMC) study (1), 27% of patients with lung adenocarcinoma had *KRAS* mutations, and as many as one-third of these patients had another carcinogenic driver. Skoulidis et al. (26) discovered three clusters based on strong expression: co-mutation with serine/threonine kinase 11 (*STK11*)/liver kinase B1 (*LKB1*) known as the KL subgroup, tumour protein 53 (TP53)(KP subgroup), and cyclin-dependent kinase inhibitor 2A/B (CDNK2A/B) inactivation plus thyroid transcription factor-1 low expression (KC subgroup). In addition, Kelch-like ECH-associated protein 1 (*KEAP1*)/Nuclear factor E2 related factor 2 (*NFE2L2*) is also a critical co-mutation, which is also enriched in the KL subgroup (2, 7). These clusters had various biological characteristics and treatment reaction: the ORR of immunotherapy for NSCLC due to *KRAS* mutations alone, KRAS co-mutations with STK11/LKB1 and TP53 was approximately 28.6%, 7.4% (because the blocking of PD-1 by immunosuppressive agents was reduced), and 35.7% (showing better efficacy), respectively (27). Patients with co-mutations in KEAP1/NFE2L2 have a significantly shorter survival (HR = 1.96; 95%CI: 1.33–2.92; p ≤ 0.001). This may be owing to the high levels of tumour-infiltrating cytotoxic $CD8^+$ cells, a significantly high overall mutation load, and high expression of PD-L1 in the KP subgroup tumours. In the KL subgroup tumours, *STK11* deletion promotes neutrophil recruitment, and the production of pro-inflammatory cytokines leads to a significant reduction in the number and function of T cells. Besides, *STK11/LKB1* inactivation reduces the expression levels of PD-L1 (24, 26, 28). KRAS-mutant NSCLC with *KEAP1* mutations were mostly immune inert tumours, with low T cell inflammation and low expression of PD-L1 ligands (7).

Blocking the PD-1/PD-L1 pathway is a promising treatment strategy for the treatment of KRAS-mutant NSCLC. Compared with immune combination chemotherapy, immunomonotherapy offers more evident PFS, ORR, and OS benefits (3, 4, 20, 21).

Cytotoxic T lymphocyte antigen-4 (CTLA-4) is considered another critical immune checkpoint, negatively regulating T cell immune responses. Ipilimumab (one of the CTLA-4 inhibitors) was widely used against melanoma (29). However, researchers are still studying the effect of CTLA-4 inhibitors on NSCLC. According to the data published by the CheckMate 227 (ClinicalTrials.gov Identifier: NCT02477826) and CheckMate 9LA (ClinicalTrials.gov Identifier: NCT03215706) studies, which included KRAS-mutant NSCLC patients, first-line treatment with nivolumab plus ipilimumab led to better survival than did chemotherapy in patients with NSCLC, regardless of PD-L1 expression level (30, 31).

In addition, tumour lymphoid-infiltrating cells are significantly cytotoxic and can accurately identify cancer cells. Therefore, therapy with these cells may be a promising new strategy.

Immunotherapy is a potential first-line treatment option for patients with KRAS-mutant NSCLC. However, because of the heterogeneity of KRAS-mutant NSCLC, especially the existence of co-mutations, individualised immunotherapy is needed.

PROGRESS IN TARGETED THERAPY FOR KRAS-MUTANT NSCLC

KRAS protein lacks a suitable "pocket" for small-molecule binding. Notably, KRAS has a very strong affinity for GTP and GDP (1000 times stronger than adenosine triphosphate [ATP]). There was very little difference between KRAS wild-type and mutant structures. Within the G or catalytic domain sequences, KRAS proteins are reportedly highly homologous with other RAS proteins, with nearly 90% similarity (10). Drugs targeting *KRAS* mutations often affect the normal KRAS. The similar structure of KRAS mutants challenges the development of effective drugs selectively targeting mutant KRAS (32).

Direct Inhibition of *KRAS*

The most common type of *KRAS* mutation is *KRAS* G12C. The mutant cysteine is located near a pocket (P2) in the switch II region. The P2 pocket only exists in the inactive GDP-binding conformation of KRAS, which can be used to make KRAS G12C irretrievable inhibitors (33). *KRAS* G12C allele inhibitors trap oncoproteins in an inactive state by inhibiting the reactivation of exchanged nucleotides, thereby blocking the proliferation of tumour cells that depend on the protein's signalling pathways

(34). AMG510 is a selective and irreversible small molecule targeting *KRAS* G12C with a mechanism similar to that described above. Preclinical studies have shown that AMG510 can inhibit almost all measurable ERK phosphorylations, a key downstream effector of KRAS, thereby enabling *KRAS* G12C mutant tumour mice to achieve long-lasting tumour regression (22). According to the latest data published by the CodeBreak 100 study (5), among the 59 patients who carry the *KRAS* G12C mutation in patients with advanced NSCLC undergoing multi-line therapy, a total of 19 patients had definite objective remission, with an ORR of 32.2% [95% CI: 20.62–45.64]; 52 patients had clear disease controVS-6766l, with a DCR of 88.1% (95% CI: 77.07–95.09). The median PFS was 6.3 months, significantly improved compared with previous second/third-line treatments for NSCLC. In terms of safety, 39 cases (66.1%) of treatment-related adverse events and 11 cases (18.6%) of adverse events of grade 3 or above were reported. The latest research data of CodeBreak 100 Phase II was announced at the 21st World Lung Cancer Conference. Among 124 patients with evaluable efficacy, the ORR was 37.1%, the DCR was 80.6%, and the median PFS was 6.8 months. In terms of safety, during treatment with AMG510, no dose-limiting side effects were observed, and no treatment-related deaths occurred. These findings indicate that AMG510 is safe, causes remission and long-lasting benefits in patients with KRAS-mutant NSCLC (35). Based on the positive results from the preliminary clinical trials, FDA has granted Sotorasib (AMG510) the title of breakthrough therapy for the treatment of locally advanced or metastatic NSCLC with *KRAS* G12C mutation on December 8, 2020. The CodeBreak 101 (ClinicalTrials.gov Identifier: NCT04185883) study investigated AMG510 monotherapy and combination therapy with anti-tumour drugs, and the CodeBreak 200 (ClinicalTrials.gov Identifier: NCT04303780, **Table 1**) study compared the effects of AMG510 in second-line treatment with standard chemotherapy. These studies have entered the clinical trial phase, and the results are promising.

A preclinical study of another oral, selective, small molecule (MRTX849) targeting *KRAS* G12C showed a broad spectrum of activity in tumours with the *KRAS* G12C mutation in *in vivo* models, resulting in significant tumour regression in most models (23). Mirati reported the latest clinical trial results of the Phase I/II clinical study of MRTX849 (6). In patients with advanced NSCLC who received chemotherapy and a PD-1/PD-L1 inhibitor, MRTX849 monotherapy has indicated up to 96% ORR and 45% DCR. Seventy percent (16/23) of patients with confirmed remission had more than 40% tumour reduction in comparison with the baseline. In terms of safety, 30% of patients experienced grade 3 or 4 treatment-related adverse events, 4.5% terminated treatment due to adverse reactions, and two patients died from treatment-related adverse events (one pneumonia and one heart failure case). The currently published data show that the efficacy of MRTX849 is slightly better than that of AMG510; however, the adverse effects are more significant, especially cardiac toxicity. The evaluation of the efficacy of these two drugs needs a larger cohort size. The Phase I/II clinical study (ClinicalTrials.gov Identifier: NCT04330664) of MRTX849 combined with the Src homology phosphortyrosyl phosphatase 2 (SHP2) inhibitors, TNO155, is underway.

Furthermore, the small-molecule *KRAS* G12C inhibitor JNJ-74699157 (ARS-3248) is in Phase I clinical trials (ClinicalTrials.gov Identifier: NCT04006301). Another newly developed small-molecule inhibitor, LY3499446, is under Phase I/II clinical study (ClinicalTrials.gov Identifier: NCT04165031) in combination with cyclin-dependent kinase (CDK) 4/6 inhibitor (abemaciclib), EGFR inhibitor (cetuximab), erlotinib, and docetaxel, respectively. A new *KRAS* G12C irreversible covalent inhibitor, GDC-6036, has also entered clinical trials (ClinicalTrials.gov Identifier: NCT04449874).

Although the emergence of KRAS G12C inhibitors has brought hope to patients with KRAS G12C mutations, the duration of response (DOR) (range 1.1 to 13.6 months) is not as good as the EGFR inhibitors (range 7.3 to 22.0 months) (35–37).

Furthermore, Mei Zeng et al. (38) have designed a library of C12 directed covalent degradation molecules (PROTACs). Although the degradants they found, in the end, cannot degrade the endogenous KRAS G12C, it provides new ideas and insights for the development of KRAS degradants.

In addition to the *KRAS* G12C mutation, mutations such as *KRAS* G12D also play an important role in the occurrence and development of tumours. The *KRAS* G12D-specific inhibitor MRTX1133, developed by Mirati, can reversibly bind to the activated and inactivated *KRAS* G12D mutants and inhibit their activity. The specificity of MRTX1133 to *KRAS* G12D is more than 1000 times that of wild-type *KRAS*, and its half-life is more than 50 hours (6). *In vitro* experiments indicated that MRTX1133 has a dose-dependent inhibition of the KRAS signalling pathway activity and significantly reduced the size of tumours with *KRAS* G12D mutations in pancreatic and colorectal cancer models compared with the control group (6).

Inhibition of the Nucleotide Exchange Cycles

The conversion of inactive KRAS-GDP to active KRAS-GTP requires GEFs, including the most common one, the Son of Sevenless (SOS) protein (39). A study (40) screened out a specific small-molecule SOS1 inhibitor, BAY-293, which can effectively destroy the mutual effect between KRAS and SOS1, prevent the formation of the KRAS-SOS1 complex, and thereby inhibit the activity of all *KRAS* mutants. Another SOS1 inhibitor, BI-1701963, is in Phase I clinical trial (ClinicalTrials.gov Identifier: NCT04111458) (41).

Inhibition of KRAS Membrane Positioning

KRAS needs to be processed by post-translational enzymes to bind to cell membranes and exert its activity, which requires the regulation of a variety of enzymes, such as farnesyltransferase, geranylgeranyltransferase, RAS-converting enzyme 1, isoprenylcysteine carboxyl methyltransferase, etc. The rate-limiting step in this series of enzymatic reactions is the isoprenylation of cysteine in the cysteine–aliphatic–aliphatic–terminal amino acid (CAAX) tetrapeptide structure mediated by

TABLE 1 | Ongoing Clinical Trials of KRAS-Mutant Lung Cancer.

NCT number	Drug code	Properties	Study Phase	Intervention Model	Allocation	Blind	Sponsor
NCT04625647	AMG 510	*KRAS* G12C inhibitor	Phase 2	Single Group Assignment: AMG 510 monotherapy	Not Applicable	None	• Southwest Oncology Group; • National Cancer Institute (NCI)
NCT04620330	VS-6766	RAF/MEK inhibitor	Phase 2	Single Group Assignment: VS-6766 monotherapy or VS-6766 in combination with defactinib	Randomised	None	• Verastem, Inc.
NCT04613596	MRTX849	*KRAS* G12C inhibitor	Phase 2	Single Group Assignment: MRTX849 in combination with Pembrolizumab	Not Applicable	None	• Mirati Therapeutics Inc.
NCT04470674	Durvalumab	Anti-PD-L1	Phase 2	Parallel Assignment: Durvalumab monotherapy vs Durvalumab plus chemotherapy	Randomised	None	• Shirish M Gadgeel; • AstraZeneca; • Henry Ford Health System; • Hoosier Cancer Research Network
NCT03808558	TVB-2640	FASN inhibitor	Phase 2	Single Group Assignment: TVB-2640 monotherapy	Not Applicable	None	• David E Gerber; • Universityof Texas Southwestern Medical Center
NCT03777124	SHR-1210; YN968D1	Anti-PD-1 antibody; VEGFR inhibitor	Phase 2	Parallel Assignment: SHR-1210 combination with apatinib vs Pemetrexed and Carboplatin	Randomised	Blind	• Jiangsu HengRui Medicine Co., Ltd.; • Shanghai Chest Hospital
NCT03693326	PDR001	Anti-PD-1 antibody	Phase 2	Single Group Assignment: PDR001 monotherapy	Not Applicable	None	• Asan Medical Center
NCT03520842	CL-14377; BAY 73-4506	antimetabolite and antifolate agent; kinase inhibitor	Phase 2	Single Group Assignment: Regorafenib in combination with Methotrexate	Not Applicable	None	• Stanford University
NCT02642042	GSK1120212	MEK Inhibitor	Phase 2	Single Group Assignment: Trametinib in combination with Docetaxel	Not Applicable	None	• National Cancer Institute (NCI)
NCT04303780	AMG 510	*KRAS* G12C inhibitor	Phase 3	Parallel Assignment: AMG 510 vs Docetaxel	Randomised	None	• Amgen
NCT02743923	carboplatin-paclitaxel-bevacizumab; cisplatin-pemetrexed	chemotherapy	Phase 3	Parallel Assignment: carboplatin-paclitaxel-bevacizumab vs cisplatin-pemetrexed	Randomised	None	• The Netherlands Cancer Institute; • Dutch Society of Physicians for Pulmonology and Tuberculosis
NCT02152631	LY2835219	CDK4/6 inhibitor	Phase 3	Parallel Assignment: LY2835219 vs Erlotinib	Randomised	None	• Eli Lilly and Company
NCT01933932	AZD6244	MEK inhibitor	Phase 3	Parallel Assignment: Selumetinib in combination with Docetaxel vs Placebo in combination with Docetaxel	Randomised	Blind	• AstraZeneca

farnesyltransferase (42). However, farnesyltransferase inhibitors (FTIs) such as tipifarnib, lonafarnib, and second-generation salirasib, did not show significant efficacy. This may be because when KRAS-mutant cells are deactivated by FTIs, farnesylation is deactivated. However, KRAS is modified by γ-glutamyl transpeptidase (GGT), a geranylgeranyl KRAS which allows its membrane positioning and signal transduction and overcomes the influence of FTIs (42). Simultaneous inhibition of farnesyltransferase and geranylgeranyltransferase may be an effective method, but it is necessary to observe toxicity levels. Another method to prevent the compensation effect of geranylgeranyltransferase on FTIs in KRAS-mutant NSCLC is to target other enzymes such as RAS-converting enzyme 1 and isoprenylcysteine carboxyl methyltransferase, whose inhibitors still need to be further studied. Phosphodiesterase-δ (PDE-δ) is an isoprene-binding protein that regulates the correct positioning and signal transmission of farnesylated KRAS. PDE-δ inhibitors interfere with the binding of mammalian PDE-δ and KRAS, change their location on the membrane, and inhibit carcinogenic KRAS signals (43). However, PDE-δ inhibitors' stability is unclear, and they may lack sufficient selectivity for KRAS protein, thus, warranting further research.

Inhibition of the Downstream Signal Pathway of KRAS

RAF-MEK-ERK pathway inhibition: Sorafenib (BAY 43-9006) is the first compound developed specifically for RAF. It is a multi-TKI (not a specific RAF kinase inhibitor) against vascular EGFR, platelet-derived growth factor receptor, and proto-oncogene tyrosine-protein kinase (44). In the BATTLE trial and the phase III MISSION trial, sorafenib did not have a noticeable therapeutic effect on KRAS-mutant NSCLC, nor did it prove *KRAS*-mutant state has predictive value for the efficacy of sorafenib (45–47). Unlike sorafenib, v-RAF murine sarcoma viral oncogene homolog B1 (BRAF) inhibitors are RAF-specific inhibitors. Currently, many BRAF inhibitors, for instance, dabrafenib, vemurafenib, and encorafenib, have been approved to target *BRAF* V600 mutations, but RAF kinase inhibitors do not perform well in *KRAS*-mutant cells (48, 49). ATP-competitive RAF inhibitors inhibit ERK signalling in mutant *BRAF* cells but enhance signal transduction in wild-type *BRAF* cells (50). The study found that type 1.5 RAF inhibitor, PLX-8394, and type II inhibitors, AZ-628 and LY3009120, had a certain inhibitory effect on *KRAS*-mutant cells and did not cause the contradictory MAPK pathway activation (49). An effective RAF inhibitor, HM95573 (belvarafenib), is under Phase I clinical study (ClinicalTrials.gov Identifier: NCT03284502).

MEK is a serine/threonine kinase, a downstream signal of KRAS and BRAF. Activated RAF activates MEK, which activates ERK and other transcription factors, in turn promoting cell cycle progression and cell proliferation. MEK inhibitors have shown potential efficacy in cancers with MEK or BRAF mutations, especially in BRAF V600E mutant tumour cell lines (50, 51). However, data from a number of studies have shown that the MEK1/MEK2 inhibitors, smeltinib (AZD6244; ARRY-142886) and trametinib (GSKll20212) cannot improve the prognosis of patients with KRAS-mutant NSCLC (52, 53). The reason may be that MEK inhibitors can induce signal feedback of the MAPK pathway in *KRAS*-mutant tumours, resulting in drug resistance to MEK inhibitors (54). HL-085 is a new ATP non-competitive MEK inhibitor in Phase I clinical trial (ClinicalTrials.gov Identifier: NCT03990077). Binimetinib (MEK162) is a selective MEK1/2 inhibitor in ongoing clinical trials (ClinicalTrials.gov Identifier: NCT01859026 and NCT02964689). Another Phase I clinical trial (ClinicalTrials.gov Identifier: NCT01986166) of the combination of the MEK inhibitor cobimetinib (GDC-0973) with MEHD7945A has not yet announced its results. Hyejin Choi et al. (55) used MEK inhibitors (MEKis) for pulsatile treatment in preclinical studies instead of continuous treatment. They found that the pulse regimen alone has a better anti-tumour effect and delayed the emergence of drug resistance. In addition, pulse MEK treatment combined with CTLA-4 blockade can prolong the survival time of KRAS-mutant tumour in mice, which may be related to T cell activation and increased CTLA-4 expression due to MEK pulse therapy.

A single application of a MEK- or RAF inhibitor for *KRAS* mutations shows no clinical efficacy. On the contrary, the combined application of a MEK inhibitor and a RAF inhibitor may be a feasible strategy. Combining the RAF inhibitor LXH254 and the MEK inhibitor trametinib is currently in Phase I clinical trial (ClinicalTrials.gov Identifier: NCT02974725). A Phase I clinical study (ClinicalTrials.gov Identifier: NCT03284502) of belvarafenib combined with cobimetinib is in progress. VS-6766 (RO5126766), a new targeted drug, whose Phase II clinical study (ClinicalTrials.gov Identifier: NCT04620330) is underway, inhibits both MEK and RAF.

SHP2 plays an indispensable role in *KRAS* mutation-driven tumours. SHP2 is involved in the downstream signal transduction of a variety of growth factors, cytokines, and integrin receptors, and its reduced activity inhibits tumour progression (56). Ruess et al. (56) reported that the combination of SHP2 with MEK inhibitors to target the xenograft models of KRAS-mutant NSCLC resulted in a synergistic effect to control tumour growth continuously. The RMC-4630 single drug Phase I clinical study (ClinicalTrials.gov Identifier: NCT03634982) and the clinical trial (ClinicalTrials.gov Identifier: NCT04418661) on its combination with pembrolizumab have been launched. TNO155 has also entered a Phase I clinical trial (ClinicalTrials.gov Identifier: NCT03114319). Notably, JAB-3312 can block the PD-1 pathway of T cells and the KRAS-MAPK pathway of tumour cells by inhibiting SHP2; thus, it plays a dual role in tumour immunity and tumour targeting. It is currently in Phase I clinical studies both in China and abroad (ClinicalTrials.gov Identifier: NCT04121286 and NCT04045496).

ERK is the final kinase in the MAPK pathway. The resistance of *KRAS*-mutated tumours to RAF or MEK inhibitors is usually caused by ERK feedback activation. Combined inhibition of ERK may be a feasible strategy to prevent drug resistance. Currently, ERK inhibitors such as JSI-1187-01, ASN007, and KO-947 are in Phase I clinical trials; ClinicalTrials.gov Identifier: NCT04418167, NCT03415126, and NCT03051035, respectively.

PI3K-AKT-mTOR pathway inhibition: PI3K is a cell effector molecule downstream of KRAS, and PI3K inhibitors BKM120, GDC0941, and XL147 have shown promising results in Phase I clinical trials (57–59). Serabelisib is a P13K catalytic subunit inhibitor and is in a Phase I/II clinical study (ClinicalTrials.gov Identifier: NCT04073680). TAS0612 is a new AKT inhibitor in Phase I clinical trial (ClinicalTrials.gov Identifier: NCT04586270). mTOR is a serine/threonine kinase downstream of PI3K in the PI3K-AKT-mTOR pathway. The mTOR inhibitor rapamycin and its analogues (CCI-779, RAD001, and AP23573), which induce cell cycle arrest in the G1 Phase, have certain anti-tumour activity in NSCLC (60). AZD2014 is a new mTOR inhibitor in Phase I/II clinical studies (ClinicalTrials.gov Identifier: NCT02583542).

Inactivation of a single MAPK or PI3K pathway has poor efficacy in *KRAS*-mutated tumours. The inhibition of the MAPK pathway activates the PI3K pathway, reducing *KRAS*-mutated cell sensitivity to MEK inhibitors (61). Therefore, the P13K-AKT-mTOR and RAF-MEK-ERK pathways were targeted simultaneously may be a promising strategy, but its toxicity should be observed.

Janus kinase-signal transducer and activator of transcription 3 (STAT3) inhibition: In KRAS-mutant NSCLC, after inhibiting MEK, STAT3 is activated *via* fibroblast growth factor receptor and Janus kinase; combined inhibition of this receptor, MEK, and Janus kinase can promote tumour regression (62).

Inhibition of *KRAS* Synergetic Genes

KRAS-mutated tumour cells can be killed by inhibiting other synergetic lethal genes responsible for their growth and survival. There are many transcription factors, including Wilms tumour 1 and GATA (A conserved sequence in a gene promoter whose core base sequence is Cys-X2-Cys-X17-Cys-X2-Cys)-binding protein 2 (GATA2) and small molecules involved in the nuclear factor kappa B (NF-κB) pathway. Wilms tumour 1 is a key regulator of ageing and proliferation downstream of oncogenic *KRAS* signalling (63). Kumar et al. (64) demonstrated that KRAS-mutant NSCLC relies on GATA2, and the deletion of GATA2 reduces the activity of KRAS-mutant NSCLC cells without affecting the wild-type cells. Bortezomib, a proteasome inhibitor that affects ubiquitin-proteasome pathways, disrupts protein homeostasis, leads to cell cycle interruption, inhibits transcription factors such as NF-κB, and produces anti-angiogenic effects, which inhibit tumour growth and proliferation, ultimately leading to apoptosis (65). In addition, the nuclear outlet receptor, exportin 1, has a strong synergetic lethal effect on *KRAS*-mutated cancer cells *in vitro* and *in vivo* (66). The exportin 1 inhibitor selinexor (KPT-330) is currently under Phase I/II clinical study (ClinicalTrials.gov Identifier: NCT03095612).

Heat shock protein 90 (HSP90) is a conservative and highly active molecular chaperone protein that stabilises the protein conformation of important signal transduction factors in the tumour pathogenesis pathway and protects the proteasome from degradation. Sos et al. (67) found that *KRAS* mutations enhanced tumour dependence on HSP90. They also found that tumours significantly regressed when treated with HSP90 inhibitors in a mouse model of lung adenocarcinoma driven by *KRAS*. Ganetespib is an HSP90 inhibitor. In a Phase II study, ganetespib monotherapy showed efficacy in KRAS-mutant NSCLC, but it was more significant in patients with anaplastic lymphoma kinase fusion (68). In a Phase II trial of ganetespib combined with docetaxel, the combination failed to improve PFS or OS in patients with KRAS-mutant NSCLC (69). AUY922 is a highly effective ATP-competitive HSP90 inhibitor. Although preclinical research results have shown that KRAS-mutant NSCLC is sensitive to AUY922, no clinical benefit of AUY922 has been observed in patients with *KRAS* mutations (70). Puyol et al. (71) found that CDK4 has a specific synthetic effect on KRAS-driven NSCLC. Abemaciclib and palbociclib (PD-0332991) are both CDK4/6 inhibitors under clinical study.

Other Therapy Options

Mesenchymal-epithelial transition factor (MET) is a transmembrane tyrosine kinase receptor involved in invasion, proliferation, angiogenesis, and metastasis and can also activate the KRAS pathway. MET amplification is discovered from approximately 4% of lung adenocarcinomas and leads to resistance to EGFR TKIs *via* activating the KRAS-PI3K-AKT-mTOR pathway. Currently, MET inhibitors include onartuzumab, a monoclonal antibody targeting the MET receptor, and tivantinib (ARQ 197), a small-molecule c-MET receptor TKI. In a Phase II study of onartuzumab combined with erlotinib, no response was observed in KRAS-mutant NSCLC (72). Another randomised Phase II study showed (73) that tivantinib combined with erlotinib did not improve prognosis in patients with unselected advanced NSCLC (PFS was 3.8 months in the ET group and 2.3 months in the EP group, respectively (HR: 0.81; 95% CI: 0.57–1.16). However, an exploratory analysis showed a significant improvement in PFS in patients with KRAS-mutant NSCLC (HR: 0.18; 95% CI: 0.05–0.70; P = 0.006).

Focal adhesion kinase (FAK) participates in the adhesion between cells and the extracellular matrix. The ERK-RAS Homolog Family Member A (RHOA) -FAK pathway is necessary to maintain KRAS-mutant lung adenocarcinoma. Inhibition of FAK can selectively induce KRAS-mutant cell death and lead to KRAS-mutant lung cancer regression (74). In a Phase II study (ClinicalTrials.gov Identifier: NCT01778803) (75) on defactinib (VS-6063; a selective oral inhibitor of FAK) treatment of advanced KRAS-mutant NSCLC, defactinib monotherapy showed moderate clinical activity. The study included 55 patients with KRAS-mutant NSCLC; 15 patients (28%) achieved a 12-week PFS endpoint, and one patient achieved partial remission with a median PFS of 45 days. Moreover, defactinib was generally well-tolerated.

Human vascular endothelial growth factor (VEGF) plays a vital role in promoting the proliferation, migration, and survival of endothelial cells (ECs); VEGF also can stimulate tumour angiogenesis. Besides, bevacizumab can directly inhibit deoxyribonucleic acid (DNA) repair in tumour cells. The reason may be that anti-angiogenic therapy can downregulate DNA repair genes, such as excision repair cross complementary gene 1 (ERCC-1) and X-ray repair of complementary cross gene 1 (XRCC-1), thereby enhancing the radiosensitivity of tumours (76). Some studies showed that bevacizumab combined with chemotherapy had no survival benefit for KRAS-mutant NSCLC (77, 78). Poly adenosine diphosphate (ADP)-ribose polymerase 1 (PARP1) plays an essential role in DNA damage repair and apoptosis, which, combined with WEE1 inhibitors, is associated with the killing of 25%-40% of KRAS-mutant NSCLC cells (79).

Many other combined inhibition therapies are available, for example, the combined inhibition of mTOR and Weel nuclear kinase (80), combined inhibition of checkpoint kinase 1 and MAPK-activated protein kinase 2 (81), and MEK/Bromodomain and extraterminal combined inhibitors (82), which have shown synergistic effects in preclinical studies and need to be demonstrated in further clinical trials.

PROSPECTS

The treatment of lung cancer has made rapid progress due to developments in medicine, particularly immunotherapy. The immunotherapy of KRAS-mutant NSCLC has shown promising efficacy. Many studies have indicated that immunotherapy can be recommended as the first-line treatment for KRAS-mutant NSCLC. However, it is also necessary to pay attention to the existence of its mutation subtypes and co-mutations and design individualised treatment. The clinical trials on AMG510 and MRTX849, inhibitors that directly target *KRAS* G12C, have shown surprising results. Nevertheless, the efficacy, duration of efficacy, and potential drug resistance of *KRAS* G12C inhibitors in treating different mutation subtypes warrant further research. Targeting KRAS downstream effector molecules (PI3K, BRAF, mTOR, MEK, etc.), especially the combined use of downstream effector molecule inhibitors, shows promising prospects. Furthermore, the combination of a variety of therapeutic drugs with different mechanisms has shown synergistic effects in preclinical studies and is a promising strategy that can improve drug efficacy and solve drug resistance. We believe that drug combinations can help patients with KRAS-mutant NSCLC bring more effective treatment.

AUTHOR CONTRIBUTIONS

MX performed the literature search, wrote the manuscript, and guaranteed its integrity. YF conceived the framework of the manuscript. XX revised the entire manuscript. All authors contributed to the article and approved the submitted version.

ACKNOWLEDGMENTS

The authors thank YF for editing the manuscript.

REFERENCES

1. El Osta B, Behera M, Kim S, Berry LD, Sica G, Pillai RN, et al. Characteristics and Outcomes of Patients With Metastatic Kras-Mutant Lung Adenocarcinomas: The Lung Cancer Mutation Consortium Experience. *J Thorac Oncol* (2019) 14(5):876–89. doi: 10.1016/j.jtho.2019.01.020
2. Ghimessy A, Radeczky P, Laszlo V, Hegedus B, Renyi-Vamos F, Fillinger J, et al. Current Therapy of KRAS-mutant Lung Cancer. *Cancer Metastasis Rev* (2020) 39(4):1159–77. doi: 10.1007/s10555-020-09903-9
3. Rittmeyer A, Barlesi F, Waterkamp D, Park K, Ciardiello F, von Pawel J, et al. Atezolizumab Versus Docetaxel in Patients With Previously Treated non-Small-Cell Lung Cancer (OAK): A Phase 3, Open-Label, Multicentre Randomised Controlled Trial. *Lancet* (2017) 389(10066):255–65. doi: 10.1016/s0140-6736(16)32517-x
4. Borghaei H, Paz-Ares L, Horn L, Spigel DR, Steins M, Ready NE, et al. Nivolumab Versus Docetaxel in Advanced Nonsquamous Non-Small-Cell Lung Cancer. *N Engl J Med* (2015) 373(17):1627–39. doi: 10.1056/NEJMoa1507643
5. Hong DS, Fakih MG, Strickler JH, Desai J, Durm GA, Shapiro GI, et al. Kras (G12c) Inhibition With Sotorasib in Advanced Solid Tumors. *N Engl J Med* (2020) 383(13):1207–17. doi: 10.1056/NEJMoa1917239
6. Therapeutics M. *Mirati Therapeutics Reports Investigational Adagrasib (MRTX849) Preliminary Data Demonstrating Tolerability and Durable Anti-Tumor Activity as Well as Initial MRTX1133 Preclinical Data* (2020). Available at: https://ir.mirati.com/news-releases/news-details/2020/Mirati-Therapeutics-Reports-Investigational-Adagrasib-MRTX849-Preliminary-Data-Demonstrating-Tolerability-and-Durable-Anti-Tumor-Activity-as-well-as-Initial-MRTX1133-Preclinical-Data/default.aspx (Accessed November 18, 2020).
7. Ferrer I, Zugazagoitia J, Herbertz S, John W, Paz-Ares L, Schmid-Bindert G. Kras-Mutant non-Small Cell Lung Cancer: From Biology to Therapy. *Lung Cancer* (2018) 124:53–64. doi: 10.1016/j.lungcan.2018.07.013
8. Friedlaender A, Drilon A, Weiss GJ, Banna GL, Addeo A. KRAS as a Druggable Target in NSCLC: Rising Like a Phoenix After Decades of Development Failures. *Cancer Treat Rev* (2020) 85:101978. doi: 10.1016/j.ctrv.2020.101978
9. Roman M, Baraibar I, Lopez I, Nadal E, Rolfo C, Vicent S, et al. KRAS Oncogene in non-Small Cell Lung Cancer: Clinical Perspectives on the Treatment of an Old Target. *Mol Cancer* (2018) 17(1):33. doi: 10.1186/s12943-018-0789-x
10. Burns T, Borghaei H, Ramalingam S, Mok T, Peters S. Kras Targeting -Mutant Non-Small-Cell Lung Cancer: One Mutation At a Time, With a Focus on Mutations. *J Clin Oncol* (2020) 38(35):4208–18. doi: 10.1200/jco.20.00744
11. Macerelli M, Caramella C, Faivre L, Besse B, Planchard D, Polo V, et al. Does KRAS Mutational Status Predict Chemoresistance in Advanced non-Small Cell Lung Cancer (NSCLC)? *Lung Cancer* (2014) 83(3):383–8. doi: 10.1016/j.lungcan.2013.12.013
12. Marabese M, Ganzinelli M, Garassino MC, Shepherd FA, Piva S, Caiola E, et al. KRAS Mutations Affect Prognosis of non-Small-Cell Lung Cancer Patients Treated With First-Line Platinum Containing Chemotherapy. *Oncotarget* (2015) 6(32):34014–22. doi: 10.18632/oncotarget.5607
13. Linardou H, Dahabreh IJ, Kanaloupiti D, Siannis F, Bafaloukos D, Kosmidis P, et al. Assessment of Somatic k-RAS Mutations as a Mechanism Associated With Resistance to EGFR-targeted Agents: A Systematic Review and Meta-Analysis of Studies in Advanced non-Small-Cell Lung Cancer and Metastatic Colorectal Cancer. *Lancet Oncol* (2008) 9(10):962–72. doi: 10.1016/s1470-2045(08)70206-7
14. Liu C, Zheng S, Jin R, Wang X, Wang F, Zang R, et al. The Superior Efficacy of anti-PD-1/PD-L1 Immunotherapy in KRAS-mutant non-Small Cell Lung Cancer That Correlates With an Inflammatory Phenotype and Increased Immunogenicity. *Cancer Lett* (2020) 470:95–105. doi: 10.1016/j.canlet.2019.10.027
15. Valero C, Lee M, Hoen D, Weiss K, Kelly DW, Adusumilli PS, et al. Pretreatment Neutrophil-to-Lymphocyte Ratio and Mutational Burden as Biomarkers of Tumor Response to Immune Checkpoint Inhibitors. *Nat Commun* (2021) 12(1):729. doi: 10.1038/s41467-021-20935-9
16. Sekine K, Kanda S, Goto Y, Horinouchi H, Fujiwara Y, Yamamoto N, et al. Change in the Lymphocyte-to-Monocyte Ratio is an Early Surrogate Marker of the Efficacy of Nivolumab Monotherapy in Advanced non-Small-Cell Lung Cancer. *Lung Cancer* (2018) 124:179–88. doi: 10.1016/j.lungcan.2018.08.012
17. Hurkmans DP, Kuipers ME, Smit J, van Marion R, Mathijssen RHJ, Postmus PE, et al. Tumor Mutational Load, CD8(+) T Cells, Expression of PD-L1 and HLA Class I to Guide Immunotherapy Decisions in NSCLC Patients. *Cancer Immunol Immunother* (2020) 69(5):771–7. doi: 10.1007/s00262-020-02506-x
18. Calles A, Liao X, Sholl LM, Rodig SJ, Freeman GJ, Butaney M, et al. Expression of PD-1 and Its Ligands, PD-L1 and PD-L2, in Smokers and Never Smokers With KRAS-Mutant Lung Cancer. *J Thorac Oncol* (2015) 10(12):1726–35. doi: 10.1097/JTO.0000000000000687
19. Huynh TG, Morales-Oyarvide V, Campo MJ, Gainor JF, Bozkurtlar E, Uruga H, et al. Programmed Cell Death Ligand 1 Expression in Resected Lung Adenocarcinomas: Association With Immune Microenvironment. *J Thorac Oncol* (2016) 11(11):1869–78. doi: 10.1016/j.jtho.2016.08.134
20. Passiglia F, Cappuzzo F, Alabiso O, Bettini AC, Bidoli P, Chiari R, et al. Efficacy of Nivolumab in Pre-Treated non-Small-Cell Lung Cancer Patients Harbouring KRAS Mutations. *Br J Cancer* (2019) 120(1):57–62. doi: 10.1038/s41416-018-0234-3
21. Herbst RS, de Marinis F, Giaccone G, Reinmuth N, Vergnenegre A, Barrios CH, et al. Lba1 Clinical Efficacy of Atezolizumab (Atezo) in Biomarker Subgroups by SP142, SP263 and 22C3 PD-L1 Immunohistochemistry (IHC) Assays and by Blood Tumour Mutational Burden (Btmb): Results From the IMpower110 Study. *Ann Oncol* (2019) 30:xi62–3. doi: 10.1093/annonc/mdz453
22. Canon J, Rex K, Saiki AY, Mohr C, Cooke K, Bagal D, et al. The Clinical KRAS (G12C) Inhibitor AMG 510 Drives Anti-Tumour Immunity. *Nature* (2019) 575(7781):217–23. doi: 10.1038/s41586-019-1694-1
23. Hallin J, Engstrom LD, Hargis L, Calinisan A, Aranda R, Briere DM, et al. The KRAS(G12C) Inhibitor MRTX849 Provides Insight Toward Therapeutic Susceptibility of KRAS-Mutant Cancers in Mouse Models and Patients. *Cancer Discovery* (2020) 10(1):54–71. doi: 10.1158/2159-8290.CD-19-1167
24. Aredo JV, Padda SK, Kunder CA, Han SS, Neal JW, Shrager JB, et al. Impact of KRAS Mutation Subtype and Concurrent Pathogenic Mutations on non-Small Cell Lung Cancer Outcomes. *Lung Cancer* (2019) 133:144–50. doi: 10.1016/j.lungcan.2019.05.015
25. Jeanson A, Tomasini P, Souquet-Bressand M, Brandone N, Boucekine M, Grangeon M, et al. Efficacy of Immune Checkpoint Inhibitors in KRAS-Mutant non-Small Cell Lung Cancer (Nsclc). *J Thorac Oncol* (2019) 14 (6):1095–101. doi: 10.1016/j.jtho.2019.01.011
26. Skoulidis F, Byers LA, Diao L, Papadimitrakopoulou VA, Tong P, Izzo J, et al. Co-Occurring Genomic Alterations Define Major Subsets of KRAS-mutant

Lung Adenocarcinoma With Distinct Biology, Immune Profiles, and Therapeutic Vulnerabilities. *Cancer Discovery* (2015) 5(8):860–77. doi: 10.1158/2159-8290.CD-14-1236
27. Skoulidis F, Goldberg ME, Greenawalt DM, Hellmann MD, Awad MM, Gainor JF, et al. Stk11/Lkb1 Mutations and PD-1 Inhibitor Resistance in KRAS-Mutant Lung Adenocarcinoma. *Cancer Discovery* (2018) 8(7):822–35. doi: 10.1158/2159-8290.CD-18-0099
28. Koyama S, Akbay EA, Li YY, Aref AR, Skoulidis F, Herter-Sprie GS, et al. Stk11/Lkb1 Deficiency Promotes Neutrophil Recruitment and Proinflammatory Cytokine Production to Suppress T-Cell Activity in the Lung Tumor Microenvironment. *Cancer Res* (2016) 76(5):999–1008. doi: 10.1158/0008-5472.CAN-15-1439
29. Havel JJ, Chowell D, Chan TA. The Evolving Landscape of Biomarkers for Checkpoint Inhibitor Immunotherapy. *Nat Rev Cancer* (2019) 19(3):133–50. doi: 10.1038/s41568-019-0116-x
30. Hellmann MD, Paz-Ares L, Bernabe Caro R, Zurawski B, Kim SW, Carcereny Costa E, et al. Nivolumab Plus Ipilimumab in Advanced non-Small-Cell Lung Cancer. *N Engl J Med* (2019) 381(21):2020–31. doi: 10.1056/NEJMoa1910231
31. Paz-Ares L, Ciuleanu T, Cobo M, Schenker M, Zurawski B, Menezes J, et al. First-Line Nivolumab Plus Ipilimumab Combined With Two Cycles of Chemotherapy in Patients With non-Small-Cell Lung Cancer (CheckMate 9LA): An International. *Randomised Open-label Phase 3 Trial* (2021) 22 (2):198–211. doi: 10.1016/s1470-2045(20)30641-0
32. Nagasaka M, Li Y, Sukari A, Ou SI, Al-Hallak MN, Azmi AS. Kras G12C Game of Thrones, Which Direct KRAS Inhibitor Will Claim the Iron Throne? *Cancer Treat Rev* (2020) 84:101974. doi: 10.1016/j.ctrv.2020.101974
33. Janes MR, Zhang J, Li LS, Hansen R, Peters U, Guo X, et al. Targeting KRAS Mutant Cancers With a Covalent G12c-Specific Inhibitor. *Cell* (2018) 172 (3):578–89.e17. doi: 10.1016/j.cell.2018.01.006
34. Lito P, Solomon M, Li LS, Hansen R, Rosen N. Allele-Specific Inhibitors Inactivate Mutant KRAS G12C by a Trapping Mechanism. *Science* (2016) 351 (6273):604–8. doi: 10.1126/science.aad6204
35. Li B, Skoulidis F, Falchook G, Sacher A, Velcheti V, Dy G, et al. CodeBreaK 100: Registrational Phase 2 Trail of Sotorasib in KRAS P.G12C Mutated non-Small Cell Lung Cancer. Abstract No. Ps01.07. In: *2020 World Conference on Lung Cancer* Singapore, Worldwide Virtual Event (2021).
36. Soria JC, Ohe Y, Vansteenkiste J, Reungwetwattana T, Chewaskulyong B, Lee KH, et al. Osimertinib in Untreated Egfr-Mutated Advanced non-Small-Cell Lung Cancer. *N Engl J Med* (2018) 378(2):113–25. doi: 10.1056/NEJMoa1713137
37. Wu YL, Saijo N, Thongprasert S, Yang JC, Han B, Margono B, et al. Efficacy According to Blind Independent Central Review: Post-hoc Analyses From the Phase III, Randomized, Multicenter, IPASS Study of First-Line Gefitinib Versus Carboplatin/Paclitaxel in Asian Patients With EGFR Mutation-Positive Advanced NSCLC. *Lung Cancer* (2017) 104:119–25. doi: 10.1016/j.lungcan.2016.11.022
38. Zeng M, Xiong Y, Safaee N, Nowak RP, Donovan KA, Yuan CJ, et al. Exploring Targeted Degradation Strategy for Oncogenic Kras(G12c). *Cell Chem Biol* (2020) 27(1):19–31.e6. doi: 10.1016/j.chembiol.2019.12.006
39. Cox AD, Fesik SW, Kimmelman AC, Luo J, Der CJ. Drugging the Undruggable RAS: Mission Possible? *Nat Rev Drug Discovery* (2014) 13 (11):828–51. doi: 10.1038/nrd4389
40. Hillig RC, Sautier B, Schroeder J, Moosmayer D, Hilpmann A, Stegmann CM, et al. Discovery of Potent SOS1 Inhibitors That Block RAS Activation Via Disruption of the RAS-SOS1 Interaction. *Proc Natl Acad Sci U S A* (2019) 116 (7):2551–60. doi: 10.1073/pnas.1812963116
41. Moore AR, Rosenberg SC, McCormick F, Malek S. RAS-Targeted Therapies: Is the Undruggable Drugged? *Nat Rev Drug Discovery* (2020) 19(8):533–52. doi: 10.1038/s41573-020-0068-6
42. Cox AD, Der CJ, Philips MR. Targeting RAS Membrane Association: Back to the Future for Anti-RAS Drug Discovery? *Clin Cancer Res* (2015) 21(8):1819–27. doi: 10.1158/1078-0432.CCR-14-3214
43. Zimmermann G, Papke B, Ismail S, Vartak N, Chandra A, Hoffmann M, et al. Small Molecule Inhibition of the KRAS-PDEdelta Interaction Impairs Oncogenic KRAS Signalling. *Nature* (2013) 497(7451):638–42. doi: 10.1038/nature12205
44. Wilhelm SM, Carter C, Tang L, Wilkie D, McNabola A, Rong H, et al. Bay 43-9006 Exhibits Broad Spectrum Oral Antitumor Activity and Targets the RAF/MEK/ERK Pathway and Receptor Tyrosine Kinases Involved in Tumor Progression and Angiogenesis. *Cancer Res* (2004) 64(19):7099–109. doi: 10.1158/0008-5472.CAN-04-1443
45. Paz-Ares L, Hirsh V, Zhang L, de Marinis F, Yang JC, Wakelee HA, et al. Monotherapy Administration of Sorafenib in Patients With Non-Small Cell Lung Cancer (Mission) Trial: A Phase III, Multicenter, Placebo-Controlled Trial of Sorafenib in Patients With Relapsed or Refractory Predominantly Nonsquamous non-Small-Cell Lung Cancer After 2 or 3 Previous Treatment Regimens. *J Thorac Oncol* (2015) 10(12):1745–53. doi: 10.1097/JTO.0000000000000693
46. Blumenschein GRJr., Saintigny P, Liu S, Kim ES, Tsao AS, Herbst RS, et al. Comprehensive Biomarker Analysis and Final Efficacy Results of Sorafenib in the BATTLE Trial. *Clin Cancer Res* (2013) 19(24):6967–75. doi: 10.1158/1078-0432.CCR-12-1818
47. Papadimitrakopoulou V, Lee JJ, Wistuba II, Tsao AS, Fossella FV, Kalhor N, et al. The BATTLE-2 Study: A Biomarker-Integrated Targeted Therapy Study in Previously Treated Patients With Advanced non-Small-Cell Lung Cancer. *J Clin Oncol* (2016) 34(30):3638–47. doi: 10.1200/JCO.2015.66.0084
48. Uprety D, Adjei AA. Kras: From Undruggable to a Druggable Cancer Target. *Cancer Treat Rev* (2020) 89:102070. doi: 10.1016/j.ctrv.2020.102070
49. Yen I, Shanahan F, Merchant M, Orr C, Hunsaker T, Durk M, et al. Pharmacological Induction of RAS-GTP Confers RAF Inhibitor Sensitivity in KRAS Mutant Tumors. *Cancer Cell* (2018) 34(4):611–25.e7. doi: 10.1016/j.ccell.2018.09.002
50. Poulikakos PI, Zhang C, Bollag G, Shokat KM, Rosen N. RAF Inhibitors Transactivate RAF Dimers and ERK Signalling in Cells With Wild-Type BRAF. *Nature* (2010) 464(7287):427–30. doi: 10.1038/nature08902
51. Yaeger R, Corcoran RB. Targeting Alterations in the RAF-MEK Pathway. *Cancer Discovery* (2019) 9(3):329–41. doi: 10.1158/2159-8290.CD-18-1321
52. Janne PA, van den Heuvel MM, Barlesi F, Cobo M, Mazieres J, Crino L, et al. Selumetinib Plus Docetaxel Compared With Docetaxel Alone and Progression-Free Survival in Patients With KRAS-Mutant Advanced Non-Small Cell Lung Cancer: The Select-1 Randomized Clinical Trial. *JAMA* (2017) 317(18):1844–53. doi: 10.1001/jama.2017.3438
53. Blumenschein GRJr., Smit EF, Planchard D, Kim DW, Cadranel J, De Pas T, et al. A Randomized Phase II Study of the MEK1/MEK2 Inhibitor Trametinib (GSK1120212) Compared With Docetaxel in KRAS-mutant Advanced non-Small-Cell Lung Cancer (NSCLC)Dagger. *Ann Oncol* (2015) 26(5):894–901. doi: 10.1093/annonc/mdv072
54. Martinelli E, Morgillo F, Troiani T, Ciardiello F. Cancer Resistance to Therapies Against the EGFR-RAS-RAF Pathway: The Role of MEK. *Cancer Treat Rev* (2017) 53:61–9. doi: 10.1016/j.ctrv.2016.12.001
55. Choi H, Deng J, Li S, Silk T, Dong L, Brea EJ, et al. Pulsatile MEK Inhibition Improves Anti-Tumor Immunity and T Cell Function in Murine Kras Mutant Lung Cancer. *Cell Rep* (2019) 27(3):806–19.e5. doi: 10.1016/j.celrep.2019.03.066
56. Ruess DA, Heynen GJ, Ciecielski KJ, Ai J, Berninger A, Kabacaoglu D, et al. Mutant KRAS-driven Cancers Depend on PTPN11/SHP2 Phosphatase. *Nat Med* (2018) 24(7):954–60. doi: 10.1038/s41591-018-0024-8
57. Bendell JC, Rodon J, Burris HA, de Jonge M, Verweij J, Birle D, et al. Phase I, Dose-Escalation Study of BKM120, an Oral Pan-Class I PI3K Inhibitor, in Patients With Advanced Solid Tumors. *J Clin Oncol* (2012) 30(3):282–90. doi: 10.1200/JCO.2011.36.1360
58. Ding X, Morrison G, Dean B, Hop CE, Tobler L, Percey S, et al. A Solid Phase Extraction-Liquid Chromatographic-Tandem Mass Spectrometry Method for Determination of Concentrations of GDC-0941, a Small Molecule Class I Phosphatidylinositide 3-Kinase Inhibitor, to Support Clinical Development. *J Pharm BioMed Anal* (2012) 61:1–7. doi: 10.1016/j.jpba.2011.11.005
59. Shapiro GI, Rodon J, Bedell C, Kwak EL, Baselga J, Brana I, et al. Phase I Safety, Pharmacokinetic, and Pharmacodynamic Study of SAR245408 (XL147), an Oral Pan-Class I PI3K Inhibitor, in Patients With Advanced Solid Tumors. *Clin Cancer Res* (2014) 20(1):233–45. doi: 10.1158/1078-0432.CCR-13-1777
60. Gridelli C, Maione P, Rossi A. The Potential Role of mTOR Inhibitors in non-Small Cell Lung Cancer. *Oncologist* (2008) 13(2):139–47. doi: 10.1634/theoncologist.2007-0171
61. Wee S, Jagani Z, Xiang KX, Loo A, Dorsch M, Yao YM, et al. PI3K Pathway Activation Mediates Resistance to MEK Inhibitors in KRAS Mutant Cancers. *Cancer Res* (2009) 69(10):4286–93. doi: 10.1158/0008-5472.CAN-08-4765

62. Lee HJ, Zhuang G, Cao Y, Du P, Kim HJ, Settleman J. Drug Resistance Via Feedback Activation of Stat3 in Oncogene-Addicted Cancer Cells. *Cancer Cell* (2014) 26(2):207–21. doi: 10.1016/j.ccr.2014.05.019
63. Vicent S, Chen R, Sayles LC, Lin C, Walker RG, Gillespie AK, et al. Wilms Tumor 1 (WT1) Regulates KRAS-driven Oncogenesis and Senescence in Mouse and Human Models. *J Clin Invest* (2010) 120(11):3940–52. doi: 10.1172/JCI44165
64. Kumar MS, Hancock DC, Molina-Arcas M, Steckel M, East P, Diefenbacher M, et al. The GATA2 Transcriptional Network is Requisite for RAS Oncogene-Driven non-Small Cell Lung Cancer. *Cell* (2012) 149(3):642–55. doi: 10.1016/j.cell.2012.02.059
65. Fanucchi MP, Fossella FV, Belt R, Natale R, Fidias P, Carbone DP, et al. Randomized Phase II Study of Bortezomib Alone and Bortezomib in Combination With Docetaxel in Previously Treated Advanced non-Small-Cell Lung Cancer. *J Clin Oncol* (2006) 24(31):5025–33. doi: 10.1200/JCO.2006.06.1853
66. Kim J, McMillan E, Kim HS, Venkateswaran N, Makkar G, Rodriguez-Canales J, et al. XPO1-Dependent Nuclear Export is a Druggable Vulnerability in KRAS-mutant Lung Cancer. *Nature* (2016) 538(7623):114–7. doi: 10.1038/nature19771
67. Sos ML, Michel K, Zander T, Weiss J, Frommolt P, Peifer M, et al. Predicting Drug Susceptibility of non-Small Cell Lung Cancers Based on Genetic Lesions. *J Clin Invest* (2009) 119(6):1727–40. doi: 10.1172/JCI37127
68. Socinski MA, Goldman J, El-Hariry I, Koczywas M, Vukovic V, Horn L, et al. A Multicenter Phase II Study of Ganetespib Monotherapy in Patients With Genotypically Defined Advanced non-Small Cell Lung Cancer. *Clin Cancer Res* (2013) 19(11):3068–77. doi: 10.1158/1078-0432.CCR-12-3381
69. Ramalingam S, Goss G, Rosell R, Schmid-Bindert G, Zaric B, Andric Z, et al. A Randomized Phase II Study of Ganetespib, a Heat Shock Protein 90 Inhibitor, in Combination With Docetaxel in Second-Line Therapy of Advanced non-Small Cell Lung Cancer (GALAXY-1). *Ann Oncol* (2015) 26(8):1741–8. doi: 10.1093/annonc/mdv220
70. Felip E, Barlesi F, Besse B, Chu Q, Gandhi L, Kim SW, et al. Phase 2 Study of the HSP-90 Inhibitor AUY922 in Previously Treated and Molecularly Defined Patients With Advanced non-Small Cell Lung Cancer. *J Thorac Oncol* (2018) 13(4):576–84. doi: 10.1016/j.jtho.2017.11.131
71. Puyol M, Martin A, Dubus P, Mulero F, Pizcueta P, Khan G, et al. A Synthetic Lethal Interaction Between K-Ras Oncogenes and Cdk4 Unveils a Therapeutic Strategy for non-Small Cell Lung Carcinoma. *Cancer Cell* (2010) 18(1):63–73. doi: 10.1016/j.ccr.2010.05.025
72. Koeppen H, Yu W, Zha J, Pandita A, Penuel E, Rangell L, et al. Biomarker Analyses From a Placebo-Controlled Phase II Study Evaluating Erlotinib +/-Onartuzumab in Advanced non-Small Cell Lung Cancer: MET Expression Levels are Predictive of Patient Benefit. *Clin Cancer Res* (2014) 20(17):4488–98. doi: 10.1158/1078-0432.CCR-13-1836
73. Sequist LV, von Pawel J, Garmey EG, Akerley WL, Brugger W, Ferrari D, et al. Randomized Phase II Study of Erlotinib Plus Tivantinib Versus Erlotinib Plus Placebo in Previously Treated non-Small-Cell Lung Cancer. *J Clin Oncol* (2011) 29(24):3307–15. doi: 10.1200/JCO.2010.34.0570
74. Konstantinidou G, Ramadori G, Torti F, Kangasniemi K, Ramirez RE, Cai Y, et al. Rhoa-FAK is a Required Signaling Axis for the Maintenance of KRAS-driven Lung Adenocarcinomas. *Cancer Discovery* (2013) 3(4):444–57. doi: 10.1158/2159-8290.CD-12-0388
75. Gerber DE, Camidge DR, Morgensztern D, Cetnar J, Kelly RJ, Ramalingam SS, et al. Phase 2 Study of the Focal Adhesion Kinase Inhibitor Defactinib (vs-6063) in Previously Treated Advanced KRAS Mutant non-Small Cell Lung Cancer. *Lung Cancer* (2020) 139:60–7. doi: 10.1016/j.lungcan.2019.10.033
76. Gao H, Xue J, Zhou L, Lan J, He J, Na F, et al. Bevacizumab Radiosensitizes non-Small Cell Lung Cancer Xenografts by Inhibiting DNA Double-Strand Break Repair in Endothelial Cells. *Cancer Lett* (2015) 365(1):79–88. doi: 10.1016/j.canlet.2015.05.011
77. Chaft JE, Rusch V, Ginsberg MS, Paik PK, Finley DJ, Kris MG, et al. Phase II Trial of Neoadjuvant Bevacizumab Plus Chemotherapy and Adjuvant Bevacizumab in Patients With Resectable Nonsquamous non-Small-Cell Lung Cancers. *J Thorac Oncol* (2013) 8(8):1084–90. doi: 10.1097/JTO.0b013e31829923ec
78. Ghimessy AK, Gellert A, Schlegl E, Hegedus B, Raso E, Barbai T, et al. Kras Mutations Predict Response and Outcome in Advanced Lung Adenocarcinoma Patients Receiving First-Line Bevacizumab and Platinum-Based Chemotherapy. *Cancers (Basel)* (2019) 11(10):1514. doi: 10.3390/cancers11101514
79. Burns TF, Borghaei H, Ramalingam SS, Mok TS, Peters S. Targeting KRAS-Mutant non-Small-Cell Lung Cancer: One Mutation At a Time, With a Focus on KRAS G12c Mutations. *Clin Oncol* (2020) 38(35):4208–18. doi: 10.1200/JCO.20
80. Hai J, Liu S, Bufe L, Do K, Chen T, Wang X, et al. Synergy of WEE1 and Mtor Inhibition in Mutant Kras-Driven Lung Cancers. *Clin Cancer Res* (2017) 23 (22):6993–7005. doi: 10.1158/1078-0432.CCR-17-1098
81. Dietlein F, Kalb B, Jokic M, Noll EM, Strong A, Tharun L, et al. A Synergistic Interaction Between Chk1- and MK2 Inhibitors in KRAS-Mutant Cancer. *Cell* (2015) 162(1):146–59. doi: 10.1016/j.cell.2015.05.053
82. Guerra SL, Maertens O, Kuzmickas R, De Raedt T, Adeyemi RO, Guild CJ, et al. A Deregulated Hox Gene Axis Confers an Epigenetic Vulnerability in KRAS-Mutant Lung Cancers. *Cancer Cell* (2020) 37(5):705–19.e6. doi: 10.1016/j.ccell.2020.03.004

4

Peripheral Lung Squamous Carcinoma with ROS1 Rearrangement Sensitive to Crizotinib

Guangdie Yang[1†], *Jie Wang*[1†], *Yinan Yao*[1†], *Jun Zhao*[1,2], *Zheyan Yu*[3], *Qiqi Gao*[4], *Jiani Ye*[1] *and Wenjiang Ma*[1*]

[1] Department of Respiratory Medicine, The First Affiliated Hospital, College of Medicine, Zhejiang University, Hangzhou, China, [2] Department of Respiratory Medicine, Zhejiang Medical & Health Group Hangzhou Hospital, Hangzhou, China, [3] Department of Respiratory and Critical Care Medicine, Shengzhou People's Hospital, Shaoxing, China, [4] Department of Pathology, The First Affiliated Hospital, College of Medicine, Zhejiang University, Hangzhou, China

***Correspondence:**
Wenjiang Ma
mwj@zju.edu.cn

†These authors have contributed equally to this work and share first authorship

ROS1 rearrangements have been identified as driver mutations, accounting for 1–2% of lung adenocarcinoma, but are extremely rare in case of lung squamous cell carcinoma. In this work, we report a lung squamous cell carcinoma in a patient with peripheral lung cancer radiological manifestation, harboring ROS1 rearrangement, with high sensitivity to crizotinib. Our findings suggest that clinicians should pay more attention toward the occurrence of ROS1 rearrangements and the application of crizotinib for lung squamous cell carcinoma treatment.

Keywords: lung squamous carcinoma, ROS1 rearrangement, crizotinib, atypical imaging manifestation, hypoalbuminemia

INTRODUCTION

In the last few decades, genetic testing and targeted therapy have resulted in survival benefits among patients with lung adenocarcinoma, although progress in the treatment of lung squamous cell carcinoma (SCC) remains stagnant. Recently, there has been a growing biological significance to identify the molecular characteristics of patients with lung SCC. ROS1 is a proto-oncogene and one among the sevenless subfamily of tyrosine kinase insulin receptor genes. ROS1 rearrangements are a known oncogenic driver in 1–2% of patients with lung adenocarcinoma, while it is widely believed that ROS1 in SCC is very rare (1). Crizotinib is a standard treatment for adenocarcinomas with ROS1 rearrangement (2), although we still have no data regarding the application of crizotinib in patients with lung SCC. Here, we report a rare case of a non-smoker female patient, diagnosed with peripheral lung SCC harboring ROS1 rearrangement, who was extremely sensitive to crizotinib.

CASE DESCRIPTION

A 47-year old woman presented with repeated fever and fatigue in the past 3 months. She had a history of idiopathic thrombocytopenic purpura (ITP) and had undergone splenectomy 5 years ago with no evidence of recurrence. She was a non-smoker. Bilateral cervical lymph nodes (LNs) were palpable, and other physical examinations showed no abnormalities. Chest computed tomography

(CT) scan showed diffuse round high-density lesions with small pleural effusion in the lungs bilaterally, accompanied by multiple enlarged LNs in the mediastinum and right supraclavicular area (**Figure 1A**). Ultrasound evaluation of the cervical LNs suggested bilateral supraclavicular lymphadenopathy (size in the right was 2.6 cm × 1. 6cm, size in the left was 2.2 cm × 1.1 cm). Abdominal CT, transvaginal ultrasound and cranial magnetic resonance (MR) imaging were normal. The results of representative serum tumor markers were as follows: CEA 7.6 ng/ml (normal < 5.0 ng/ml), CYFRA21 >100.0 ng/ml (normal < 3.3 ng/ml), NSE 17.6 ng/ml (normal < 30 ng/ml), SCCA >70.0 ng/ml (normal < 1.5 ng/ml). Positron emission tomography (PET)–CT showed no distal metastasis, which showed similar lesions with increased Fluorodeoxyglucose (FDG) uptake as chest CT in the lung and LNs (N2, N3) (**Figure 2**). Therefore, she underwent ultrasound-guided biopsy of the lung and right supraclavicular LNs. Tissue histopathology by hematoxylin and eosin (HE) staining revealed lung SCC. Immunohistochemical staining confirmed the diagnosis of SCC with positive P40 and CK5/6, negative transcription factor-1 (TTF-1), and napsin A (**Figure 3**). The patient was clinically diagnosed with stage IVA lung SCC, T4N3M1a. Genetic status, including EGFR, ALK, ROS1, KRAS, BRAF, RET, MET, HER2, NRAS, and PI3KA presence, was detected by amplification refractory mutation system (ARMS) with AmoyDx Mutations Detection Kit (Amoy Diagnostics Co., Ltd., Xiamen, China), revealing that the tumor harbored ROS1 rearrangement (**Figure 3**).

The patient was treated with crizotinib (250 mg twice daily) from August 3, 2020. After 3 weeks of treatment, a chest CT scan showed an obvious reduction in tumor size and metastasis (**Figure 1B**), quickly resulting in partial response (PR) according to the Response Evaluation Criteria for Solid Tumors (RECIST, version 1.1) (3). The patient continued receiving crizotinib and developed mild treatment-related adverse events (TRAEs), such as rashes, nausea, and anemia. She stopped molecular targeted therapy for 2 weeks because of severe hypoalbuminemia and secondary bilateral pleural effusion which might be relative to crizotinib (**Figure 1C**). After returning to baseline, crizotinib treatment was reinitiated. The tumor lesions and enlarged LNs further reduced after 4 months (**Figure 1D**). We are still following up with the patient, and she has remained PR for 9 months till the last follow-up (**Figure 1E**).

DISCUSSION

We report a rare case of a woman diagnosed with lung SCC harboring ROS1 rearrangements, who was extremely sensitive to crizotinib. The ROS1 rearrangements occurred in only 1–2% of patients with non-small cell lung cancer (NSCLC), mainly with adenocarcinoma (2). To date, only six cases of lung SCC with ROS1 have been reported (one was ALK and ROS1 double-rearranged) (1, 2, 4–6). ROS1 rearrangement is very rare in lung SCC (7). Chest CT scans of two previous patients with lung SCC

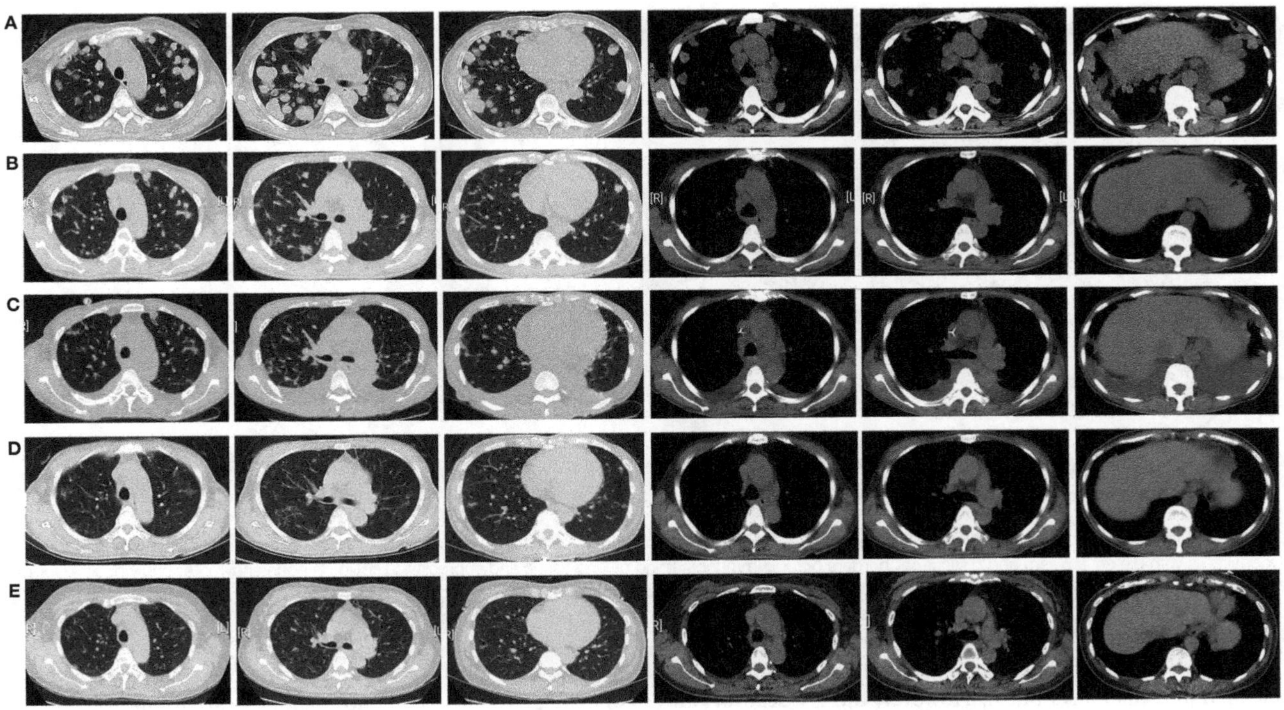

FIGURE 1 | Timeline of the patient's chest CT scan showed the obvious remission of the patient' s diffused lesions in the bilateral lung and enlarged lymph nodes after crizotinib treatment: **(A)** 7 July, 2020 (baseline), **(B)** 24 August, 2020, **(C)** 22 September, 2020, **(D)** 14 December, 2020, **(E)** 25 April, 2021.

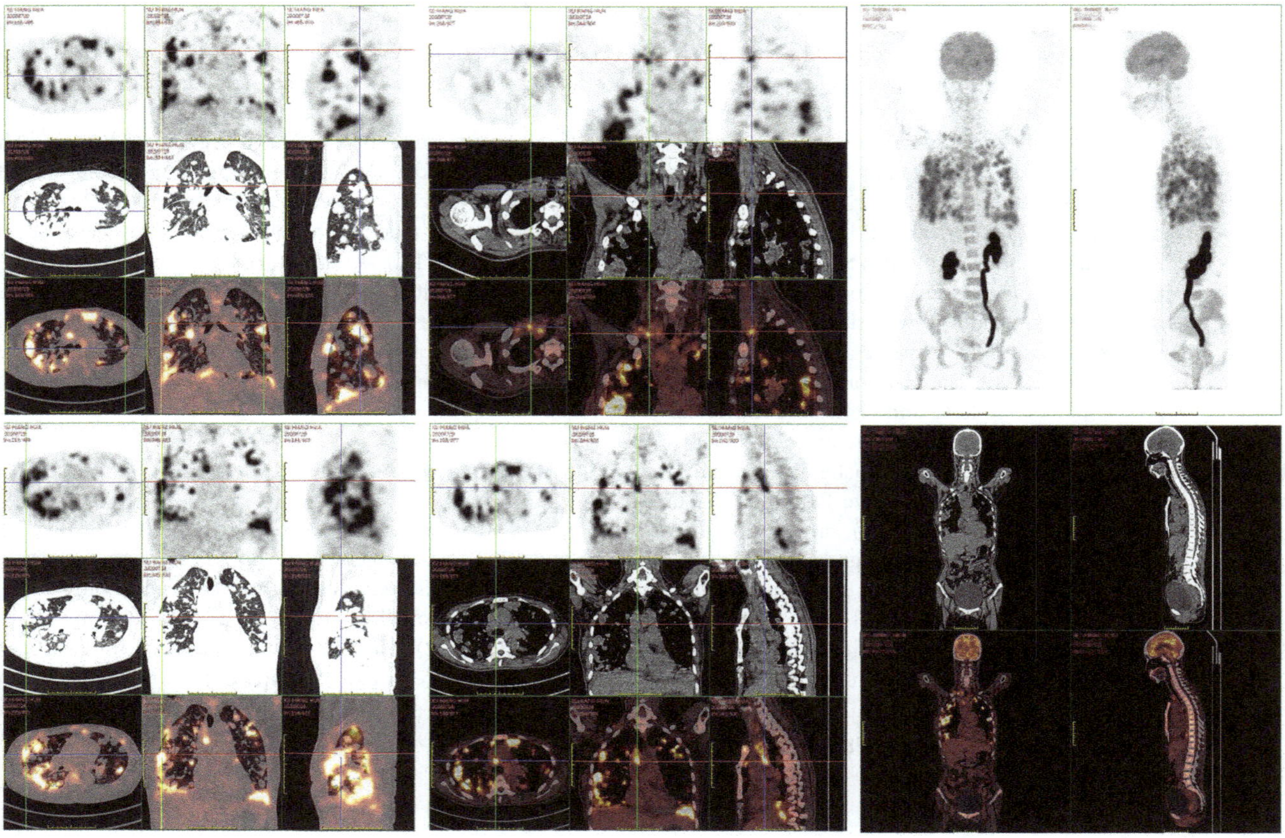

FIGURE 2 | The patient' s PET/CT scan showed diffused lesions with increased FDG uptake like chest CT located in the lung and LNs without distal metastasis.

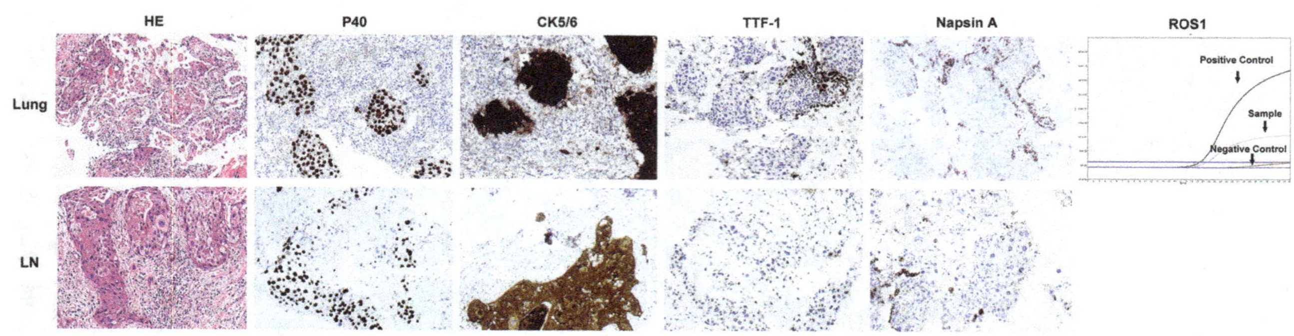

FIGURE 3 | Pathological and molecular examinations of the case. HE staining showed the microscopic appearance of squamous cell carcinoma with nests of polygonal cells with pink cytoplasm and distinct cell borders (×200). Immunostaining of lung tissue and supraclavicular lymph node showed strongly positive for p40 and CK5/6, and negative for TTF-1 and Napsin A (×200). ARMS assay of lung tissue showed ROS1 rearrangement.

were typical, both presenting a central mass, enlarged mediastinal and hilar LNs (4, 5). However, the CT scan of our patients showed diffuse nodules in the bilateral lung, which we initially suspected as lung adenocarcinoma or lung metastasis from other cancers. We excluded other malignant tumors, mainly by PET–CT. Although we could not completely rule out the possibility of adenosquamous carcinoma, we confirmed the diagnosis of squamous carcinoma based on histopathology of double specimens, immunohistochemistry, and sensitivity of the lesions to crizotinib.

Crizotinib has been approved for the treatment of NSCLC patients with ROS1 rearrangements. As reported in PROFILE 1001 study, crizotinib showed an objective response rate (ORR) of 72%, median progression free survival (PFS) of 19.3 months, median overall survival (OS) of 51.4 months, and 48-months survival probability of 51% in 53 advanced NSCLC patients with ROS1 rearrangements, and TRAEs were mainly grade 1 or 2 per CTCAE v3.0 (8). The efficacy and safety of crizotinib were also confirmed in a phase II OxOnc Study in East Asian patients, with an ORR of 71.7%, median PFS of 15.9 months, and median OS of 32.5 months; most TRAEs were grade 1 or 2 in severity (9). Both two studies showed that the ORR of crizotinib in the treatment of ROS1 rearrangement in NSCLC exceeded 70%. In fact, studies on crizotinib in the treatment of ROS1 rearrangement NSCLC have focused on lung adenocarcinoma since the vast majority of ROS1 mutations occur in the adenocarcinoma subtype. Significantly, the patient in our case was diagnosed with peripheral lung SCC and surprisingly showed a remarkable shrinkage of both tumor lesions and enlarged LNs and has remained PR for 9 months after receiving crizotinib treatment until now. The most commonly reported TRAEs (occurring in more than 25% of patients) of crizotinib in clinical trials were visual disturbances, gastrointestinal toxicities, edema, and elevated ALT/AST, mostly assessed as grade 1/2 in severity (10, 11). Hypoalbuminemia is an uncommon TRAE that was quite severe in this patient. The patient was treated with an albumin infusion. Fortunately, when she resumed crizotinib treatment, severe TRAEs did not recur and she remained PR for a long time. Among the six previous cases, two patients received crizotinib as the first line (5, 6) and two patients received crizotinib as the second line treatment (2, 4). Compared patients with lung SCC receiving first-line treatment with crizotinib, our patient had a better treatment effect and a longer PFS.

CONCLUSION

In conclusion, we presented the case of a lung SCC patient with an atypical imaging manifestation and molecular pathology, suggesting that rare ROS1 rearrangement could also unexpectedly occur in patients with lung SCC and is a sensitive target of crizotinib in lung SCC.

AUTHOR CONTRIBUTIONS

GY, JW, and YY designed the study and wrote the original draft of the manuscript. JZ, ZY, and QG contributed to the data collections. JY revised the manuscript. WM supervised the study and revised the manuscript. All authors contributed to the article and approved the submitted version.

REFERENCES

1. Davies KD, Le AT, Theodoro MF, Skokan MC, Aisner DL, Berge EM, et al. Identifying and Targeting ROS1 Gene Fusions in Non-Small Cell Lung Cancer. *Clin Cancer Res* (2012) 18(17):4570–9. doi: 10.1158/1078-0432.Ccr-12-0550
2. Shaw AT, Ou SH, Bang YJ, Camidge DR, Solomon BJ, Salgia R, et al. Crizotinib in ROS1-Rearranged Non-Small-Cell Lung Cancer. *N Engl J Med* (2014) 371(21):1963–71. doi: 10.1056/NEJMoa1406766
3. Eisenhauer EA, Therasse P, Bogaerts J, Schwartz LH, Sargent D, Ford R, et al. New Response Evaluation Criteria in Solid Tumours: Revised RECIST Guideline (Version 1.1). *Eur J Cancer (Oxford Engl: 1990)* (2009) 45 (2):228–47. doi: 10.1016/j.ejca.2008.10.026
4. Gibelin C, Avrillon V, de la Fouchardiere A, Mc Leer-Florin A, Lantuejoul S, Fayette J. Clinical Relevance of ROS1 Rearrangements Detection in Advanced Squamous Cell Carcinomas. *Lung Cancer (Amsterdam Neth)* (2016) 102:42–3. doi: 10.1016/j.lungcan.2016.10.005
5. Ju L, Han M, Su J, Wu C, Dong Z. A Lung Squamous Carcinoma Patient With ROS1 Rearrangement Sensitive to Crizotinib. *Cancer Chemother Pharmacol* (2018) 82(3):561–4. doi: 10.1007/s00280-018-3660-2
6. Li Q, Wu J, Yan LX, Huang JW, Zhang Z, Zhang JE, et al. ALK and ROS1 Double-Rearranged Lung Squamous Cell Carcinoma Responding to Crizotinib Treatment: A Case Report. *J Thorac Oncol* (2017) 12(12):e193–e7. doi: 10.1016/j.jtho.2017.08.021
7. Zhao W, Choi YL, Song JY, Zhu Y, Xu Q, Zhang F, et al. Alk, ROS1 and RET Rearrangements in Lung Squamous Cell Carcinoma Are Very Rare. *Lung Cancer (Amsterdam Neth)* (2016) 94:22–7. doi: 10.1016/j.lungcan.2016.01.011
8. Shaw AT, Riely GJ, Bang YJ, Kim DW, Camidge DR, Solomon BJ, et al. Crizotinib in ROS1-Rearranged Advanced Non-Small-Cell Lung Cancer (NSCLC): Updated Results, Including Overall Survival, From PROFILE 1001. *Ann Oncol* (2019) 30(7):1121–6. doi: 10.1093/annonc/mdz131
9. Wu YL, Yang JC, Kim DW, Lu S, Zhou J, Seto T, et al. Phase II Study of Crizotinib in East Asian Patients With ROS1-Positive Advanced Non-Small-Cell Lung Cancer. *J Clin Oncol* (2018) 36(14):1405–11. doi: 10.1200/jco.2017.75.5587
10. Shaw AT, Kim DW, Nakagawa K, Seto T, Crinó L, Ahn MJ, et al. Crizotinib Versus Chemotherapy in Advanced ALK-positive Lung Cancer. *N Engl J Med* (2013) 368(25):2385–94. doi: 10.1056/NEJMoa1214886
11. Frampton JE. Crizotinib: A Review of its Use in the Treatment of Anaplastic Lymphoma Kinase-Positive, Advanced Non-Small Cell Lung Cancer. *Drugs* (2013) 73(18):2031–51. doi: 10.1007/s40265-013-0142-z

5

The Efficacy and Safety of Anlotinib Combined with PD-1 Antibody for Third-Line or Further-Line Treatment of Patients with Advanced Non-Small-Cell Lung Cancer

Chongya Zhai†, Xiaoling Zhang†, Lulu Ren, Liangkun You, Qin Pan, Hongming Pan* and Weidong Han**

Department of Medical Oncology, Sir Run Run Shaw Hospital, College of Medicine, Zhejiang University, Hangzhou, China

Correspondence:
Weidong Han
hanwd@zju.edu.cn
Hongming Pan
panhongming@zju.edu.cn
Qin Pan
tianpanqin@yeah.net

†These authors have contributed equally to this work

Background: Both anlotinib and programmed death 1 (PD-1) monoclonal antibody (mAb) have been approved for the third line treatment of metastatic non-small cell lung cancer (NSCLC). However, the combination of these two standard therapies has not been investigated in third-line or further-line treatment of patients with advanced NSCLC.

Methods: We reviewed 22 patients with NSCLC who received anlotinib combined with PD-1 mAb therapy from July 2018 to October 2019 at Sir Run Run Shaw Hospital. Based on the baseline characteristics, PD-L1 expression and EGFR mutation status, we retrospectively analyzed the efficacy and safety of this combination therapy by RESIST 1.1 and CTCAE 5.0.

Results: The combination treatment of anlotinib and PD-1 mAb in 22 NSCLC patients gained a median PFS of 6.8 months and a median OS of 17.3 months. The disease control rate (DCR) was 90.9%, and the objective response rate (ORR) was 36.4%, where 1 (4.6%) patient achieved complete response (CR) and 7 (31.8%) patients achieved partial response (PR). The median time to response was 3.9 months, and the median duration of the response was 6.8 months. The common grades 1–2 adverse events were fatigue 10/22 (45.5%), decreased appetite 9/22 (40.9%), hypertension 10/22 (45.5%); the common grades 3–4 adverse events were hypertension 2/22 (9.1%) and mouth ulceration 2/22 (9.1%).

Conclusion: Anlotinib combined with PD-1 mAb showed promising efficacy in third-line or further-line treatment of NSCLC, and its adverse effects is tolerable.

Keywords: NSCLC, anlotinib hydrochloride, third line of therapy, TP53, EGFR

INTRODUCTION

Lung cancer is the leading cause of cancer-related morbidity and mortality, non-small-cell lung cancer (NSCLC) is the most prevalent subtype with a poor prognosis owing to the presence of locally advanced or wide metastasis in the majority of patients at the time of diagnosis or postoperative recurrence (1). Significant progress has been made in the treatment of advanced

NSCLC in the past 10 years. In patients with positive drive mutation, the drugs represented by EGFR-TKI achieved nearly 3-year overall survival (2). For patients with negative drive mutation, PD-1 mAb can significantly improve the therapeutic efficacy and prolong the overall survival (3). In the first-line treatment, it can be used alone or combined with chemotherapy, while the second-line treatment is recommended to use PD-1 mAb alone (4). When PD-1 mAb is used alone, the overall response rate and PFS are not satisfactory (5–7). Some patients even suffered from hyper-progression with single immunotherapy due to high metastatic burden (8).

Anlotinib is a multi-target drug approved for the third line treatment of advanced NSCLC, which could inhibit the vascular endothelial growth factor (VEGFR) 1-3, platelet-derived growth factor (PDGFR) α, PDGFRβ, C-proto-oncogenic receptor tyrosine kinase (C-KIT) and RET. It represses the tumor angiogenesis by down-regulating major pro-angiogenic factors, such as VEGF, PDGF-BB and fibroblast growth factor (FGF). Surprisingly, anlotinib used in the third line treatment of NSCLC gained a median PFS of 5.4 months (9). Interestingly, one study has shown that anlotinib could enhance the ratio of CD8/FoxP3$^+$ T cell in tumor tissues thus altering the tumor microenvironment (10). Moreover, anlotinib was proved to promote the infiltration of natural killer (NK) cells, M1-like tumor-associated macrophage (TAM) and dendritic cells in lung cancer mouse model, and the combination of anlotinib with immune checkpoint inhibitor gained better therapeutic response (11). These results suggest that anlotinib is involved in the regulation of tumor immune microenvironment, and the combination therapy with PD-1 mAb may be the future exploration direction.

There have been many reports on the treatment of NSCLC with PD-1 mAb combined with anti-angiogenetic agents. In patients with disease progression after first-line treatment, Sintilimab combined with bevacizumab showed unexpected efficiency. The combination therapy achieved a median PFS of 6 months, and the patients were well tolerated (12). Besides, Sintilimab combined with anlotinib in 22 patients of NSCLC at first line treatment gained an ORR of 68.2% and DCR of 100%, 2 grade 3 treatment-related adverse events (TRAEs) occurred with no grade 4/5 observation, however, the PFS and OS was not available due to the short follow-up time (13). Taken together, Angiogenesis inhibitors combined with immune check point inhibitors in the treatment of advanced lung cancer has achieved preliminary clinical validation.

Anti-angiogenesis agents and PD-1 mAb can cooperate to alter the microenvironment of the tumor. The expression of PD-1 was up-regulated in relapsed tumor after the anti-VEGFR2 agent treatment (14). Studies have shown that PD-1 mAb and anti-VEGFR2 agent combination treatment could promote tumor vessel normalization and induce high endothelial venules (HEVs), which promoted lymphocyte infiltration and activity through the activation of lymphotoxin β receptor (LTβR) signaling (15). In addition, anti-angiogenesis therapy could restore the response of effector T lymphocytes by breaking the tumor vessel barrier, and subsequent anti-PD-1 treatment further improved the activity of T lymphocytes, thereby synergistically leading to tumor shrinkage (16).

In this real-world evidence-based retrospective clinical study, we analyzed the efficacy and safety of anlotinib combined with PD-1 mAb for the third-line or further-line treatment of NSCLC patients. The results show that it has a good clinical application prospect and is worthy of further study.

METHODS

Data Source

We reviewed the records of a prospectively collected database of 22 patients with NSCLC who received anlotinib combined with PD-1 mAb, including sintilimab, nivolumab, pembrolizumab, toripalimab, and camrelizumab for the third-line or further treatment over the period of 1 year from July 2018 to October 2019 at Sir Run Run Shaw Hospital, College of Medicine, Zhejiang University, Hangzhou, China.

We retrospectively analyzed the baseline characteristics, PD-L1 expression, epithelial growth factor (EGFR) mutation status and prior and later treatment lines. All data were obtained by follow-up visits, telephone, electronic medical records, and letters. This study was approved by the Ethics Committee of Sir Run Run Shaw Hospital.

Patient Selection

The target samples included patients who received anlotinib and PD-1 mAb at Sir Run Run Shaw Hospital from July 2018 to October 2019. A definite histological or cytological diagnosis was required for the patients with NSCLC. The expected survival time was more than 3 months, and normal hematopoietic, hepatic, and renal function were prerequisite for enrollment. Exclusion criteria included patients with a history of autoimmune diseases or patients treated with steroids at a dose equivalent to or more than 10 mg prednisone daily or other immunosuppressive drugs. Patients with central squamous cell carcinoma were also excluded. The selection flow chart was shown in the **Figure 1**.

Study Variables

The clinical response to anti-PD-1 mAb combined with anlotinib treatment was evaluated according to the Response Evaluation Criteria in Solid Tumors (RECIST) version 1.1. Every 2 or 3 cycles after the combined therapy was established, and short-term efficacy was evaluated. The percentage of patients having achieved a complete response (CR: the disappearance of all target lesions) plus partial response (PR: at least a 30% reduction in the sum of the diameters of the target lesions) recorded in the medical system were defined as the objective response rate (ORR). At least a 20% increase in the sum of the diameters of the target lesions were evaluated as PD, the lesions cannot be classified as PR or PD was evaluated as SD (stable disease). The percentage of patients with CR, PR or SD was defined as the disease control rate (DCR). PFS was calculated as the time from the initiation of treatment with anti-PD-1 mAb combined with anlotinib therapy to progressive disease (PD) or death. OS referred to the time from the start of combination treatment to death from any cause.

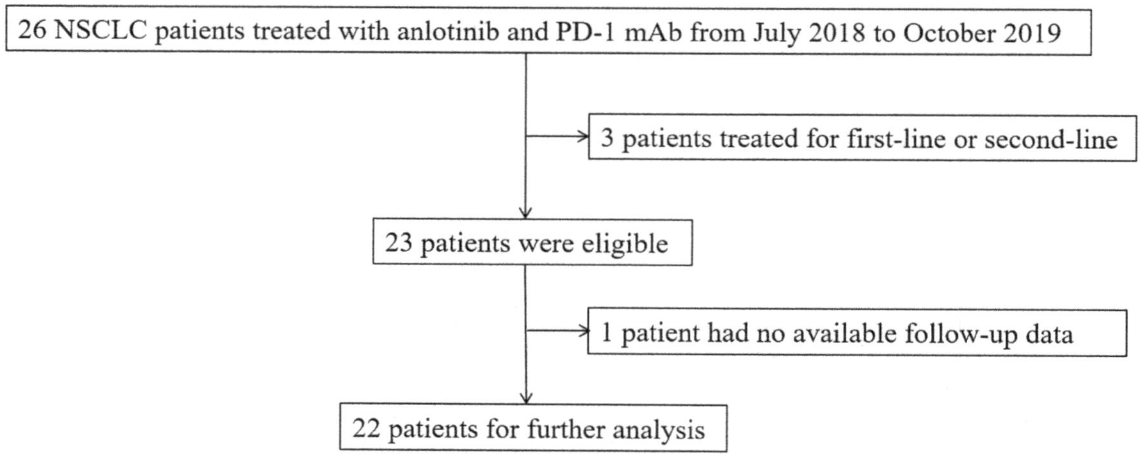

FIGURE 1 | The patients selection flow chart.

Statistical Analysis

Descriptive statistics (percentages, means, medians) were used to describe baseline characteristics and clinical features of the sample of patients with NSCLC. ORR, PFS and OS were calculated to analyze the efficacy and clinical features of the patients treated with combination therapy. Statistical analyses were performed using SPSS statistical software (version 20.0; SPSS, IBM Corporation).

RESULTS

From July 2018 to October 2019, 22 patients with NSCLC were enrolled in this real-world study. Baseline demographics and clinical characteristics were exhibited in **Table 1**. In the final eligible sample, the median age of the patients was 65 years. Of 22, 10 (45.4%) patients were current or former smokers; 11 (50%), never smokers; and 1 (4.6%), unknown smoking status. Notably, 2 (9.1%) patients were with ECOG status of 0, and 20 (90.9%) patients had ECOG status of 1 at the time of diagnosis. 10 (45.4%) patients were current or former smokers, and 11 (50%) patients were never smoker. The smoking status was unknown in 1 (4.6%) patient. Patients with non-squamous histology predominated: 15 (68.2%) had adenocarcinoma, seven (31.8%) had squamous cell carcinoma. Fourteen (63.6%) patients had metastasis organ number more than 3 and eight (36.4%) patients had metastasis organ number below 3. As for the PD-1 mAb treatment, a numbers of patients received nivolumab, pembrolizumab, Sintilimab, toripalimab, or camrelizumab treatment were 6 (27.3%), 2 (9.1%), 5 (22.7%), 5 (22.7%) and 4 (18.2%), respectively. In addition, two (9.1%) patients had PD-L1 tumor proportion score (TPS) above 50%; seven (31.8%), below 1%; nine (40.9%), between 1% and 49%; four (18.2%), unknown PD-L1 TPS. The efficacy of PD-1 mAb was related to the basic EGFR mutation status. In this study, 12 (54.6%) patients had negative EGFR mutation status, followed by unknown EGFR mutation status (7, 31.8%), positive EGFR mutation (3, 13.6%), EGFR exon19 mutation (2, 9.1%), and EGFR L858/T790M mutation (1, 4.5%). 7 (31.8%) patients had radiotherapy previously and 3 (13.6%) patients ever received target therapy. The patients receiving 12 mg or 10 mg anlotinib dose numbered 6 (27.3%) and 16 (72.7%), respectively. The anlotinib dose was given after fully assessment of the tolerance and other basic physical status of the patients. The detailed anlotinib dose and treatment lines were listed in the **Supplementary Table 1**.

Patients response to anlotinib combined with PD-1 mAb was displayed in the **Table 2**. One (4.6%) patient got CR; seven (31.8%) patients got PR; 12 (54.5%) patients remained SD; and two (9.1%) patients had disease progressed. The ORR was 36.4% and the DCR was 90.9%. The median time to response was 3.9 months, and the median duration of the response was 6.8 months. The median PFS (**Figure 2A**) of the combination therapy was 6.8 months (95%CI: 3.4, 9.8), and the median OS (**Figure 2B**) of the treatment was 17.3 months (95%CI: 16.1, 18.5). For each patient, the percent change in the sum of the longest diameter of target lesions diameter from the baseline was graphed in a waterfall plot (based on the treatment lines and patient's response, **Figures 3A, B**) and spider plot (**Figure 4**). For patients with brain metastasis subgroup analysis, six patients had brain metastasis, the median PFS was 4.7 months (95% CI:2.3–7.1 months), 16 patients had no brain metastasis, the median PFS was 10.5 months (95%CI:6.8–14.3 months), the *p* value is 0.053 between two groups using the log-rank survival analysis.

The adverse events during the combination treatment were listed in the **Table 3**. The most common grade 1-2 TRAEs were fatigue 10/22 (45.5%), decreased appetite 9/22 (40.9%), and hypertension 10/22 (45.5%). The less common mild adverse events were nausea 3/22 (13.6%), cough 2/22 (9.1%) and hepatic function abnormal 3/22 (13.6%). The grades 3–4 adverse events were rash 2/22 (9.1%), hypertension 2/22 (9.1%), diarrhea 1/22 (4.6%), mouth ulceration 2/22 (9.1%), and pneumonitis 2/22 (4.6%).

TABLE 1 | Population characteristics.

Baseline Characteristics	All patients (n=22)
Age	
Median(range), years	65 (46–82)
Gender, n(%)	
Male	14 (63.6)
Female	8 (36.4)
ECOG score at the time of diagnosis, n(%)	
0	2 (9.1)
1	20 (90.9)
Histological subtype, n(%)	
Adenocarcinoma	15 (68.2)
Squamous cell carcinoma	7 (31.8)
Smoking status, n(%)	
Never smoked	11 (50.0)
Current or former smoker	10 (45.5)
Unknown	1 (4.5)
No.of prior systemic regimens, n(%)	
2	15 (68.2)
3	4 (18.2)
≥4	3 (13.6)
No.of organs of metastasis, n(%)	
≥3	14 (63.6)
<3	8 (36.4)
Anlotinib treatment dose, n(%)	
12mg	6 (27.3)
10mg	16 (72.7)
Anti-PD-1 mAbs, n(%)	
Nivolumab	6 (27.3)
Pembrolizumab	2 (9.1)
Sintilimab	5 (22.7)
Toripalimab	5 (22.7)
Camrelizumab	4 (18.2)
PD-L1 TPS, n(%)	
≥50%	2 (9.1)
1-49%	9 (40.9)
<1%	7 (31.8)
Unknown	4 (18.2)
EGFR mutation status, n(%)	
Negative	12 (54.6)
Positive	3 (13.6)
Unknown	7 (31.8)
Chemotherapy regimens, n(%)	
1	5 (22.7)
2	11 (50.0)
≥3	6 (27.3)
Previous radiotherapy treatment, n(%)	
No	15 (68.2)
Yes	7 (31.8)
Previous target treatment, n(%)	
No	19 (86.4)
Yes	3 (13.6)

Anti-PD-1, anti-programmed death-1; EGFR, epidermal growth factor receptor; ECOG, Eastern Cooperative Oncology Group; PD-L1, programmed death ligand-1; TPS, tumor proportion score.

TABLE 2 | Efficacy of Anlotinib combined with Anti-PD-1 mAbs in third-line or further treatment of NSCLC patients.

Efficacy	All patients (n=22)
Complete response, n(%)	1 (4.6)
Partial response, n(%)	7 (31.8)
Stable disease, n(%)	12 (54.5)
Progressive disease, n(%)	2 (9.1)
ORR (%, CR+PR)	36.4
DCR (%, CR+PR+SD)	90.9
Time to response(m)	
Media(range)	3.9 (1.6, 7.7)
Duration of response(m)	
Media	6.8
ongoing, n/N(%)	4/8 (50.0)
PFS(m)	
Media (95% CI)	6.8 (3.4, 9.8)
OS(m)	
Media (95% CI)	17.3 (16.1, 18.5)

CR, complete response; PR, partial response; SD, stable disease; PD, Progressive disease; ORR, objective response rate; DCR, disease control rate.

DISCUSSION

From the retrospective summary of the anlotinib combined with the PD-1 mAb treatment, the efficacy was promising and unexpected. The third-line treatment of sole anlotinib in NSCLC gained a median PFS of 5.4 months and the median OS of 9.6 months (9), whereas combination treatment exhibited a median PFS of 6.8 months, median OS of 17.3 months and the ORR of 36.4%, providing an extra 1.4 months PFS and 7.7 months OS benefit compared with anlotinib alone. In comparison with sole PD-1 mAb treatment, the combination treatment also provided survival benefit. The median OS of nivolumab ranged from 9.2 months to 12.2 months in CheckMate 017 and CheckMate 057 clinical trials; 12.7 months of pembrolizumab in Keynote 010 clinical trial; for atezolizumab, the median OS ranged from 12.6 months to 13.8 months in OAK (third line therapy) and POPLAR clinical trial (6, 17). Therefore, the combination treatment gained an encouraging OS. This favorable OS was achieved for several reasons. The different treatment lines between Checkmate017, Checkmate057 (second-line) and our cohort (third line) were part of the reason for the prolonged OS, meanwhile, in standard third line treatment, anlotinib alone gained a favorable survival time, PD-1 mAb also prolonged the survival time compared with chemotherapy. Besides, the adverse events were tolerable for patients with combination treatment, few patients withdrew the clinical trial due to the TRAEs. With no doubt, the combination of PD-1 mAb and anlotinib can gained a longer survival benefit *via* a synergistic way. The mechanism may be that anlotinib altered the tumor immune microenvironment and PD-1 mAb improved the vessel normalization, which leads to the mutual sensitization between these two drugs (15). For instance, anlotinib treatment increased the INF-γexpression in $CD4^+$ T cells and upregulated the tumor-infiltrating NK cells (11). Besides, anlotinib can inhibit PD-L1 expression on vascular endothelial cells so as to break through "immune tolerance barrier", it also promotes $CD8^+$ T cell infiltration and improves the balance of CD8/Foxp3 (10). Many pro-angiogenic factors are derived from immune cells, such as M2-like TAMs, immature dendritic cells, myeloid-derived suppressor cells (MDSCs), Trges and so on. These cells play various roles in the regulation of tumor angiogenesis (18). PD-1 mAb can suppress the activity of the immunosuppressive cells, indirectly down-regulate the angiogenic factors, and alleviate the abnormalities of tumor vessel (19, 20). In line with this, a number of experimental studies have confirmed that anti-angiogenesis agents combined with PD-1 mAb can reduce the tumor volume of tumor bearing mice (21, 22).

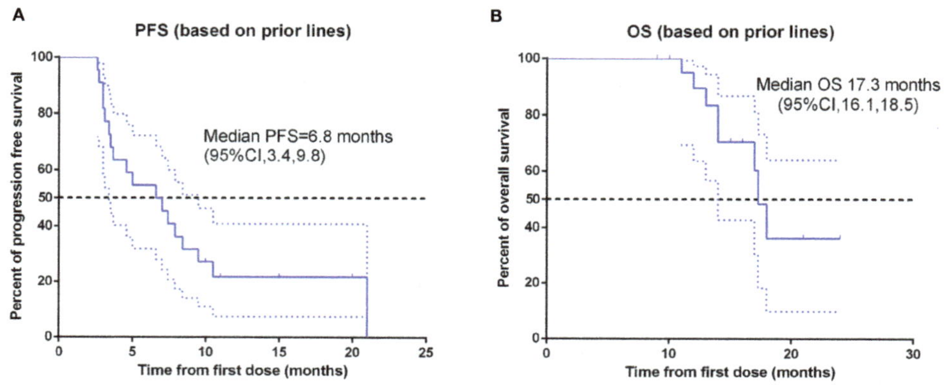

FIGURE 2 | Kaplan-Meier survival curve of progression-free survival **(A)** and overall survival **(B)** in 22 non-small cell lung cancer patients. PFS, progression-free survival; OS, over survival; CI, confidence interval.

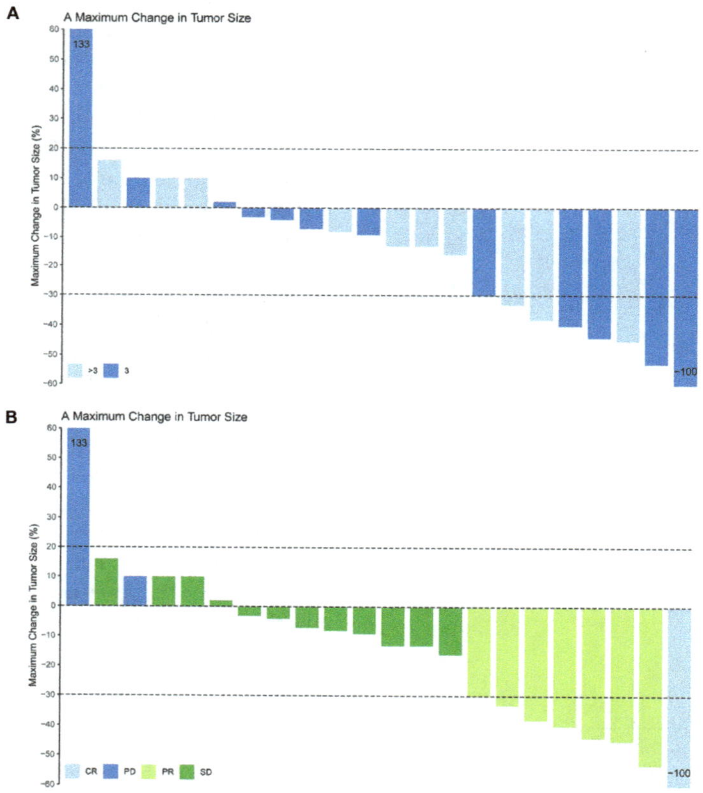

FIGURE 3 | Maximum change in tumor size based on the treatment lines **(A)** and tumor response **(B)** in 22 non-small cell lung cancer patients. CR, complete response; PR, partial response; SD, stable disease; PD, Progressive disease; ORR, objective response rate.

The median time to response (TTR) and the duration of response (DOR) of pembrolizumab in KEYNOTE 001 was 2.1 months and 18 months, respectively, and 101/495 (20.4%) patients in this clinical trial were treatment naïve (23). In camrelizumab (PD-1 mAb) combined with apatinib treatment, the TTR was 3.7 months and DOR was 5.3 months (24). While in our study, the TTR was 3.9 months, which is longer than the results of both above studies, probably because that most patients in this study were third line or above line and 63.6% (14/22) patients were with three or more organ metastases. Although the TTR was longer in our study, however, the DOR of our study is 6.8 months, which was lengthened than the camrelizumab

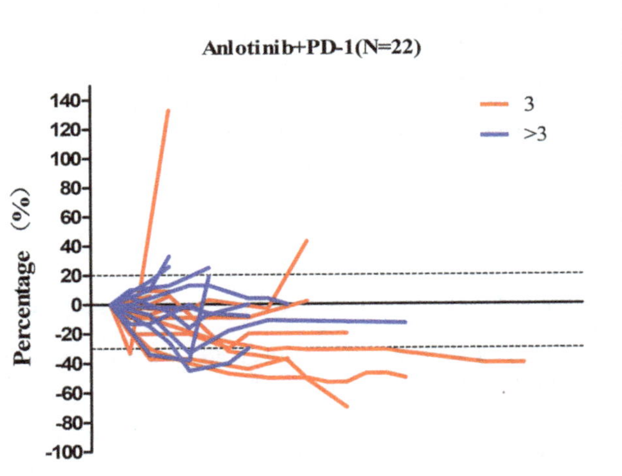

FIGURE 4 | The percent change in the sum of the longest diameter of target lesions diameter from the baseline in 22 non-small cell lung cancer patients.

combined with apatinib treatment. The results indicated that anlotinib combined with PD-1 mAb could also achieve long-term benefits.

It is worth noting that one patient achieved a CR response and had PFS for more than 20 months. The patient had complex mixed mutations, including K-RAS exon 2 missense mutation, TP53 exon 9 frameshift mutation, TAPBPL (TAP binding protein like) exon 2 missense mutation and SMARCA4 (SEI/SNF related, matrix associated, actin dependent regulator of chromatin, subfamily a, member 4) exon 20 missense mutation. Consistent with our findings, In Keynote 001, the median PFS of patients with K-RAS mutation and TP53 mutation treated with pembrolizumab was 14.7 months, much higher than that of 3.5 months in the wild-type group of K-RAS (25). Interestingly, it has been reported that a squamous-cell NSCLC patient with TP53 and KRAS co-mutation was treated with pembrolizumab combined with gemcitabine. The therapeutic effect reached PR and PFS was more than 7 months (26). The K-RAS mutation status may be an indicator of good response to the PD-1 mAb, the TP53 mutation patients also showed good response to anlotinib (27). So clinical trial like combination of anlotinib and PD-1 mAb may be promising in patients with K-RAS mutation and TP53 mutation co-existed. In addition, recently, it is generally believed that PD-L1 high expression is correlated with good prognosis in patients treated with PD-1 mAb (28, 29). In keynote 024, the patients whose PD-L1 TPS score >50% treated with pembrolizumab gained a median OS of 30 months (30), and in keynote-042 (TPS>50% Subgroup),the median OS is 20 months (31). It is impressive that in keynote 024, three patients treated with single pembrolizumab achieved CR (30, 32). In our study the CR patient also had a PD-L1 TPS above 50%. Therefore, among the three factors of K-RAS mutation, TP53 mutation and high score of PD-L1 TPS, which was the real prognostic factor is still uncertain. More clinical trials or experience should be focused on the factors.

For patients with brain metastasis, the prognosis was worse than the patients without brain metastasis, but the only 22 patients was included in our cohort, it may not be convincing enough until more prospective studies were conducted.

The adverse events of the combination treatment were tolerable in our patients, so the combination was safe and could be popularized in the future. The most common grade 1-2 adverse events were hypertension and fatigue (33), which were in line with the ALTER-0303 clinical trial. However, the thyroid stimulating hormone (TSH) elevation and hypertriglyceridemia were less common in our center, which might due to a limited number of cases. The common adverse events of PD-1 mAb were diarrhea, rash, decreased appetite, nausea, anemia and neutropenia (34). The organ specific immune-related adverse events were hypothyroidism, pneumonitis, colitis, hepatitis and hypophysitis (35). In our study, four (18.2%) patients had mild hypothyroidism, and four (18.2%) patients had grades 1–2 pneumonitis. These adverse events were consistent with the previous clinical trial. However, it should be noted that the median time to follow up was 384 days (95%CI: 298 days, 469 days), some immune related adverse event can occur later, for example, the hepatitis can occur after 34 weeks exposed to nivolumab treatment (36). The median time to onset of late-immune-related adverse events was 16.6 months in a multi-center study (37). So the immune-related adverse events need to follow up later.

Our study has obvious limitations because only 22 patients were included, resulting in the inability to carry out univariate or multivariate analysis. The anlotinib dose, different pathology types, number of metastasis organs, treatment lines and other factors may affect the efficacy of combination treatment. More clinical trials or clinical experience are needed to identify the beneficial patient group. In addition, retrospective study may lose some detailed information of the patients, like the gene mutation and PD-L1 of some patients were unknown; besides, multi PD-1 mAb were used in our center, which might produce diverse efficacy. In this study, three patients with EGFR mutation had a history of target therapy, the PFS of three patients were very different (3, 5, and 10.5 months, respectively). So we cannot come to a conclusion right now, this requires more data based on these subtype of patients. To

TABLE 3 | Treatment-related adverse events.

AEs	Grade 1-2, n (%)	Grade 3-4, n (%)
Fatigue	10 (45.5)	0
Decreased appetite	9 (40.9)	0
Nausea	3 (13.6)	0
Weight decrease	4 (18.2)	0
Rash	8 (36.4)	1 (4.6)
Hypertension	10 (45.5)	2 (9.1)
Diarrhea	7 (31.8)	1 (4.6)
Mouth ulceration	5 (22.7)	2 (9.1)
Dysphonia	4 (18.2)	0
Pneumonitis	4 (18.2)	1 (4.6)
Cough	2 (9.1)	0
Hepatic function abnormal	3 (13.6)	0
Hypothyroidism	4 (18.2)	0
proteinuria	5 (22.7)	0
Palmar-plantar erythrodysaesthesia syndrome	4 (18.2)	0

AEs, adverse events.

sum up, our retrospective analysis shows that the efficacy and safety of the combination therapy of anlotinib and PD-1 mAb are encouraging and worthy of further clinical trials.

AUTHOR CONTRIBUTIONS

CZ: Data curation, Methodology, Investigation. XZ: Data curation, Methodology, Writing original draft. LR: Data curation, Writing-review and editing. LY: Data curation, Methodology. QP: Methodology, Supervision. HP: Methodology, Supervision. WH: Methodology, Supervision, Writing-review and editing. All authors contributed to the article and approved the submitted version.

REFERENCES

1. Herbst RS, Morgensztern D, Boshoff C. The biology and management of non-small cell lung cancer. *Nature* (2018) 553(7689):446–54. doi: 10.1038/nature25183
2. Ramalingam SS, Vansteenkiste J, Planchard D, Cho BC, Gray JE, Ohe Y, et al. Overall Survival with Osimertinib in Untreated, EGFR-Mutated Advanced NSCLC. *N Engl J Med* (2020) 382(1):41–50. doi: 10.1056/NEJMoa1913662
3. Borghaei H, Paz-Ares L, Horn L, Spigel DR, Steins M, Ready NE, et al. Nivolumab versus Docetaxel in Advanced Nonsquamous Non-Small-Cell Lung Cancer. *N Engl J Med* (2015) 373(17):1627–39. doi: 10.1056/NEJMoa1507643
4. Doroshow DB, Sanmamed MF, Hastings K, Politi K, Rimm DL, Chen L, et al. Immunotherapy in Non-Small Cell Lung Cancer: Facts and Hopes. *Clin Cancer Res* (2019) 25(15):4592–602. doi: 10.1158/1078-0432.CCR-18-1538
5. Rizvi NA, Mazières J, Planchard D, Stinchcombe TE, Dy GK, Antonia SJ, et al. Activity and safety of nivolumab, an anti-PD-1 immune checkpoint inhibitor, for patients with advanced, refractory squamous non-small-cell lung cancer (CheckMate 063): a phase 2, single-arm trial. *Lancet Oncol* (2015) 16(3):257–65. doi: 10.1016/S1470-2045(15)70054-9
6. Rittmeyer A, Barlesi F, Waterkamp D, Park K, Ciardiello F, von PJ, et al. Atezolizumab versus docetaxel in patients with previously treated non-small-cell lung cancer (OAK): a phase 3, open-label, multicentre randomised controlled trial. *Lancet* (2017) 389(10066):255–65. doi: 10.1016/S0140-6736(16)32517-X
7. Sheng Z, Zhu X, Sun Y, Zhang Y. The efficacy of anti-PD-1/PD-L1 therapy and its comparison with EGFR-TKIs for advanced non-small-cell lung cancer. *Oncotarget* (2017) 8(34):57826–35. doi: 10.18632/oncotarget.18406
8. Kim JY, Lee KH, Kang J, Borcoman E, Saada-Bouzid E, Kronbichler A, et al. Hyperprogressive Disease during Anti-PD-1 (PDCD1) / PD-L1 (CD274) Therapy: A Systematic Review and Meta-Analysis. *Cancers (Basel)* (2019) 11 (11):1699. doi: 10.3390/cancers11111699
9. Han B, Li K, Wang Q, Zhang L, Shi J, Wang Z, et al. Effect of Anlotinib as a Third-Line or Further Treatment on Overall Survival of Patients With Advanced Non-Small Cell Lung Cancer: The ALTER 0303 Phase 3 Randomized Clinical Trial. *JAMA Oncol* (2018) 4(11):1569–75. doi: 10.1001/jamaoncol.2018.3039
10. Liu S, Qin T, Liu Z, Wang J, Jia Y, Feng Y, et al. anlotinib alters tumor immune microenvironment by downregulating PD-L1 expression on vascular endothelial cells. *Cell Death Dis* (2020) 11(5):309. doi: 10.1038/s41419-020-2511-3
11. Yang Y, Li L, Jiang Z, Wang B, Pan Z. Anlotinib optimizes anti-tumor innate immunity to potentiate the therapeutic effect of PD-1 blockade in lung cancer. *Cancer Immunol Immunother* (2020) 69(12):2523–32. doi: 10.1007/s00262-020-02641-5
12. Zhang Y, Zhao M, Cao S, Zhang X, Du Y. Unexpected favorable outcome to sintilimab plus bevacizumab in an EGFR-mutated non-small cell lung cancer patient: A case report. *Thorac Cancer* (2020) 11(9):2717–22. doi: 10.1111/1759-7714.13569
13. Han TCB, Zhong R. Efficacy and safety of Sinitilimab with Anlotinib as first-line therapy for advanced Non-Small Cell Lung Cancer(NSCLC). *J Thorac Oncol* (2019) 14(10):S439. doi: 10.1016/j.jtho.2019.08.269
14. Cai X, Wei B, Li L, Chen X, Liu W, Cui J, et al. Apatinib enhanced anti-PD-1 therapy for colon cancer in mice via promoting PD-L1 expression. *Int Immunopharmacol* (2020) 88:106858. doi: 10.1016/j.intimp.2020.106858
15. Allen E, Jabouille A, Rivera LB, Lodewijckx I, Missiaen R, Steri V, et al. Combined antiangiogenic and anti-PD-L1 therapy stimulates tumor immunity through HEV formation. *Sci Transl Med* (2017) 9(385):eaak9679. doi: 10.1126/scitranslmed.aak9679
16. Lanitis E, Irving M, Coukos G. Targeting the tumor vasculature to enhance T cell activity, Curr. *Opin Immunol* (2015) 33:55–63. doi: 10.1016/j.coi.2015.01.011
17. Fehrenbacher L, Spira A, Ballinger M, Kowanetz M, Vansteenkiste J, Mazieres J, et al. Atezolizumab versus docetaxel for patients with previously treated non-small-cell lung cancer (POPLAR): a multicentre, open-label, phase 2 randomised controlled trial. *Lancet* (2016) 387(10030):1837–46. doi: 10.1016/S0140-6736(16)00587-0
18. Lee WS, Yang H, Chon HJ, Kim C. Combination of therapy and immune checkpoint blockade normalizes vascular-immune crosstalk to potentiate cancer immunity. *Exp Mol Med* (2020) 52(9):1475–85. doi: 10.1038/s12276-020-00500-y
19. Huang Y, BYS K, Chan CK, Hahn SM, Weissman IL, Jiang W. Improving immune-vascular crosstalk for cancer immunotherapy. *Nat Rev Immunol* (2018) 18(3):195–203. doi: 10.1038/nri.2017.145
20. Rahma OE, Hodi FS. The Intersection between Tumor Angiogenesis and Immune Suppression. *Clin Cancer Res* (2019) 25(18):5449–57. doi: 10.1158/1078-0432.CCR-18-1543
21. Zhao S, Ren S, Jiang T, Zhu B, Li X, Zhao C, et al. Low-Dose Apatinib Optimizes Tumor Microenvironment and Potentiates Antitumor Effect of PD-1/PD-L1 Blockade in Lung Cancer. *Cancer Immunol Res* (2019) 7(4):630–43. doi: 10.1158/2326-6066.CIR-17-0640
22. Schmittnaegel M, Rigamonti N, Kadioglu E, Cassará A, Wyser RC, Kiialainen A, et al. Dual angiopoietin-2 and VEGFA inhibition elicits antitumor immunity that is enhanced by PD-1 checkpoint blockade. *Sci Transl Med* (2017) 9(385):eaak9670. doi: 10.1126/scitranslmed.aak9670
23. Garon EB, Hellmann MD, Rizvi NA, Carcereny E, Leighl NB, Ahn MJ, et al. Five-Year Overall Survival for Patients With Advanced Non-Small-Cell Lung Cancer Treated With Pembrolizumab: Results From the Phase I KEYNOTE-001 Study. *J Clin Oncol* (2019) 37(28):2518–27. doi: 10.1200/JCO.19.00934
24. Zhou C, Gao G, Wang YN, Zhao J, Chen G, Liu Z, et al. Efficacy of PD-1 monoclonal antibody SHR-1210 plus apatinib in patients with advanced nonsquamous NSCLC with wild-type EGFR and ALK. *J Clin Oncol* (2019) 37(15_suppl):9112–9112.
25. Dong ZY, Zhong WZ, Zhang XC, Su J, Xie Z, Liu SY, et al. Potential Predictive Value of TP53 and KRAS Mutation Status for Response to PD-1 Blockade Immunotherapy in Lung Adenocarcinoma. *Clin Cancer Res* (2017) 23 (12):3012–24. doi: 10.1016/j.jtho.2016.11.504
26. Fang C, Zhang C, Zhao WQ, Hu WW, Wu J, Ji M. Co-mutations of TP53 and KRAS serve as potential biomarkers for immune checkpoint blockade in squamous-cell non-small cell lung cancer: a case report. *BMC Med Genomics* (2019) 12(1):136. doi: 10.1186/s12920-019-0592-6
27. Fang S, Cheng W, Zhang M, Yang R. Association of TP53 Mutations with Response to Anlotinib Treatment in Advanced Non-Small Cell Lung Cancer. *Onco Targets Ther* (2020) 13:6645–50. doi: 10.2147/OTT.S257052
28. Lin H, Wei S, Hurt EM, Green MD, Zhao L, Vatan L, et al. Host expression of PD-L1 determines efficacy of PD-L1 pathway blockade-mediated tumor regression. *J Clin Invest* (2018) 128(4):1708. doi: 10.1172/JCI120803
29. Shen X, Zhao B. Efficacy of PD-1 or PD-L1 inhibitors and PD-L1 expression status in cancer: meta-analysis. *BMJ* (2018) 362:k3529. doi: 10.1136/bmj.k3529
30. Reck M, Rodríguez-Abreu D, Robinson AG, Hui R, Csőszi T, Fülöp A, et al. Updated Analysis of KEYNOTE-024: Pembrolizumab Versus Platinum-Based Chemotherapy for Advanced Non-Small-Cell Lung Cancer With PD-L1

Tumor Proportion Score of 50% or Greater. *J Clin Oncol* (2019) 37(7):537–46. doi: 10.1200/JCO.18.00149

31. TSK M, Wu YL, Kudaba I, Kowalski DM, Cho BC, Turna HZ, et al. Pembrolizumab versus chemotherapy for previously untreated, PD-L1-expressing, locally advanced or metastatic non-small-cell lung cancer (KEYNOTE-042): a randomised, open-label, controlled, phase 3 trial. *Lancet* (2019) 393(10183):1819–30. doi: 10.1016/S0140-6736(18)32409-7
32. Reck M, Rodríguez-Abreu D, Robinson AG, Hui R, Csőszi T, Fülöp A, et al. Pembrolizumab versus Chemotherapy for PD-L1-Positive Non-Small-Cell Lung Cancer. *N Engl J Med* (2016) 375(19):1823–33. doi: 10.1056/NEJMoa1606774
33. Si X, Zhang L, Wang H, Zhang X, Wang M, Han B, et al. Management of anlotinib-related adverse events in patients with advanced non-small cell lung cancer: Experiences in ALTER-0303. *Thorac Cancer* (2019) 10(3):551–6. doi: 10.1111/1759-7714.12977
34. Hellmann MD, Paz-Ares L, Bernabe CR, Zurawski B, Kim SW, Carcereny CE, et al. Nivolumab plus Ipilimumab in Advanced Non-Small-Cell Lung Cancer. *N Engl J Med* (2019) 381(21):2020–31. doi: 10.1056/NEJMoa1910231
35. Baxi S, Yang A, Gennarelli RL, Khan N, Wang Z, Boyce L, et al. Immune-related adverse events for anti-PD-1 and anti-PD-L1 drugs: systematic review and meta-analysis. *BMJ* (2018) 360:k793. doi: 10.1136/bmj.k793
36. Imafuku K, Yoshino K, Yamaguchi K, Tsuboi S, Ohara K, Hata H. Successful Treatment of Sudden Hepatitis Induced by Long-Term Nivolumab Administration. *Case Rep Oncol* (2017) 10(1):368–71. doi: 10.1159/000471480
37. Nigro O, Pinotti G, De Galitiis F, Di Pietro FR, Giusti R, Filetti M, et al. Late immune-related adverse events in long-term responders to PD-1/PD-L1 checkpoint inhibitors: A multicentre study. *Eur J Cancer* (2020) 134:19–28. doi: 10.1093/annonc/mdz449.009

6

Peripheral Blood Autoantibodies Against to Tumor-Associated Antigen Predict Clinical Outcome to Immune Checkpoint Inhibitor-Based Treatment in Advanced Non-Small Cell Lung Cancer

Juan Zhou[1†], Jing Zhao[1†], Qingzhu Jia[2†], Qian Chu[3†], Fei Zhou[1], Xiangling Chu[1], Wencheng Zhao[1], Shengxiang Ren[1], Caicun Zhou[1] and Chunxia Su[1]*

[1] Department of Oncology, Shanghai Pulmonary Hospital & Thoracic Cancer Institute, Tongji University School of Medicine, Shanghai, China, [2] Department of Oncology, Xinqiao Hospital, Third Military Medical University, Chongqing, China, [3] Department of Oncology, Tongji Hospital of Tongji Medical College, Huazhong University of Science and Technology, Wuhan, China

***Correspondence:**
Chunxia Su
susu_mail@126.com

†These authors have contributed equally to this work

Background: Peripheral blood biomarkers to immunotherapy have attracted more and more attentions owing to noninvasive nature. This study was designed to identify a panel of tumor associated autoantibodies (TAAbs) in plasma to predict the clinical outcome of ICIs-based treatment in advanced NSCLC patients and correlation between TAAbs and checkpoint inhibitor pneumonitis (CIP) would also be investigated.

Materials and Methods: Baseline plasma was collected from patients with advanced NSCLC before receiving ICIs-based treatment. ELISA was used to detect concentration of autoantibodies. Clinical efficacy was evaluated according to RECIST v1.1.

Results: We have identified a panel of five-TAAbs to predict responses of ICIs-based treatment in a discovery cohort (n = 37), and confirmed its predictive value in a validation cohort (n = 129). In the validation cohort, the positivity of this 5-TAAbs panel was significantly associated with better response (ORR: 44.4% vs. 13.6%, $P < 0.001$) and longer PFS (7.6 vs. 3.3m, $P < 0.001$). This significant association was remained in subgroup of patients treated with combination therapy (ORR: 43.8% vs. 13.7%, $P = 0.004$,PFS: 6.7 vs. 3.7m, $P = 0\ .017$). Furthermore, this 5-TAAs panel worked better in patients who received subsequent-line treatment (ORR: 42.4% vs. 7.7%, $P = 0.001$, PFS: 6.2 vs. 3.0m, $P = 0.004$) than those received first-line treatment (ORR: 46.7% vs. 35.7%, $P = 0.345$, PFS: NR vs. 10.48m, $P = 0.146$). In addition, the CIP incidence in patients with 5-TAAbs positive was significantly higher comparing to negative patients (20.4% vs. 5.9%, $P = 0.015$).

Conclusion: Our 5-TAAbs panel is a potential predictive biomarker for responses and toxicities to ICIs-based treatment in patients with advanced NSCLC.

Keywords: biomarker, autoantibody, tumor-associated antigen, immune checkpoint inhibitor, lung cancer

INTRODUCTION

Immune checkpoint inhibitors (ICIs), targeting programmed cell death-1 (PD-1) and its ligand PD-L1, have significantly prolonged overall survival (OS) of patients with advanced non-small cell lung cancer (NSCLC) (1, 2). However, only around 20% of patients responded to ICIs monotherapy. Combining checkpoint inhibitors with other therapeutics like chemotherapy or anti-angiogenesis therapy has improved objective response rate (ORR) to 47.6%~63.5% (3–6). Therefore, exploring efficacy biomarkers for ICIs-based therapy has been being an essential hotspot in current clinical practice. PD-L1 has been recognized as the current standard biomarker for immunotherapy. However, even in a highly selected population (PD-L1 tumor proportion score≥50%), ORR was only 44.8% for monotherapy, while around 60% for combination therapy in the first-line setting (3, 4, 7). Besides, differences in testing platforms, the various cut-off values for different immunotherapy agents, and the heterogenous nature of PD-L1 expression within tumors have all been points of criticism. Tumor mutational burden (TMB) has been highlighted as another important biomarker irrelative to PD-L1. But it remains great controversial as the OS data from CheckMate 227 revealed a statistically nonsignificant benefit of ipilimumab with nivolumab in patients with high TMB (7). Peripheral blood biomarkers have attracted more and more attentions owing to the relative ease and less invasive nature. Studies suggested that the neutrophil-to-lymphocyte ratio, number of HLA-DR monocytes, activity or number of NK cells, lactate dehydrogenase, and so forth in blood were related to clinical outcome of ICIs-based therapy (8–11). However, the predictive value of these biomarkers needs to be further verified and many other parameters in peripheral blood remain to be clarified to better understand antitumor immune response.

Autoantibodies are produced by activated B cells in response to autologous antigens which are generated by altered protein expression and defect in immune tolerance or inflammation. Autoantibodies have been considered as attractive blood biomarkers for predicting efficacy and toxicity of cancer immunotherapy since they play an important role in the maintenance of host homeostasis. Gowen et al. provided the first evidence that pre-treatment serum antibody profiles were associated with severe immune-related adverse events (irAEs) for anti-CTLA-4 or anti-PD-1 treatment in melanoma (12). de Moel et al. found that autoantibodies developed in 19.2% of patients who were autoantibody-negative pretreatment and autoantibody development following ipilimumab treatment predisposed patients to irAEs under subsequent anti–PD-1 therapy, but patients who developed autoantibodies showed a trend for better survival (Hazard ratio (HR) for all-cause death: 0.66; 95% CI, 0.34–1.26) and therapy response (odds ratio, 2.64; 95% CI, 0.85–8.16) (13). Toi et al. reported that the presence of preexisting antibodies was associated with clinical benefit and development of irAEs in patients with NSCLC treated with nivolumab or pembrolizumab monotherapy (14). Notably, all the above studies have focused on the autoantibodies against to self-antigen like anti-thyroid antibody, antinuclear antibodies, rheumatoid factor, etc. Autoantibody production could also be triggered by tumor associated antigens (TAAs) in cancer patients, which are referred as tumor associated autoantibodies (TAAbs) in the present study. The production of TAAbs is believed to reflect greater immunologic reactivity in cancer patients and enhanced immune surveillance for cancer cells. Two recent studies reported that preexisting TAAbs such as antibody against to NY-ESO-1, XAGE1, and SIX2 correlated with clinical responses to anti-PD-1 monotherapy in NSCLC (15, 16). However, the clinical utility of TAAbs for monitoring efficacy and toxicity to ICIs-based treatment especially combination therapy in lung cancer is less conclusive. In the present study, we aimed to identify a panel of TAAbs to predict the clinical outcome of ICIs-based treatment in advanced NSCLC patients and correlation between TAAbs and irAE occurrence would also be investigated.

MATERIALS AND METHODS

Patients

Patients who have advanced NSCLC with metastatic/recurrent or unresectable stages were enrolled into this study from three medical centers (Shanghai Pulmonary Hospital, Xinqiao Hospital, and Tongji Hospital of Tongji Medical College) between May 2018 and November 2019. Inclusion criteria are as follows: 1) confirmed NSCLC by pathology; 2) staged IIIB/IV according to the eighth edition of the TNM classification for lung cancer; 3) ECOG performance status 0–2. 3) measurable lesions according to Response Evaluation Criteria in Solid Tumors version 1.1 (RECIST v1.1); and 4) received PD-1 inhibitor-based treatment. Exclusion criteria included: 1) autoimmune diseases; 2) received other immunotherapy including but not limiting vaccines and adoptive cellular immunotherapy; 3) active multiple primary malignancies; and 4) receiving intensive immunosuppressive agents.

Specimen Characteristics

We collected 10 ml peripheral blood of each patient before initiation of ICIs-based treatment within a week, and then centrifuged it to obtain plasma. Plasma was stored at −80 centigrade degree before detection.

Assay Methods

We used enzyme-linked immunosorbent assay (ELISA) to determine the reactivity of TAAbs. Briefly, TAAs were expressed in *E. coli* and purified *via* multiple steps including affinity chromatography and size exclusion chromatography. The immuno maxisorp 96-well plate (Thermo scientific, #456537) was pre-immobilized with 50 ul of 10 ug/ml of bovine serum albumin (BSA)-biotin (Thermo scientific, #29130). Each TAA protein used in this study contain both streptavidin and Myc tag for purification and quantification purpose. Then, 50 ul of each antigen at a concentration of 150nM was added into microwells and incubated for 1.5 h before assaying for autoantibody level in serum or plasma.

A negative control antigen that contained both streptavidin and Myc tag was immobilized in a separate microwell as the background signal. Plasma samples were diluted with phosphate-buffered saline [1:109] and added to the microwells (50 ml/well) for binding of the TAAbs to their respective TAAs. After washing off the extra proteins with washing buffer, horseradish peroxidase -conjugated anti-human IgG was added to each well to bind TAAbs. ELISA substrate 3,3',5,5'-tetramethylbenzidine was added for color development followed by the addition of stopping solution (1N HCl), and the absorbance was read at optical density (OD) 450 nm on a spectrometer. All incubations were carried out with shaking at room temperature and plates were washed three times with PBS containing Tween 20 (0.1% v/v; Sigma, Poole, UK) between each step. The autoantibody levels by OD measurements were compared to the cutoff OD value determined using healthy control subjects. The cutoff OD value for positive result was calculated as the average plus two times of standard deviation of OD values in healthy control subjects (data did not show). The reliability of this method was confirmed in our previous study (17). A minimal of 95% of specificity in control subjects was observed for five antigens in this study.

Study Design

This study was retrospectively designed and performed to identify a panel of TAAbs to predict clinical responses and patient survival with ICIs-based treatment, according to the Reporting Recommendations for Tumor Marker Prognostic Studies' criteria as listed in the guideline.

ICIs-based treatment with monotherapy or combination therapy was administered according to the decision of physicians. When ORR was 30% overall and at least 60% in the TAAbs-positive patients (10, 11), and when the TAAbs-positive proportion was 50% which was indicated in the discovery cohort, the required sample size was 24 in the independent validation set. It was calculated in *a priori* power analysis for Fisher's exact test with the power level of 0.8 and the significance level of 0.05 by G*Power calculator. Recapitulatory, the whole study was divided into two independent parts, a discovery cohort including 37 patients who received ICIs-based treatment at first-line and a validation cohort including 129 patients treated with ICIs-based treatment at any-line.

The primary endpoint in this study was ORR and progression-free survival (PFS) to ICIs-based treatment, and the secondary endpoint was the incidence of irAEs. To reduce bias of retrospective data, only checkpoint inhibitor pneumonitis (CIP) was selected to be further investigated since it's occurrence could be traced through computerized tomography images. Efficacy was evaluated according to RECIST v1.1. ORR was complete response plus partial response (PR). Disease control rate (DCR) was complete response plus partial response plus stable disease (SD). PFS was defined as the interval from the initiation of ICIs-based treatment to confirmed disease progression or death of any cause. If disease progression did not occur before the analysis' deadline or last follow up date, the data would be censored. CIP was diagnosed by experienced oncologists and confirmed by three experienced radiologists independently. The date of CIP diagnosis and highest ICI-pneumonitis grade [according to the fourth Common Toxicity Criteria for Adverse Events (CTCAE) classification] were recorded. If CIP did not occur, the end-time would be censored at last follow up date.

The institutional review board of Shanghai pulmonary hospital approved the study and informed consent of patients were obtained.

Statistical Analysis

Statistical analyses were performed using SPSS version 22.0. Intergroup comparisons were performed using the Mann–Whitney U test for continuous variables, and Pearson's $\chi2$ or Fisher's exact tests for categorical variables. PFS and OS were estimated by Kaplan–Meier method and compared by log-rank test in univariate analyses. Factors with *P*-value < 0.1 in univariate analysis were included to multivariate analysis by the Cox proportional hazards model, which was also used to calculate the HR and corresponding 95% CI. Two-sided *P*-value < 0.05 was considered significant.

RESULTS

Characteristics of Study Population

A total of 166 patients with advanced NSCLC who received ICIs-based treatment were enrolled into this study, including a discovery cohort (n = 37) and a validation cohort (n = 129). Baseline characteristics were summarized in **Table 1**. The TAAbs positivity rate in two groups were 51.4% and 48.8%, respectively. In the discovery cohort, patients with squamous lung cancer were inclined to be positive for TAAbs (90% vs. 37%, *P* = 0.008), which was consistant to previously reported data (10, 13). In the validation cohort, patients with only intrathoracic metastases had a lower positivity rate comparing to those with extrathoracic metastases (35.6% vs. 66.1%, *P* = 0.001). Thirty-four patients with EGFR mutation were also included, 2 (4.5%) into the discovery cohort and 32 (25.0%) into the validation cohort. Positivity rates for TAAbs were similar among patients with EGFR mutation, other gene alteration or wild type (37.5% vs. 61.1% vs. 50.6%, *P* = 0.254). In addition, Patients receiving first-line ICIs-based treatment had a higher TAAbs positivity rate than those receiving subsequent-line treatment (68.2% vs. 38.8%, *P* = 0.002). Other clinical factors, such as median age, gender, smoking history, stage, PD-L1 expression level, and treatment regimen were not observed to be significantly correlated with TAAbs positivity.

Determination of the Reactivity of the 5-Tumor-Associated Autoantibodies in the Discovery Cohort

We first evaluated TAAbs in a set of serum samples from advanced NSCLC patients together with healthy control subjects (data not shown). The 43 TAA proteins, which showed high enough sensitivity (>5%) and specificity (93.6%), were then selected to test in the discovery cohort (**Supplement Table**). These TAAs were categorized based on the correlation of their "positive" score of corresponding autoantibody measurement and clinical response of patients who received ICIs-based treatment. Three categories were classified: 1. "positive correlation": more than twice patients with PR

TABLE 1 | Baseline characteristics of patients.

Characteristics	Discovery cohort (n = 37)				Validation cohort (n = 129)			
	all	positive	negative	*P*-value	all	positive	negative	*P*-value
Age,yr								
Median, range	63(26-79)	64(49-79)	61(26-73)	0.408	62(30-82)	62.5(36-82)	62(30-76)	0.938
Gender								
male	32(86.5)	16(84.2)	16(88.9)	1.000	93(72.1)	48(76.2)	45(68.2)	0.333
female	5(13.5)	3(15.8)	2(11.1)		36(27.9)	15(23.8)	21(31.8)	
Smoking#1								
no/light	27(73.0)	14(73.7)	13(72.2)	1.000	84(65.1)	37(58.7)	47(71.2)	0.145
heavy	10(27.0)	5(26.3)	5(27.8)		45(34.9)	26(41.3)	19(28.8)	
ECOG								
0-1	36(97.3)	19(100.0)	17(94.4)	0.486	123(95.3)	59(93.7)	64(97.0)	0.433
2	1(2.7)	0	1(5.6)		6(4.7)	4(6.3)	2(3.0)	
Histology								
non-squa	27(73.0)	10(52.6)	17(94.4)	0.008	96(74.4)	44(69.8)	52(78.8)	0.244
squa	10(27.0)	9(47.4)	1(5.6)		33(25.6)	19(30.2)	14(21.2)	
Stage								
IIIB-IIIC	8(21.6)	6(31.6)	2(11.1)	0.232	14(10.9)	7(11.1)	7(10.6)	0.927
IV	29(78.4)	13(68.4)	16(88.9)		115(89.1)	56(88.9)	59(89.4)	
Metastatic site#2								
intrathoracic	21(56.8)	9(47.4)	12(66.7)	0.236	73(56.6)	26(41.3)	47(71.2)	0.001
bone	10(27.0)	6(31.6)	4(22.2)	0.714	29(22.5)	16(25.4)	13(19.7)	0.438
brain	3(8.1)	1(5.3)	2(11.1)	0.604	27(20.9)	15(23.8)	12(18.2)	0.432
liver	1(2.7)	1(5.3)	0	1.000	12(9.3)	5(7.9)	7(10.6)	0.602
others	5(13.5)	2(10.5)	3(16.7)	0.660	37(28.7)	20(31.7)	17(25.8)	0.452
PD-L1								
≥50%	6(30.0)	2(22.3)	4(36.3)	0.850	15(26.8)	9(28.1)	6(25.0)	1.000
1-49%	5(25.0)	3(33.3)	2(18.2)		15(26.8)	8(25.0)	7(29.2)	
negative	9(45.0)	4(44.4)	5(45.5)		26(46.4)	15(46.9)	11(45.8)	
unknown	17	10	7		73	31	42	
Gene type								
EGFR mutation	2(5.4)	1(5.3)	1(5.6)	0.230	32(24.8)	12(19.0)	20(30.3)	0.254
other alteration	3(8.1)	3(15.8)	0		18(14.0)	11(17.5)	7(10.6)	
Wild type	32(86.5)	15(78.9)	17(94.4)		79(61.2)	40(63.5)	39(59.1)	
ICIs Line								
1	37(100.0)	19(100.0)	18(100.0)	/	44(34.1)	30(47.6)	14(21.2)	0.002
≥2	0	0	0		85(65.9)	33(52.4)	52(78.8)	
Treatment								
mono	6(16.2)	2(10.5)	4(22.2)	0.405	30(23.3)	15(23.8)	15(22.7)	1.000
combination	31(83.8)	17(89.5)	14(77.8)		99(76.7)	48(76.2)	51(77.3)	
ICI agent								
Nivolumab	4(10.8)	3(15.8)	1(5.6)	0.649	13(10.1)	6(9.5)	7(10.6)	0.798
Pembrolizumab	19(51.4)	10(52.6)	9(50.0)		33(25.6)	18(28.6)	15(22.7)	
Others#3	14(37.8)	6(31.6)	8(44.4)		83(64.3)	39(61.9)	44(66.7)	

The number (outside the parentheses) and percentage (in the parentheses) of patients in each subgroup were listed in this table. ***#1:*** *unit: package*year.* ***#2:*** *What were listed here were the number and percentage of patients with corresponding distant metastatic site. "Intrathoracic" means metastases tumor were confined in thoracic including contralateral pulmonary or pleura metastasis; "bone/brain/liver/others" means whether patient had metastases in these respective organs.* ***#3:*** *other ICI agents mainly referred to Chinese domestic PD-1 inhibitors, including camrelizumab, toripalimab, sintilimab, and tislelizumab. yr, year; squa, squamous; mono, monotherapy.*

than PD were positive for these autoantibodies (**Figure 1A**). 2. "negative correlation": more than twice patients with PD than PR were positive for these autoantibodies. 3. "no correlation": these did not meet the above two conditions. Antigens in "positive correlation" category included Claudin2, BRCA2, HUD, P53, Annexin1, MAGE-A4, Trim21, TTC14, IMP2, GAGE7, NY-ESO-2, NY-ESO-1; Antigens in "negative correlation" category included ETHE1, AKAP4, PRAME, HSP105, MAGE-A3, KRT8, KRAS, RALA, FEZF1, TTC14, PRAME. Finally, we evaluated the correlation of these 12 antigens from "positive correlation" category with survival in discovery cohort and five TAAbs (p53, BRCA2, HUD, TRIM21, and NY-ESO-1) that performed best were selected.

Consistent with published data, the sensitivity of a single autoantibody was low, ranging from 5% to 20%. Therefore, a panel of 5-TAAbs was selected, and the detection result was considered being positive if at least one autoantibody was positive. In contrast, the result was regarded as negative if none of the 5 TAAbs were positive.

As shown in **Figure 1B**, positive results among the antibodies panel in the discovery cohort predicted 47.4% of patients as "PR", while only 15.8% of patients as "PD". The sensitivity and specificity of 5-TAAbs for response were 0.643 and 0.565, respectively. The positivity of this 5-TAAbs panel was also associated with better PFS (not reached vs. 5.32 m, P = 0.05, HR = 0.383, 95% CI: 0.140–1.046) (**Figure 1C**).

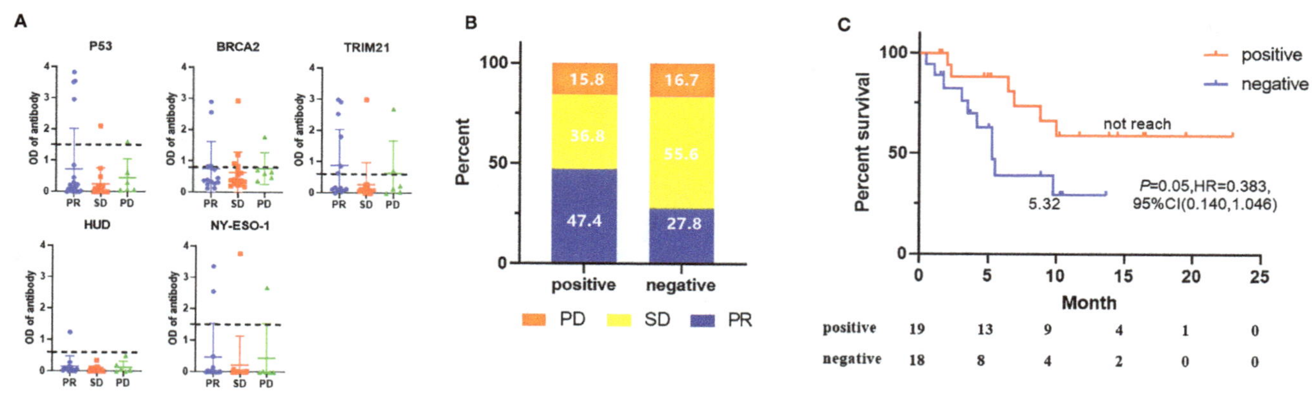

FIGURE 1 | In the discovery cohort, screening results of five "positive correlation" biomarkers **(A)**, A negative value was generated when no corresponding autoantibody signal existed in serum, while the complex matrix effect of serum gave more OD signals in background control well than the well immobilized with a TAAs protein. ORR **(B)** and PFS **(C)** comparison of patients with 5-AABs positive or negative. ORR were compared by fisher's exact tests and PFS were compared by log-rank test. Two-sided P-value < 0.05 was considered significant.

Predictive Value of the 5-Tumor-Associated Autoantibody Panel in the Validation Cohort

To confirm the predictive value of the 5-TAAbs panel in heterogeneous patients at clinical setting, we have evaluated how this panel worked in an independent validation cohort which included 129 patients who received ICIs-based treatment at any-line from three hospitals and patients with EGFR mutation were also permitted. In the validation cohort, the positivity of this 5-TAAbs panel was significantly associated with better response (ORR: 44.4% vs. 13.6%, P = 0.001; DCR 84.1% vs. 59.1%, P = 0.002) and longer PFS (7.6 vs. 3.3 m, P < 0.001, HR = 0.394,95% CI: 0.245-0.634) (**Figures 2A, B**). In the subgroup of patients treated with ICIs monotherapy, better response and longer PFS were also observed in TAAbs-positive patients (ORR: 46.7% vs. 13.3%, P = 0.003, PFS: 19.7 vs. 2.2 m, P < 0.001, HR = 0.198, 95% CI: 0.076–0.511) (**Figures 3A, B**). Furthermore, the 5-TAAbs panel remained to be a good predictive biomarker for patients treated with combination therapy (ORR: 43.8% vs. 13.7%, P = 0.004, PFS: 6.7 vs. 3.7m, P = 0.017, HR = 0.509, 95% CI: 0.303-0.857) (**Figures 3C, D**). Regarding to treatment-line, subgroup analysis indicated that this 5-TAAs panel worked better in patients who received subsequent-line ICIs-based treatment (ORR: 42.4% vs. 7.7%, P = 0.001, PFS: 6.2 vs. 3.0 m, P = 0.004, HR = 0.481, 95%CI: 0.295-0.785) (**Figures 3G, H**). Similar responses to first-line treatment (ORR: 46.7% vs. 35.7%, P = 0.345, PFS: NR vs. 10.48m, P = 0.146) between patients with positive or negative 5-TAAs might be mainly contributed by high proportion of combination therapy and small sample size (**Figures 3E, F**). In addition, for patients with EGFR mutation (n = 34), patients with 5-TAAbs positive has relatively longer median PFS and better responses than negative patients (6.2 vs. 3.7m, P = 0.196, HR = 0.527, 95% CI: 0.196–1.419, ORR: 20.0% vs. 9.1%, P = 0.572; DCR: 70.0% vs. 68.2%, P = 1.000) (**Supplement Figure**), though the differences did not reach the statistical significance. Univariate and multivariate analysis suggested that the 5-TAAbs positivity was an independent factor for PFS (**Table 2**).

Association Between 5-Tumor Associated Autoantibody Panel and CIP

For all patients included into the current study and followed up for more than 3 months (n = 122), CIP occurrence rate was 12.3%. The median onset time was 2.3 months (range 1.3–4.2 months). Comparing to negative patients, the CIP incidence in patients with 5-TAAbs positive was significantly higher (20.4% vs. 5.9%, P = 0.015) (**Figure 2C**). However, for all patients with CIP, the grades were similar between patients with positive and negative 5-TAAbs (**Figure 2D**). Significant higher risk of CIP occurrence was also observed in patients with positive 5-TAAbs (HR = 3.504, P = 0.032) (**Figure 2E**).

DISCUSSION

Predictive biomarkers of immunotherapy remain to be explored. Here, we identified a 5-TAAbs panel in a discovery cohort and subsequently confirmed its predictive value in a validation cohort. Like the recent study from Ohue and colleagues (15) that reported a strong correlation between serum antibodies (NY-ESO-1 and XAGE1) and clinical response to anti–PD-1 monotherapy for NSCLC, we have demonstrated the predictive value of 5-TAAbs panel for responses to both ICIs monotherapy and ICIs-based combination therapy for NSCLC in our study. While only 20%–25% of subjects in their study showed positive autoantibody results, our 5-TAAbs panel showed that about 50% of subjects were positive indicating a larger beneficial population would be covered. Besides, consistent with their results, we also did not observe a significant correlation between PD-L1 expression and TAAbs positivity. This

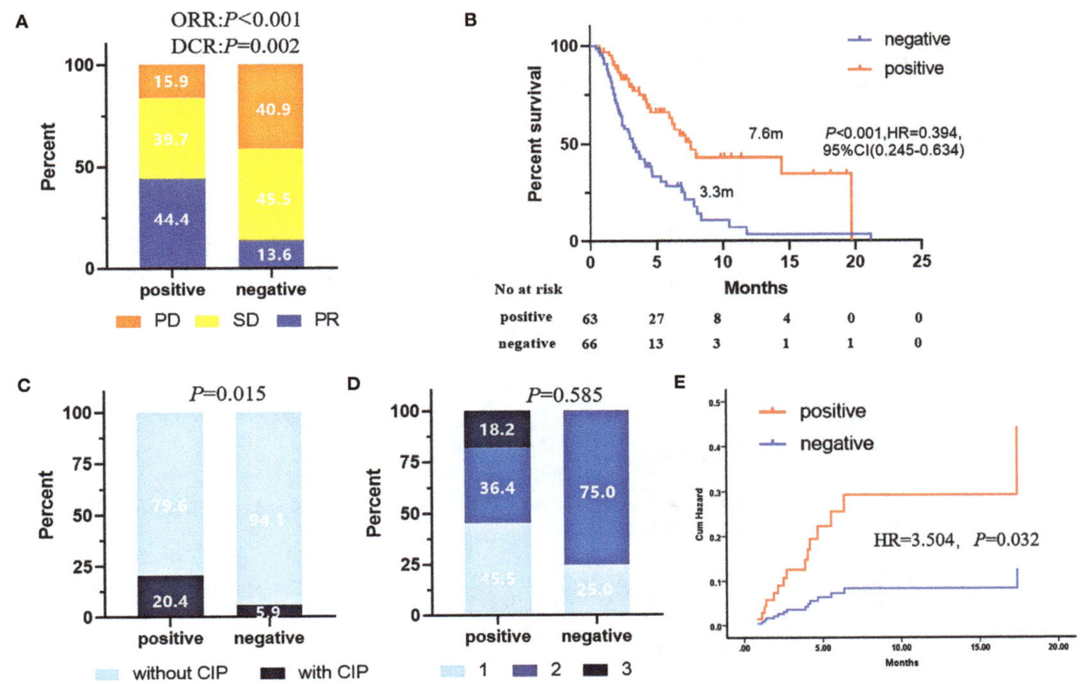

FIGURE 2 | In the validation cohort, ORR **(A)**, PFS **(B)**, CIP incidence **(C)**, CIP grades **(D)**, and risks **(E)** comparison of patients with 5-AABs positive or negative. Pearson's $\chi 2$ test was used to compare ORR, Fisher's exact tests was used to compare CIP and CIP grades. and PFS were compared by log-rank test. CIP risks were compared by Hazard function of Cox regression. Two-sided P-value < 0.05 was considered significant.

may reflect two sets of predictive biomarkers with independent mechanistic pathways. One drawback of this study was that PD-L1 expression were detected by antibodies from different commercial companies, and other biomarkers such as TMB and tumor infiltration lymphocytes were not available for this study.

An explanation for the predictive role of autoantibody is that positivity of these TAAbs represented the high immunogenicity of corresponding TAAs, leading to antigen-specifical CD8+ T cells activation and checkpoint molecule-mediated strong immunosuppression, exactly as Ohue et al. isolated NY-ESO-1–

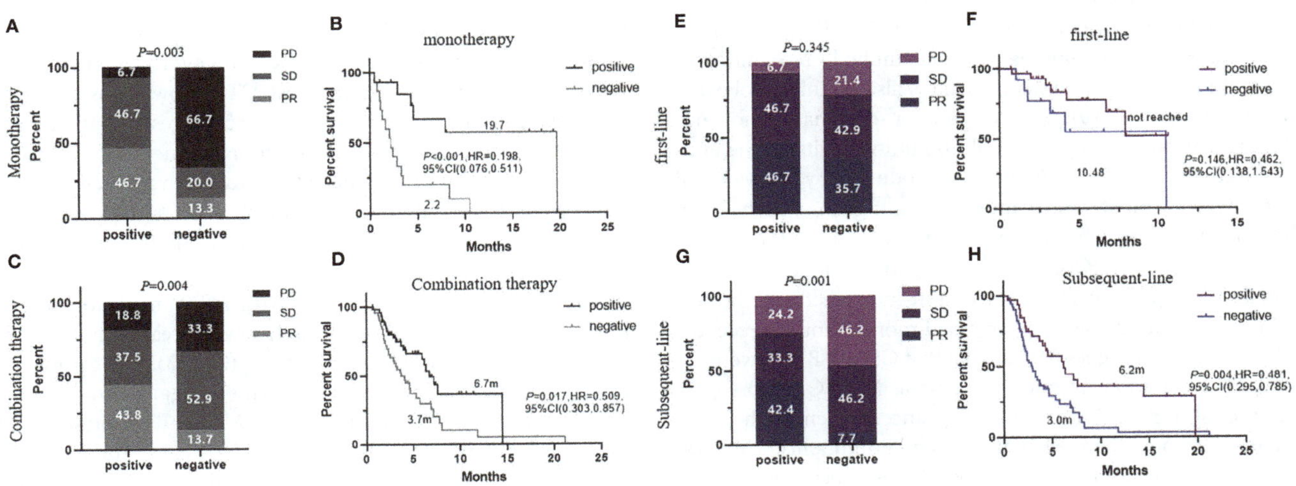

FIGURE 3 | ORR and PFS comparison of patients with 5-AABs positive or negative in subgroup of patients who received ICI monotherapy **(A, B)** and ICI-based combination therapy **(C, D)**, or patients who received immunotherapy at first-line **(E, F)** and subsequent-line **(G, H)**. ORR were compared by fisher's exact tests and PFS were compared by log-rank test. Two-sided P-value < 0.05 was considered significant.

TABLE 2 | Univariate and multivariate analyses of clinical parameters of PFS in validation cohort.

Factors	Univariate analysis			Multivariate analysis		
	HR	95%CI	*P*	HR	95%CI	*P*
Age,yr						
≤63/>63	1.296	0.815-2.059	0.273			
Gender						
male/female	0.932	0.571-1.523	0.780			
Smoking						
heavy/no,light	0.944	0.561-1.589	0.828			
ECOG						
0-1/2-3	0.402	0.145-1.114	0.080	0.208	0.070-0.622	0.005
Histology						
non-squa/suq	0.958	0.562-1.632	0.875			
Stage						
IIIB-IIIC/IV	0.768	0.367-1.609	0.484			
Metastasis						
intrathoracic yes/no	1.017	0.636-1.627	0.943			
bone yes/no	1.552	0.880-2.738	0.129			
brain yes/no	1.238	0.709-2.162	0.454			
liver yes/no	1.791	0.942-3.403	0.075	1.843	0.953-3.564	0.069
others yes/no	0.930	0.561-1.541	0.777			
PD-L1						
1-49%/negative	0.593	0.245-1.436	0.247			
≥50%/negative	0.547	0.212-1.408	0.211			
Genetype						
EGFRm/WT	1.327	0.802-2.195	0.271			
ICIs Lines						
1/≥2	0.414	0.227-0.755	0.004	0.461	0.241-0.882	0.019
Treatment						
combination/mono	1.015	0.600-1.716	0.956			
Autoantibodies						
positive/negative	0.394	0.245-0.634	<0.001	0.413	0.253-0.675	<0.001

specifical CD8+ T cell from peripheral blood of patient with NY-ESO-1 positive and speculated that antibody titers reflected cytotoxic activity levels of antigen-specific CD8+ T cell (15). Nonetheless, not all tumor antigens could elicit CD8+ T-cell responses. A previous study reported that mutant p53 peptides elicited CD4+ T cell and humoral, but not CD8+ T-cell responses (18). Tripartite motif-containing protein 21 (TRIM21) is an intracellular Fc receptor linking cytosolic antibody recognition to the ubiquitin proteasome system, which is also mainly involved in humoral immunity (19). Hence, another explanation for our finding is that pre-existing humoral immunity facilitated the anti-tumor activity of ICIs. TAAbs are produced by activated B lymphocytes stimulated by tumor autoantigens, which is an indication of active humoral immune response. Although for patients treated with ICIs, T cell-mediated immune reactive is considered as a prerequisite factor of anti-tumor activity, the role of humoral immunity has also been paid more attentions recently. Stankovic B and colleagues have shown that CD19+ B cells were the second most common immune cell type in NSCLC tumors (20). Suyama et al. reported a case of lung cancer patient with PR to nivolumab for more than seven months and immunohistochemical analysis of the metastatic lymph node biopsy specimen showed prominent accumulation of plasma cells and immunoglobulin G (21). These findings, together with our results suggested that pre-existing humoral immunity may be worth considering as a candidate therapeutic biomarker of ICIs in lung cancer patients.

Furthermore, unlike other studies focused on autoantibodies against to self-antigen, the current study was the first to report that autoantibodies against to TAAs was associated with CIP occurrence, which suggested that the preexisting active humoral response would also lead to excessive immune-attack and damage to self-tissue (12–14). However, as this was a retrospective study, periodic chest CT follow-up was difficult for every patient and thus certain percentages of patients with pneumonitis, especially with asymptomatic pneumonitis, may be neglected. Hence, our data need to be further validated in a large and perspective study. In addition, this 5-TAAbs panel had a trend in predicting clinical response of ICIs-based therapy among patients with EGFR mutations (25.0%) included in this study. As we all known, patients with EGFR mutations derives limited clinical benefits from ICIs-based treatment and even brought detrimental adverse reaction (22, 23). Up to now, the resistance mechanism is not clarified clearly and existing research attributed it to the low TMB and immune desert tumor microenvironment (24, 25). However, there are still some data suggest that some of these patients do respond to ICIs (26, 27). Although our results did not show statistical significance, which may attribute to the small sample size of this subgroup and possible different role for each antibody in such patients, we think that as a potential stratification biomarker, TAAbs, not limited to these 5 TAAbs in the present study, is worthy of further large-scale studies in EGFR mutant lung cancer patients.

In conclusion, we have identified a panel of 5-TAAbs and proved that this panel could predict clinical benefits of ICIs-based treatment in three centers from different regions of China. A diagnostic kit using this 5-TAAbs panel as a biomarker has been under development. The limitations of the present study were the small number of patients included, the short follow-up time after ICIs-based treatment and the lack of correlation analysis with other well-known biomarkers. Large clinical studies and further mechanistic research are needed to confirm the usefulness and rationality of the 5-TAAbs panel as a predictive biomarker for responses and toxicity to ICIs-base treatment.

AUTHOR CONTRIBUTIONS

CS conceptualized the study and acquired the funding. JuZ, JiZ, QJ, and QC conducted the data curation and performed the formal analysis. JiZ, QJ, FZ, WZ, and XC acquired the clinical data and clinical samples. JuZ, JiZ, SR, CZ, and CS wrote, reviewed, and/or revised the manuscript. All authors contributed to the article and approved the submitted version.

ACKNOWLEDGMENTS

We would like to give the special thanks to Hangzhou Kaipaul Biotechnology Company for the great supporting and contribution to this study.

REFERENCES

1. Arbour KC, Riely GJ. Systemic Therapy for Locally Advanced and Metastatic Non-Small Cell Lung Cancer: A Review. *JAMA* (2019) 322(8):764–74. doi: 10.1001/jama.2019.11058
2. Garon EB, Hellmann MD, Rizvi NA, Carcereny E, Leighl NB, Ahn MJ, et al. Five-Year Overall Survival for Patients With Advanced Non-Small-Cell Lung Cancer Treated With Pembrolizumab: Results From the Phase I KEYNOTE-001 Study. *J Clin Oncol* (2019) 37(28):2518–27. doi: 10.1200/JCO.19.00934
3. Gandhi L, Rodríguez-Abreu D, Gadgeel S, Esteban E, Felip E, De Angelis F, et al. Pembrolizumab plus Chemotherapy in Metastatic Non-Small-Cell Lung Cancer. *N Engl J Med* (2018) 378(22):2078–92. doi: 10.1056/NEJMoa1801005
4. Paz-Ares L, Luft A, Vicente D, Tafreshi A, Gümüş M, Mazières J, et al. Pembrolizumab plus Chemotherapy for Squamous Non-Small-Cell Lung Cancer. *N Engl J Med* (2018) 379(21):2040–51. doi: 10.1056/NEJMoa1810865
5. West H, McCleod M, Hussein M, Morabito A, Rittmeyer A, Conter HJ, et al. Atezolizumab in combination with carboplatin plus nab-paclitaxel chemotherapy compared with chemotherapy alone as first-line treatment for metastatic non-squamous non-small-cell lung cancer (IMpower130): a multicentre, randomised, open-label, phase 3 trial. *Lancet Oncol* (2019) 20 (7):924–37. doi: 10.1016/S1470-2045(19)30167-6
6. Socinski MA, Jotte RM, Cappuzzo F, Orlandi F, Stroyakovskiy D, Nogami N, et al. Atezolizumab for First-Line Treatment of Metastatic Nonsquamous NSCLC. *N Engl J Med* (2018) 378(24):2288–301. doi: 10.1056/NEJMoa1716948
7. Hellmann MD, Paz-Ares L, Bernabe Caro R, Zurawski B, Kim SW, Carcereny Costa E, et al. Nivolumab plus Ipilimumab in Advanced Non-Small-Cell Lung Cancer. *N Engl J Med* (2019) 381(21):2020–31. doi: 10.1056/NEJMoa1910231
8. Li Y, Zhang Z, Hu Y, Yan X, Song Q, Wang G, et al. Pretreatment Neutrophil-to-Lymphocyte Ratio (NLR) May Predict the Outcomes of Advanced Non-small-cell Lung Cancer (NSCLC) Patients Treated With Immune Checkpoint Inhibitors (ICIs). *Front Oncol* (2020) 10:654. doi: 10.3389/fonc.2020.00654
9. Möller M, Turzer S, Schütte W, Seliger B, Riemann D. Blood Immune Cell Biomarkers in Patient With Lung Cancer Undergoing Treatment With Checkpoint Blockade. *J Immunother* (2020) 43(2):57–66. doi: 10.1097/CJI.0000000000000297
10. Cho YH, Choi MG, Kim DH, Choi YJ, Kim SY, Sung KJ, et al. Natural Killer Cells as a Potential Biomarker for Predicting Immunotherapy Efficacy in Patients with Non-Small Cell Lung Cancer. *Target Oncol* (2020) 15(2):241–7. doi: 10.1007/s11523-020-00712-2
11. Zhang Z, Li Y, Yan X, Song Q, Wang G, Hu Y, et al. Pretreatment lactate dehydrogenase may predict outcome of advanced non small-cell lung cancer patients treated with immune checkpoint inhibitors: A meta-analysis. *Cancer Med* (2019) 8(4):1467–73. doi: 10.1002/cam4.2024
12. Gowen MF, Giles KM, Simpson D, Tchack J, Zhou H, Moran U, et al. Baseline antibody profiles predict toxicity in melanoma patients treated with immune checkpoint inhibitors. *J Transl Med* (2018) 16(1):82. doi: 10.1186/s12967-018-1452-4
13. de Moel EC, Rozeman EA, Kapiteijn EH, Verdegaal EME, Grummels A, Bakker JA, et al. Autoantibody Development under Treatment with Immune-Checkpoint Inhibitors. *Cancer Immunol Res* (2019) 7(1):6–11. doi: 10.1158/2326-6066.CIR-18-0245
14. Toi Y, Sugawara S, Sugisaka J, Ono H, Kawashima Y, Aiba T, et al. Profiling Preexisting Antibodies in Patients Treated With Anti-PD-1 Therapy for Advanced Non-Small Cell Lung Cancer. *JAMA Oncol* (2019) 5(3):376–83. doi: 10.1001/jamaoncol.2018.5860
15. Ohue Y, Kurose K, Karasaki T, Isobe M, Yamaoka T, Futami J, et al. Serum Antibody Against NY-ESO-1 and XAGE1 Antigens Potentially Predicts Clinical Responses to Anti-Programmed Cell Death-1 Therapy in NSCLC. *J Thorac Oncol* (2019) 14(12):2071–83. doi: 10.1016/j.jtho.2019.08.008
16. Tan Q, Wang D, Yang J, Xing P, Yang S, Li Y, et al. Autoantibody profiling identifies predictive biomarkers of response to anti-PD1 therapy in cancer patients. *Theranostics* (2020) 10(14):6399–410. doi: 10.7150/thno.45816
17. Ren S, Zhang S, Jiang T, He Y, Ma Z, Cai H, et al. Early detection of lung cancer by using an autoantibody panel in Chinese population. *Oncoimmunology* (2017) 7(2): e1384108. doi: 10.1080/2162402X.2017.1384108
18. Tsuji T, Gnjatic S. Split T-cell tolerance as a guide for the development of tumor antigen-specific immunotherapy. *Oncoimmunology* (2012) 1(3):405–7. doi: 10.4161/onci.19310
19. Rhodes DA, Isenberg DA. TRIM21 and the Function of Antibodies inside Cells. *Trends Immunol* (2017) 38(12):916–26. doi: 10.1016/j.it.2017.07.005
20. Stankovic B, Bjørhovde HAK, Skarshaug R, Aamodt H, Frafjord A, Müller E, et al. Immune Cell Composition in Human Non-small Cell Lung Cancer. *Front Immunol* (2019) 9:3101. doi: 10.3389/fimmu.2018.03101
21. Suyama T, Fukuda Y, Soda H, Ogawara D, Iwasaki K, Hara T, et al. Successful treatment with nivolumab for lung cancer with low expression of PD-L1 and prominent tumor-infiltrating B cells and immunoglobulin G. *Thorac Cancer* (2018) 9(6):750–3. doi: 10.1111/1759-7714.12644
22. Oxnard GR, Yang JC, Yu H, Kim SW, Saka H, Horn L, et al. TATTON: a multi-arm, phase Ib trial of osimertinib combined with selumetinib, savolitinib, or durvalumab in EGFR-mutant lung cancer. *Ann Oncol* (2020) 31(4):507–16. doi: 10.1016/j.annonc.2020.01.013
23. Lee CK, Man J, Lord S, Links M, Gebski V, Mok T, et al. Checkpoint Inhibitors in Metastatic EGFR-Mutated Non-Small Cell Lung Cancer-A Meta-Analysis. *J Thorac Oncol* (2017) 12(2):403–7. doi: 10.1016/j.jtho.2016.10.007
24. Santaniello A, Napolitano F, Servetto A, De Placido P, Silvestris N, Bianco C, et al. Tumour Microenvironment and Immune Evasion in EGFR Addicted NSCLC: Hurdles and Possibilities. *Cancers (Basel)* (2019) 11(10):1419. doi: 10.3390/cancers11101419
25. Soo RA, Lim SM, Syn NL, Teng R, Soong R, Mok TSK, et al. Immune checkpoint inhibitors in epidermal growth factor receptor mutant non-small cell lung cancer: Current controversies and future directions. *Lung Cancer* (2018) 115:12–20. doi: 10.1016/j.lungcan.2017.11.009
26. Gettinger S, Hellmann MD, Chow LQM, Borghaei H, Antonia S, Brahmer JR, et al. Nivolumab Plus Erlotinib in Patients With EGFR-Mutant Advanced NSCLC. *J Thorac Oncol* (2018) 13(9):1363–72. doi: 10.1016/j.jtho.2018.05.015

7

Molecular Characteristics of Genes and the Immune Microenvironment of a Rare Chest Malignant Tumor (Pulmonary Clear Cell Sarcoma)

Xiaoling Xu[1,2]*, Ding Wang*[3]*, Wei Wu*[4] *and Hongyang Lu*[1,2,5*]

[1] *Department of Thoracic Oncology, Cancer Hospital of the University of Chinese Academy of Sciences (Zhejiang Cancer Hospital), Hangzhou, China,* [2] *Institute of Cancer and Basic Medicine (IBMC), Chinese Academy of Sciences, Hangzhou, China,* [3] *Department of Thoracic Surgery, Cancer Hospital of the University of Chinese Academy of Sciences (Zhejiang Cancer Hospital), Hangzhou, China,* [4] *Department of Pathology, Cancer Hospital of the University of Chinese Academy of Sciences (Zhejiang Cancer Hospital), Hangzhou, China,* [5] *Zhejiang Key Laboratory of Diagnosis & Treatment Technology on Thoracic Oncology (Lung and Esophagus), Cancer Hospital of the University of Chinese Academy of Sciences (Zhejiang Cancer Hospital), Hangzhou, China*

***Correspondence:**
Hongyang Lu
luhy@zjcc.org.cn

Pulmonary clear cell sarcoma is a rare malignant tumor that has rarely been reported and is challenging to diagnose, especially when differentiating from malignant melanoma. Currently, EWSR1-ATF1 is the key marker for distinguishing clear cell sarcoma from melanoma, but IHC has diagnostic limitations. We report a patient diagnosed with pulmonary clear cell sarcoma, in which an NGS was used to help with the pathological diagnosis. The exposure to the immune microenvironment in pulmonary clear cell sarcoma suggests that TIGIT-related drugs may be a new and effective treatment for this rare disease. Immune microenvironment-related markers, including PD-L1, CD8, TIM3, LAG3, and CD163, were negatively expressed in pulmonary clear cell sarcoma.

Keywords: clear cell sarcoma, next-generation sequencing, lung, EWS-ATF1, PD-L1, TIGIT

INTRODUCTION

Enzinger first described a rare soft tissue tumor of clear cell sarcoma (CCS) in 1965 that arose from the abnormal differentiation of pigment cells (1), previously known as soft tissue malignant melanoma. CCS cases account for approximately 1% of rare tumors originating from stromal cells (2). CCS is most common in young men and women between the ages of 20 and 40 years. CCS usually arises on the distal extremities, especially on the tendons and aponeurosis of the foot and ankle and on the arms, hands, and trunk, as reported by Goh et al. (3). At present, EWSR1-ATF1 is used as a key marker to distinguish melanoma from CCS (4). This disease has a slow course, and the average age of CCS diagnosis is 39 years. According to Gonzaga et al., at diagnosis, CCS is usually advanced and locally aggressive, with a high rate of recurrence and metastasis (up to 50%). The most common site of distant metastases is the lung; the overall 5- and 10-year survival rates are approximately 50 and 38%, respectively, with no significant differences in survival rates between males and females (5). Although surgical treatment may be beneficial for the patient, new molecular targeted therapy should be implemented to improve the oncologic outcome in early- and late-stage disease (2, 6). Hence, we report a patient with pulmonary CCS, in which NGS was used to help with the diagnosis and explore molecular characteristics of genes and the immune microenvironment of pulmonary CCS in this patient.

CASE DESCRIPTION

A 51-year-old Chinese woman visited the hospital because of chest tightness for 10 days. Her chest CT showed a 2.3 cm × 2 cm nodule in her left lung. Multiple plaques were seen on the left pleura. Pleural effusion, compression atelectasis, and swollen hilar lymphadenopathy in the left lung can be seen on contrast-enhanced CT (**Figure 1A**). From November 19, 2018, after admission to the hospital, obvious tumor cells could not be found in the repeated pleural effusion tests (**Figure 2A**). Additionally, bronchoscopy, neck lymph nodes, and brain CT showed no apparent abnormalities. A biopsy of the left pleural mass was performed on November 20, 2018. The histopathologic findings revealed an epithelioid tumor with fibrous vascular nests and strands surrounding it. Some cells were hyaline, and mitotic figures were seen. Positive staining for Ki-67 (approximately 40%), Sy, Melan-A, Hmb45, and S-100 was detected by immunohistochemistry using monoclonal antibodies (**Figure 2B**). The patient had no previous skin lesions and had no history of previous excision of the skin or other lesions. We used bevacizumab 200 mg for left intrathoracic treatment on December 7, 2018, for patients with self-reported chest tightness improved with this treatment. Because this primary pathological type of lung disease is rare, we sent a pleural biopsy sample for the next-generation sequencing of tissue samples to FoundationOne CDX on December 14, 2018; NGS revealed an EWSR1-ATF1 fusion, CDKN2A/b loss, and MTAP loss (**Table 1**). We also confirmed that PD-L1 as a target by immunohistochemistry using an anti-PD-L1 IHC 22C3 pharmDx (Dako) antibody (**Figures 2C, D**). Because the PD-L1 target did not perform as expected, we performed immunofluorescence analysis (**Figure 3**) with the OPAL™ Multiplex IHC (Akoya) Kit. Immune microenvironment-related markers, including CD8, TIM3, PD-L1, LAG3, CD163, and TIGIT, were examined to find a new therapeutic target. Only TIGIT was observed in positive cells ≥1%, and there were <1% positive cells for the other markers. CD8 and TIM3 showed colocalization, but no colocalization was identified between the other markers. TIGIT is one of the most promising and potential targets in the new generation of immunotherapy drugs, and several anti-TIGIT monoclonal antibodies have been studied. The outcome of the PET-CT scan on December 20, 2018, showed

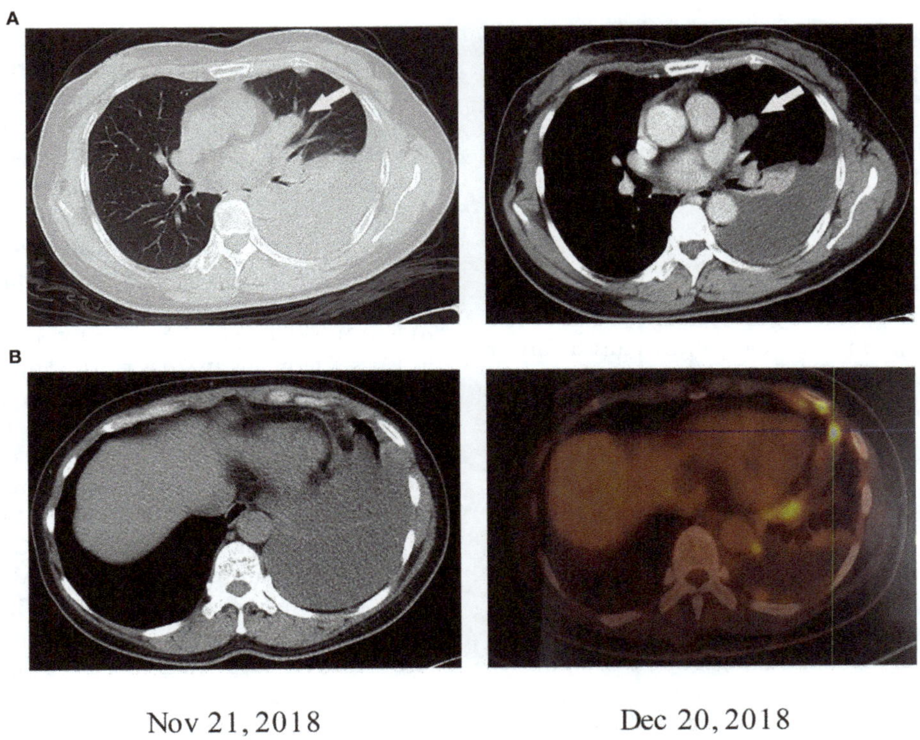

FIGURE 1 | **(A)** The lung windows show 2.3 cm × 2 cm nodules with uniform density next to the heart margin of the left lung segment. Contrast-enhanced CT of mediastinal windows shows that the nodules were uniformly strengthened. **(B)** The PET-CT results of the patient on December 20, 2018, showed a decrease in pleural effusion compared to the PET-CT results on November 21, 2018.

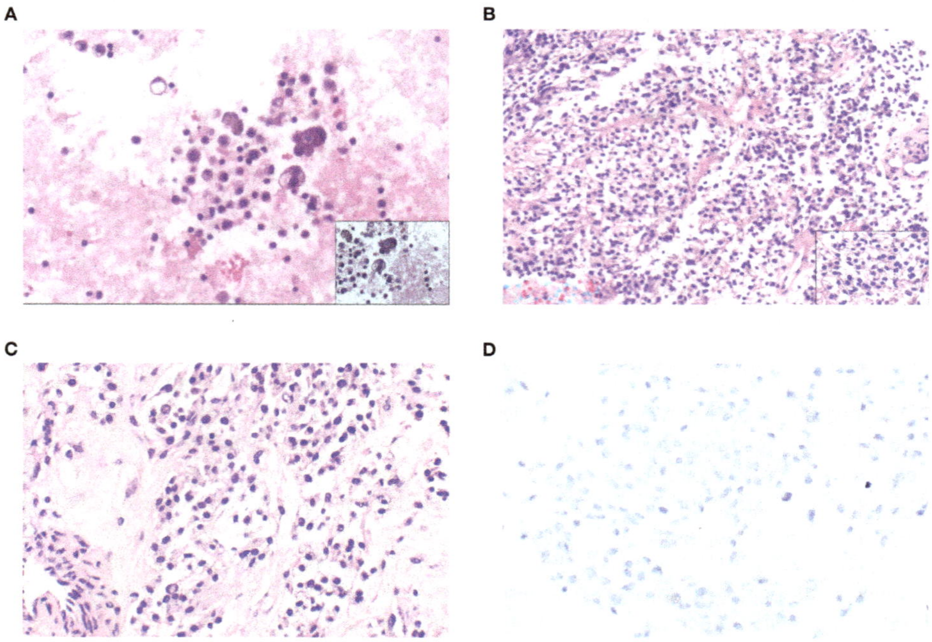

FIGURE 2 | **(A)** Scattered lymphocytes, tissue cells, mesothelial cells, and individual atypical cells (H&E staining: original magnification ×100). **(B)** Epithelioid tumor cells distributed in nests and sheets around fibers and blood vessels; some of the cells have transparent cytoplasm with nuclear division (H&E staining: original magnification ×100). **(C)** PD-L1 control (H&E staining: original magnification ×100). **(D)** PD-L1-negative staining.

TABLE 1 | NGS panel findings.

Genomic findings	Lung tissue results	Biomarker findings	Lung tissue results
EWSR1	EWSR1-ATF1 fusion	Tumor mutational burden	TMB-low (3 mutations/Mb)
CDKN2A/B	Loss	Microsatellite status	MS-stable
MTAP	Loss		

that the patient's pleural effusion improved after bevacizumab treatment (**Figure 1B**). However, the patient refused further treatment after the diagnosis of pulmonary CCS. Follow-up until her death on June 27, 2019.

DISCUSSION

CCS is a rare stromal soft tissue tumor similar to melanoma and soft tissue sarcoma but has a different genetic history. The clinical features of CCS lack specificity, which often manifests as slow painless local growth of the mass, and patients can experience local pain, itching, movement restrictions, easy postoperative recurrence, or metastasis (1, 7, 8). CT and MRI have limited diagnostic value for CCS, and CCS is confirmed by biopsy pathology and IHC staining; its variants often need molecular testing. The classic histological feature of soft tissue CCS is a small cluster of polygonal cells and spindle cells, characterized by hyaline to slightly basophilic cytoplasm and vesicular nuclei with prominent nucleoli separated by fine fibers (1, 9). Both CCS and malignant melanoma originate from melanocyte differentiation, so they are positive for common melanocyte markers such as S-100, HMB-45, MelanA, and NKI/C3 (2). We cannot easily distinguish them by immunohistochemistry. Hence, the use of fluorescence *in situ* hybridization or reverse transcription-polymerase chain reaction (RT-PCR) is essential for diagnosing CCS and distinguishing CCS from primary and metastatic melanoma (2). The cytogenetic feature of CCS is t (12; 22) (q13; q12), resulting in a chimeric EWSR1/ATF1 gene in which the EWS 3' terminus at 22q is replaced by the ATF1 3' terminus at 12q. Therefore, EWSR1/ATF1 can be used as a marker to distinguish CCS from melanoma (4). In this case, NGS was a feasible method to help pathologically diagnose CCS as the diagnosis was difficult to determine after biopsy and immunohistochemistry. The EWSR1-ATF1 fusion also supported the diagnosis of pulmonary CCS.

Yasmin Aghajan reported a case in which a novel EWSR1-ATF1 gene fusion was revealed using next-generation sequencing analysis, but FLI-1 immunohistochemical results were negative, suggesting that NGS has the advantage of showing the CCS EWSR1-ATF1 fusion (10). NGS was finally used to help diagnose this rare disease. Compared with traditional biopsy pathology and immunohistochemistry, NGS has unique advantages; NGS not only improves the diagnostic accuracy but also provides more possibilities for follow-up treatment strategies (11). Whereas the workload of NGS is still

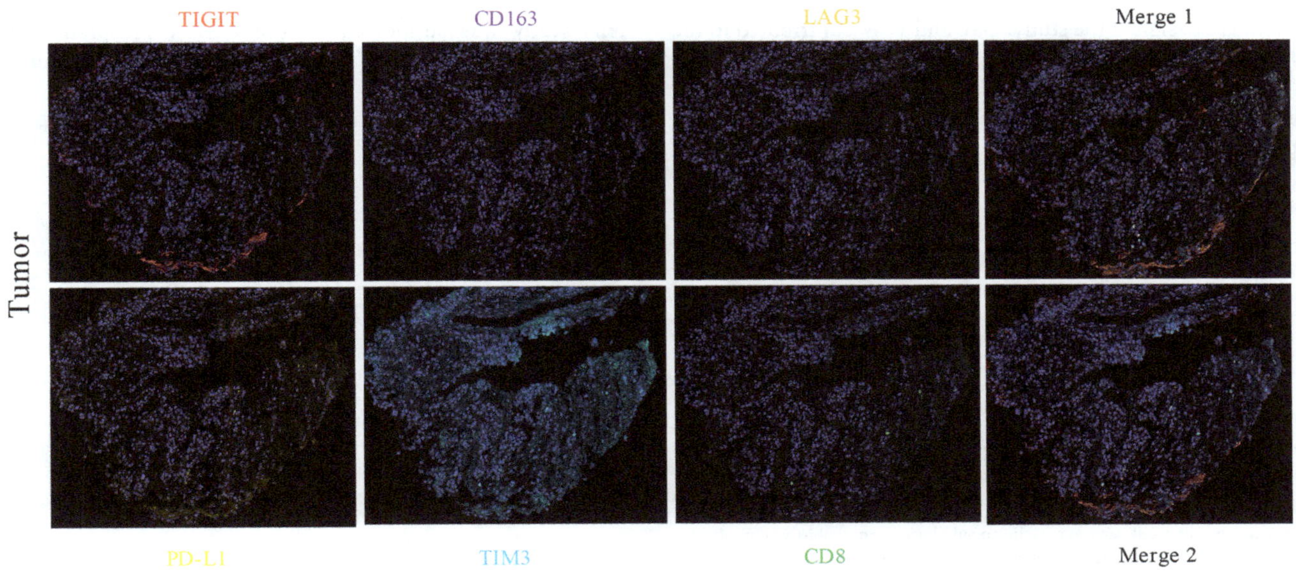

FIGURE 3 | The expression levels of CD8 (green), TIM3 (light blue), PD-L1 (yellow), LAG3 (orange), CD163 (purple), and TIGIT (red) in lung CCS were detected by multiple immunofluorescence assays. The number of positive cells was estimated as follows: TIGIT ≥1%, other indexes <1%. CD8 and TIM3 colocalized, and there was no colocalization with other indexes.

large, and the cost is still high. And the technical defects of NGS can also affect the final test result. In this study, the patient had a previously unknown CCS mutation, CDKN2AB, which was identified with NGS, and the absence of CDKN2AB may lead to hyperimmune progression (12). Moreover, we examined the PD-L1 expression and the immune microenvironment of this patient, which is the first time these were studied in CCS in the chest. However, this study also has obvious limitations. After the patient was diagnosed, we strongly recommended chemotherapy or immunotherapy, but the patient refused for economic reasons; therefore, we did not observe the patient's efficacy. However, this study suggests that bevacizumab appears to have some effect in treating pleural effusion within the cavity with CCS.

Currently, the most effective treatment for most patients with CCS remains surgical resection, with only a small fraction of patients benefiting from conventional cytotoxic chemotherapy (6). Some of the latest potential therapeutic targets of CCS, such as MET, PDGFRA/B, and HDAC, have been identified. Due to the identification of these targets, some small molecules and monoclonal antibodies, such as sunitinib, sorafenib, and crizotinib, are in clinical trials. These treatments offer new hope for improving the prognosis of patients with this rare invasive disease (2, 13).

The immunophenotype of CCS is similar to that of melanoma, so CCS may have similar immunotherapy targets at similar immune checkpoints. PD-1- and PD-L1-associated antibodies have a wide range of antitumor effects and have been shown to benefit melanoma patients (14). The PD-L1 antibody as a potential immunotherapy for CCS was not favorable in our patient, suggesting that CCS may lack relevant immune checkpoints. In the meantime, we further explored the tumor microenvironment of the pulmonary CCS to search for more effective therapeutic targets with immunofluorescence. The results suggest that drugs that target TIGIT could become a new treatment for CCS. In 2009, TIGIT was first discovered by Xin Yu (15). TIGIT is considered a desirable target for cancer treatment because it can hinder the cancer immunity cycle's multiple steps. Pre-clinical studies indicated that TIGIT blockade might protect against multiple solid and hematological cancers was confirmed in Pre-clinical studies (16). Several clinical trials (Phase 1, 2) of human anti-TIGIT mAbs are tested to treat advanced solid cancers, and its combination with PD-1 blockade enhances the antitumor effect (17). In the meantime, with the continuous advancement of clinical trials and our increasing understanding of the mechanism of TIGIT-mediated immune response regulation, more effective treatment strategies for cancer patients will emerge.

CONCLUSION

In summary, pulmonary CCS is a rare soft tissue malignant tumor that occurs in young adults and has rarely been reported. In our study, a new NGS technique was used to help pathologically diagnose PCCS, thereby improving the diagnostic strategy, especially the differential diagnosis between CCS and malignant melanoma. Exploring the molecular characteristics of genes and the immune microenvironment of pulmonary CCS will be an essential for the clinical treatment of this rare disease

AUTHOR CONTRIBUTIONS

XX and HL designed the study. DW and WW contributed to the data curation. HL supervised the study. XX and DW wrote the original draft of the manuscript. HL wrote, reviewed, and edited the manuscript. All authors contributed to the article and approved the submitted version.

REFERENCES

1. Enzinger FM. Clear-cell sarcoma of tendons and aponeuroses. An analysis of 21 cases. *Cancer* (1965) 18:1163–74. doi: 10.1002/1097-0142(196509)18:9<1163::AID-CNCR2820180916>3.0.CO;2-0
2. Cornillie J, van Cann T, Wozniak A, Hompes D, Schöffski P. Biology and management of clear cell sarcoma: state of the art and future perspectives. *Expert Rev Anticancer Ther* (2016) 16:839–45. doi: 10.1080/14737140.2016.1197122
3. Goh GH, Teh M, Vanecek T, Moran C, Petersson F. Primary pulmonary clear cell sarcoma-the first two reported cases. *Virchows Arch* (2016) 469:111–7. doi: 10.1007/s00428-016-1943-8
4. Hantschke M, Mentzel T, Rütten A, Palmedo G, Calonje E, Lazar AJ, et al. Cutaneous clear cell sarcoma: a clinicopathologic, immunohistochemical, and molecular analysis of 12 cases emphasizing its distinction from dermal melanoma. *Am J Surg Pathol* (2010) 34:216–22. doi: 10.1097/PAS.0b013e3181c7d8b2
5. Gonzaga MI, Grant L, Curtin C, Gootee J, Silberstein P, Voth E. The epidemiology and survivorship of clear cell sarcoma: a National Cancer Database (NCDB) review. *J Cancer Res Clin Oncol* (2018) 144:1711–6. doi: 10.1007/s00432-018-2693-6
6. Bianchi G, Charoenlap C, Cocchi S, Rani N, Campagnoni S, Righi A, et al. Clear cell sarcoma of soft tissue: A retrospective review and analysis of 31 cases treated at Istituto Ortopedico Rizzoli. *Eur J Surg Oncol* (2014) 40:505–10. doi: 10.1016/j.ejso.2014.01.016
7. Lucas DR, Nascimento AG, Sim FH. Clear cell sarcoma of soft tissues. Mayo Clinic experience with 35 cases. *Am J Surg Pathol* (1992) 16:1197–204. doi: 10.1097/00000478-199212000-00006
8. Chung EB, Enzinger FM. Malignant melanoma of soft parts. A reassessment of clear cell sarcoma. *Am J Surg Pathol* (1983) 7:405–13. doi: 10.1097/00000478-198307000-00003
9. Hisaoka M, Ishida T, Kuo T-T, Matsuyama A, Imamura T, Nishida K, et al. Clear cell sarcoma of soft tissue: a clinicopathologic, immunohistochemical, and molecular analysis of 33 cases. *Am J Surg Pathol* (2008) 32:452–60. doi: 10.1097/PAS.0b013e31814b18fb
10. Aghajan Y, Malicki DM, Levy ML, Crawford JR. Atypical central neurocytoma with novel EWSR1-ATF1 fusion and MUTYH mutation detected by next-generation sequencing. *BMJ Case Rep* (2019) 12:1. doi: 10.1136/bcr-2018-226455
11. Fernandez-Marmiesse A, Gouveia S, Couce ML. NGS Technologies as a Turning Point in Rare Disease Resea rch, Diagnosis and Treatment. *Curr Med Chem* (2018) 25:404–32. doi: 10.2174/0929867324666170718101946
12. Giusti R, Mazzotta M, Filetti M, Marinelli D, Di Napoli A, Scarpino S, et al. CDKN2A/B gene loss and MDM2 alteration as a potential molecular signature for hyperprogressive disease in advanced NSCLC: A next-generation-sequencing approach. *JCO* (2019) 37:e20628-8. doi: 10.1200/JCO.2019.37.15_suppl.e20628
13. Mir O, Boudou-Rouquette P, Larousserie F, Babinet A, Dumaine V, Anract P, et al. Objective response to sorafenib in advanced clear-cell sarcoma. *Ann Oncol* (2012) 23:807–9. doi: 10.1093/annonc/mds005
14. Mahoney KM, Freeman GJ, McDermott DF. The Next Immune-Checkpoint Inhibitors: PD-1/PD-L1 Blockade in Melanoma. *Clin Ther* (2015) 37:764–82. doi: 10.1016/j.clinthera.2015.02.018
15. Yu X, Harden K, Gonzalez LC, Francesco M, Chiang E, Irving B, et al. The surface protein TIGIT suppresses T cell activation by promoting the generation of mature immunoregulatory dendritic cells. *Nat Immunol* (2009) 10:48–57. doi: 10.1038/ni.1674
16. Harjunpää H, Guillerey C. TIGIT as an emerging immune checkpoint. *Clin Exp Immunol* (2020) 200:108–19. doi: 10.1111/cei.13407
17. Chauvin J-M, Zarour HM. TIGIT in cancer immunotherapy. *J Immunother Cancer* (2020) 8:4. doi: 10.1136/jitc-2020-000957

ACKNOWLEDGMENTS

This study was supported by the Cancer Hospital of the University of Chinese Academy of Sciences (Zhejiang Cancer Hospital).

8

Clinical Relevance of PD-L1 Expression and CD8+ T Cells' Infiltration in Patients with Lung Invasive Mucinous Adenocarcinoma

Xiaoling Xu[1,2,3†], *Na Li*[2,3†], *Ding Wang*[3], *Wei Chen*[2] *and Yun Fan*[1,2,3*]

[1] Key Laboratory of Head & Neck Cancer Translational Research of Zhejiang Province, Cancer Hospital of the University of Chinese Academy of Sciences (Zhejiang Cancer Hospital), Hangzhou, China, [2] Institute of Cancer and Basic Medicine (IBMC), Chinese Academy of Sciences, Hangzhou, China, [3] Department of Medical Oncology, The Second Clinical Medical College of Zhejiang Chinese Medical University, Hangzhou, China

***Correspondence:**
Yun Fan
fanyun1218@163.com

[†]These authors have contributed equally to this work and share first authorship

Background: Invasive mucinous adenocarcinoma (IMA) of the lung is a rare and distinct subtype of adenocarcinoma. At present, people have no idea whether IMA patients can benefit from immunotherapy and target therapy; thus there is an urgent need to clarify the immune microenvironment and genetic characteristics of this cohort.

Methods: A total of 31 IMA patients matched with 27 non-mucinous adenocarcinoma (non-IMA) patients were enrolled in this study, and clinical data was collected. The expression of PD-L1, CD8+ tumor-infiltrating lymphocytes (TILs) and ALK was determined by immunohistochemistry. Polymerase Chain Reaction was used to determine the mutations of EGFR. The Chi-square test, Kaplan–Meier method and Cox proportional hazard regression model were used to explore the correlations between these clinicopathological variables, survival and identify risk factors.

Results: Of the patients with IMA 9.7% (3/31) revealed positive PD-L1 expression and 35.5% (11/31) showed CD8+ TIL infiltration, which were markedly lower than that of non-IMA group [PD-L1: 48.1% (13/27); CD8: 81.5% (22/27)]. Moreover, five (16.1%) patients in IMA group and 10 (37.0%) patients in non-IMA group had EGFR mutations, and nine (29.0%) patients in IMA group and zero (0.0%) patient in non-IMA group had ALK rearrangements. Additionally, we observed that IMA patients with CD8+ TIL infiltration had a worse prognosis than CD8-negative group (P = 0.024). Multivariate analyses showed that CD8 was an independent prognostic factor for patient's survival (HR = 5.60, 95% CI: 1.35–23.22, P = 0.017).

Conclusion: Patients with IMA have down-regulated expression of PD-L1 and less CD8+ TIL infiltration in tumor microenvironment. Besides, a lower frequency of EGFR mutations was detected in patients with IMA than non-IMA patients while a higher rate of ALK rearrangements was found. Our results provide important reference for therapy of lung IMA.

Keywords: invasive mucinous adenocarcinoma, lung cancer, PD-L1 expression, CD8+ T cells, tumor microenvironment, genetic characteristics, treatment

INTRODUCTION

Lung cancer remains the leading cause of cancer-related mortality worldwide which can be pathologically classified into two major subtypes, non-small cell lung cancer (NSCLC) and small cell lung cancer (SCLC) (1). Lung adenocarcinoma (ADC) is the most frequent type of NSCLC. According to the new classification proposed by the European Respiratory Society (ERS), American Thoracic Society (ATS) and International Association for the Study of Lung Cancer (IASLC) in 2011, invasive mucinous adenocarcinoma of the lung (IMA) is a rare and unique lung ADC subtype, about 2–5% (2). IMA is histologically characterized by goblet and/or columnar cells with basal nuclei and abundant cytoplasmic mucin (3). As for prognosis, IMA is related with poor prognosis mainly owing to airway propagation mode (4). In addition, pathological parameters, including tumor cell spread size, invasive size, and mucin spread size, were also adverse prognostic factors for IMA (5). As a subtype of lung ADC, the same therapeutic regimen as for other ADCs was usually applied for treating patients with IMA. However, neither platinum-based chemotherapy nor targeted therapy has been demonstrated to be obviously effective against IMA (6, 7). Thus, new therapeutic approach for IMA is necessary.

IMA has a special gene expression profiling. Recent research studies have proved that KRAS mutation was the most frequent oncogenic driver mutations in IMA (63–90%) followed by NRG1 fusions (7–27%) (8–11). Compared with non-mucinous adenocarcinoma (non-IMA), IMA has a lower rate of EGFR mutations (only 0–5%) and a higher rate of ALK rearrangements (2.2%) and ERBB2 mutations (1.2%) (6, 12, 13). In addition, rare gene mutations, such as HER2, BRAF, and PI3KA mutations, and rare gene fusions, such as TRIM4-BRAF, VAMP2-NRG1, and CD74-NRG1fusions, were observed in IMA patients with KRAS-negative (8). However, owing to the rarity of treatable mutations, IMA patients are usually ineligible for target therapy (6).

Recently, immune checkpoint inhibitors (ICIs) have greatly changed the treatment landscape of patients with non-small cell lung cancer (14). However, due to the rarity of IMA, the studies of immune-checkpoint expression in patients with IMA have been limited, and no specific immune checkpoint therapy has been established for IMA yet (15). Nakagomi et al. (7) found that PD-L1 expression tended to be lower in the IMA group (6.1%) compared to the conventional ADC group (59.7%). Another study (16) detect PD-L1 expression in NSCLC including various adenocarcinoma subtypes. Out of the 90 samples, only four were IMA and none of them expressed PD-L1. In general, the PD-L1 expression in IMA patients was rather low and, in fact, whether IMA patients can benefit from ICIs still needs further investigation. Moreover, B7-H3 expressed highly in IMA group (42.4%), which maybe a potential and promising immunotherapeutic target.

Based on the available literature, although IMA is a variant of lung ADC, it has specific genetic profiles and immune-checkpoint status, which means that innovative therapies are needed for this subgroup. Unfortunately, there are only a few studies relevant. In our study, by reviewing the clinicopathological features, genetic mutations, tumor microenvironment (TME), and survival of 31 IMA patients, we aimed to clarify PD-L1 expression and tumor-infiltrating lymphocytes (TILs) in IMA, the correlation between these factors and patient's survival, and the potential of targeted therapy and immunotherapy in IMA patients.

MATERIALS AND METHODS

Study Population

A total of 9,260 patients with lung cancer were reviewed; only 148 patients with lung IMA were confirmed from January 2010 to December 2015 at Zhejiang Cancer Hospital. IMA patients who satisfied all of the following criteria were enrolled: (1) All collected tumor samples must be pathologically diagnosed as IMA; (2) All patients had complete clinical and follow-up information; (3) All patients did not receive any anti-tumor treatment; and (4) All patients signed informed consent. As a control group, NSCLC patients with non-IMA were also included. The clinical characteristics of the participants are listed in **Table 1**. The study was conducted in accordance with the ethical standards of the Ethics Committee of Zhejiang Cancer Hospital, and informed consent for the use of tumor specimens was obtained.

Immunohistochemistry

Immunohistochemistry (IHC) assay was performed in tumor samples comprising 41 surgical samples and 17 biopsies. The 4-μm tissue sections were cut from formalin-fixed paraffin-embedded (FFPE) tumor tissues. After deparaffinization and rehydration, slides were stained in an automated system (Leica Biosystems, Wetzlar, Germany). Antibodies used were rabbit anti-PD-L1 (1:100, clone SP142, cat# ZA-0629, Beijing zhongshan Jinqiao Biotechnology Co., Ltd, Beijing, China), mouse anti-CD8 (1:100, clone ES05, cat# IR079, Dako, Agilent Technologies, Santa Clara, CA, USA), and rabbit anti-ALK (1:100, clone D5F3, cat# 3633S, Cell Signaling Technology, MA, USA).

PD-L1 expression was evaluated by the tumor proportion score (TPS), defined as the percentage of tumor cells observed as partial or complete membrane staining. The cut-off for PD-L1 positive expression was set at ≥1%. The positivity of CD8+ T cells of all nucleated cells in the intercellular substance was defined as ≥10%. PD-L1+/CD8+ expression was defined as both positive expression of PD-L1 and CD8+ T cell.

ALK expression was determined using binary interpretation. We defined ALK positivity as any percentage of presence of strong granular cytoplasmic staining in the tumor cells; otherwise, the absence of strong cytoplasmic staining was deemed ALK negative. IHC assay was performed according to the manufacturer's protocols, and two pathologists independently scored staining with blind assessments.

EGFR Mutation Analyses

DNA was extracted from the FFPE tumor tissues using Amoydx FPE DNA Kit (Amoy Diagnostics, Xiamen, China) according to

TABLE 1 | Clinicopathological characteristics of the 58 patients with lung adenocarcinoma.

	All case (n = 58)	IMA (n = 31)	non-IMA (n = 27)	*P*-value
Sex				
Male	27 (46.6%)	15 (48.4%)	11 (40.7%)	0.408
Female	31 (53.4%)	16 (51.6%)	16 (59.3%)	
Age				
<65	47 (81.0%)	25 (80.6%)	22 (81.5%)	0.935
≥65	11 (19.0%)	6 (19.4%)	5 (18.5%)	
Smoking status				
Never	36 (62.1%)	19 (61.3%)	17 (63.0%)	0.896
Ever/current	22 (37.9%)	12 (38.7%)	10 (37.0%)	
Clinical stage				
I–III	45 (77.6%)	27 (87.1%)	18 (66.7%)	0.063
IV	13 (22.4)	4 (12.9%)	9 (33.3%)	
EGFR status				
Mutation	15 (25.9%)	5 (16.1%)	10 (37.0%)	0.070
Wild	43 (74.1%)	26 (83.9%)	17 (63.0%)	
ALK status				
Mutation	9 (15.5%)	9 (29.0%)	0 (0.0%)	***0.002****
Wild	49 (82.8%)	22 (71.0%)	27 (100.0%)	
PD-L1 expression				
+ (≥1%)	16 (27.6%)	3 (9.7%)	13 (48.1%)	***0.001****
− (<1%)	42 (72.4%)	28 (90.3%)	14 (51.9%)	
CD8 expression				
+ (≥10%)	33 (56.9%)	11 (35.5%)	22 (81.5%)	***<0.001****
− (<10%)	25 (43.1%)	20 (64.5%)	5 (18.5%)	

**P-value < 0.05 in Chi-square test.*
In bold: P < 0.05.

protocols. Polymerase chain reaction (PCR) was performed at the Mx3000PTM real-time PCR system (Strata gene, La Jolla, USA). EGFR mutations were detected by EGFR 29 Mutations Detection Kit (Amoy Diagnostics, Xiamen, China). We used ΔCt method to quantify the amplification. If ΔCt values were higher than 2.0, the patient was identified as "EGFR mutant"; otherwise, the patient was identified as "EGFR wild-type".

Statistical Analyses

To compare categorical characteristics, the Chi-square test was performed. Survival analyses were performed by plotting Kaplan–Meier curves with the log-rank test, and the hazard ratio (HR) was determined by multivariable Cox proportional hazard regression model. Variables included in this model were sex, age, smoking status, clinical stage, EGFR and ALK status, PD-L1, and CD8 expression. P value ≤0.05 was considered statistically significant. The data were statistically analyzed by using SPSS software, GraphPad Prism (version 5), and version 22.0 for Windows (Chicago, IL, USA).

RESULTS

Patient Characteristics

From a screened population of 9,260 patients with lung cancer, a total of 31 IMA patients were identified; see flow chart in **Figure 1**. The non-IMA group consisting of 27 individuals was matched with the IMA group for age, sex, and smoking status. The median age of patients at diagnosis was 58 years (range: 29–85 years); 27 (46.6%) were men and 31 (53.4%) were women. Among them, 81.0% (47 patients) were <65 years, 37.9% (22 patients) were have a history of smoking, and 22.4% (13 patients) were diagnosed at stage IV. There were no significant differences between the IMA and non-IMA groups in terms of sex, age, smoking, and clinical stage. Five (16.1%) patients in IMA group, and 10 (37.0%) patients in non-IMA group had EGFR mutations, and nine (29.0%) patients in IMA group and zero (0.0%) patient in non-IMA group had ALK rearrangements. The ALK rearrangements rate were significantly higher in the IMA group (P = 0.002). Clinical and pathological characteristics of this cohort were presented in **Table 1**.

Correlation With the Clinicopathology and Prognosis of PD-L1 Expression and CD8+ TIL Status

Figure 2 presents the representative images for PD-L1 expression on the membrane of tumor cells and CD8+ TILs. As shown in **Table 1**, 9.7% (3/31) of the IMA patients had positive expression of PD-L1, and 35.5% (11/31) showed positive CD8 staining, which were markedly lower than that of non-IMA group [PD-L1: 48.1% (13/27); CD8: 81.5% (22/27)]. Differences between the groups were statistically significant (P < 0.001). Neither the PD-L1 expression nor CD8+ staining showed the association with other clinical factors (**Tables S1, S2**). The median OS was significantly shorter in patients with CD8+ staining than in those obscene (47.3 *vs* 60.2 months, P = 0.024, **Figure 3A**). As presented in **Table 2**, CD8 TIL status was correlated with poor OS (HR = 4.32, 95% CI: 1.08–17.34, P = 0.039) by the univariate analyses. Furthermore, after adjusting for clinicopathological factors, multivariate analysis

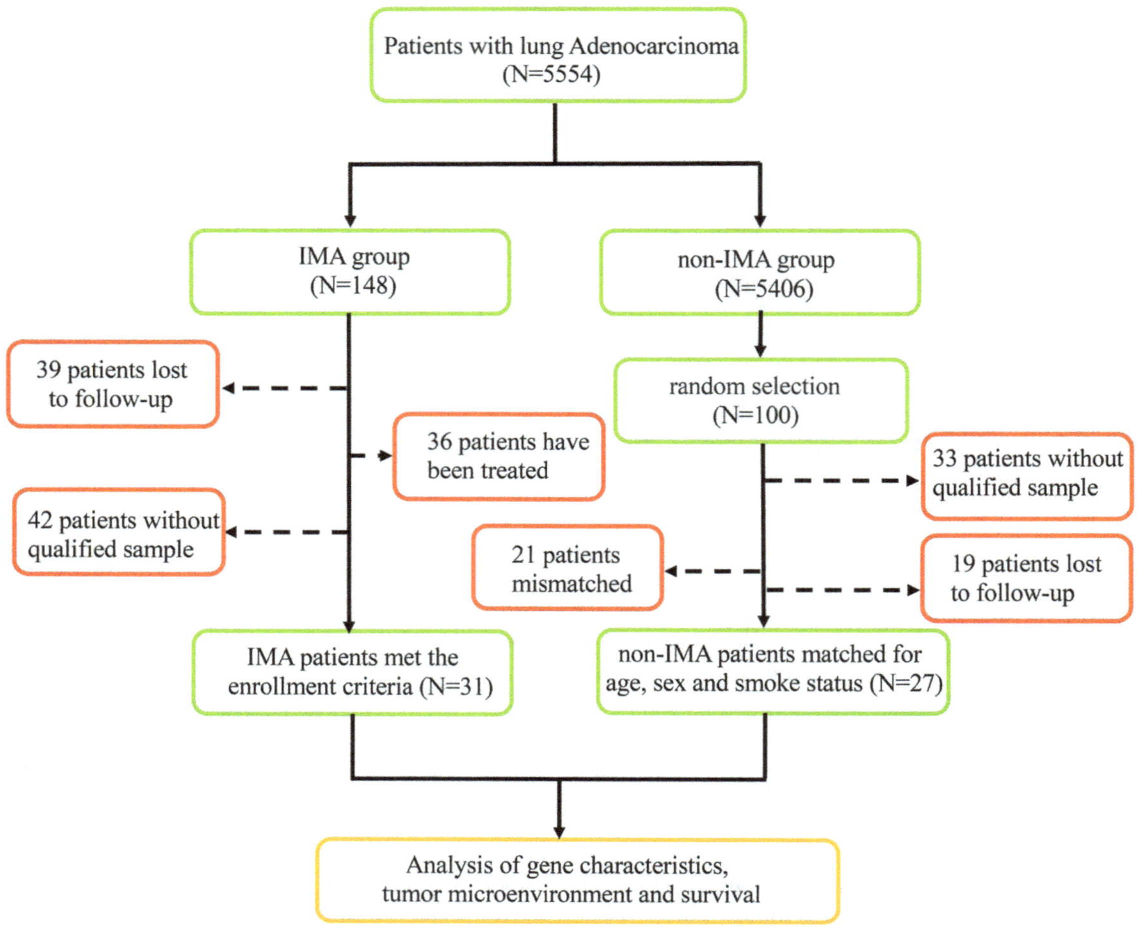

FIGURE 1 | Flow chart of the protocol followed for patients' enrollment.

suggested that CD8 was an independent prognostic factor for survival (HR = 5.60, 95% CI: 1.35–23.22, P = 0.017). Neither the PD-L1 expression nor the mutations of EGFR, ALK showed prognostic value (P > 0.05). Neither the PD-L1 expression nor the mutations of EGFR, ALK showed prognostic value (P > 0.05, **Figures 3B–D**).

Response to Immunotherapy of IMA

To evaluate the clinical efficacy of checkmate inhibitor based on TME status, we collected clinical data of a patient with IMA of the lung who was treated with PD-1 inhibitors. As shown in **Figure 4**, the patient was a 32-year-old young woman with lung ADC with pleural metastases (cT2bN2M1a, stage IVA). The IHC of her biopsy sample showed positive PD-L1 expression (50%) and strong CD8+ staining (40%). After four cycles of pembrolizumab plus pemetrexed–platinum regimen, the patient exhibited partial response (PR), with obviously shrunken pulmonary lesions (**Figure 4**). This patient then continued to receive pembrolizumab monotherapy and experienced a disease stabilization. Ultimately, after six cycles of pembrolizumab monotherapy, the patient developed disease progression due to a relapse with lung lesions; PFS was of 11.9 months.

DISCUSSION

As ICIs have dramatically changed anticancer strategies recently, there is a great need to better understand the immune axis and crosstalk with the TME in tumors. To our knowledge, this is the first study to evaluate the expression of PD-L1 and the infiltration of lymphocytes in patients with IMA. By reviewing the clinicopathological data of 31 IMA patients, we mainly investigate the immunophenotypic characteristics and their clinical relevance in IMA patients.

First, our study found a statistically significant decrease in PD-L1 expression and CD8+ TIL infiltration in IMA patients compared to non-IMA patients. Similar to our results, previous studies have also shown a low level of PD-L1 expression in IMA group (7, 17, 18). However, studies regarding TIL abundance in

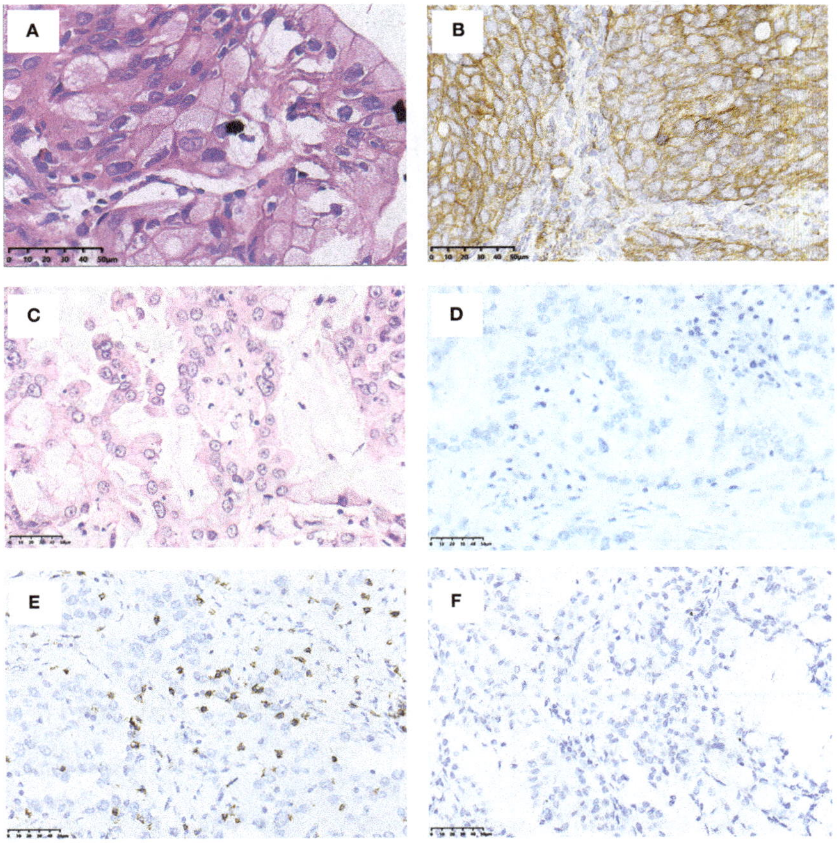

FIGURE 2 | Representative images of PD-L1 and CD8 immuno-staining (×400 original magnification). H&E **(A)** and PD-L1 **(B)** staining of patients with PD-L1+; H&E **(C)** and PD-L1 **(D)** staining of patients with PD-L1−; **(E)** presence of CD8+ TILs; and **(F)** absence of CD8 + TILs.

patients with IMA have not been carried out yet, which need to be verified by experiments with large sample sizes. As far as we know, interferon-γ (IFN-γ) can up-regulate PD-L1 expression through the JAK2–STAT1 and PI3K–AKT pathways in NSCLC (19, 20). Considering that CD8+ TILs could produce IFN-γ and induce PD-L1 expression (21), we speculate that the decrease of PD-L1 expression in IMA patients is associated with low levels of CD8+ TIL infiltration by inhibiting IFN-γ production. However, the mechanism underlying low CD8+ TIL infiltration in IMA needs further investigations.

Moreover, in the present study, 16.1% of IMA patients have EGFR mutations and 29.0% with ALK rearrangement, which was consistent with previous studies indicating that IMA patients have a lower frequency of EGFR mutations and a higher frequency of ALK rearrangements than non-IMA patients (8, 9, 12). Our former next-generation sequencing (NGS)-based study using a panel of 425 genes has identified that KRAS mutations were the most frequent oncogenic driver mutations in IMAs (23.1% in pure-IMA group and 4.0% in mixed-IMA group) (22). However, owing to the rarity or absence of targetable mutations, there are few studies on the target therapy of IMA (23). Several studies have suggested that KRAS mutations, ERBB2 mutations, and ALK rearrangements could be targeted for therapeutic intervention; however, its efficacy for IMA patients has not be verified in clinical practice yet (24, 25). Since NRG1 fusions are in a high proportion of lung IMA, multiple studies have demonstrated that afatinib, an irreversible ErbB family inhibitor, is effective in NSCLC patients with NRG1 fusions, which maybe a potential therapeutic strategy to IMA patients (26–28). Hence there is an urgent need to determine the molecular mechanisms driving IMA and identify novel target therapy.

Second, we observed that the CD8-negative group exhibited longer overall survival (OS) than CD8+ TIL group, and CD8 was an independent prognostic factor for IMA patients' survival. Contrary to our results, CD8+ T lymphocytes are thought to be the dominant cytotoxic immune cells that are able to eliminate tumor cells (29). Recently, elevated levels of cytotoxic CD8+ T cells in the TME have been linked with positive anti-tumor effects in various cancers, indicating a good prognosis in patients with elevated cytotoxic CD8+ TILs (30–32). Researchers have found that CD8+ TILs at different tumor sites have diverse clinical attributes and a number of factors in the TME, such as the activation of inhibitory checkpoint pathways, abnormal

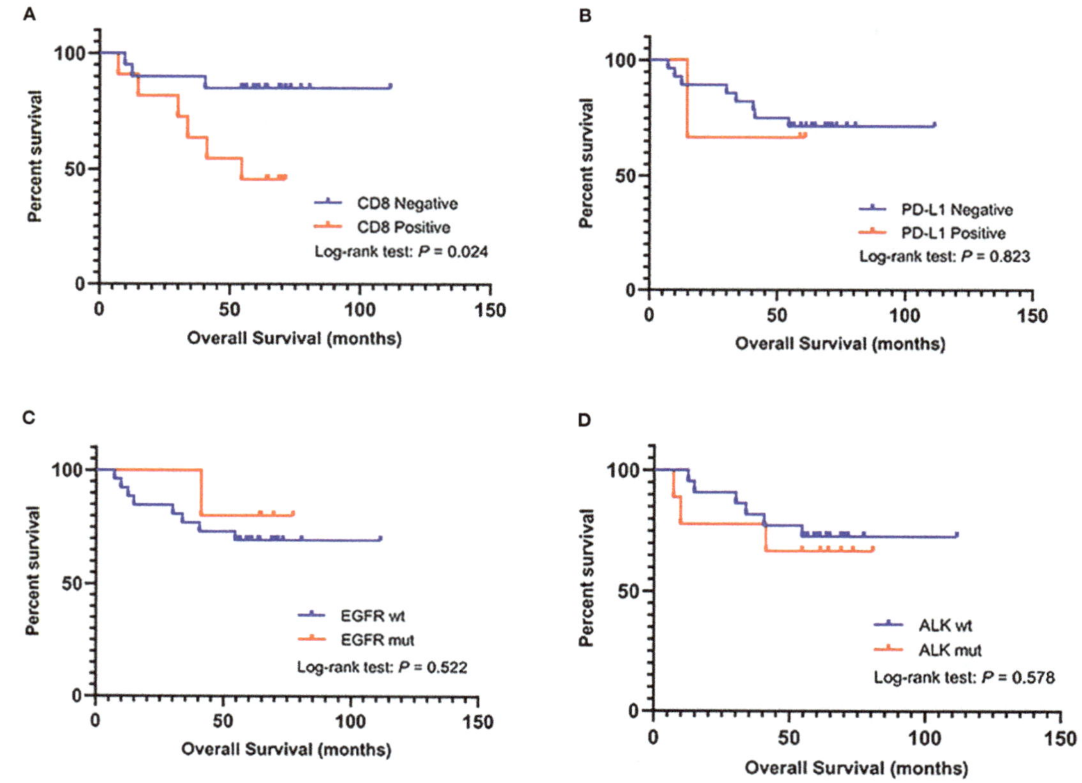

FIGURE 3 | (A) Kaplan–Meier analysis of overall survival (OS) in IMA patients based on CD8+ TIL infiltration. **(B)** Kaplan–Meier analysis of OS in IMA patients based on PD-L1 expression. **(C)** Kaplan–Meier analysis of OS in IMA patients based on EGFR mutations. **(D)** Kaplan–Meier analysis of OS in IMA patients based on ALK mutations.

TABLE 2 | Univariate and multivariate Cox regression analyses of prognostic factors for survival in patients with IMA.

	Univariate analysis		**Multivariate analysis**	
	HR (95% CI)	***P*-value**	**HR (95% CI)**	***P*-value**
Sex				
Male	1.00	0.825	1.00	0.794
Female	1.16 (0.31–4.32)		0.81 (0.18–3.79)	
Age				
<65	1.00	0.444	1.00	0.290
≥65	0.44 (0.06–3.55)		0.31 (0.03–2.74)	
EGFR status				
Wild	1.00	0.586	1.00	0.620
Mutation	0.56 (0.70–4.49)		0.58 (0.07–4.90)	
ALK status				
Wild	1.00	0.658	1.00	0.646
Mutation	1.37 (0.34–5.48)		1.46 (0.29–7.30)	
PD-L1 expression				
+ (≥1%)	1.00	0.824	1.00	0.534
- (<1%)	0.79 (0.10–6.33)		0.49 (0.05–4.65)	
CD8 expression				
+ (≥10%)	1.00	***0.039****	1.00	***0.017****
- (<10%)	4.32 (1.08–17.34)		5.60 (1.35–23.22)	

HR, hazard ratio; CI, confidence interval.
**P-value < 0.05 in Cox proportional hazard model.*
In bold: P < 0.05.

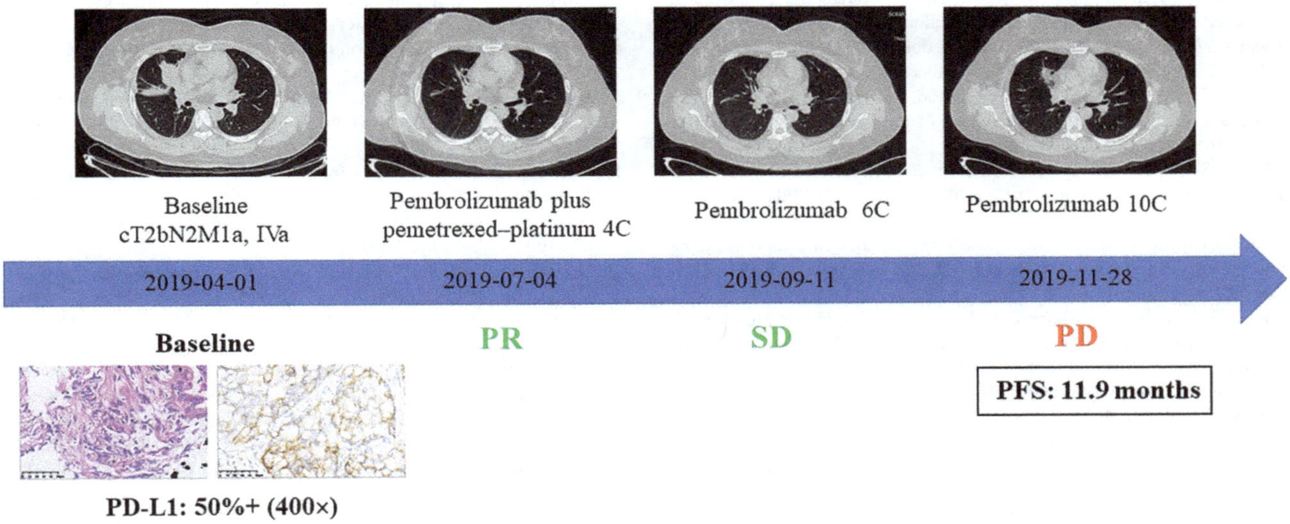

FIGURE 4 | The clinical response to immune checkpoint inhibitors combined with chemotherapy in an IMA patient with PD-L1 expression and CD8+ TIL infiltration.

tumor angiogenesis, and chemokine secretions, can exactly suppress the function of CD8+ TILs (33). Thus, we speculate that IMA patients have a special TME that affect CD8+ TILs.

Our results showed that IMA patients have low PD-L1 expression and less CD8+ infiltration, which indicated poorer response rates to checkmate inhibitors (34, 35). Therefore, we considered that patients with IMA cannot benefit from ICI monotherapy; surgery and platinum-based conventional chemotherapy are still the main therapeutic modalities. In our study, one female patient with strong PD-L1 expression (50%) and abundant CD8+ T cell infiltration (40%) experienced PR to ICIs combined with chemotherapy. We speculate that the combination of immunotherapy and chemotherapy may be a new therapeutic direction for advanced IMA patients. In addition, the favorable clinical efficacy of ICIs is also associated with positive PD-L1 expression and CD8+ T cell infiltration in the tumor tissue, as sufficient CD8+ TILs in the TME is the foundation of anti-tumor effect activated by ICIs (36). However, the potential of PD-L1 and CD8 as predictive biomarkers to immunotherapy in IMA patients remains to be further investigated.

Our study has several limitations. First, the number of patients enrolled in this study was relatively small due to the rarity of IMA. Second, the IMA group was not further divided into pure-IMA and mixed-IMA subgroups, leading to the possible heterogeneity of the IMA group which may influence the expression of PD-L1 and CD8+ TILs. Third, some patients were diagnosed at an early stage, and the median OS in the IMA group was unavailable. Fourth, because of insufficient samples, ALK rearrangement was not reconfirmed by fluorescence *in situ* hybridization (FISH) assay. Finally, as the samples used in study were obtained years ago, the PD-L1 expression may be underestimated because the expression of PD-L1 might be dynamic with time going.

In conclusion, we demonstrated that IMA patients might have lower levels of PD-L1 expression and CD8+ TIL infiltration than non-IMA patients. We also observed a lower frequency of EGFR mutations and a higher frequency of ALK rearrangements and KRAS mutations in IMA patients. Moreover, patients with CD8+ TIL infiltration had shorter OS and worse prognosis, and CD8 was an independent prognostic factor of IMA patients' survival. Based on the characteristics of gene and immune microenvironment, target therapy and immunotherapy in IMA patients are limited, which needs further investigation.

AUTHOR CONTRIBUTIONS

Conceptualization: YF. Methodology: XX and DW. Investigation: NL. Bioinformatics analysis: XX and NL. Writing, original draft: NL. Writing, review, and editing: WC. Funding acquisition: XX. Supervision: YF. All authors contributed to the article and approved the submitted version.

REFERENCES

1. Siegel RL, Miller KD, Jemal A. Cancer Statistics, 2020. *CA Cancer J Clin* (2020) 70:7–30. doi: 10.3322/caac.21590
2. Travis WD, Brambilla E, Noguchi M, Nicholson AG, Geisinger KR, Yatabe Y, et al. International Association for the Study of Lung Cancer/American Thoracic Society/European Respiratory Society International Multidisciplinary Classification of Lung Adenocarcinoma. *J Thoracic Oncol* (2011) 6:244–85. doi: 10.1097/JTO.0b013e318206a221
3. Travis WD, Brambilla E, Nicholson AG, Yatabe Y, Austin JHM, Beasley MB, et al. The 2015 World Health Organization Classification of Lung Tumors: Impact of Genetic, Clinical and Radiologic Advances Since the 2004 Classification. *J Thorac Oncol* (2015) 10:1243–60. doi: 10.1097/JTO.0000000000000630

4. Lee MA, Kang J, Lee HY, Kim W, Shon I, Hwang NY, et al. Spread Through Air Spaces (STAS) in Invasive Mucinous Adenocarcinoma of the Lung: Incidence, Prognostic Impact, and Prediction Based on Clinicoradiologic Factors. *Thorac Cancer* (2020) 11:3145–54. doi: 10.1111/1759-7714.13632
5. Saito T, Tsuta K, Honda O, Ishida M, Yamaka R, Tanaka N, et al. Prognostic Impact of Mucin Spread, Tumor Cell Spread, and Invasive Size in Invasive Mucinous Adenocarcinoma of the Lung. *Lung Cancer* (2020) 146:50–7. doi: 10.1016/j.lungcan.2020.05.030
6. Cha YJ, Shim HS. Biology of Invasive Mucinous Adenocarcinoma of the Lung. *Transl Lung Cancer Res* (2017) 6:508–12. doi: 10.21037/tlcr.2017.06.10
7. Nakagomi T, Goto T, Hirotsu Y, Shikata D, Yokoyama Y, Higuchi R, et al. Genomic Characteristics of Invasive Mucinous Adenocarcinomas of the Lung and Potential Therapeutic Targets of B7-H3. *Cancers (Basel)* (2018) 10:478. doi: 10.3390/cancers10120478
8. Shim HS, Kenudson M, Zheng Z, Liebers M, Cha YJ, Hoang Ho Q, et al. Unique Genetic and Survival Characteristics of Invasive Mucinous Adenocarcinoma of the Lung. *J Thorac Oncol* (2015) 10:1156–62. doi: 10.1097/JTO.0000000000000579
9. Hwang DH, Sholl LM, Rojas-Rudilla V, Hall DL, Shivdasani P, Garcia EP, et al. KRAS and NKX2-1 Mutations in Invasive Mucinous Adenocarcinoma of the Lung. *J Thorac Oncol* (2016) 11:496–503. doi: 10.1016/j.jtho.2016.01.010
10. Fernandez-Cuesta L, Plenker D, Osada H, Sun R, Menon R, Leenders F, et al. CD74-NRG1 Fusions in Lung Adenocarcinoma. *Cancer Discovery* (2014) 4:415–22. doi: 10.1158/2159-8290.CD-13-0633
11. Guo M, Tomoshige K, Meister M, Muley T, Fukazawa T, Tsuchiya T, et al. Gene Signature Driving Invasive Mucinous Adenocarcinoma of the Lung. *EMBO Mol Med* (2017) 9:462–81. doi: 10.15252/emmm.201606711
12. Nakaoku T, Tsuta K, Ichikawa H, Shiraishi K, Sakamoto H, Enari M, et al. Druggable Oncogene Fusions in Invasive Mucinous Lung Adenocarcinoma. *Clin Cancer Res* (2014) 20:3087–93. doi: 10.1158/1078-0432.CCR-14-0107
13. Jurmeister P, Vollbrecht C, Behnke A, Frost N, Arnold A, Treue D, et al. Next Generation Sequencing of Lung Adenocarcinoma Subtypes With Intestinal Differentiation Reveals Distinct Molecular Signatures Associated With Histomorphology and Therapeutic Options. *Lung Cancer* (2019) 138:43–51. doi: 10.1016/j.lungcan.2019.10.005
14. Madden K, Kasler MK. Immune Checkpoint Inhibitors in Lung Cancer and Melanoma. *Semin Oncol Nurs* (2019) 35:150932. doi: 10.1016/j.soncn.2019.08.011
15. Beck KS, Sung YE, Lee KY, Han DH. Invasive Mucinous Adenocarcinoma of the Lung: Serial CT Findings, Clinical Features, and Treatment and Survival Outcomes. *Thorac Cancer* (2020) 11:3463–72. doi: 10.1111/1759-7714.13674
16. Miyazawa T, Marushima H, Saji H, Kojima K, Hoshikawa M, Takagi M, et al. PD-L1 Expression in Non-Small-Cell Lung Cancer Including Various Adenocarcinoma Subtypes. *Ann Thorac Cardiovasc Surg* (2019) 25:1–9. doi: 10.5761/atcs.oa.18-00163
17. Ng Kee Kwong F, Laggner U, McKinney O, Croud J, Rice A, Nicholson AG. Expression of PD-L1 Correlates With Pleomorphic Morphology and Histological Patterns of Non-Small-Cell Lung Carcinomas. *Histopathology* (2018) 72:1024–32. doi: 10.1111/his.13466
18. Shimizu K, Okita R, Saisho S, Maeda A, Nojima Y, Nakata M. Clinicopathological and Immunohistochemical Features of Lung Invasive Mucinous Adenocarcinoma Based on Computed Tomography Findings. *Onco Targets Ther* (2017) 10:153–63. doi: 10.2147/OTT.S121059
19. Lingling Z, Jiewei L, Li W, Danli Y, Jie Z, Wen L, et al. Molecular Regulatory Network of PD-1/PD-L1 in Non-Small Cell Lung Cancer. *Pathol Res Pract* (2020) 216:152852. doi: 10.1016/j.prp.2020.152852
20. Kythreotou A, Siddique A, Mauri FA, Bower M, Pinato DJ. Pd-L1. *J Clin Pathol* (2018) 71:189–94. doi: 10.1136/jclinpath-2017-204853
21. Lin Z, Gu J, Cui X, Huang L, Li S, Feng J, et al. Deciphering Microenvironment of NSCLC Based on CD8+ TIL Density and PD-1/PD-L1 Expression. *J Cancer* (2019) 10:211–22. doi: 10.7150/jca.26444
22. Cai L, Wang J, Yan J, Zeng J, Zhu L, Liang J, et al. Genomic Profiling and Prognostic Value Analysis of Genetic Alterations in Chinese Resected Lung Cancer With Invasive Mucinous Adenocarcinoma. *Front Oncol* (2020) 10:603671. doi: 10.3389/fonc.2020.603671
23. Cha YJ, Kim HR, Lee HJ, Cho BC, Shim HS. Clinical Course of Stage IV Invasive Mucinous Adenocarcinoma of the Lung. *Lung Cancer* (2016) 102:82–8. doi: 10.1016/j.lungcan.2016.11.004
24. Ku BM, Jho EH, Bae YH, Sun JM, Ahn JS, Park K, et al. BYL719, a Selective Inhibitor of Phosphoinositide 3-Kinase Alpha, Enhances the Effect of Selumetinib (AZD6244, ARRY-142886) in KRAS-Mutant Non-Small Cell Lung Cancer. *Invest New Drugs* (2015) 33:12–21. doi: 10.1007/s10637-014-0163-9
25. Zhao J, Xia Y. Targeting HER2 Alterations in Non–Small-Cell Lung Cancer: A Comprehensive Review. *JCO Precis Oncol* (2020) 4:411–25. doi: 10.1200/PO.19.00333
26. Laskin J, Liu SV, Tolba K, Heining C, Schlenk RF, Cheema P, et al. NRG1 Fusion-Driven Tumors: Biology, Detection, and the Therapeutic Role of Afatinib and Other ErbB-targeting Agents. *Ann Oncol* (2020) 31:1693–703. doi: 10.1016/j.annonc.2020.08.2335
27. Drilon A, Somwar R, Mangatt BP, Edgren H, Desmeules P, Ruusulehto A, et al. Response to ERBB3-Directed Targeted Therapy in NRG1-Rearranged Cancers. *Cancer Discovery* (2018) 8:686–95. doi: 10.1158/2159-8290.CD-17-1004
28. Gay ND, Wang Y, Beadling C, Warrick A, Neff T, Corless CL, et al. Durable Response to Afatinib in Lung Adenocarcinoma Harboring NRG1 Gene Fusions. *J Thorac Oncol* (2017) 12:e107–10. doi: 10.1016/j.jtho.2017.04.025
29. Farhood B, Najafi M, Mortezaee K. CD8(+) Cytotoxic T Lymphocytes in Cancer Immunotherapy: A Review. *J Cell Physiol* (2019) 234:8509–21. doi: 10.1002/jcp.27782
30. Kim PS, Ahmed R. Features of Responding T Cells in Cancer and Chronic Infection. *Curr Opin Immunol* (2010) 22:223–30. doi: 10.1016/j.coi.2010.02.005
31. Kmiecik J, Poli A, Brons NH, Waha A, Eide GE, Enger PO, et al. Elevated CD3+ and CD8+ Tumor-Infiltrating Immune Cells Correlate With Prolonged Survival in Glioblastoma Patients Despite Integrated Immunosuppressive Mechanisms in the Tumor Microenvironment and at the Systemic Level. *J Neuroimmunol* (2013) 264:71–83. doi: 10.1016/j.jneuroim.2013.08.013
32. Piersma SJ, Jordanova ES, van Poelgeest MI, Kwappenberg KM, van der Hulst JM, Drijfhout JW, et al. High Number of Intraepithelial CD8+ Tumor-Infiltrating Lymphocytes Is Associated With the Absence of Lymph Node Metastases in Patients With Large Early-Stage Cervical Cancer. *Cancer Res* (2007) 67:354–61. doi: 10.1158/0008-5472.CAN-06-3388
33. Maimela NR, Liu S, Zhang Y. Fates of CD8+ T Cells in Tumor Microenvironment. *Comput Struct Biotechnol J* (2019) 17:1–13. doi: 10.1016/j.csbj.2018.11.004
34. Fumet JD, Richard C, Ledys F, Klopfenstein Q, Joubert P, Routy B, et al. Prognostic and Predictive Role of CD8 and PD-L1 Determination in Lung Tumor Tissue of Patients Under Anti-PD-1 Therapy. *Br J Cancer* (2018) 119:950–60. doi: 10.1038/s41416-018-0220-9
35. Jiang L, Su X, Zhang T, Yin X, Zhang M, Fu H, et al. PD-L1 Expression and Its Relationship With Oncogenic Drivers in Non-Small Cell Lung Cancer (NSCLC). *Oncotarget* (2017) 8:26845–57. doi: 10.18632/oncotarget.15839
36. Chen DS, Mellman I. Elements of Cancer Immunity and the Cancer-Immune Set Point. *Nature* (2017) 541:321–30. doi: 10.1038/nature21349

9

The Effect of Asymptomatic and/or Treated Brain Metastases on Efficacy of Immune Checkpoint Inhibitors in Metastatic Non–Small Cell Lung Cancer

Sihan Li[1†], Hongwei Zhang[1†], Tingting Liu[2], Jun Chen[3] and Jun Dang[1]*

[1] *Department of Radiation Oncology, The First Affiliated Hospital of China Medical University, Shenyang, China,* [2] *Department of Radiation Oncology, Anshan Cancer Hospital, Anshan, China,* [3] *Department of Radiation Oncology, Shenyang Chest Hospital, Shenyang, China*

***Correspondence:**
Jun Dang
dangjunsy@163.com

†These authors have contributed equally to this work

Background: To assess the effect of asymptomatic and/or treated brain metastases (BMs) on the efficacy of immune checkpoint inhibitors (ICIs) in metastatic non-small cell lung cancer (NSCLC).

Patients and Methods: PubMed, Embase, Cochrane Library, Web of Science, and recent meetings were searched for randomized controlled trials (RCTs). The primary outcomes of interest were overall survival (OS) and progression-free survival (PFS).

Results: Seventeen articles reporting 15 RCTs with 10,358 patients (1,199 with and 9,159 without BMs) were eligible. ICIs were associated with longer OS and PFS than those in chemotherapy either in patients with (hazard ratio [HR], 0.65; 95% confidence interval [CI], 0.51–0.82 and HR, 0.60; 95% CI, 0.45–0.79) or without BMs (HR, 0.74; 95% CI, 0.70–0.78 and HR, 0.70; 95% CI, 0.57–0.86); no significant difference in the pooled HRs for OS ($P_{interaction}$ = 0.29) and PFS ($P_{interaction}$ = 0.37) was observed between the two patient populations. Subgroup analyses revealed that either ICI monotherapy or combination therapy significantly improved OS and PFS compared with those in chemotherapy both for patients with and without BMs. Superior OS benefit from ICI combination therapy than that in monotherapy was observed in patients with BMs (HR, 0.49 *vs.* 0.81, $P_{interaction}$ = 0.005) but not in patients without BMs (HR, 0.71 *vs.* 0.76, $P_{interaction}$ = 0.27).

Conclusion: There was no compelling statistical evidence that the efficacy of ICIs in metastatic NSCLC was modified by the presence of asymptomatic and/or treated BMs. Patients with BMs were likely to obtain more OS benefit from ICI combination therapy than that from monotherapy.

Keywords: immune checkpoint inhibitors, chemotherapy, non-small cell lung cancer, brain metastases, meta-analysis

INTRODUCTION

Brain metastases (BMs) are a common complication of advanced lung cancer with poor prognosis, occurring in 20% to 40% of patients with non-small cell lung cancer (NSCLC) (1). Currently, tyrosine kinase inhibitors (TKIs), especially third-generation TKIs, such as osimertinib and alectinib, have been recommended for epidermal growth factor receptor (EGFR) or anaplastic lymphoma kinase (ALK) mutations in NSCLC patients with BMs (2). However, for patients without these genetic aberrations, there are few satisfactory systemic treatment options. Recently, immune checkpoint inhibitors (ICIs) have changed the therapeutic landscape of metastatic NSCLC patients lacking EGFR or ALK alteration. However, the majority of ICIs trials systematically excluded patients with untreated/unstable BMs. Some recent RCTs (3–19) have included a small number of patients with asymptomatic and/or treated BMs but with inconsistent results. In CheckMate-057 (9), -078 (10), and a pooled analysis of KEYNOTE-010 and -024 and -042 trials (20), patients with baseline asymptomatic or treated BMs had similar OS with ICIs or chemotherapy (CT). Conversely, CheckMate-227 (11, 12), -9LA (13), and a pooled analysis of KEYNOTE-021 and -189 and -407 trials (21) showed that ICIs significantly improved survival compared with that in CT.

To date, no randomized-controlled trial (RCT) has specifically addressed the role of ICIs in NSCLC patients with BMs. Whether the presence of asymptomatic and/or treated BMs can affect the efficacy of ICIs remains uncertain. In light of this important issue, we conducted a meta-analysis to assess the efficacy of ICIs relative to CT in NSCLC patients with asymptomatic and/or treated BMs. In addition, differences in survival benefit from ICIs between patients with and without asymptomatic and/or treated BMs were also evaluated.

MATERIALS AND METHODS

Literature Search Strategy

This meta-analysis was conducted in accordance with the Preferred Reporting Items for Systematic Reviews and Meta-analysis (PRISMA) criteria (22) (**Supplementary File, Table S1**). A systematic literature search of PubMed, Embase, Cochrane Library, and Web of Science up to November 10, 2020, was performed by two authors (LD and JQ) independently. Abstracts of recent international scientific meetings, including the American Society of Clinical Oncology (ASCO), European Society for Medical Oncology (ESMO), and World Conference on Lung Cancer (WCLC), were also inspected. The reference lists of relevant studies were checked for additional articles. The detailed search strategy is shown in **Supplementary File, Table S2**.

Inclusion and Exclusion Criteria

Studies were included if they met the following criteria: (1) phase II and III trials in metastatic NSCLC; (2) compared ICIs (alone or in combination with other agents) with CT; (3) data regarding patients with and without BMs could be retrieved, respectively; (4) reported overall survival (OS) or progression-free survival (PFS) data in each arm; and (5) published in English. Retrospective studies were not considered eligible. If studies had multiple publications, the most recent one was used. Conference abstracts could be included in the meta-analysis if they reported OS and/or PFS data according to patients' BMs status.

Data Extraction

Two authors (SL and HZ) independently extracted the following information from each included trial: trial name/first author, design, region, number of patients with and without BMs, interventions, hazard ratios (HRs), and their 95% confidence intervals (CIs) of OS and PFS.

Quality Assessment

The risk of bias of individual studies was assessed by two authors (SL and HZ) independently, using the Cochrane Risk of Bias Tool (23), which consists of the following domains: sequence generation, allocation concealment, blinding, incomplete data, and selective reporting. The studies were finally classified as low (all domains indicated as low risk), high (one or more domains indicated as high risk), and unclear risk of bias (more than three domains indicated as unclear risk).

Statistical Analysis

Statistical analysis was performed using the software Review Manager 5.3 (Cochrane Collaboration, Oxford, UK). The primary outcomes of interest were OS and PFS. HRs and their 95% CIs were used as summary statistics. A statistical test for heterogeneity was conducted using the Chi-square (χ^2) and I-square (I^2) test with significance set at $P < 0.10$ and/or $I^2 > 50\%$. If significant heterogeneity existed, a random-effects analysis model was used; otherwise, a fixed-effects model was used. In addition, we performed subgroup analyses according to ICI monotherapy, ICI combination therapy, first-line treatment with ICIs, and subsequent-line treatment with ICIs. The differences in the effect of ICIs were assessed using the χ^2 test and expressed as P for interaction. The stability of the pooled results was evaluated by a sensitivity analysis in which the data of an individual study were removed each time. The funnel plot, Begg's test (24), and Egger's linear regression test (25) were performed to investigate any potential publication bias. *P*-values < 0.05 were generally considered statistically significant. However, for multiple interaction tests in subgroup analyses, a *P*-value of 0.05÷K (K, number of subgroups) was used as the threshold for significance in light of the correction for multiplicity (26).

RESULTS

Literature Search and Study Selection

A total of 1,161 studies were identified from the initial literature search (n = 173 for PubMed, n = 511 for Embase, n = 104 for

Web of science, n = 170 for Cochrane Library, and n = 203 for meetings), and 41 potentially eligible reports were retrieved for detailed review (**Figure 1**). The relevant references were also reviewed for missed studies. Finally, 17 eligible articles (3–19) reporting 15 RCTs (14 phase 3 and 1 phase 2 trials) with 10,358 patients (1,199 with and 9,159 without asymptomatic/treated BMs) were included in the meta-analysis. Most of the RCTs (3, 5–9, 11–18) stated clearly that patients with meningeal metastasis were excluded, whereas the other three trials (4, 10, 19) did not provide information for whether patients with meningeal metastasis were excluded. The clinical and demographic characteristics of included studies are shown in **Table 1** and **Supplementary File**: **Table S3**. Twelve studies provided OS data, and 13 studies reported PFS data. Given that two studies (20, 21) provided pooled data of KEYNOTE-010 (3), -024 (4), and -042 (5) trials, and KEYNOTE-021 (6), -189 (7), and -407 (8) trials, respectively, the pooled data were used instead of data from the individual trials in this meta-analysis. The median sample sizes of BMs and non-BMs arms were 72 participants (range: 15–152) and 514 participants (range: 277–1204), respectively.

Assessment of Included Studies and Publication Bias

The risk of bias in included RCTs is summarized in **Supplementary File, Figure S1**. Only one trial (19) was judged as having an unclear risk of bias, as it had more than three domains for indicating them an unclear risk. The remaining trials were rated with a low risk of bias. The Begg's and Egger's test results indicated no publication bias in OS (P = 0.71 and P = 0.57) and PFS (P = 0.12 and P = 0.99). The funnel plot is shown in **Supplementary File, Figure S2**.

Effect of ICIs on OS and PFS in Patients With and Without BMs

ICIs were associated with significantly longer OS and PFS than those in CT either in patients with (n = 1048; HR, 0.65; 95% CI, 0.51–0.82 and n = 961; HR, 0.60; 95% CI, 0.45–0.79) or without BMs (n = 7952; HR, 0.74; 95% CI, 0.70–0.78 and n = 7038; HR, 0.70; 95% CI, 0.57–0.86); no significant differences were observed in the pooled HRs for OS ($P_{interaction}$ = 0.29) and PFS ($P_{interaction}$ = 0.37) between the two patient populations (**Figure 2**). Heterogeneity was observed for OS (I^2 = 53%, P = 0.04) and PFS (I^2 = 58%, P = 0.01) in patients with BMs and for PFS in patients without BMs (I^2 = 88%, P < 0.0001) (**Figure 2**).

Subgroup Analyses

Results of ICI efficacy in patients with and without BMs according to subgroups are shown in **Figure 3**. ICI monotherapy, ICI combination therapy, and first-line treatment with ICIs significantly improved OS and PFS compared with that in CT both for patients with and without

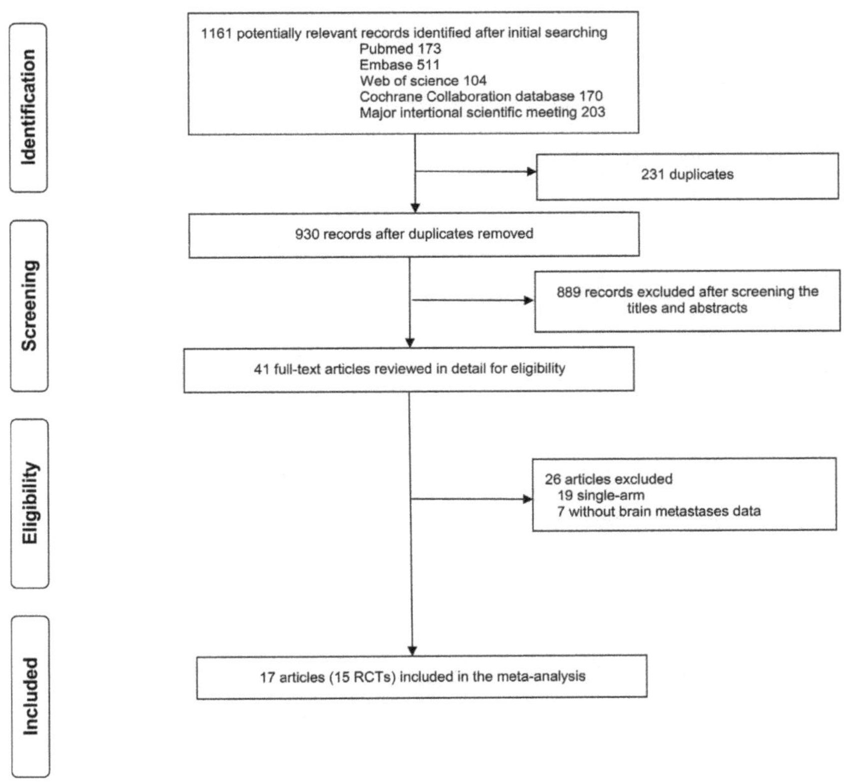

FIGURE 1 | Literature search and selection. RCTs, randomized control trials.

TABLE 1 | Clinical characteristics of included trials.

Trial/Year	Phase	Treatment line	Primary endpoint	Median follow-up (months)	Treatment	Size (with/ without BMs)	ICIs class	With BMs		Without BMs	
								OS	PFS	OS	PFS
								HR (95% CI)	HR (95% CI)	HR (95% CI)	HR (95% CI)
Keynote-010/ 2016 (3)	3	≥2	OS, PFS	13·1	Pembrolizumab	104/586	Anti-PD-1	0.83 (0.62–1.10)	0.96 (0.73–1.25)	0.78 (0.71–0.85)	0.91 (0.84–0.99)
					Doctaxel	48/295					
Keynote-024/ 2016 (4)	3	1	PFS	11.2	Pembrolizumab	18/136	Anti-PD-1	0.83 (0.62–1.10)	0.96 (0.73–1.25)	0.78 (0.71–0.85)	0.91 (0.84–0.99)
					PP/GP/PC	10/141					
Keynote-042/ 2019 (5)	3	1	OS	12.8	Pembrolizumab	35/602	Anti-PD-1	0.83 (0.62–1.10)	0.96 (0.73–1.25)	0.78 (0.71–0.85)	0.91 (0.84–0.99)
					PC/PP	35/602					
Keynote-021/ 2016 (6)	2	1	ORR	10.6	Pembrolizumab+ PP	9/51	Anti-PD-1	0.48 (0.32–0.70)	0.44 (0.31–0.62)	0.63 (0.53–0.75)	0.55 (0.48–0.63)
					PP	6/57					
Keynote-189/ 2018 (7)	3	1	OS, PFS	10.5	Pembrolizumab+ PP	73/337	Anti-PD-1	0.48 (0.32–0.70)	0.44 (0.31–0.62)	0.63 (0.53–0.75)	0.55 (0.48–0.63)
					PP	35/171					
Keynote-407/ 2018 (8)	3	1	OS, PFS	7.8	Pembrolizumab+ PC/CnP	20/258	Anti-PD-1	0.48 (0.32–0.70)	0.44 (0.31–0.62)	0.63 (0.53–0.75)	0.55 (0.48–0.63)
					PC/CnP	24/257					
CheckMate-057/ 2015 (9)	3	≥2	OS	13.2	Nivolumab	34/258	Anti-PD-1	1.04 (0.62–1.76)	0.80 (0.47–1.36)	0.71 (0.58–0.88)	0.92 (0.76–1.12)
					Doctaxel	34/256					
CheckMate-078/ 2019 (10)	3	≥2	OS	8.8	Nivolumab	45/293	Anti-PD-1	0.82 (0.42–1.60)	0.62 (0.35–1.10)	0.70 (0.53–0.92)	0.79 (0.62–1.00)
					Doctaxel	27/139					
CheckMate-227/ 2019 (11, 12)	3	1	OS	28.3	Nivolumab+ Ipilimumab	64/519	Anti-PD-1+ Anti-CTLA-4	0.64 (0.42–0.98)	NR	0.75 (0.64–0.88)	NR
					Platinum-based	52/532					
CheckMate-9LA/ 2020 (13)	3	1	OS	8·1	Nivolumab+ Ipilimumab+CT	65/296	Anti-PD-1+ Anti-CTLA-4	0.38 (0.24–0.61)	NR	0.75 (0.61–0.92)	NR
					CT	57/301					
OAK/2019 (14, 15)	3	≥2	OS	21	Atezolizumab	61/364	Anti-PD-L1	0.74 (0.49–1.13)	0.38 (0.16–0.91)	0.74 (0.63-0.88)	0.99 (0.50–1.97)
					Doc	62/363					
SHR-1210-303/ 2019 (16)	3	1	PFS	11.9	Camrelizumab+ PC	10/194	Anti-PD-1	NR	0.14 (0.01–0.88)	NR	0.61 (0.46–0.81)
					PC	6/201					
ORIENT-11/ 2020 (17)	3	1	PFS	8.9	Sintilimab+PP	36/230	Anti-PD-1	NR	0.58 (0.28–1.18)	NR	0.47 (0.34–0.64)
					PP	22/109					
EMPOWER-Lung1/2020 (18)	3	1	PFS、OS	10.8	Cemiplimab	44/312	Anti-PD-1	0.44 (0.19–1.07)	0.49 (0.27–0.90)	0.71 (0.54-0.92)	0.62 (0.51–0.76)

(Continued)

TABLE 1 | Continued

Trial/Year	Phase	Treatment line	Primary endpoint	Median follow-up (months)	Treatment	Size (with/ without BMs)	ICIs class	With BMs		Without BMs	
								OS	PFS	OS	PFS
								HR (95% CI)	HR (95% CI)	HR (95% CI)	HR (95% CI)
					CT	39/315					
Lee/2020 (19)	3	1	PFS	7.4	Nivolumab+PC+ Bev	36/239	Anti-PD-1	NR	0.65 (0.36–1.18)	NR	NR
					PC+Bev	41/234					

OS, overall survival; PFS, progression-free survival; ORR, objective response rate; HR, hazard ratio; 95%CI, confidence interval; ICIs, immune checkpoint inhibitors; BMs, brain metastases; CT, chemotherapy; PP, pemetrexed-cisplatin/carboplatin; PC, paclitaxel-carboplatin; CnP, paclitaxel-nanoparticle albumin-bound-carboplatin; GP, gemcitabine-cisplatin; Bev, bevacizumab; NR, not reported.

BMs (with the HR and upper limit of the 95% CI smaller than 1 for each comparison). Subsequent-line treatment with ICIs was correlated with significant improvement in OS for patients without BMs (HR, 0.72; 95% CI, 0.64–0.82) but not for those with BMs (HR, 0.84; 95% CI, 0.63–1.13), whereas significant improvement in PFS was observed for patients with BMs (HR, 0.64; 95% CI, 0.45–0.91), but not for those without BMs (HR, 0.87; 95% CI, 0.75–1.01). As there were four subgroups either for OS or PFS, a *P-value* < 0.013 (0.05÷4) was considered to be statistically significant for interaction tests. As such, there was no significant difference in OS and PFS benefit between patients with and without BMs in each subgroup, including ICI combination therapy (OS: HR, 0.49 *vs.* 0.71; $P_{interaction}$ = 0.02; PFS: HR, 0.48 *vs.* 0.55; $P_{interaction}$ = 0.41), ICI monotherapy (OS: HR, 0.81 *vs.* 0.76; $P_{interaction}$ = 0.53; PFS: HR, 0.69 *vs.* 0.82; $P_{interaction}$ = 0.36), first-line treatment with ICIs (OS: HR, 0.56 *vs.* 0.74; $P_{interaction}$ = 0.1; PFS: HR, 0.58 *vs.* 0.62; $P_{interaction}$ = 0.75), and subsequent-line treatment with ICIs (OS: HR, 0.84 *vs.* 0.72; $P_{interaction}$ = 0.35; PFS: HR, 0.64 *vs.* 0.87; $P_{interaction}$ = 0.12). There was also no significant difference in OS benefit in subgroups of ICI monotherapy with PD-1 inhibitors, ICI monotherapy in patients with PD-L1 expression ≥1%, dual ICIs combination (**Supplementary File**: **Figure S3**).

Subgroup analyses in patients with and without BMs are detailed in **Figure 4**. As there were two subgroups for OS or PFS in patients with or without BMs, a *P-value* < 0.025 (0.05÷2) was considered to be statistically significant for interaction tests. For patients with BMs, a greater OS benefit from ICI combination therapy than that from ICI monotherapy was observed (HR, 0.49 *vs.* 0.81; $P_{interaction}$ = 0.005). No significant difference in OS benefit between first-line treatment with ICIs and subsequent-line treatment with ICIs was observed (HR, 0.56 *vs.* 0.84; $P_{interaction}$ = 0.07). There were also no significant differences in PFS benefit between ICI combination therapy and ICI monotherapy (HR, 0.49 *vs.* 0.69; $P_{interaction}$ = 0.13), and first-line treatment with ICIs and subsequent-line treatment with ICIs (HR, 0.58 *vs.* 0.64; $P_{interaction}$ = 0.71).

For patients without BMs, no significant differences in OS benefit from ICIs were observed between ICI combination therapy and ICI monotherapy (HR, 0.71 *vs.* 0.76; $P_{interaction}$ = 0.27), and first-line treatment with ICIs and subsequent-line treatment with ICIs (HR, 0.75 *vs.* 0.72; $P_{interaction}$ = 0.64). However, ICI combination therapy achieved superior PFS compared with that in ICI monotherapy (HR, 0.55 *vs.* 0.82; $P_{interaction}$ < 0.0001). There were no significant differences in PFS benefit between first-line and subsequent-line treatment with ICIs (HR, 0.62 *vs.* 0.87; $P_{interaction}$ = 0.04).

Sensitivity Analysis

Results of sensitivity analysis are shown in **Supplementary File, Figure S4**. When individual studies were removed one at a time from the analyses for OS and PFS, the corresponding pooled HRs were not markedly altered by any single study (HR lies between 0.61 and 0.70 for OS, and between 0.53 and 0.66 for PFS), indicating q relatively good stability of the presented results.

DISCUSSION

Currently, ICIs have been the standard first-line treatments for metastatic NSCLC lacking sensitizing EGFR or ALK or other druggable mutations. However, whether the presence of asymptomatic and/or treated can decrease the survival benefit from ICIs remains uncertain. This is a comprehensive meta-analysis focusing on the effect of asymptomatic and/or treated BMs on the efficacy of ICIs in metastatic NSCLC. This study included 15 RCTs involving 10358 patients (1,199 with and 9,159 without BMs). It showed that ICIs were associated with longer OS and PFS than that in CT either in patients with or without BMs; no significant differences in the pooled HRs for OS (HR, 0.65 *vs.* 0.60; $P_{interaction}$ = 0.29) and PFS (HR, 0.74 *vs.* 0.70; $P_{interaction}$ = 0.37) were observed, suggesting a comparable efficacy of ICIs for the two patient populations.

The exact mechanism of action of ICIs in the central nervous system (CNS) is yet to be determined; however, It is likely related to modified immune cell activity rather than direct action in the brain (27), and immune cell trafficking (28) and T-cell priming in the extracranial compartment could be essential for producing an effective immune response in the CNS (29). Moreover, lymphatic vessels in the dura mater were found to be potentially capable of allowing CNS antigen presentation in the peripheral lymph nodes (30), which might be another potential

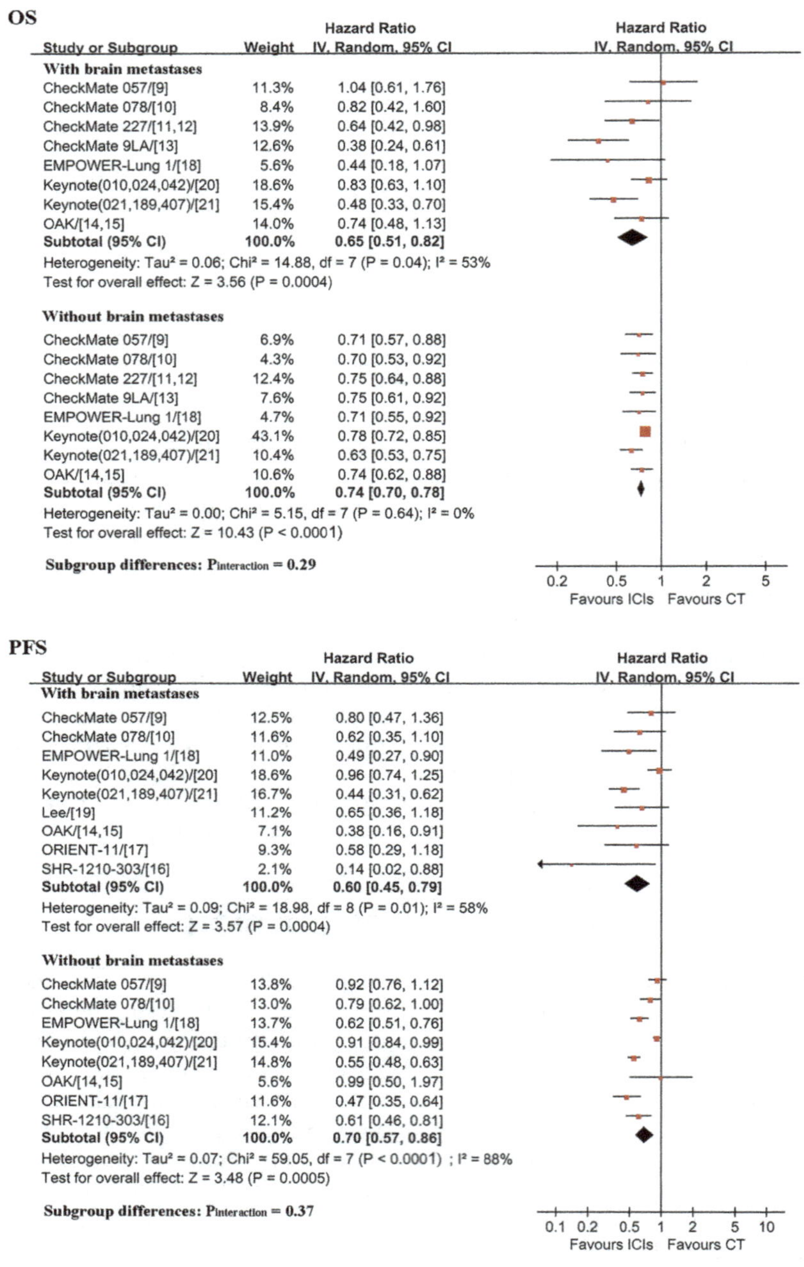

FIGURE 2 | Comparison of ICIs efficacy between patients with and without brain metastases. OS, overall survival; PFS, progression-free survival; ICIs, immune checkpoint inhibitors; CT, chemotherapy; HR, hazard ratio; CI, confidence interval.

mechanism of action. Recently, several studies have reported a good activity of ICIs in CNS (31, 32). In a phase II trial, pembrolizumab resulted in a 33% objective CNS response rate in NSCLC patients with untreated BMs (31). An exploratory analysis of the phase III OAK study in patients with asymptomatic/treated BMs showed that new brain lesion-free probability at 24 months was 76.6% for atezolizumab and 0% for docetaxel (15). The additional intracranial activity of ICIs might be an explanation for our finding that patients with asymptomatic and/or treated BMs could obtain similar survival benefits from ICIs to patients without BMs.

The choice of monotherapy or combination therapy is an important factor that could affect the efficacy of ICIs in metastatic NSCLC. Current NCCN guidelines have recommended ICI monotherapy only for patients with high PD-L1 level, such as tumor proportion score (TPS) ≥50%, whereas ICIs in combination with CT is recommended, regardless of PD-L1 expression (2). However, PD-L1 expression of BMs sites can be different from

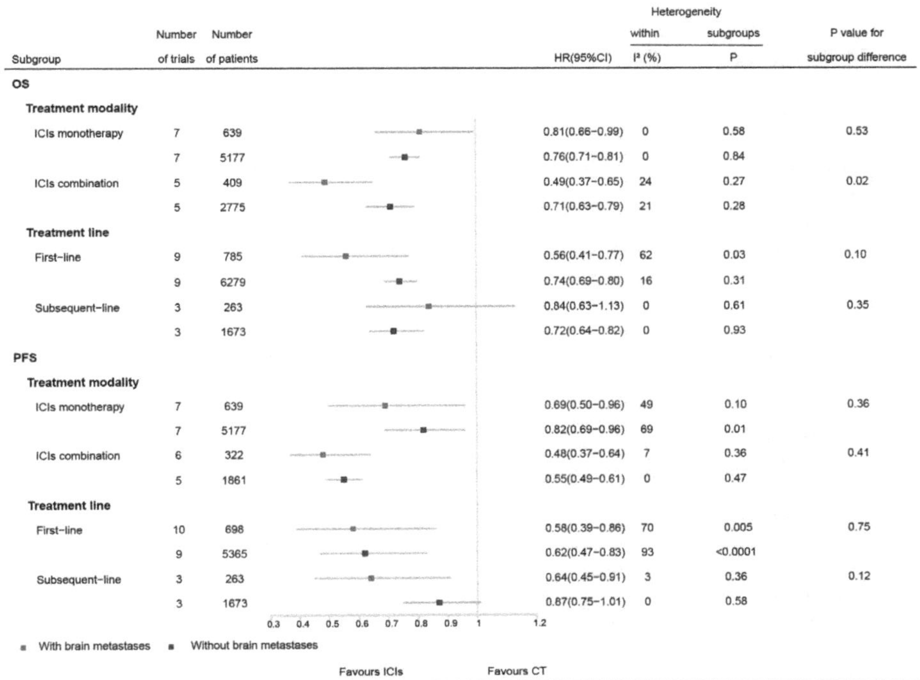

FIGURE 3 | Comparison of ICIs efficacy between patients with and without brain metastases by subgroups. OS, overall survival; PFS, progression-free survival; ICIs, immune checkpoint inhibitors; CT, chemotherapy; HR, hazard ratio; CI, confidence interval.

primary lung tumors because of the distinct immune microenvironment of CNS (33). Whether the PD-L1 level of the primary tumor can work as a predictor of the efficacy of ICIs in patients with BMs remains uncertain. In a phase 2 trial of pembrolizumab in NSCLC or melanoma patients with untreated BMs, 29.7% of patients with PD-L1 expression ≥1% had a brain metastasis response, but no responses were observed in those with PD-L1 expression <1% or unevaluable (32). In a pooled analysis of KEYNOTE-010 and -024 and -042 trials (20), although pembrolizumab improved clinical outcomes compared with that in CT in PD-L1 positive patients (TPS ≥1%), no survival benefits were observed for those with asymptomatic/treated BMs at baseline. Our study did not assess the correlation between PD-L1 expression and the efficacy of ICIs due to few studies reporting PD-L1 status for patients with BMs. In subgroup analyses of treatment modality, both ICI monotherapy and combination therapy achieved significantly longer OS and PFS compared with that in CT in patients with BMs, whereas a greater OS benefit from combination therapy was observed (HR, 0.49 *vs.* 0.81; $P_{interaction}$ = 0.005). Unexpectedly, we also found that patients with BMs could obtain more OS benefits from ICI combination therapy than that in patients without BMs. Despite our inability to provide a satisfactory explanation for this result, ICI combination therapy was likely to be the optimal choice for patients with asymptomatic and/or treated BMs based on the results above. Nevertheless, these findings need to be confirmed in large phase III trials.

Besides the first-line treatment with ICIs, several trials investigated the efficacy of ICI monotherapy as a subsequent-line treatment in NSCLC patients with treated BMs. Two phase III trials demonstrated that nivolumab achieved superior OS compared with that in docetaxel in previously treated advanced NSCLC, but the OS benefit was not observed in the subgroup of patients with treated, stable BMs at baseline (9, 10). However, in the exploratory analyses of the phase III OAK study (15), subsequent-line treatment with atezolizumab gained a trend OS benefit compared with that in docetaxel (HR, 0.74; 95% CI, 0.49–1.13) in patients with a history of asymptomatic or treated BMs. In our meta-analysis, subsequent-line treatment with ICIs significantly improved PFS compared with that in CT but failed to show a significant OS benefit in patients with asymptomatic and/or treated BMs. Whether subsequent-line treatment with combinations of immunotherapy, such as dual ICI combination or ICIs in combination with antiangiogenic agents, could be more effective in this patient population requires further investigation.

The selection of PD-1 or PD-L1 inhibitors might be another factor that influences the efficacy of ICIs. Results of a more recent meta-analysis showed that anti-PD-1 achieved superior OS and PFS compared with those in anti-PD-L1 in cancer patients (34). However, whether there is a difference in intracranial activity between the two ICI classes in NSCLC patients with BMs remains unclear. Since there was only one included trial providing information on PD-L1 inhibitors, we did not compare the efficacy of PD-1 with PD-L1 inhibitors for this patient population.

In fact, our meta-analysis included two types of BMs: previously treated or untreated asymptomatic BMs, and previously treated and stable symptomatic BMs. For patients

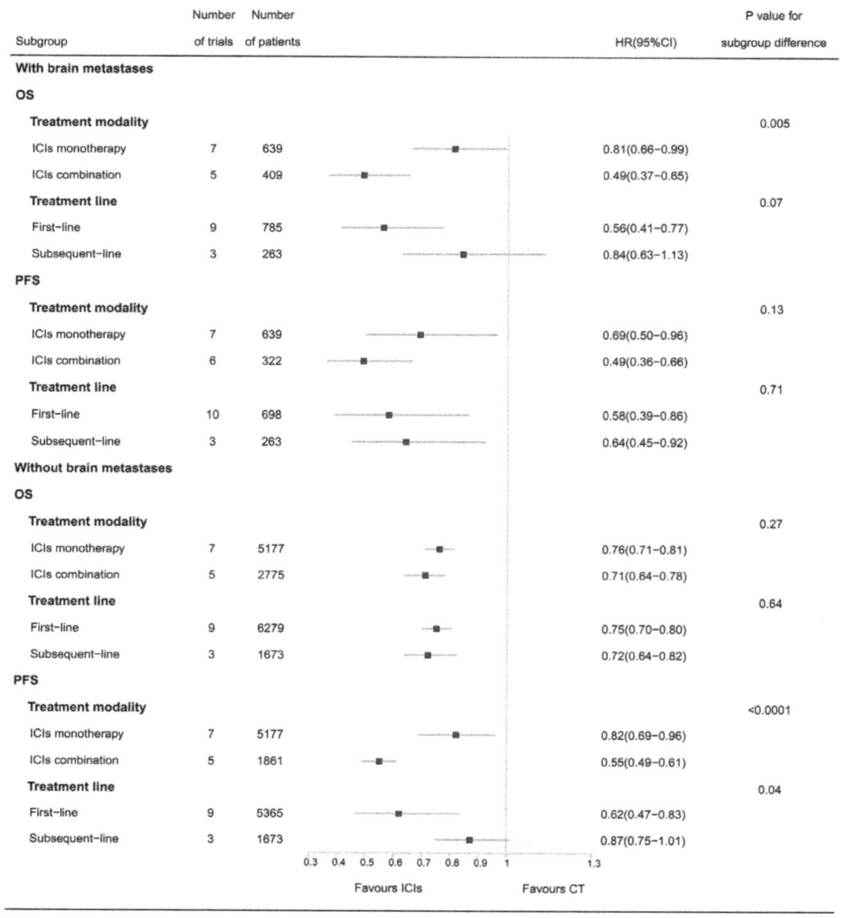

FIGURE 4 | Subgroup analyses of ICIs efficacy in patients with and without brain metastases. OS, overall survival; PFS, progression-free survival; ICIs, immune checkpoint inhibitors; CT, chemotherapy; HR, hazard ratio; CI, confidence interval.

with asymptomatic BMs, whether upfront brain irradiation before the start of ICI therapy is needed remains unclear because of the paucity of clinical trials assessing this. In a recent retrospective study on PD-L1, in ≥ 50% of advanced NSCLC patients treated with first-line pembrolizumab (35), a high intracranial response rate (iRR) of 67.5% was observed in patients with BMs. Of note, 80.0% (32/40) of the patients with BMs received brain irradiation prior to treatment with pembrolizumab, which might contribute to the high iRR. However, an iRR of 75% (6/8) was still observed in those without prior brain irradiation because their BMs were asymptomatic. In addition, Wakuda et al. also retrospectively reviewed NSCLC patients with PD-L1 ≥ 50% receiving first-line pembrolizumab (36). In their study, the BM group was divided into patients who previously received radiation for BMs before pembrolizumab (BM-T group) and those with no prior radiation for BMs (BM-not T group); and there were 53% (7/13) and 100% (10/10) patients with asymptomatic BMs in BM-T and BM-not T groups, respectively. They found that there was no significant difference in treatment efficacy between the BM-T and BM-not T groups. These findings suggest that upfront brain irradiation before first-line treatment with pembrolizumab may be spared for PD-L1 ≥ 50% NSCLC patients with asymptomatic BMs, whereas this strategy needs to be confirmed in phase 3 trials. Meanwhile, there is also a need to assess the value of brain irradiation prior to ICI therapy for asymptomatic BMs with low/negative PD-L1 expression in further trials.

A recently published pooled analysis of metastatic NSCLC patients (including 255 patients with BMs) from seven European centers investigated predictors of the efficacy of ICIs in patients with BMs (37). Active BMs (defined as patients with previously untreated BMs or patients with brain involvement that have progressed after previous local therapy), lower disease-specific Graded Prognostic Assessment (ds-GPA) score, and use of corticosteroids at the start of ICIs treatment were associated with poorer OS in multivariate analysis in the BMs subgroup (37). The patients with active BMs had brain PD significantly more often than that in patients with stable BMs (54.2% *vs.* 30%, p <0.001). Among patients with active BMs, PD-L1 expression ≥1% was associated with a higher intracranial RR: 35.7% *vs.* 11.1% in PD-

L1-negative patients (37). These results may help clinicians in the decision of whether to administer ICIs to a patient with NSCLC who has BMs. Nevertheless, given the retrospective nature of this analysis, the findings need to be confirmed by more robust clinical trials.

Currently, there are still insufficient unified criteria to assess the intracranial response in patients with BMs undergoing ICIs. Conventional methods, such as RECIST and WHO, evaluate tumor response only depending on the tumor shrinkage within a few weeks of initiating treatment (38). However, immunotherapy might demonstrate a delay in response, transient enlargement followed by tumor shrinkage, stable size, or the appearance of new lesions (39). Unlike the WHO and RECIST criteria, the modified immune-related Response Criteria (irRC) and immune-Related RECIST (irRECIST) criteria take the delayed response and new measurable lesions into account (39). Nevertheless, the two new criteria are mainly used for solid tumors of the whole body. RANO-BM was developed for assessing the therapeutic response of brain metastasis only. Intracranial response evaluation is based on a combination of tumor measurements, clinical status, and corticosteroid use (40). The use of immunotherapy in metastatic brain tumors leads to modifications in the RANO-BM criteria for these patients (iRANO-BM) (41). iRANO-BM is now thought to be a representative assessment criterion considering intracranial pseudoprogression after immunotherapy (41, 42).

Several previous meta-analyses (43–45) of metastatic NSCLC also investigated the efficacy of ICIs in patients with asymptomatic and/or treated BMs in subgroup analyses. However, a maximum of three trials was included in those studies for assessing this subgroup of patients, which would result in poor accuracy. Our meta-analysis specifically addressed this subject and included 11 additional RCTs (including six more recent phase 3 trials presented at the meeting of the ESMO/ASCO/WCLC in 2019 and 2020). Moreover, we performed subgroup analyses of ICI monotherapy, ICI combination therapy, first-line treatment with ICIs, and subsequent-line treatment with ICIs and compared the efficacy of ICIs between patients with and without BMs. The present meta-analysis would be more comprehensive in assessing the effect of asymptomatic and/or treated BMs on the efficacy of ICIs in metastatic NSCLC.

Nevertheless, our meta-analysis has several limitations. First, despite all included studies being RCTs and most of them being phase III trials, all data of patients with and without BMs were extracted from subgroup analyses of these RCTs, which might result in a potential imbalance in baseline characteristics between the two sets of patients. Second, some RCTs, such as IMpower series studies (46–50) and CheckMate 017 (51) and 026 (52), were excluded from our study because of the non-reporting of survival information of patients with BMs. This might result in a selection bias to some extent. Third, heterogeneity was observed for OS and PFS in patients with BMs, and for PFS in patients without BMs. Results of subgroup analyses suggested that treatment line and treatment modality may be two potential sources of heterogeneity. In addition, chemotherapy regimens were inconsistent among studies, which might also lead to heterogeneity. Finally, this study only assessed patients with asymptomatic and/or treated BMs; therefore, the conclusion should be interpreted with caution for patients with symptomatic, untreated brain disease.

In conclusion, there was no compelling statistical evidence that the efficacy of ICIs in metastatic NSCLC was modified by the presence of asymptomatic and/or treated BMs. Patients with BMs were likely to obtain more OS benefits from ICI combination therapy than that from monotherapy. Further RCTs specifically on this subject are needed to confirm these findings.

AUTHOR CONTRIBUTIONS

Conception and design: JD. Collection and assembly of data: SL and HZ. Data analysis and interpretation: all authors. All authors contributed to the article and approved the submitted version.

REFERENCES

1. Barnholtz-Sloan JS, Sloan AE, Davis FG, Vigneau FD, Lai P, Sawaya RE. Incidence Proportions of Brain Metastases in Patients Diagnosed (1973 to 2001) in the Metropolitan Detroit Cancer Surveillance System. *J Clin Oncol* (2004) 22:2865–72. doi: 10.1200/JCO.2004.12.149
2. National Comprehensive Cancer Network. *NCCN Clinical Practice Guidelines in Oncology for Non-Small Cell Lung Cancer* (2020). Available at: www.nccn.org/patients.
3. Herbst RS, Baas P, Kim DW, Felip E, Pérez-Gracia JL, Han JY, et al. Pembrolizumab Versus Docetaxel for Previously Treated, PD-L1-Positive, Advanced Non-Small-Cell Lung Cancer (KEYNOTE-010): A Randomised Controlled Trial. *Lancet* (2016) 387:1540–50. doi: 10.1016/S0140-6736(15)01281-7
4. Reck M, Rodríguez-Abreu D, Robinson AG, Hui R, Csőszi T, Fülöp A, et al. KEYNOTE-024 Investigators. Pembrolizumab Versus Chemotherapy for PD-L1-Positive Non-Small-Cell Lung Cancer. *N Engl J Med* (2016) 375:1823–33. doi: 10.1056/NEJMoa1606774
5. Mok TSK, Wu YL, Kudaba I, Kowalski DM, Cho BC, Turna HZ, et al. Pembrolizumab Versus Chemotherapy for Previously Untreated, PD-L1-expressing, Locally Advanced or Metastatic Non-Small-Cell Lung Cancer (KEYNOTE-042): A Randomised, Open-Label, Controlled, Phase 3 Trial. *Lancet* (2019) 393:1819–30. doi: 10.1016/S0140-6736(18)32409-7
6. Langer CJ, Gadgeel SM, Borghaei H, Papadimitrakopoulou VA, Patnaik A, Powell SF, et al. Carboplatin and Pemetrexed With or Without Pembrolizumab for Advanced, Non-Squamous Non-Small-Cell Lung Cancer: A Randomised, Phase 2 Cohort of the Open-Label KEYNOTE-021 Study. *Lancet Oncol* (2016) 17:1497–508. doi: 10.1016/S1470-2045(16)30498-3
7. Gandhi L, Rodríguez-Abreu D, Gadgeel S, Esteban E, Felip E, De Angelis F, et al. Pembrolizumab Plus Chemotherapy in Metastatic Non-Small-Cell Lung Cancer. *N Engl J Med* (2018) 378:2078–92. doi: 10.1056/NEJMoa1810865
8. Paz-Ares L, Luft A, Vicente D, Tafreshi A, Gümüş M, Mazières J, et al. Pembrolizumab Plus Chemotherapy for Squamous Non-Small-Cell Lung Cancer. *N Engl J Med* (2018) 379:2040–51. doi: 10.1056/NEJMoa1810865
9. Borghaei H, Paz-Ares L, Horn L, Spigel DR, Steins M, Ready NE, et al. Nivolumab Versus Docetaxel in Advanced Nonsquamous Non-Small-Cell Lung Cancer. *N Engl J Med* (2015) 373:1627 39. doi: 10.1056/NEJMoa1507643
10. Wu YL, Lu S, Cheng Y, Zhou C, Wang J, Mok T, et al. Nivolumab Versus Docetaxel in a Predominantly Chinese Patient Population With Previously Treated Advanced NSCLC: CheckMate 078 Randomized Phase III Clinical Trial. *J Thorac Oncol* (2019) 14:867–75. doi: 10.1016/j.jtho.2019.01.006

11. Hellmann MD, Paz-Ares L, Bernabe Caro R, Zurawski B, Kim SW, Carcereny Costa E, et al. Nivolumab Plus Ipilimumab in Advanced Non-Small-Cell Lung Cancer. *N Engl J Med* (2019) 381:2020–31. doi: 10.1056/NEJMoa1910231
12. Peters S, Ramalingam S, Paz-Ares L, Caro B, Zurawski B, Kim S, et al. Nivolumab + Low Dose Ipilimumab Versus Platinum Doublet Chemotherapy as First Line Treatment for Advanced Non Small Cell Lung Cancer: CheckMate 227 Part 1 Final Analysis. *Paper Presented at Meeting ESMO;* (2019) Abstract7128. doi: 10.1093/annonc/mdz394.075
13. Paz-Ares L, Ciuleanu TE, Cobo M, Schenker M, Zurawski B, Menezes J, et al. First-Line Nivolumab Plus Ipilimumab Combined With Two Cycles of Chemotherapy in Patients With Non-Small-Cell Lung Cancer (CheckMate 9LA): An International, Randomised, Open-Label, Phase 3 Trial. *Lancet Oncol* (2021) 22:198–211. doi: 10.1016/S1470-2045(20)30641-0
14. Rittmeyer A, Barlesi F, Waterkamp D, Park K, Ciardiello F, von Pawel J, et al. Atezolizumab Versus Docetaxel in Patients With Previously Treated Non-Small-Cell Lung Cancer (OAK): A Phase 3, Open-Label, Multicentre Randomised Controlled Trial. *Lancet* (2017) 389:255–65. doi: 10.1016/S0140-6736(16)32517-X
15. Gadgeel SM, Lukas RV, Goldschmidt J, Conkling P, Park K, Cortinovis D, et al. Atezolizumab in Patients With Advanced Non-Small Cell Lung Cancer and History of Asymptomatic, Treated Brain Metastases: Exploratory Analyses of the Phase III OAK Study. *Lung Cancer* (2019) 128:105–12. doi: 10.1016/j.lungcan.2018.12.017
16. Zhou C, Chen G, Huang Y, Zhou J, Lin L, Feng J, et al. Camrelizumab Plus Carboplatin and Pemetrexed Versus Chemotherapy Alone in Chemotherapy-Naive Patients With Advanced Non-Squamous Non-Small-Cell Lung Cancer (CameL): A Randomised, Open-Label, Multicentre, Phase 3 Trial. *Lancet Respir Med* (2021) 9:305–14. doi: 10.1016/S2213-2600(20)30365-9
17. Yang Y, Wang Z, Fang J, Yu Q, Han B, Cang S, et al. Efficacy and Safety of Sintilimab Plus Pemetrexed and Platinum as First-Line Treatment for Locally Advanced or Metastatic Nonsquamous NSCLC: A Randomized, Double-Blind, Phase 3 Study (Oncology pRogram by InnovENT Anti-PD-1-11). *J Thorac Oncol* (2020) 15:1636–46. doi: 10.1016/j.jtho.2020.07.014
18. Sezer A, Kilickap S, Gümüş M, Bondarenko I, Özgüroğlu M, Gogishvili M, et al. Cemiplimab Monotherapy for First-Line Treatment of Advanced Non-Small-Cell Lung Cancer With PD-L1 of at Least 50%: A Multicentre, Open-Label, Global, Phase 3, Randomised, Controlled Trial. *Lancet* (2021) 397:592–604. doi:10.1016/S0140-6736(21)00228-2
19. Lee J, Sugawara S, Kang JH, Kim HR, Inui N, Hida T, et al. Randomized Phase III Trial of Nivolumab in Combination With Carboplatin, Paclitaxel, and Bevacizumab as First-Line Treatment for Patients With Advanced or Recurrent Non-Squamous NSCLC. *Paper Presented at Meeting ESMO* (2020) Abstract LBA54. doi:10.1016/j.annonc.2020.08.2287
20. Mansfield AS, Herbst RS, Castro J Jr, Hui R, Peled N, Kim DW, et al. Outcomes With Pembrolizumab (Pembro) Monotherapy in Patients (Pts) With PD-L1–Positive NSCLC With Brain Metastases: Pooled Analysis of KEYNOTE-001, -010, -024, and -042. *Paper Presented at Meeting ESMO;* (2019) Abstract4580. doi: 10.1093/annonc/mdz260.004
21. Powell SF, Rodriguez Abreu D, Langer CJ, Tafreshi A, Paz–Ares L, Kopp HG, et al. Pembrolizumab (Pembro) Plus Platinum-Based Chemotherapy (Chemo) in NSCLC With Brain Metastases: Pooled Analysis of KEYNOTE-021, 189, and 407. *Paper Presented at Meeting ESMO;* (2019) 4597. doi: 10.1093/annonc/mdz260.005
22. Moher D, Liberati A, Tetzlaff J, Altman DG. Preferred Reporting Items for Systematic Reviews and Meta-Analyses: The PRISMA Statement. *Int J Surg* (2010) 8:336–41. doi: 10.1016/j.ijsu.2010.02.007
23. Higgins JP, Altman DG, Gøtzsche PC, Jüni P, Moher D, Oxman AD, et al. The Cochrane Collaboration's Tool for Assessing Risk of Bias in Randomised Trials. *BMJ* (2011) 343:d5928. doi: 10.1136/bmj.d5928
24. Begg CB, Mazumdar M. Operating Characteristics of a Rank Correlation Test for Publication Bias. *Biometrics* (1994) 50:1088–101. doi: 10.2307/2533446
25. Egger M, Davey Smith G, Schneider M, Minder C. Bias in Meta-Analysis Detected by a Simple, Graphical Test. *BMJ* (1997) 315:629–34. doi: 10.1136/bmj.315.7109.629
26. Wang R, Lagakos SW, Ware JH, Hunter DJ, Drazen JM. Statistics in Medicine–Reporting of Subgroup Analyses in Clinical Trials. *N Engl J Med* (2007) 357:2189–94. doi: 10.1056/NEJMsr077003
27. Eguren-Santamaria I, Sanmamed MF, Goldberg SB, Kluger HM, Idoate MA, Lu BY, et al. Pd-1/Pd-L1 Blockers in NSCLC Brain Metastases: Challenging Paradigms and Clinical Practice. *Clin Cancer Res* (2020) 26:4186–97. doi: 10.1158/1078-0432.CCR-20-0798
28. Crinò L, Bronte G, Bidoli P, Cravero P, Minenza E, Cortesi E, et al. Nivolumab and Brain 577 Metastases in Patients With Advanced Non-Squamous Non-Small Cell Lung Cancer. *Lung Cancer* (2019) 129:35–40. doi: 10.1016/j.lungcan.2018.12.025
29. Taggart D, Andreou T, Scott KJ, Williams J, Rippaus N, Brownlie RJ, et al. Anti-PD-1/Anti-CTLA-4 Efficacy in Melanoma Brain Metastases Depends on Extracranial Disease and Augmentation of CD8+ T Cell Trafficking. *Proc Natl Acad Sci* (2018) 115:E1540–49. doi: 10.1073/pnas.1714089115
30. Engelhardt B, Vajkoczy P, Weller RO. The Movers and Shapers in Immune Privilege of the CNS. *Nat Immunol* (2017) 18:123–31. doi: 10.1038/ni.3666
31. Goldberg SB, Gettinger SN, Mahajan A, Chiang AC, Herbst RS, Sznol M, et al. Pembrolizumab for Patients With Melanoma or Non-Small-Cell Lung Cancer and Untreated Brain Metastases: Early Analysis of a Non-Randomised, Open-Label, Phase 2 Trial. *Lancet Oncol* (2016) 17:976–83. doi: 10.1016/S1470-2045(16)30053-5
32. Goldberg SB, Schalper KA, Gettinger SN, Mahajan A, Herbst RS, Chiang AC, et al. Pembrolizumab for Management of Patients With NSCLC and Brain Metastases: Long-Term Results and Biomarker Analysis From a Non-Randomised, Open-Label, Phase 2 Trial. *Lancet Oncol* (2020) 21:655–63. doi: 10.1016/S1470-2045(20)30111-X
33. Mansfield AS, Aubry MC, Moser JC, Harrington SM, Dronca RS, Park SS, et al. Temporal and Spatial Discordance of Programmed Cell Death-Ligand 1 Expression and Lymphocyte Tumor Infiltration Between Paired Primary Lesions and Brain Metastases in Lung Cancer. *Ann Oncol* (2016) 27:1953–58. doi: 10.1093/annonc/mdw289
34. Duan J, Cui L, Zhao X, Bai H, Cai S, Wang G, et al. Use of Immunotherapy With Programmed Cell Death 1 *vs* Programmed Cell Death Ligand 1 Inhibitors in Patients With Cancer: A Systematic Review and Meta-Analysis. *JAMA Oncol* (2020) 6:375–84. doi: 10.1001/jamaoncol.2019.5367
35. Metro G, Banna GL, Signorelli D, Gili A, Galetta D, Galli G, et al. Efficacy of Pembrolizumab Monotherapy in Patients With or Without Brain Metastases From Advanced Non-Small Cell Lung Cancer With a PD-L1 Expression ≥50%. *J Immunother* (2020) 43:299–306. doi: 10.1097/CJI.0000000000000340
36. Wakuda K, Yabe M, Kodama H, Nishioka N, Miyawaki T, Miyawaki E, et al. Efficacy of Pembrolizumab in Patients With Brain Metastasis Caused by Previously Untreated Non-Small Cell Lung Cancer With High Tumor PD-L1 Expression. *Lung Cancer* (2021) 151:60–8. doi: 10.1016/j.lungcan.2020.11.009
37. Hendriks LEL, Henon C, Auclin E, Mezquita L, Ferrara R, Audigier–Valette C, et al. Outcome of Patients With Non-Small Cell Lung Cancer and Brain Metastases Treated With Checkpoint Inhibitors. *J Thorac Oncol* (2019) 14:1244–54. doi: 10.1016/j.jtho.2019.02.009
38. Majd N, Dasgupta P, de Groot J. Cancer Imaging in Immunotherapy. *Adv Exp Med Biol* (2020) 1244:309–24. doi: 10.1007/978-3-030-41008-7_18
39. Wolchok JD, Hoos A, O'Day S, Weber JS, Hamid O, Lebbé C, et al. Guidelines for the Evaluation of Immune Therapy Activity in Solid Tumors: Immune-Related Response Criteria. *Clin Cancer Res* (2009) 15:7412. doi: 10.1158/1078-0432.CCR-09-1624
40. Wen PY, Chang SM, Van den Bent MJ, Vogelbaum MA, Macdonald DR, Lee EQ. Response Assessment in Neuro-Oncology Clinical Trials. *J Clin Oncol* (2017) 35:2439. doi: 10.1200/JCO.2017.72.7511
41. Okada H, Weller M, Huang R, Finocchiaro G, Gilbert MR, Wick W, et al. Immunotherapy Response Assessment in Neuro-Oncology: A Report of the RANO Working Group. *Lancet Oncol* (2015) 16(15):e534–42. doi: 10.1016/S1470-2045(15)00088-1
42. Chukwueke U, Wen P. Use of the Response Assessment in Neuro-Oncology (RANO) Criteria in Clinical Trials and Clinical Practice. *CNS Oncol* (2019) 8:28. doi: 10.2217/cns-2018-0007
43. Yang K, Li J, Bai C, Sun Z, Zhao L. Efficacy of Immune Checkpoint Inhibitors in Non-Small-Cell Lung Cancer Patients With Different Metastatic Sites: A Systematic Review and Meta-Analysis. *Front Oncol* (2020) 10:1098. doi: 10.3389/fonc.2020.01098
44. Lee CK, Man J, Lord S, Cooper W, Links M, Gebski V, et al. Clinical and Molecular Characteristics Associated With Survival Among Patients Treated With Checkpoint Inhibitors for Advanced Non-Small Cell Lung Carcinoma: A Systematic Review and Meta-Analysis. *JAMA Oncol* (2018) 4:210–16. doi: 10.1001/jamaoncol.2017.4427

45. El-Osta H, Jafri S. Predictors for Clinical Benefit of Immune Checkpoint Inhibitors in Advanced Non-Small-Cell Lung Cancer: A Meta-Analysis. *Immunotherapy* (2019) 11:189–99. doi: 10.2217/imt-2018-0086
46. West H, McCleod M, Hussein M, Morabito A, Rittmeyer A, Conter HJ, et al. Atezolizumab in Combination With Carboplatin Plus Nab-Paclitaxel Chemotherapy Compared With Chemotherapy Alone as First-Line Treatment for Metastatic Non-Squamous Non-Small-Cell Lung Cancer (Impower130): A Multicentre, Randomised, Open-Label, Phase 3 Trial. *Lancet Oncol* (2019) 20:924–37. doi: 10.1016/S1470-2045(19)30167-6
47. Jotte R, Cappuzzo F, Vynnychenko I, Stroyakovskiy D, Rodríguez-Abreu D, Hussein M, et al. Atezolizumab in Combination With Carboplatin and Nab-Paclitaxel in Advanced Squamous NSCLC (Impower131): Results From a Randomized Phase III Trial. *J Thorac Oncol* (2020) 15:1351–60. doi: 10.1016/j.jtho.2020.03.028
48. Nishio M, Barlesi F, West H, Ball S, Bordoni R, Cobo M, et al. Atezolizumab Plus Chemotherapy for First-Line Treatment of Non-Squamous Non-Small Cell Lung Cancer: Results From the Randomized Phase III Impower132 Trial. *J Thorac Oncol* (2021) 16:653–64. doi: 10.1016/j.jtho.2020.11.025
49. Herbst RS, Giaccone G, de Marinis F, Reinmuth N, Vergnenegre A, Barrios CH, et al. Atezolizumab for First-Line Treatment of PD-L1-Selected Patients With NSCLC. *N Engl J Med* (2020) 383:1328–39. doi: 10.1056/NEJMoa1917346
50. Socinski MA, Jotte RM, Cappuzzo F, Orlandi F, Stroyakovskiy D, Nogami N, et al. Impower150 Study Group. Atezolizumab for First-Line Treatment of Metastatic Nonsquamous Nsclc. *N Engl J Med* (2018) 378:2288–301. doi: 10.1056/NEJMoa1716948
51. Brahmer J, Reckamp KL, Baas P, Crinò L, Eberhardt WE, Poddubskaya E, et al. Nivolumab Versus Docetaxel in Advanced Squamous-Cell Non-Small-Cell Lung Cancer. *N Engl J Med* (2015) 373:123–35. doi: 10.1056/NEJMoa1504627
52. Carbone DP, Reck M, Paz-Ares L, Creelan B, Horn L, Steins M, et al. First-Line Nivolumab in Stage IV or Recurrent Non-Small-Cell Lung Cancer. *N Engl J Med* (2017) 376:2415–26. doi: 10.1056/NEJMoa1613493

10

PD-L1 Test-Based Strategy with Nivolumab as the Second-Line Treatment in Advanced NSCLC: A Cost-Effectiveness Analysis in China

Qiao Liu[1], Xia Luo[1], Zhen Zhou[2], Liubao Peng[1], Lidan Yi[1], Xiaomin Wan[1], Chongqing Tan[1] and Xiaohui Zeng[3*]*

[1] *Department of Pharmacy, The Second Xiangya Hospital of Central South University, Changsha, China,* [2] *Menzies Institute for Medical Research, University of Tasmania, Hobart, TAS, Australia,* [3] *Department of Nuclear Medicine/PET Image Center, The Second Xiangya Hospital of Central South University, Changsha, China*

Correspondence:
Xiaohui Zeng
zengxiaohui2008@csu.edu.cn
Chongqing Tan
tanchongqing@csu.edu.cn

Objective: Our previous economic assessment found that nivolumab was not cost-effective for Chinese patients with advanced non-small cell lung cancer (NSCLC) and without *EGFR* mutations or *ALK* translocations, when compared with the standard second-line drug docetaxel. However, a greater survival benefit with nivolumab was observed for patients with 1% or greater tumor programmed death ligand 1 (PD-L1) expression. In view of this, we designed the present analysis to explore whether it is cost-effective to use the PD-L1 test to guide second-line nivolumab treatment in China.

Material and Methods: A Markov model was established to project the lifetime costs and quality-adjusted life-years (QALYs) of three second-line treatment strategies: nivolumab and docetaxel (strategies without a PD-L1 test) and PD-L1 test-based strategy. Deterministic and probabilistic sensitivity analyses were performed to examine the robustness of our results. Additional price reduction and willingness-to-pay (WTP) threshold scenario analyses were performed to explore the impact of economic and health policies with Chinese characteristics on our results.

Results: The PD-L1 test-based strategy costs approximately CNY 194,607 (USD 28,210) or more and yielded an additional 0.27 QALYs compared to the docetaxel strategy without a PD-L1 test, equating an incremental cost-effectiveness ratio (ICER) of CNY 731,089 (USD 105,978)/QALY. Deterministic sensitivity analyses showed that the price of nivolumab was the strongest source of variation in the ICERs. Probability sensitivity analysis showed that the probability for the PD-L1 test-based strategy being cost-effective increases with the increase of WTP thresholds.

Conclusion: From the perspective of the Chinese healthcare system, using a PD-L1 test to guide second-line nivolumab treatment was not cost-effective. The National Healthcare Security Administration negotiation on the price reduction of nivolumab was found to be the most effective action to improve its cost-effectiveness in China.

Keywords: cost-effectiveness, NSCLC, nivolumab, PD-L1 test, China

INTRODUCTION

Lung cancer remains a major public health problem and the most commonly diagnosed cancer in China that contributes to 27% of all cancer-related deaths (1). Non-small cell lung cancer (NSCLC) accounts for approximately 85% of lung cancer cases, and most of them are advanced cases (2). In the pre-immunotherapy era, the prognosis of advanced NSCLC was generally poor, and the 5-year survival rate was less than 5.5% (3). The popularity of immunotherapy for treating advanced NSCLC has significantly prolonged the overall survival of patients with advanced NSCLC (4, 5). Since 2018, immune checkpoint inhibitors (ICIs) have been successively approved by the Chinese government as the standard treatment for advanced NSCLC, and the new therapeutic classes have presented favorable treatment efficacy and safety (6).

>Nivolumab as the first programmed death 1 (PD-1) ICI, was officially authorized by the Chinese State Food and Drug Administration (SFDA) as a second-line therapy for NSCLC in June 2018 (7). The crucial evidence underpinning the approval of nivolumab was yielded from the CheckMate 078 Phase III clinical trials, in which nivolumab was found that significantly improved the overall survival (OS) in NSCLC patients compared with docetaxel (the median OS: 12.0 vs 9.6 months) (8). In addition, this study found that the nivolumab therapy was more effective in treating advanced NSCLC with a programmed death ligand 1 (PD-L1) tumor proportion score (TPS) ≥1% (the median OS: 12.3) (8). Although the National Comprehensive Cancer Network (NCCN) guidelines of the United States recommend routine testing for PD-L1 expression in patients with diagnosed advanced NSCLC, and PD-L1 expression has been demonstrated as a reliable biomarker to predict benefits from immunotherapy (9, 10), there is lack of such recommendation in relevant Chinese treatment guidelines (11).

In 2015, China reported 733,300 new lung cancer cases, of which nearly 60% were advanced NSCLCs (1). From a Chinese healthcare system perspective, our previous cost-effectiveness analysis revealed that second-line nivolumab was unlikely to be cost-effective compared with docetaxel in patients with advanced NSCLC, despite the subgroup analysis showing the improved cost-effectiveness of nivolumab in the patients with PD-L1TPS ≥1% (12). Although this finding did not concur with the cost-effectiveness analyses conducted in other countries showing a favorable cost-effectiveness of nivolumab versus docetaxel in previously treated advanced NSCLC patients regardless of PD-L1 expression (13, 14), different perspectives, trial source used for analysis, and approach to modeling used between these studies have to be highlighted that may explain the inconsistency. Considering that nivolumab is recommended as the preferred second-line treatment for advanced NSCLC patients without *ALK* or *EGFR* mutations regardless of their PD-L1 expression in China, evidence regarding the impact of PD-L1 test results on the comparative cost-effectiveness of second-line nivolumab versus docetaxel from a Chinese health system perspective is urgently needed to inform Chinese healthcare policy making.

MATERIALS AND METHODS

Model Structure

This economic evaluation used aggregate data from the CheckMate-078 trial and was therefore exempted from institutional research ethics board approval. The model design followed the guidelines for pharmacoeconomic evaluation in China (15).

We established a Markov model consisting of three health states: progression-free survival state (PFS state), progressed survival state (PS state), and death to simulate the treatment and survival process for a cohort of Chinese NSCLC patients (**Figure 1**). The cost and effectiveness associated with the second-line treatments were estimated according to the transfer probability between different health states, and the medical expenses and health outcomes assigned to each health state. Our economic evaluation was conducted from the perspective of the Chinese healthcare system.

The target population was confirmed pre-treated advanced NSCLC patients who were negative for the *EGFR* mutation or *ALK* mutation. All patients started in the PFS state and could move to another health state according to transition probabilities. For two strategies without a PD-L1 test, nivolumab (A) and docetaxel (B) were randomly assigned to patients regardless of their PD-L1 expression. For the PD-L1 test-based strategy, patients were treated according to their PD-L1 status (C): patients with a PD-L1TPS ≥1% were assigned to receive nivolumab (C-Niv), and those who had a TPS <1% were assigned to receive docetaxel (C-Doc). We assumed that 55% of patients had a PD-L1TPS ≥1% (8). Second-line treatment regimens and dosages in the model followed those detailed in the CheckMate078 trial (**Supplementary Table 1**) (8). The primary analysis was preformed to compare (1) the PD-L1 test-based strategy (C) with docetaxel (A); (2) the PD-L1 test-based strategy (C) with nivolumab (B); and (3) the nivolumab (B) and docetaxel (A).

Medication schemes for nivolumab and docetaxel were adjusted to fit a 3-week model cycle. A lifetime horizon was used to project cancer treatment-related costs and health outcomes for this analysis. In this model, patients in PFS state were assumed to receive second-line nivolumab or docetaxel until disease progression, or discontinuation owing to toxicity. Subsequent therapy included chemotherapy, targeted therapy and immunotherapy was assigned to 42% of the patients in the treatment groups whose disease progressed. Other patients were recommended for the best supportive care (BSC) according to current clinical guidelines in China (16).

The principal output of our model was the incremental cost-effectiveness ratios (ICERs) between treatment strategies under comparison, which were calculated as the incremental costs per quality-adjusted life year (QALY) gained. A discount rate of 5% per year was recommended by the Guidelines for Pharmacoeconomic Evaluation in China (15). All the costs were reported in 2019 Chinese yuan and US dollars. Since there is no recommended willing-to-pay (WTP) threshold in Chinese pharmacoeconomic guidelines, we used three times the

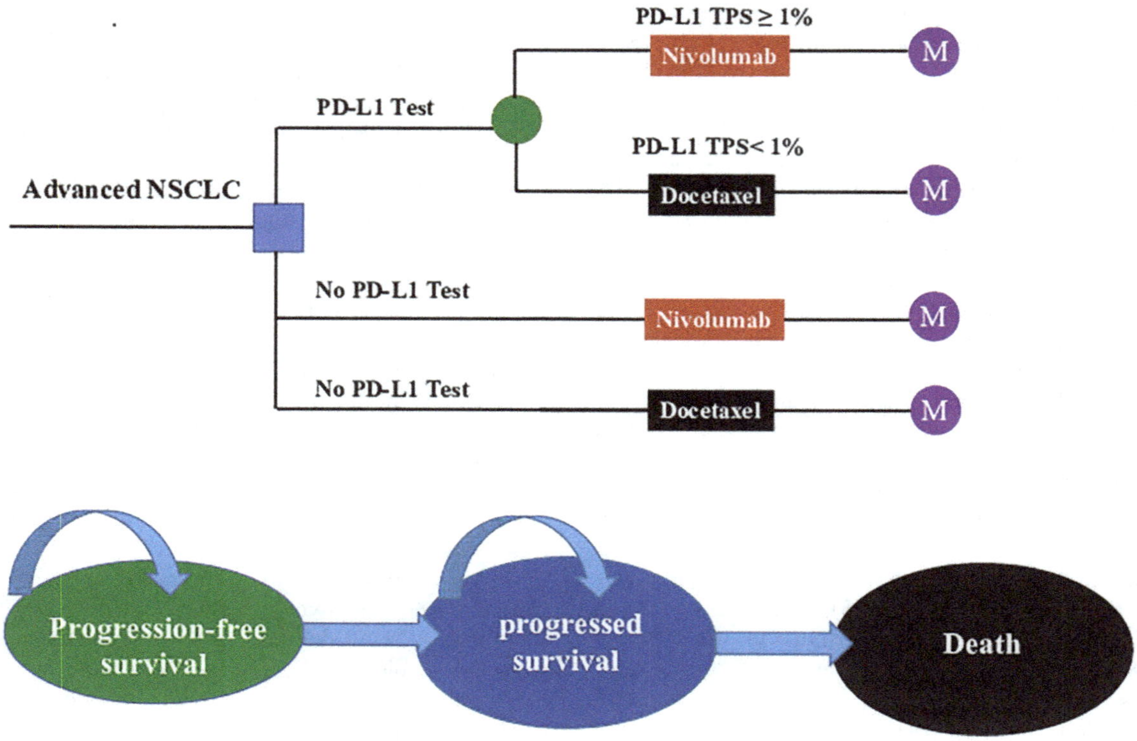

FIGURE 1 | The Markov state transition model. NSCLC, non-small cell lung cancer; PD-L1, programmed death ligand 1; TPS, tumor proportion score; M, Markov node.

gross domestic product (GDP) as the WTP threshold according to the recommendation from the World Health Organization (WHO). In light of the imbalance in economic development among different regions in China, we compared ICERs with two WTP thresholds: CNY 212,667 (USD 30,828)/QALY [3 × the per capita gross domestic product (GDP) value of China in 2019] for general regions and CNY 492,656 (USD 71,415)/QALY (3 × the per capita GDP value of Beijing city in 2019) for affluent regions (17). In our study, all the analyses were performed with TreeAge Pro 2018 software (https://www.treeage.com/).

Clinical Inputs

For the two strategies without PD-L1 test, we digitized the PFS and OS curves from the CheckMate 078 trial (ClinicalTrials.gov: NCT02613507) to extract clinical efficacy data points (8, 18). To minimize the impact of statistical fluctuations on our results, we constructed the pseudo-individual patient data based on Hoyle et al.'s algorithm (19). Then, the PFS and OS projections were modeled by fitting pseudo-individual patient data with four commonly used parameter distributions, namely, exponential, Weibull, log-logistic, and log-normal distributions.

For the PD-L1 test-based strategy, we digitized the OS curves for subgroups of nivolumab-treated patients with a PD-L1 TPS ≥1% and docetaxel-treated patients with a PD-L1 TPS <1% from the CheckMate 078 trial to extract clinical efficacy data points, and then fitted and extrapolated data points with the four commonly used parameter distributions. However, the PFS curves by tumor PD-L1 expression have not yet been published along with the results of the CheckMate 078 trial. Therefore, we assumed that the PFS data of these two subgroups were similar to those of the whole trial population corresponding to nivolumab or docetaxel treatment.

The final log-logistic variables, theta (θ), and kappa (k) listed in **Table 1**, were estimated using R software (version 3.3.1, http://www.r-project.org). In this study, log-logistic distribution was chosen based on the result of goodness of fit test using the Akaike's information criterion (AIC) and Bayesian information criterion (BIC) (**Supplementary Tables 2, 3**). For the validation purposes, the predicted OS and PFS curves were compared with the investigated Kaplan–Meier (KM) curves (**Figure 2**).

The time-dependent transition probabilities of death were calculated according to the following formula:

$$tp_{die} = 1 - \frac{1 + \exp(\theta_{OS})(t-1)^{k_{OS}}}{1 + \exp(\theta_{OS})t^{k_{OS}}} \quad (k > 0),$$

The transition probabilities of PFS were calculated from the following formula:

$$tp_{pfs} = \frac{1 + \exp(\theta_{pfs})(t-1)^{k_{pfs}}}{1 + \exp(\theta_{pfs})t^{k_{pfs}}} / (1 - tp_{die})$$

where t represents the current number of Markov model cycles (27).

TABLE 1 | Model parameters: baseline values, ranges, and distributions for sensitivity analysis.

Parameter	Value	Range	Distribution	Ref
Survival				
The PD-L1 test-based strategy (C)				
Log-logistic OS survival of nivolumab (C-Niv)	Theta = 0.01532; kappa = 1.45712	–	–	(18)
Log-logistic OS survival of docetaxel (C-Doc)	Theta = 0.01816; kappa = 1.52881	–	–	(18)
Log-logistic PFS survival of nivolumab (C-Niv)	Theta = 0.01502; kappa = 1.49269	–	–	(8)
Log-logistic PFS survival of docetaxel (C-Doc)	Theta = 0.01925; kappa = 1.55954	–	–	(8)
No PD-L1 test strategy				
Log-logistic PFS survival of nivolumab (B)	Theta = 0.1402; kappa = 1.3017	–	–	(8)
Log-logistic PFS survival of docetaxel (A)	Theta = 0.1001; kappa = 1.7305	–	–	(8)
Log-logistic OS survival of nivolumab (B)	Theta = 0.01502; kappa = 1.49269	–	–	(8)
Log-logistic OS survival of docetaxel (A)	Theta = 0.01925; kappa = 1.55954	–	–	(8)
Costs (CNY)				
Nivolumab (4.5 mg/kg per cycle)	413.9	124.2–413.9	Fixed in PSA	Local charge
Docetaxel (75 mg/m^2 per cycle)[a]	38.6	31.0–46.2	Fixed in PSA	Local charge
PD-L1 test	322.2	258.0–386.3	Lognormal	Local charge
Routine follow-up per cycle[b]	383.6	287.7–478.8	Lognormal	(20)
Subsequent therapy in PS state per cycle[c]	5,892.0	4,873.8–6,846.1	Lognormal	(21)
BSC per cycle[d]	2,328.2	1,862.6–2,793.9	Lognormal	(20)
Death-associated costs[e]	18,127.9	15,810.0–20,465.1	Lognormal	(21)
Neutropenia per event	3,183.7	2,865.6–3,502.4	Lognormal	(22)
Anemia per event	3,667.9	3,300.9–4,034.9	Lognormal	(22)
Fatigue per event	796.1	716.1–875.4	Lognormal	(22)
Rash per event	37.9	30.4–45.5	Lognormal	(23)
Utilities				
PFS state	0.768	0.614–0.922	Beta	(24)
PS state	0.703	0.562–0.844	Beta	(24)
Disutility for neutropenia	0.200	0.160–0.240	Beta	(25)
Disutility for fatigue	0.070	0.060–0.080	Beta	(25)
Disutility for rash	0.100	0.080–0.120	Beta	(25)
Risk for treatment-related AEs				
Neutropenia in nivolumab arm	0.003	0.002–0.004	Beta	(8)
Neutropenia in docetaxel arm	0.147	0.118–0.177	Beta	(8)
Anemia in nivolumab arm	0.003	0.002–0.004	Beta	(8)
Anemia in docetaxel arm	0.019	0.015–0.023	Beta	(8)
Fatigue in nivolumab arm	0.008	0.007–0.011	Beta	(8)
Fatigue in docetaxel arm	0.032	0.025–0.038	Beta	(8)
Rash in nivolumab arm	0.008	0.007–0.011	Beta	(8)
Rash in docetaxel arm	–	–	–	(8)
Other				
The proportion of PD-L1 TPS ≥1% (%)	0.55	0.44–0.66	Beta	(8)
Discount rate (%)	5	0–8	Fixed in PSA	(15)
Patient weight (kg)	65	52–78	Normal	(26)
body surface area (m^2)	1.72	1.38–2.07	Normal	(26)

PD-L1, programmed death ligand 1; OS, overall survival; PFS, progression-free survival; PS, progressed survival; BSC, best supportive care; AEs, adverse effects; TPS, tumor proportion score.
[a]Docetaxel has been included in the category B list of the Chinese basic medical insurance drug list, the drug expenses incurred by treating advanced non-small-cell lung cancer patients with docetaxel need only be paid at 5% by the patients themselves, and the remaining 95% is paid by medical insurance.
[b]The cost of routine follow-up included the cost of outpatient physician visit, laboratory tests and examinations.
According to CheckMate 078 trial, subsequent therapy referred to the treatment after disease progression, including chemotherapy, targeted therapy and immunotherapy.
BSC referred to the intervention of clinical symptoms caused by cancer, the treatment of complications of anti-tumor treatment, and the rehabilitation treatment after the whole treatment.
Death-associated costs referred to the cost of palliative end-of-life.

Cost Estimates

Costs associated with cancer treatment in the analysis only covered direct medical costs, namely, drug acquisition, PD-L1 test, treating major adverse events (AEs), routine follow-up, subsequent therapy, BSC, and death-associated costs (12, 28). The cost of nivolumab was obtained from the Chinese health industry big data service platform (https://db.yaozh.com/). The cost of docetaxel was calculated based on the local bid-winning price and the payment ratio of the Chinese basic medical insurance (see **Table 1** for details). In calculating dosage amounts, a mean body weight of 65 kg (range, 52–78 kg) and a body surface area of 1.72 m^2 (range, 1.38–2.07 m^2) were assumed in the model (26).

As per our previous study, costs for managing AEs associated with rash, fatigue, anemia, and neutropenia were considered in this economic analysis (12). Costs estimates for these AEs were derived from published studies (22, 23), and the risks were obtained from the CheckMate 078 trial (**Supplementary Table 4**). The costs of the PD-L1 test, as well as other costs related to cancer treatment were collected from the National

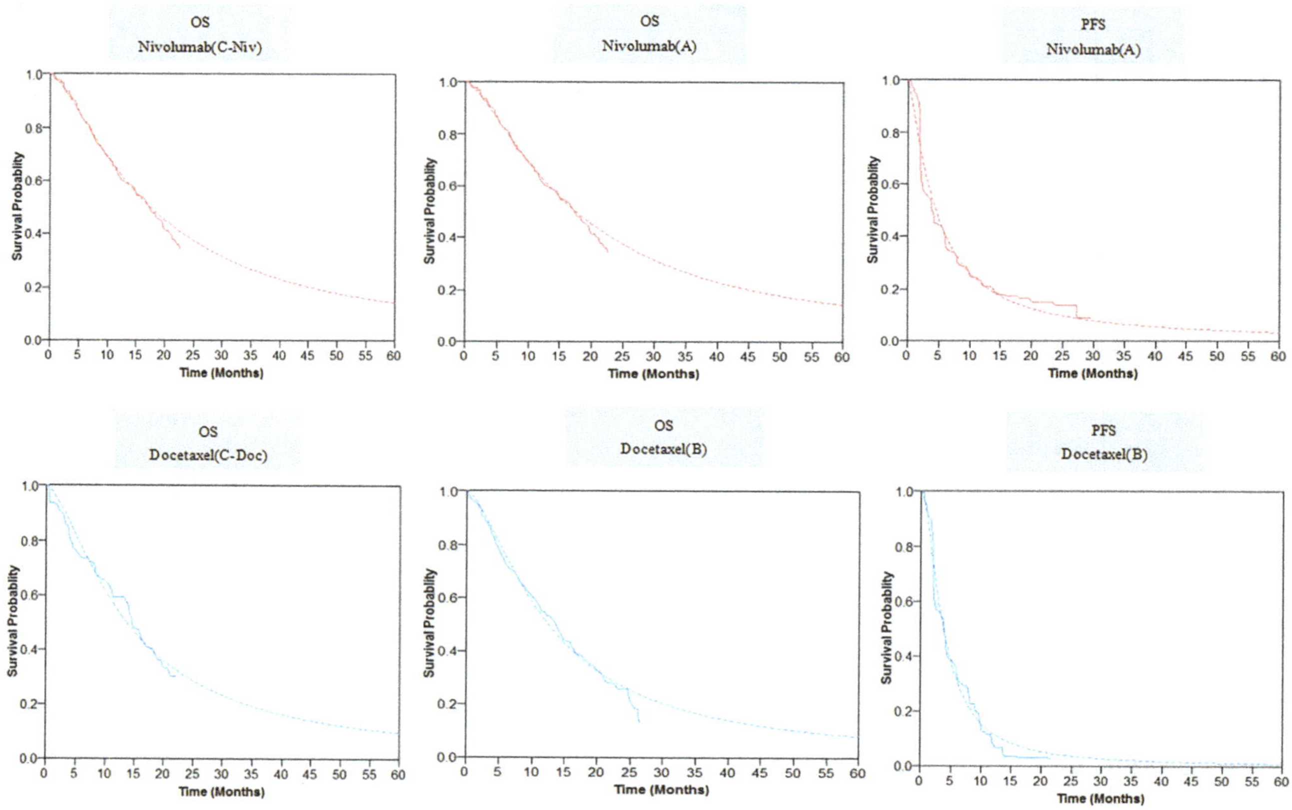

FIGURE 2 | Parametric survival distributions fitted and extrapolated for OS and PFS data. The solid lines represented the observed data for each strategy; the dotted lines represented the fitted data for each strategy. OS, overall survival; PFS, progression-free survival.

Development and Reform Commission of China (29), local hospitals or published studies (20, 21). The cost inputs used in the model are detailed in **Table 1**.

Utility Estimates

PFS and PS health state utilities were obtained from a published study that measured health utilities in Chinese NSCLC patients (24). The decrease in utility caused by treatment-related grade III/IV toxicities was considered in our model (25). Therefore, the utility value for PFS state in the economic evaluation was weighted by the risk of AEs reported in the CheckMate 078 trial, and the corresponding utility decreases. The utility values used in the model are listed in **Table 1**.

Statistical Analysis

One-way deterministic sensitivity analyses (DSA) were conducted to determine the influence of uncertainties in individual input variables on our results. In general, model variables were tested within 95% confidence intervals quoted from the published literature or assumed to vary within ±20% of the base-case value (**Table 1**). Probabilistic sensitivity analyses (PSA) were performed by running 1,000 iterations to generate 1,000 estimates of costs and QALYs for each treatment strategy to test the robustness of our findings. For each iteration, model inputs varied simultaneously and were randomly sampled from appropriate statistical distributions (**Table 1**). The PSA results were presented by a cost-effectiveness acceptability curve (CEAC).

To explore the impact of economic and health policies with Chinese characteristics on our results, we conducted the following two scenario analyses. First, China has a large population and is a rapidly developed developing country, thus the imbalance in economic development among different province-level administrative units is an objective fact. The China Statistical Yearbook 2019 showed that the per capita GDP in the Chinese mainland varied widely from CNY 33,058 (USD 4,792) in Gansu Province to CNY 164,220 (USD 23,805) in Beijing city (17). Against such economic background, we explored the probability that the PD-L1 test-based strategy (C) is cost-effective when compared with alternative treatment strategies under different WTPs (3 × per capita GDP value of each province-level administrative unit). Second, to alleviate the economic burden on cancer patients, since 2017, the price of many cancer drugs has been reduced by 30–70% through the National Healthcare Security Administration (NHSA) negotiations over cancer drugs in China. Therefore, we paid more attention to the impact of the NHSA negotiations on our results. Scenario analyses were performed based on the 30 to 70% reduction in nivolumab price.

RESULTS

Base-Case Analysis

In the PD-L1 test base case, the model projected a mean cost of CNY334,301 (USD 48,460) and a mean survival of 1.22 QALYs per patient for the PD-L1 test-based strategy (C), and the ICERs for the PD-L1 test-based strategy (C) vs docetaxel (A) and vs nivolumab (B), were estimated to be CNY 731,089 (USD 105,978) per QALY and CNY 2165,577 (USD 313,920) per QALY, respectively. The higher total direct medical costs associated with nivolumab were mainly attributed to the higher drug acquisition costs, which were significantly impacted by the improved PFS.

In the no PD-L1 test base case, the model projected a mean cost of CNY 459,833 (USD 66,657) and a mean survival of 1.27 QALYs per patient for nivolumab (B), while a mean cost of CNY 139,701 (USD 20,251) and the mean survival of 0.95 per patient for docetaxel (A), yielded an ICER of CNY 987,618 (USD 143,016)/QALY for nivolumab (B) vs docetaxel (A). The predicted mean costs and effectiveness related to each strategy are listed in **Table 2** for comparison.

In our WTP threshold scenario analysis, the estimated ICERs between the PD-L1 test-based strategy (C) and docetaxel (A) were higher than the WTPs defined based on the different per capita GDP in Chinese mainland. In our price reduction scenario analysis, we found that reducing the price of nivolumab decreased the total medical costs for nivolumab-treated patients, therefore, to a great extent, significantly lowered the ICERs between nivolumab-treated arm and docetaxel-treated arm. **Supplementary Tables 5, 6** show the results of price reduction and WTP scenario analyses.

Sensitivity Analyses

Deterministic Sensitivity Analysis

The DSA results were visualized by tornado diagrams. The price of nivolumab was a main driver for the variation in ICERs. The ICERs decreased to a greater extent with the lower limit of the nivolumab price. In the PD-L1 test base case, the ICER between the PD-L1 test-based strategy (C) and docetaxel (A) dropped below the WTPs for affluent regions, when the reduction in the price of nivolumab exceeded 39% (**Figure 3**). In the no PD-L1 test base case, the ICER between nivolumab (B) and docetaxel (A) dropped below the WTPs for affluent regions, when the reduction in the price of nivolumab exceeded 54% (**Supplementary Figure 1**).

The patient weight, utility for PFS state, discount rate, proportion of patients with a PD-L1 TPS ≥1%, and the utility for the PS state also had considerable influences on the ICERs. Other variables, namely, the risk of AEs, costs other than drug acquisition cost, and decreased utility related to grade III/IV AEs had minimal influence on the ICERs. The results indicated that the lower or upper limits of any tested variable failed to result in the ICERs for the PD-L1 test-based strategy (C) vs docetaxel (A) to be lower than the WTP for general regions. However, the lower limits of the cost of nivolumab (4.5 mg/kg per cycle) produced an ICER below the WTP for affluent regions.

Probabilistic Sensitivity Analysis

In performing the PSA for the PD-L1 test base case, compared with docetaxel (A), the cost-effective probabilities of PD-L1

TABLE 2 | Summary base case results.

Model outputs	No PD-L1 test strategy		The PD-L1 test-based strategy			Incremental		
	Docetaxel (A)	Nivolumab (B)	Overall[a] (C)	Docetaxel (C-Doc)	Nivolumab (C-Niv)	B vs A	C vs A	C vs B
LYs	1.33	1.75	1.69	1.46	1.87	0.42	0.36	−0.06
PFS state	0.42	0.68	0.57	0.42	0.69	0.26	0.15	−0.11
PS state	0.91	1.07	1.13	1.05	1.19	0.16	0.22	0.06
QALYs	0.95	1.27	1.22	1.04	1.36	0.32	0.27	−0.06
PFS state	0.31	0.52	0.43	0.31	0.52	0.21	0.12	−0.09
PS state	0.64	0.75	0.79	0.74	0.83	0.11	0.15	0.04
Cost (CNY)	139,699	459,836	334,302	158,262	478,335	320,137	194,607	−125,532
PD-L1 test cost	0	0	324	324	324	0	324	324
Drug acquisition cost	442	297,794	165,143	442	299,898	297,353	164,702	−132,644
Routine follow-up cost	3,365	3,932	3,235	2,345	3,960	1,587	890	−697
AEs management cost	566	28	269	566	28	−538	−297	241
Subsequent therapy cost[b]	91,460	107,348	112,528	104,754	118,882	15,715	20,889	5,174
BSC cost	36,210	42,419	44,468	41,398	46,979	6,209	8,258	2,042
Death-associated cost	8,499	8,313	8,340	8,444	8,258	−186	−159	28
ICER (CNY)								
Cost per LY						762,229	547,410	1,946,253
Cost per QALY						987,618	731,089	2,165,577

LY, life-year; QALY, quality-adjusted life-year; ICER, incremental cost-effectiveness ratio; PFS, progression-free survival; PS, progressed survival; PD-L1, programmed death ligand 1; AEs, adverse effects; BSC, best supportive care.

[a]The total mean costs and QALYs of overall patients in the PD-L1 test-based strategy were calculated by multiplying the proportion of patients with a PD-L1 TPS ≥1% (reported in the CheckMate 078 trial) by the mean cost and QALYs of nivolumab-treated patients, plus the proportion of patients with a PD-L1 TPS <1% (reported in the CheckMate 078 trial) multiplied by the mean cost and QALY of docetaxel-treated patients.

[b]Subsequent therapy costs in PS state were estimated based on the proportion of patients received subsequent after disease progressed reported in the CheckMate 078 trial.

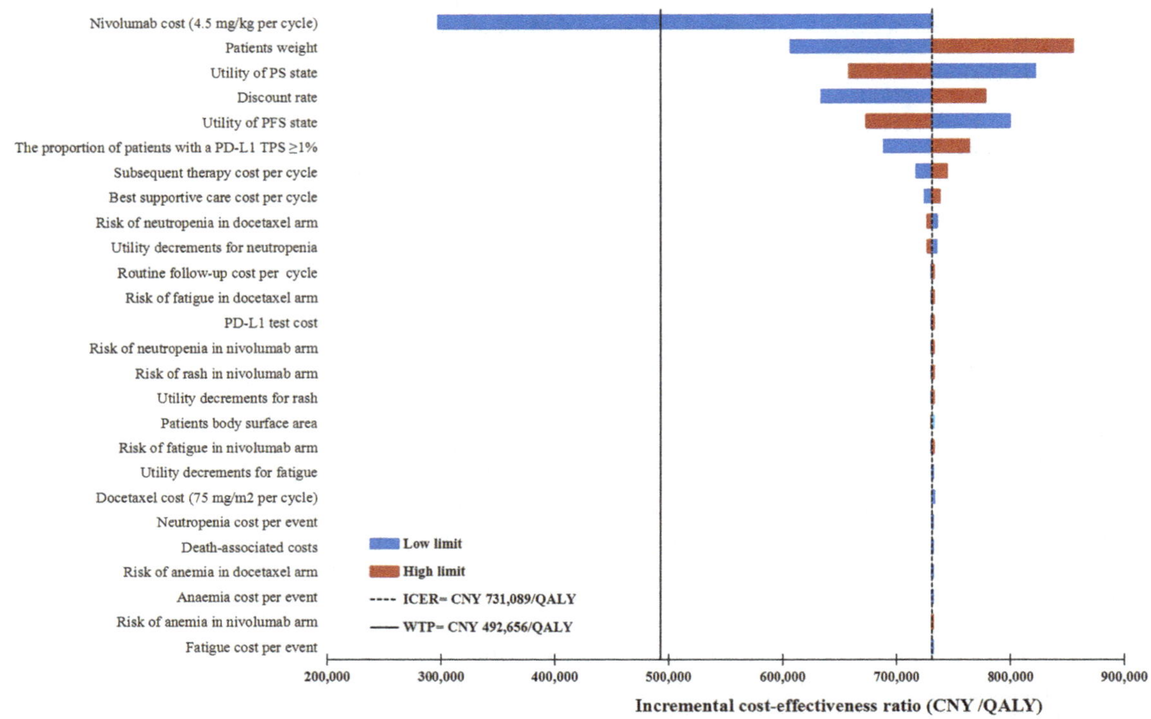

FIGURE 3 | The result of one-way deterministic sensitivity analysis for the PD-L1 test-based strategy (C) versus docetaxel (A). ICER, incremental cost-effectiveness ratio; WTP, willingness-to-pay; QALY, quality-adjusted life-year; PFS, progression-free survival; PS, progressed survival; PD-L1, programmed death ligand 1; TPS, tumor proportion score.

test-based strategy (C) were 16 and 4% when the WTP was CNY 212,667 (USD 30,828)/QALY and CNY 492,656 (USD 71,415)/QALY, respectively (**Figure 4**).

In performing the PSA for the no PD-L1 test base case, compared with docetaxel (A), cost-effective probabilities of nivolumab (B) were nearly 14% when WTP was CNY 492,656 (USD 71,415)/QALY, and zero when WTP was CNY 212,667 (USD 30,828)/QALY (**Figure 4**).

In the price reduction scenario, the possibility of the nivolumab strategy being cost-effective increased as the nivolumab price decreased. In the PD-L1test base case, a 50% reduction in the price of nivolumab increased the cost-effective probability of the PD-L1 test-based strategy (C) to up to 26 and 6%, respectively, at the WTPs of CNY492,656 (USD 71,415)/QALY and CNY 212,667 (USD 30,828)/QALY. In the no PD-L1test base case, a 50% reduction in the price of nivolumab increased the cost-effective probability of nivolumab (B) to up to 19 and 4% at the WTPs of CNY492,656 (USD 71,415)/QALY and CNY 212,667 (USD 30,828)/QALY, respectively (**Figure 5**).

DISCUSSION

Our study was the first economic evaluation investigating the costs and health outcomes of using the PD-L1 test to guide second-line nivolumab treatment for Chinese advanced NSCLC patients with no *EGFR* mutations or *ALK* translocations. Our results demonstrated that compared with docetaxel (A), the PD-L1 test-based strategy (C) extended survival in PFS and PS states by 0.12 QALYs and 0.15 QALYs, respectively (see detail in **Table 2**). Using two WTPs in this study, we found that the incremental costs of the PD-L1 test-based strategy (C) [CNY334,301 (USD 48,460) vs CNY139,702 (USD 20,251)] were not commensurate with the modest survival benefits it can provide, when compared with the docetaxel (A). As a result, the ICERs were not in favor of the PD-L1 test-based strategy (C).

The expert consensus on immunosuppressive therapy for NSCLC in China (2019) recommends nivolumab monotherapy as the preferred second-line treatment for advanced NSCLC with no *EGFR* mutations or *ALK* translocations, regardless of PD-L1 expression (30). Despite this, the expression of PD-L1 was found to be related to the efficacy of nivolumab (8). Hence, in this study, we aimed to advance the discussion around whether employing the PD-L1 test to guide second-line nivolumab therapy is cost-effective. The PD-L1 test-based strategy (C) was associated with greater survival benefits than nivolumab (B), mainly because that the nivolumab is more effective in advanced NSCLC with high levels of PD-L1 expression (8). Although we concluded that the PD-L1 test-based strategy (C) was not cost-effective compared with docetaxel (A), it produced a lower ICER than nivolumab (B). These results suggested that selecting patients for second-line nivolumab based on the PD-L1 test result improved

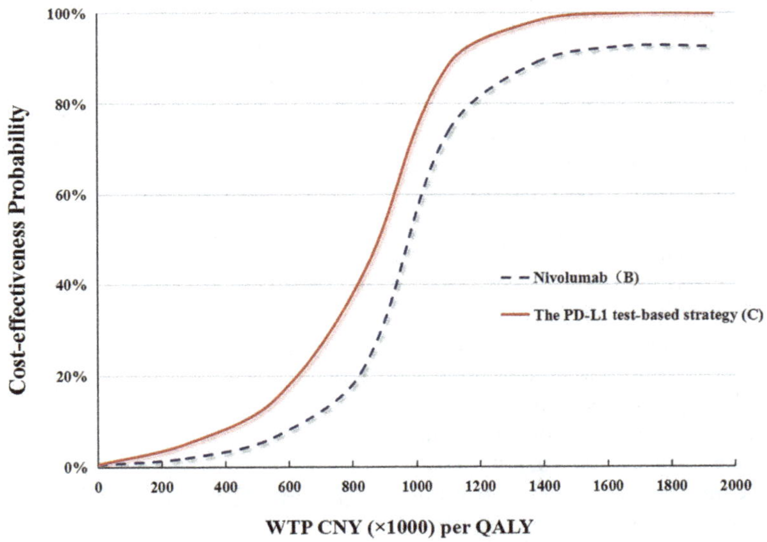

FIGURE 4 | **(A)** The cost-effectiveness probability achieved by the PD-L1 test-based strategy (C) and nivolumab (B) compared to docetaxel (A) at different WTP thresholds. QALY, quality adjusted life-year; WTP, willingness-to-pay; PD-L1, programmed death ligand.

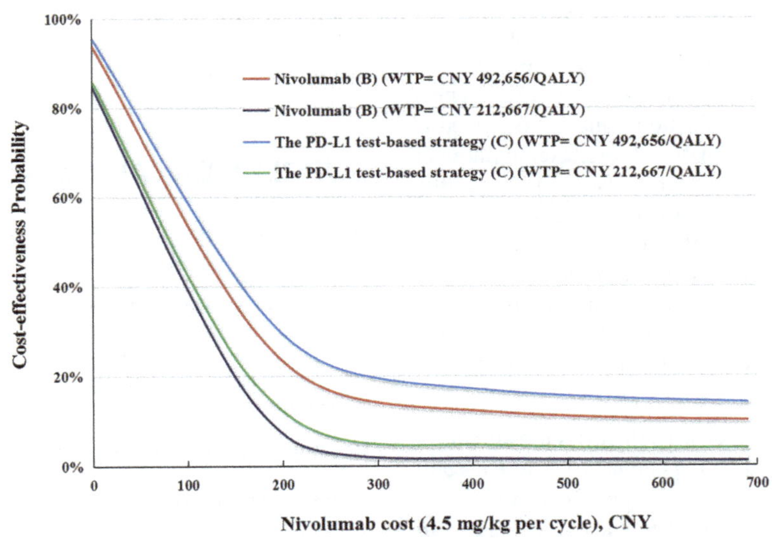

FIGURE 5 | The cost-effectiveness probability achieved by the PD-L1 test-based strategy (C) and nivolumab (B) compared to docetaxel (A) at different nivolumab prices. QALY, quality adjusted life-year; WTP, willingness-to-pay; PD-L1, programmed death ligand.

its cost-effectiveness. The current study did not evaluate the cost-effectiveness of nivolumab in patients with higher PD-L1 expression, due to the lack of relevant clinical data.

Comprehensive sensitivity analyses were performed to assess the robustness of our model. Reducing the price of nivolumab was found to be the most realistic action to push the PD-L1 test-based strategy (C) toward cost-effectiveness. In recent years, great efforts have been paid to reduce the price of anticancer drugs through the negotiation with pharmaceutical companies held by the NHSA in China, and as a result, the prices of many anticancer drugs have dropped by 30 to 70% (31). Therefore, negotiation over nivolumab might be an effective way to promote the cost-effectiveness of the PD-L1 test-based strategy (C) in China. In the long run, the NHSA negotiation, which enables patients to obtain better treatment at lower cost, will be the most attainable approach for optimizing medical resource allocation in China. Moreover, the WTP threshold scenario analysis showed that with the increase of the WTP threshold value, the

PD-L1 test-based strategy (C) were more cost-effective in China, which were generally consistent with our previous study (12). To reflect China's regional economic disequilibrium, two WTP thresholds were selected for general regions and affluent regions in the current analyses, respectively.

Pharmacoeconomic evaluation evidence regarding the PD-L1 test was rather limited. Only one study from the Swiss healthcare setting assessed the impact of the PD-L1 test on the cost-effectiveness of nivolumab (32). This analysis used the CheckMate-057 trial as the source for clinical inputs and reported an ICER of CHF 124,891/QALY for nivolumab in patients with a TPS ≥10%. Our results cannot be directly compared with it because the different clinical inputs sources and different study perspectives were used. However, they concluded that the cost-effectiveness of nivolumab was improved by selecting patients according to the consequences of the PD-L1 test. This finding was consistent with ours. Additionally, our previous analysis assessing the cost-effectiveness of CheckMate 078 comparators reported an ICER of CNY 643,678 (USD 93,307)/QALY for second-line nivolumab vs docetaxel, which is much lower than our current results (12). The inconsistency of the ICERs might result from the fact that our current study used the latest 2-year follow-up data from CheckMate 078 (16), which were not available in our previous study.

Our study has the following strengths. First, we synthesized the latest 2-year follow-up data of the CheckMate 078 trial through economic modeling to project the costs and health outcomes associated with second-line nivolumab and docetaxel, bolstering the reliability of these cost-effectiveness results. Second, our economic evaluation considered the cost-effectiveness of second-line nivolumab and docetaxel in different PD-L1 statuses that provided comprehensive and accurate economic profiles of the two therapies. We applied two WTP thresholds in the model, reflecting the cost-effectiveness of the PD-L1 test-based strategy (C) in both high-income and resource-constrained regions of China. By contrasting and discussing our analysis results, this paper presents proposals for the PD-L1 test-based strategy (C) to serve the patients most likely to benefit from it.

Our study has several limitations. *First*, KM survival curves obtained from the CheckMate 078 trial clinical trial were used to project survivals. Any biases in this trial, if existed, would have inevitably been reflected in our model. *Second*, a potential bias in our Markov model was that the local data on the prevalence of PD-L1 TPS ≥1% were not available due to the lack of relevant studies in China. *Third*, as previously mentioned, we only considered the costs of grade III/IV AEs affecting ≥10% of patients reported in the CheckMate 078 trial, which might lead to an uncertainty in the estimation of AE costs. However, DSA, performed by varying model inputs within a broad range, found that the ICERs were not quite sensitive to AE costs. *Fourth*, the current study did not consider other ICIs, such as pembrolizumab, which is a potential comparator for advanced NSCLC without *EGFR* and *ALK* mutations. One reason is the lack of head-to-head clinical trials. The second reason is that in China, nivolumab is limited to the second-line treatment for advanced NSCLC patients, while pembrolizumab is not. *Fifth*, there is an uncertainty in the long-term survival projection beyond the trial period, more mature data are needed to validate our model against longer-term survival data. *Finally*, generalizing our study findings to other countries/regions might be difficult.

In conclusion, for pretreated advanced NSCLC patients with no EGFR mutations or ALK translocations, using the PD-L1 test to guide second-line nivolumab treatment might not be considered cost-effective from the perspective of the Chinese healthcare system. Reducing the price of nivolumab was found to be the most realistic action to push nivolumab strategies toward cost-effectiveness.

AUTHOR CONTRIBUTIONS

XZ and QL had full access to all the data in the study and take responsibility for the integrity of the data and the accuracy of the data analysis. Concept and design: QL, XZ, and CT. Acquisition, analysis, or interpretation of data: All authors. Drafting of the manuscript: QL, XZ, and CT. Critical revision of the manuscript for important intellectual content: All authors. Statistical analysis: QL. Obtained funding: QL. Supervision: XZ and CT. All authors contributed to the article and approved the submitted version.

SUPPLEMENTARY MATERIAL

Supplementary Figure 1 | The result of one-way deterministic sensitivity analysis. The tornado diagram revealed the influence of uncertainty in individual model input variables on the ICERs between nivolumab **(B)** versus docetaxel **(A)**. The black dotted line represented the ICERs estimated from our base case analysis, and the black solid line represented the WTP of CNY492,656 (71,415 USD)/QALY for affluent regions in China. ICER, incremental cost-effectiveness ratio; WTP, willingness-to-pay; QALY, quality-adjusted life-year; PFS, progression-free survival; PS, progressed survival.

Supplementary Table 1 | Second-line treatment regimens and dosage in the Model.

Supplementary Table 2 | Parametric survival distributions fitted for OS data.

Supplementary Table 3 | Parametric survival distributions fitted for PFS data.

Supplementary Table 4 | Incidence of treatment-Related grade III/IV Adverse Events considered in the model.

Supplementary Table 5 | The results of WTP threshold scenario analysis. The WTP threshold values used in the scenario analyses were set on the basis of the per capita gross domestic product (GDP) of different province-level administrative unit in Mainland Chinese.

Supplementary Table 6 | The results of the price reduction scenario analysis. The price reduction scenario analyses were conducted based on the price of nivolumab discounted ranging from 30% and 70%.

REFERENCES

1. Chen W, Zheng R, Baade PD, Zhang S, Zeng H, Bray F, et al. Cancer Statistics in China, 2015. *CA Cancer J Clin* (2016) 66(2):115–32. doi: 10.3322/caac.21338
2. Reck M, Rabe KF. Precision Diagnosis and Treatment for Advanced Non-Small-Cell Lung Cancer. *N Engl J Med* (2017) 377(9):849–61. doi: 10.1056/NEJMra1703413
3. Siegel RL, Miller KD, Jemal A. Cancer Statistics, 2019. *CA Cancer J Clin* (2019) 69(1):7–34. doi: 10.3322/caac.21551
4. Kanda S, Ohe Y, Goto Y, Horinouchi H, Fujiwara Y, Nokihara H, et al. Five-Year Safety and Efficacy Data From a Phase Ib Study of Nivolumab and Chemotherapy in Advanced Non-Small-Cell Lung Cancer. *Cancer Sci* (2020) 111(6):1933–42. doi: 10.1111/cas.14410
5. Garon EB, Hellmann MD, Rizvi NA, Carcereny E, Leighl NB, Ahn MJ, et al. Five-Year Overall Survival for Patients With Advanced NonSmall-Cell Lung Cancer Treated With Pembrolizumab: Results From the Phase I KEYNOTE-001 Study. *J Clin Oncol* (2019) 37(28):2518–27. doi: 10.1200/JCO.19.00934
6. Guidelines Working Committee of Chinese Society of Clinical Oncology. Guidelines of Chinese society of clinical oncology (CSCO) for Non-small cell lung cancer [M] 2020 edition. Beijing: People's Medical Publishing House (2020) p. 173.
7. National Medical Products Administration. *The First PD-1 Monoclonal Antibody Drug on the Market in China* (2018). Available at: https://www.cn-healthcare.com/article/20180616/content-504767.html (Accessed 23 Jul 2020).
8. Wu YL, Lu S, Cheng Y, Zhou C, Wang J, Mok T, et al. Nivolumab Versus Docetaxel in a Predominantly Chinese Patient Population With Previously Treated Advanced NSCLC: CheckMate 078 Randomized Phase III Clinical Trial. *J Thorac Oncol* (2019) 14(5):867–75. doi: 10.1016/j.jtho.2019.01.006
9. Herbst RS, Soria JC, Kowanetz M, Fine GD, Hamid O, Gordon MS. Etal. Predictive Correlates of Response to the Anti-PD-L1 Antibody MPDL3280A in Cancer Patients. *Nature* (2014) 515(7528):563–7. doi: 10.1038/nature14011
10. Taube JM, Klein A, Brahmer JR, Xu H, Pan X, Kim JH, et al. Association of PD-1, PD-1 Ligands, and Other Features of the Tumor Immune Microenvironment With Response to Anti-PD-1 Therapy. *Clin Cancer Res* (2014) 20(19):5064–74. doi: 10.1158/1078-0432.CCR-13-3271
11. Ettinger DS, Wood DE, Aggarwal C, Aisner DL, Akerley W, Bauman JR, et al. NCCN Guidelines Insights: Non-Small Cell Lung Cancer, Version 1.2020. *J Natl Compr Canc Netw* (2019) 17(12):1464–72. doi: 10.6004/jnccn.2019.0059
12. Liu Q, Luo X, Peng L, Yi L, Wan X, Zeng X, et al. Nivolumab Versus Docetaxel for Previously Treated Advanced Non-Small Cell Lung Cancer in China: A Cost-Effectiveness Analysis. *Clin Drug Invest* (2020) 40(2):129–37. doi: 10.1007/s40261-019-00869-3
13. Rothwell B, Kiff C, Ling C, Brodtkorb TH. Cost Effectiveness of Nivolumab in Patients With Advanced, Previously Treated Squamous and Non-Squamous Non-Small-Cell Lung Cancer in England. *Pharmacoecon Open* (2021) 5 (2):251–60. doi: 10.1007/s41669-020-00245-4
14. Chaudhary MA, Holmberg C, Lakhdari K, Smare C, Theriou C, Dale P, et al. Cost-Effectiveness of Nivolumab in Squamous and Non-Squamous Non-Small Cell Lung Cancer in Canada and Sweden: An Update With 5-Year Data. *J Med Econ* (2021) 24(1):607–19. doi: 10.1080/13696998.2021.1917139
15. Chinese Society of Clinical Oncology (CSCO). *Guidelines for Pharmacoeconomic Evaluation in China* (2020). Available at: http://www.doc88.com/p-87516994700123.html (Accessed 23 Jul 2020).
16. Chinese Society of Clinical Oncology (CSCO). *Primary Lung Cancer Treatment Guidelines* (2018). Available at: http://guide.medlive.cn/guideline/16783 (Accessed 23 Jul 2020).
17. National Bureau Of Statistics Of China. *National Bureau of Statistics of China: China Statistical Yearbook 2019* (2020). Available at: http://data.stats.gov.cn/english/index.htm (Accessed 24 March 2020).
18. Lu S, Wang J, Cheng Y, Mok T, Chang J, Zhang L, et al. Nivolumab Versus Docetaxel in a Predominantly Chinese Patient Population With Previously Treated Advanced Non-Small Cell Lung Cancer: 2-Year Follow-Up From a Randomized, Open-Label, Phase 3 Study (CheckMate 078). *Lung Cancer* (2021) 152:7 14. doi: 10.1016/j.lungcan.2020.11.013
19. Hoyle MW, Henley W. Improved Curve Fits to Summary Survival Data: Application to Economic Evaluation of Health Technologies. *BMC Med Res Methodol* (2011) 11:139. doi: 10.1186/1471-2288-11-139
20. Zeng X, Karnon J, Wang S, Wu B, Wan X, Peng L. The Cost of Treating Advanced Non-Small Cell Lung Cancer: Estimates From the Chinese Experience. *PloS One* (2012) 7(10):e48323. doi: 10.1371/journal.pone.0048323
21. Wu B, Li T, Cai J, Xu Y, Zhao G. Cost-Effectiveness Analysis of Adjuvant Chemotherapies in Patients Presenting With Gastric Cancer After D2 Gastrectomy. *BMC Cancer* (2014) 14:984. doi: 10.1186/1471-2407-14-984
22. Wu B, Dong B, Xu Y, Zhang Q, Shen J, Chen H, et al. Economic Evaluation of First-Line Treatments for Metastatic Renal Cell Carcinoma: A Cost-Effectiveness Analysis in a Health Resource-Limited Setting. *PloS One* (2012) 7(3):e32530. doi: 10.1371/journal.pone.0032530
23. Zhang C, Zhang H, Shi J, Wang D, Zhang X, Yang J, et al. Trial-Based Cost-Utility Analysis of Icotinib Versus Gefitinib as Second-Line Therapy for Advanced Non-Small Cell Lung Cancer in China. *PloS One* (2016) 11(3): e0151846. doi: 10.1371/journal.pone.0151846
24. Shen Y, Wu B, Wang X, Zhu J. Health State Utilities in Patients With Advanced Non-Small-Cell Lung Cancer in China. *J Comp Eff Res* (2018) 7 (5):443–52. doi: 10.2217/cer-2017-0069
25. Nafees B, Lloyd AJ, Dewilde S, Rajan N, Lorenzo M. Health State Utilities in Non-Small Cell Lung Cancer: An International Study. *Asia Pac J Clin Oncol* (2017) 13(5):e195–203. doi: 10.1111/ajco.12477
26. Lu S, Yu Y, Fu S, Ren H. Cost-effectiveness of ALK testing and first-line crizotinib therapy for Non-small-cell lung cancer in China. *PloS One* (2018) 13(10):e0205827. doi: 10.1371/journal.pone.0205827
27. Zeng X, Li J, Peng L, Wang Y, Tan C, Chen G, et al. Economic Outcomes of Maintenance Gefitinib for Locally Advanced/Metastatic Non-Small-Cell Lung Cancer With Unknown EGFR Mutations: A Semi-Markov Model Analysis. *PloS One* (2014) 9(2):e88881. doi: 10.1371/journal.pone.0088881
28. Wan X, Zhang Y, Tan C, Zeng X, Peng L. First-Line Nivolumab Plus Ipilimumab vs Sunitinib for Metastatic Renal Cell Carcinoma: A Cost-Effectiveness Analysis. *JAMA Oncol* (2019) 5(4):491–6. doi: 10.1001/jamaoncol.2018.7086
29. *National Development and Reform Commission of China* (2020). Available at: https://www.ndrc.gov.cn/wapindex/ (Accessed 23 Jul 2020).
30. Zhou CC, Wang J, Wang BC, Cheng Y, Wang ZH, Lu Y, et al. Expert Consensus on Immunosuppressive Therapy for Non-Small Cell Lung Cancer in China (2020 Edition). *Chin J Lung Cancer* (2020) 24(4):217–35. doi: 10.3779/j.issn.1009-3419.2020.02.01
31. National Healthcare Security Administration. *Notice on Reimbursement Decisions on Including 17 Cancer Drugs in National Reimbursement Drug List by National Healthcare Security Administration* (2018). Available at: http://www.gov.cn/xinwen/2018-10/10/content_5328891.htm (Accessed 13 March 2020).
32. Matter-Walstra K, Schwenkglenks M, Aebi S, Dedes K, Diebold J, Pietrini M, et al. A Cost-Effectiveness Analysis of Nivolumab versus Docetaxel for Advanced Nonsquamous NSCLC Including PD-L1 Testing. *J Thorac Oncol* (2016) 11(11):1846–55. doi: 10.1016/j.jtho.2016.05.032

11

Pre-Treatment Tumor Growth Rate Predicts Clinical Outcomes of Patients with Advanced Non-Small Cell Lung Cancer Undergoing Anti-PD-1/PD-L1 Therapy

Li-na He[1,2,3†], *Xuanye Zhang*[1,2,3†], *Haifeng Li*[1,2,3†], *Tao Chen*[1,2,4†], *Chen Chen*[1,2,5], *Yixin Zhou*[1,2,6], *Zuan Lin*[1,2,7], *Wei Du*[1,2,3], *Wenfeng Fang*[1,2,3], *Yunpeng Yang*[1,2,3], *Yan Huang*[1,2,3], *Hongyun Zhao*[1,2,7], *Shaodong Hong*[1,2,3*†] and *Li Zhang*[1,2,3*†]

[1] State Key Laboratory of Oncology in South China, Guangzhou, China, [2] Collaborative Innovation Center for Cancer Medicine, Guangzhou, China, [3] Department of Medical Oncology, Sun Yat-sen University Cancer Center, Guangzhou, China, [4] Department of Nuclear Medicine, Sun Yat-sen University Cancer Center, Guangzhou, China, [5] Department of Radiation Oncology, Sun Yat-sen University Cancer Center, Guangzhou, China, [6] Department of VIP Region, Sun Yat-sen University Cancer Center, Guangzhou, China, [7] Department of Clinical Research, Sun Yat-sen University Cancer Center, Guangzhou, China

***Correspondence:**
Shaodong Hong
hongshd@sysucc.org.cn
Li Zhang
zhangli6@mail.sysu.edu.cn

[†]These authors have contributed equally to this work

Tumor growth rate (TGR; percent size change per month [%/m]) is postulated as an early radio-graphic predictor of response to anti-cancer treatment to overcome limitations of RECIST. We aimed to evaluate the predictive value of pre-treatment TGR (TGR_0) for outcomes of advanced non-small cell lung cancer (aNSCLC) patients treated with anti-PD-1/PD-L1 monotherapy. We retrospectively screened all aNSCLC patients who received PD-1 axis inhibitors in Sun Yat-Sen University Cancer Center between August 2016 and June 2018. TGR_0 was calculated as the percentage change in tumor size per month (%/m) derived from two computed tomography (CT) scans during a "wash-out" period before the initiation of PD-1 axis inhibition. Final follow-up date was August 28, 2019. The X-tile program was used to identify the cut-off value of TGR_0 based on maximum progression-free survival (PFS) stratification. Patients were divided into two groups per the selected TGR_0 cut-off. The primary outcome was the difference of PFS between the two groups. The Kaplan-Meier methods and Cox regression models were performed for survival analysis. A total of 80 eligible patients were included (54 [67.5%] male; median [range] age, 55 [30-74] years). Median (range) TGR_0 was 21.1 (-33.7-246.0)%/m. The optimal cut-off value of TGR_0 was 25.3%/m. Patients with high TGR_0 had shorter median PFS (1.8 months; 95% CI, 1.6 - 2.1 months) than those with low TGR_0 (2.7 months; 95% CI, 0.5 - 4.9 months) (P = 0.005). Multivariate Cox regression analysis revealed that higher TGR_0 independently predicted inferior PFS (hazard ratio [HR] 1.97; 95% CI, 1.08-3.60; P = 0.026). Higher TGR_0 was also significantly associated with less durable clinical benefit rate (34.8% vs. 8.8%, P = 0.007). High pre-treatment TGR was a reliable predictor of inferior PFS and clinical benefit in aNSCLC patients undergoing anti-PD-1/PD-L1 monotherapy. The findings highlight the role of TGR_0 as an early biomarker to predict benefit from immunotherapy and could allow tailoring patient's follow-up.

Keywords: progression-free survival, non-small cell lung cancer, NSCLC, anti-PD-1/PD-L1 therapy, immunotherapy, tumor growth rate

INTRODUCTION

In recent years, immune checkpoint inhibitors (ICIs), including anti-programmed cell death 1 (PD-1) or anti-programmed cell death ligand 1 (PD-L1) therapies, have revolutionized the treatment modalities of advanced non-small cell lung cancer (aNSCLC) (1–5). However, only a small subset of patients have durable response to anti-PD-1/PD-L1 monotherapy and its clinical application was challenged by its atypical response patterns such as hyperprogressive disease (HPD), delayed response, mixed response and pseudoprogressive disease (6, 7). Numerous studies have been conducted to explore early biomarkers to predict response and survival outcomes in patients undergoing ICI treatment (8).

The Response Evaluation Criteria in Solid Tumors (RECIST) criteria provide an objective and standardized response evaluation benchmark for anticancer therapies (9). However, RECIST-based treatment response evaluation does not take into account the tumor growth kinetics (10). Therefore, the RECIST criteria can only be reliably used to compare progression-free survival (PFS) in patients with relatively uniform tumor growth rate when the radiographic evaluation intervals are fixed. Furthermore, RECIST-defined objective response does not always conform the clinical benefit from anticancer treatment (11–15). Also, the RECIST criteria do not provide pre-treatment parameters for earlier prediction of clinical benefit. Thus, it is of clinical relevance to identify other early and inexpensive predictors of benefit from ICI treatment to overcome the limitations of RECIST criteria.

Uncontrolled growth is one of the hallmarks of malignant cells. Fast-growing tumors are associated with the aggressiveness of the tumor, larger tumor bulk, relatively higher sensitivity to cytotoxic agents, significant aberrant neoangiogenesis and altered immune microenvironment (16). Tumor growth rate (TGR) provides quantitative assessment of change in tumor volume over time according to RECIST-defined sum of the longest diameters of the target lesions (SLD) from two computed tomography (CT) scans and time interval between them (17). Previous studies have showed that TGR was correlated with treatment response or clinical outcomes in patients with neuroendocrine carcinoma, renal cell carcinoma, or hepatocellular carcinoma treated with angiogenesis inhibitors or transarterial chemoembolization (18–23). These findings suggested that TGR could serve as an early radiological biomarker to predict patient's survival outcomes and to tailor radiological follow-up strategies and patients' management.

To our knowledge, no previous studies had illustrated the association of pre-treatment TGR with clinical outcomes of aNSCLC patients treated with ICI. Considering that the natural tumor growth kinetics might significantly impact the tumor microenvironment, we hypothesized that pre-treatment TGR could predict PFS of aNSCLC patients undergoing anti-PD-1/PD-L1 immunotherapy.

METHODS

Data Source

We conducted a retrospective review of electronic medical records from all aNSCLC patients undergoing ICI therapy (N = 172) at Sun Yat-Sen University Cancer Center (SYSUCC) between August 2016 and June 2018. Eligible patients should have two consecutive computed tomography (CT) scans before the initiation of ICI treatment (termed "wash-out period") and receiving no anti-cancer treatment between the two scans (**Figure 1**). Exclusion criteria were as follows: lacking available pre-treatment CT scan; time interval between pre-treatment (defined as the time prior to baseline) and baseline (defined as the time of ICI initiation) CT scans shorter than 2 weeks or longer than 3 months (tumor growth kinetics should be assessed during a proper period) (24); lacking measurable lesions by RECIST version 1.1 (RECIST 1.1) at baseline CT scans; having received local anti-cancer therapy such as radiotherapy and radiofrequency ablation during ICI treatment or follow-up. The study was approved by the Institutional Review Board of SYSUCC and written informed consent was waived due to the retrospective nature of the study. Our study followed the Strengthening the Reporting of Observational Studies in Epidemiology (STROBE) reporting guideline (25).

TGR is expressed as the percentage change in tumor size per month (%/m) and calculated based on a published formula (17,

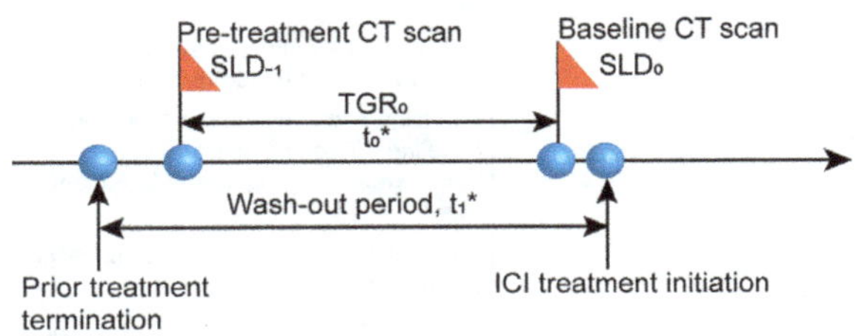

FIGURE 1 | Diagram of computed tomography (CT) scan timepoints. SLD_{-1}, sum of the longest diameters of the target lesions at pre-treatment CT scan; SLD_0, sum of the longest diameters of the target lesions at baseline CT scan; t_0, time interval between pre-treatment and baseline CT scans, 2 weeks$\leq t_0 \leq$ 3 months; t_1, wash-out period before the initiation of ICI treatment without any anti-cancer treatment.

21): TGR = 100 * [exp (TG) – 1]; TG= (3 * log(D_2/D_1))/t, where t = ($date_2$ – $date_1$ + 1)/30.44, indicating the time interval in months between two CT imaging evaluations, and TG is the growth rate. Tumor size (D) derives from the sum of the longest diameters (SLD) of the target lesions according to RECIST 1.1. D_1 = tumor size at $date_1$; D_2 = tumor size at $date_2$. We simplified the formula into this form: TGR = 100 * $((D_2/D_1)^{1.303/t} - 1)$.

For all patients, we collected data including demographic characteristics, clinical and radiological information: sex, age; previous lines of systemic therapies, smoking status, histology, clinical stage, Eastern Cooperative Oncology Group (ECOG) performance status (PS), alterations in driver genes including epidermal growth factor receptor (EGFR) and anaplastic lymphoma kinase (ALK); date of CT scans, SLD, status of non-measurable lesions and new lesions. The same assessment method and same technique (CT) were used at each imaging assessment point. For patients had disease progression with new lesions, tumor size was determined by target lesions only, while the occurrence of new lesions was recorded. In case of multiple alternative pre-baseline images, we selected the latest one to baseline for analysis. Missing data were recorded as not available.

Response and Endpoint Evaluation

All response and outcome evaluation were determined as per RECIST 1.1 by two senior radiologists blinded to patients' information. Discrepancy was solved by consensus. Follow-up CT scans were performed according to the physicians' discretion without predetermined intervals. Patients underwent tumor assessment until immunotherapy termination due to any reasons. The primary endpoint was PFS, defined as time from ICI initiation to radiologically-defined progression or death from any causes. The secondary endpoints were durable clinical benefit (DCB) rate, overall response rate (ORR) and overall survival (OS). DCB was defined as achieving any one of complete response (CR), partial response (PR) or stable disease (SD) that lasted for at least 6 months from baseline. The data cut-off date was August 28, 2019.

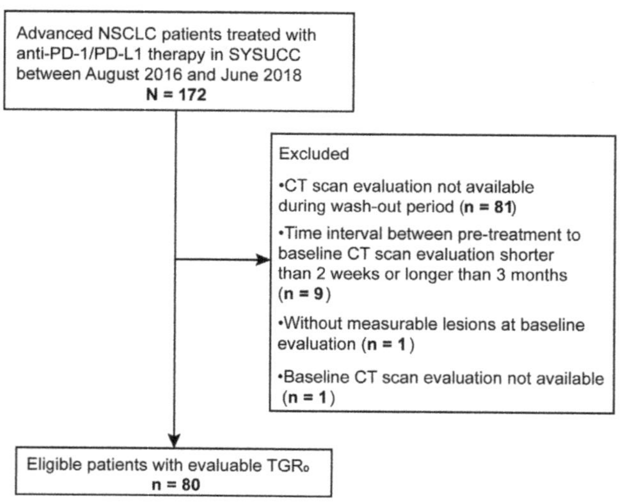

FIGURE 2 | Flowchart of patient screening process.

TABLE 1 | Patient characteristics at baseline (n = 80).

Patient characteristics	No. (%)
Age, years	
Median (range)	55 (30-74)
< 55	40 (50.0)
≥ 55	40 (50.0)
Gender	
Male	54 (67.5)
Female	26 (32.5)
ECOG PS	
0	31 (38.7)
1	45 (56.3)
2-3	4 (5.0)
Smoking status	
Never smoker	48 (60.0)
Current or former smoker	32 (40.0)
Histology	
Squamous cell carcinoma	31 (38.7)
Nonsquamous cell carcinoma	49 (61.3)
No. of prior treatment lines	
0-1	49 (61.3)
≥2	31 (38.7)
No. of metastatic sites	
1-2	44 (55.0)
≥3	36 (45.0)
Prior radiotherapy	
Yes	19 (23.8)
No	61 (76.2)
Type of ICI	
Pembrolizumab	34 (42.5)
Atezolizumab	7 (8.7)
Nivolumab	18 (22.5)
Camrelizumab	21 (26.3)
EGFR mutation status	
Positive	10 (12.5)
Negative	51 (63.7)
Not available	19 (23.8)
ALK translocation	
Positive	4 (5.0)
Negative	52 (65.0)
Not available	24 (30.0)
SLD_0, mm	
Median (range)	74 (17-231)
≤ 130	70 (87.5)
> 130	10 (12.5)
t_0, months	
Median (range)	1.0 (0.5-3.0)
TGR_0, %/m	
Median (range)	21.1 (-33.7-246.0)
≤ 25.3	46 (57.5)
> 25.3	34 (42.5)
RECIST response	
PR	10 (12.5)
SD	19 (23.7)
PD	46 (57.5)
NE	5 (6.3)

ECOG PS, Eastern Cooperative Oncology Group performance status; ICI, immune checkpoint inhibitor; EGFR, epidermal growth factor receptor; ALK, anaplastic lymphoma kinase; SLD_0, sum of the longest diameters of the target lesions at baseline; t_0, time interval from pre-treatment to baseline CT evaluation; TGR_0, pre-treatment tumor growth rate; RECIST, Response Evaluation Criteria in Solid Tumors; PR, partial response; SD, stable disease; PD, progressive disease, NE, not evaluable.

Statistical Analysis

We used the X-tile program (Yale University School of Medicine, New Haven, CT, USA) to determine the optimal cut-off values of TGR_0 and baseline SLD (SLD_0) to maximize PFS differentiation (26). According to the TGR_0 cut-off point, patients were divided into two groups, and baseline characteristics between the two groups were compared. Continuous variables were expressed as median (range) and analyzed using Mann-Whitney U-test or independent t-test depending on the normality of distribution; categorical variables were expressed as number (%) and analyzed using Fisher's exact test or Chi-square test as appropriate. PFS and OS survival curves were generated using Kaplan-Meier method and the differences were compared using the log-rank test. Investigation of the effect of TGR_0 and other baseline parameters on treatment outcomes was performed using univariate and multivariate Cox regression analyses. Two-sided *P*-value of less than 0.05 was considered statistically significant. All statistical analyses were performed using the R software version 3.6.1.

RESULTS

Patient Characteristics

Of the 172 patients screened, 80 met the eligible criteria (**Figure 2**). The median follow-up time was 23.6 months (95% confidence interval [CI], 13.5 - 33.7 months). Baseline characteristics of all patients were depicted in **Table 1**. The median (range) age was 55 (30 - 74) years. 54 (67.5%) were male, 48 (60.0%) were non-smokers, 31 (38.7%) had squamous histology, 19 (23.8%) had previously received radiotherapy and 36 (45.0%) had three or more metastatic sites. 31 patients (38.7%) had an ECOG PS of 0, with 4 (5.0%) patients scoring at 2 or 3. The median (range) duration between pre-treatment and baseline CT scans was 1.0 (0.5 - 3.0) months. The median (range) SLD_0 was 74 (17 - 231) mm, and the median (range) TGR_0 was 21.1(-33.7 - 246.0) %/m. At data cut-off, 42 out of 80 (53.5%) patients died.

As per RECIST 1.1, 10 (12.5%) patients achieved PR as best overall response, 19 (23.7%) achieved SD, 46 (57.5%) had PD and 5 (6.3%) had non-evaluable response. Overall response rate (ORR) was 12.5%, and DCB rate was 23.8%. The median PFS and OS were 2.1 months (95% CI, 1.8 - 3.1 months) and 23.6 months (95% CI, 14.8 - not reached months), respectively.

Cut-Off Points by X-Tile Program

The optimal cut-off points of SLD_0 and TGR_0 based on PFS separation were 130 mm ($\chi^2 = 22.995$, $P < 0.001$) and 25.3%/m ($\chi^2 = 7.546$, $P = 0.112$), respectively (**Figure 3**). Both cut-off points showed the maximum prognostic effects in predicting PFS. According to the TGR_0 cut-off point, we divided patients into two groups: low group, $TGR_0 \leq 25.3\%/m$ (n = 46); high group, $TGR_0 > 25.3\%/m$ (n = 34). The clinicopathological

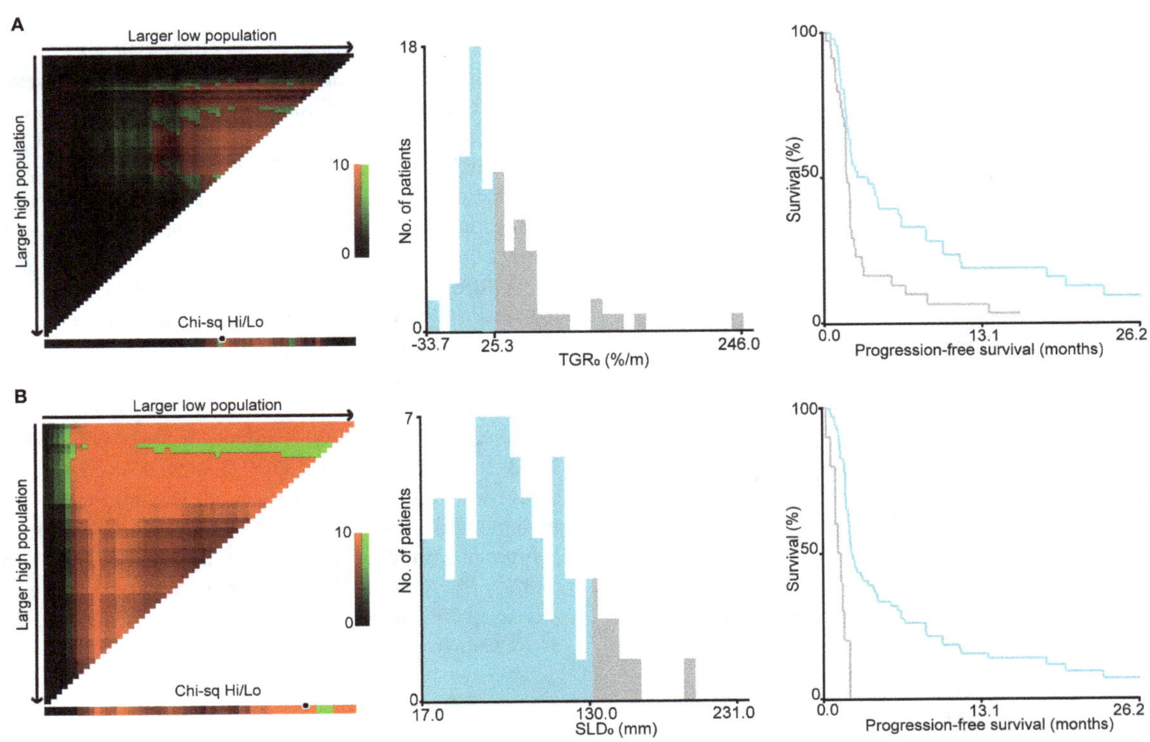

FIGURE 3 | Identification of cut-off values based on progression-free survival by X-tile analysis. **(A)** The optimal cut-off value for sum of the longest diameters of target lesions at baseline (SLD_0) was 130 mm ($\chi^2 = 22.995$, $P < 0.001$). **(B)** The optimal cut-off value for pre-treatment tumor growth rate (TGR_0) based on PFS was 25.3%/m ($\chi^2 = 7.546$, $P = 0.112$).

characteristics of TGR_0 strata were shown in **Table 2**. Low TGR_0 was significantly associated with positive smoking history (P = 0.034) and RECIST-defined best response (P = 0.028). There was no significant association between TGR_0 and other factors including age, gender, ECOG PS, histology, number of prior therapy lines, number of metastatic sites, history of prior radiotherapy, EGFR and ALK status (all with $P > 0.05$).

Association of TGR_0 With Clinical Outcomes

Kaplan-Meier survival analyses revealed that patients with high TGR_0 experienced inferior median PFS (1.8 months; 95% CI, 1.6 - 2.1 months) compared with those with low TGR_0 (2.7 months; 95% CI, 0.5 - 4.9 months) (log-rank P = 0.005) (**Figure 4A**). The 12-month PFS rate was 5.9% vs. 17.4% in patients with high vs. low TGR_0. Univariate analyses revealed that the following factors were significantly associated with inferior PFS: higher TGR_0 (hazard ratio [HR] 1.97; 95% CI, 1.21 - 3.21; P = 0.006), larger SLD_0 (HR 5.79, 95% CI, 2.64 - 12.73; $P < 0.001$), two or more lines of prior therapy for advanced disease (HR 2.98; 95% CI, 1.76 - 5.02; $P < 0.001$), three or more metastatic sites (HR 2.52; 95% CI, 1.55 - 4.10; $P < 0.001$), ECOG PS of 2 to 3 (HR 3.35; 95% CI, 1.14 - 9.80; P = 0.027) and ALK rearrangement (HR 4.69; 95% CI, 1.61 - 13.70; P = 0.005) (**Figures 4A–D, Table 3**). Patients with EGFR mutant tumor also exhibited shorter PFS, with borderline significance (HR 2.00; 95% CI, 0.98 - 4.06; P = 0.056). In multivariate Cox model included all analyzed factors in univariate analyses, we found that higher TGR_0 (HR 1.97; 95% CI, 1.08 - 3.60; P = 0.026), larger SLD_0 (HR 10.70; 95% CI, 4.20 - 27.23; $P < 0.001$) and two or more lines of prior therapy (HR 3.36; 95% CI, 1.58 - 7.15; P = 0.002) remained significantly associated with shorter PFS (**Table 3**). Negative history of prior radiotherapy (HR 1.92; 95% CI, 0.96 - 3.83; P = 0.066) and three or more metastatic sites (HR 1.97; 95% CI, 1.00 - 3.88; P = 0.051) also tended to predict inferior PFS (**Table 3**).

To further validate the effect of TGR_0 on PFS, we performed subgroup analysis based on specific baseline parameters. TGR_0 predicted efficacy of ICI in NSCLC patients across almost all the subgroups including age, ECOG PS of 0 or 1, male, never smoker, histology, prior treatment lines, 1 or 2 metastatic sites, negative history of prior radiotherapy and small SLD_0 (**Figure 5**). In the histology subgroup, 43 were histologically conformed lung adenocarcinomas. Among them, 25 had low TGR_0 level, with 18 grouped into high TGR_0 strata. High TGR_0 also tended to predicted shorter PFS (HR 1.75; 95% CI, 0.91 - 3.37), though not statistically significant (P = 0.097). However, in patients with metastatic sites of ≥ 3, ECOG PS of 2 to 3, positive history of prior radiotherapy and those with large SLD_0, TGR_0 did not have impact on PFS.

TGR_0 did not have impact on OS (HR 1.24; 95% CI, 0.64-2.39; log-rank P = 0.519) (**Figure S1**). In multivariate Cox regression analysis, ECOG PS of 1 (HR 2.65; 95% CI 1.14 - 6.19; P = 0.024), ECOG PS of 2 to 3 (HR 30.62; 95% CI 3.61 - 260.01; P = 0.002), two or more prior treatment lines (HR 2.65; 95% CI 1.14 - 6.16; P = 0.024), without EGFR mutation (HR 7.12; 95% CI 1.32 - 38.53; P = 0.023), larger SLD_0 (HR 8.24; 95% CI 2.84 - 23.85; $P <$ 0.001) were significantly associated with poorer OS (**Table S1**). Patients with low TGR_0 achieved significantly higher DCB rate compared with those with high TGR_0 (16 of 46 [34.8%] vs. 3 of 34 [8.8%], P = 0.007). However, there was only a trend towards increased ORR in patients with low TGR_0 (7 of 46 [15.2%] vs. 3 of 34 [8.8%]; P = 0.505).

TABLE 2 | Association of TGR_0 with other parameters (n = 80).

	$TGR_0 \le$ 25.3%/m (n=46) No. (%)	$TGR_0 >$ 25.3%/m (n=34) No. (%)	P-value
Age			0.873
Median (range)	56 (33-77)	52 (30-74)	
Gender			0.056
Male	35 (64.8)	19 (35.2)	
Female	11 (42.3)	15 (57.7)	
ECOG PS			0.932
0	17 (54.8)	14 (45.2)	
1	27 (60.0)	18 (40.0)	
2-3	2 (50.0)	2 (50.0)	
Smoking status			0.034
Never smoker	23 (47.9)	25 (52.1)	
Current or former smoker	23 (71.9)	9 (28.1)	
Histology			0.935
Squamous cell carcinoma	18 (58.1)	13 (41.9)	
Nonsquamous cell carcinoma	28 (57.1)	21 (42.9)	
No. of prior treatment lines			0.935
0-1	28 (57.1)	21 (42.9)	
≥2	18 (58.1)	13 (41.9)	
No. of metastatic sites			0.220
1-2	28 (63.6)	16 (36.4)	
≥3	18 (50.0)	18 (50.0)	
Prior radiotherapy			0.623
Yes	10 (52.6)	9 (47.4)	
No	36 (59.0)	25 (41.0)	
EGFR mutation status			0.983
Positive	6 (60.0)	4 (40.0)	
Negative	29 (56.9)	22 (43.1)	
Not available	11 (57.9)	8 (42.1)	
ALK translocation			0.390
Positive	1 (25.0)	3 (75.0)	
Negative	32 (61.5)	20 (38.5)	
Not available	13 (54.2)	11 (45.8)	
SLD_0, mm			0.368
Median (range)	72 (17-158)	76 (19-231)	
RECIST response			0.028
PR	7 (70.0)	3 (30.0)	
SD	15 (78.9)	4 (21.1)	
PD	20 (43.5)	26 (56.5)	
NE	4 (80.0)	1 (20.0)	

ECOG PS, Eastern Cooperative Oncology Group performance status; EGFR, epidermal growth factor receptor; ALK, anaplastic lymphoma kinase; SLD_0, sum of the longest diameters of the target lesions at baseline; RECIST, Response Evaluation Criteria in Solid Tumors; PR, partial response; SD, stable disease; PD, progressive disease; NE, not evaluable.

DISCUSSION

Early prediction of response to anti-cancer therapy is important for selecting patients that are more likely to benefit from such

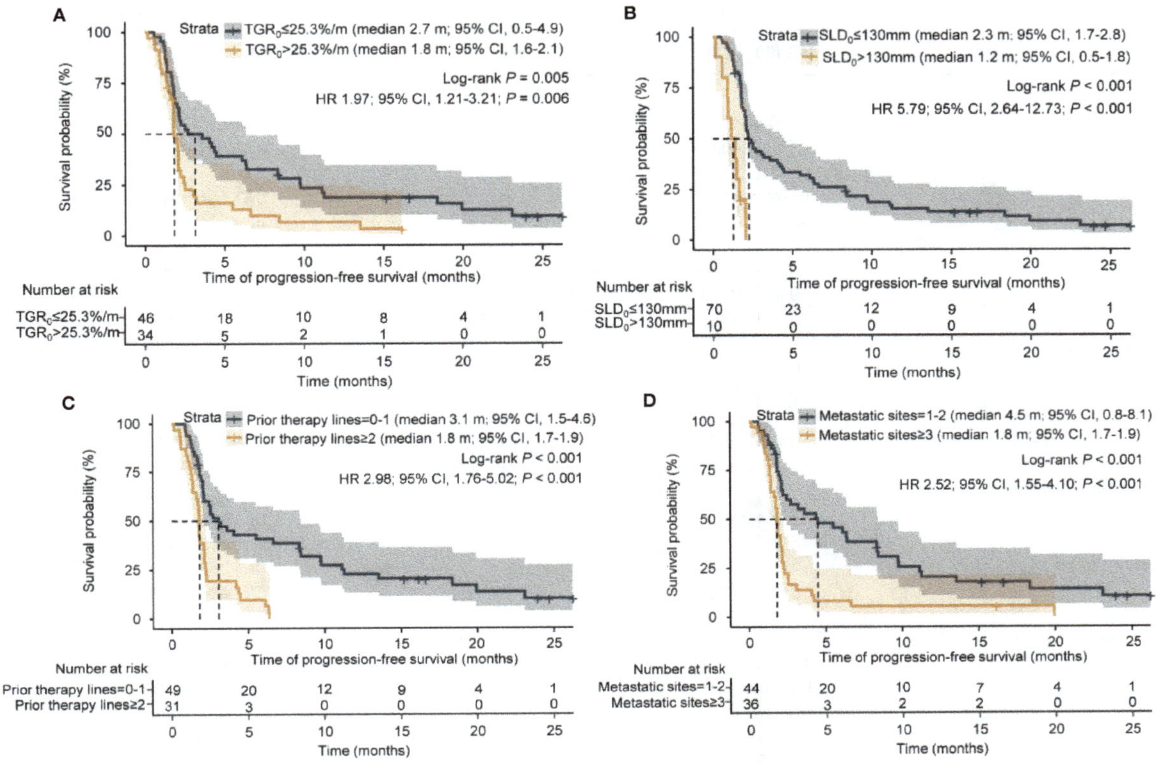

FIGURE 4 | Kaplan-Meier analysis of progression-free survival. **(A)** Progression-free survival by pre-treatment tumor growth rate. **(B)** Progression-free survival by sum of the longest diameters of the target lesions at baseline. **(C)** Progression-free survival by number of prior therapy lines. **(D)** Progression-free survival by number of metastatic sites.

treatment and optimizing radiological follow-up strategies. The results from our study suggested that higher pre-treatment tumor growth rate (TGR_0) played a role in predicting inferior PFS for aNSCLC patients treated with anti-PD-1/PD-L1 monotherapy. Patients with higher TGR_0 was also significantly associated with less durable clinical benefit.

Our findings resonated with some previous studies. A *post hoc* analysis from a phase II study revealed that higher pre-treatment TGR tended to be associated with shorter PFS in grade 1 or 2 gastroenteropancreatic neuroendocrine tumors (GEP-NETs) receiving lanreotide (27), and the CLARINET study further validated this finding (18). A TGR_0 < 4%/m predicted inferior PFS in G1 or G2 NET patients regardless of treatment modalities (21). Similarly, patients with higher pre-treatment tumor growth rate——measured as specific growth rate (SGR) experienced worse PFS in locally advanced NSCLC undergoing definitive chemoradiation therapy (CRT) (28). It was postulated that tumor growth rate may be more biologically and clinically relevant for predicting patient's clinical outcomes than the RECIST did. The GREPONET study found that TGR_{3m} provide more useful information in predicting patients' outcomes and had less variability than $RECIST_{3m}$ (21). Another study enrolling 58 aNSCLC patients showed that the deceleration in TGR at first follow-up after the start of ICI therapy was significantly associated with superior OS (29). It is worthy of note that the median (range) of TGR_0 from these 58 aNSCLC patients and our cohort was comparable (28.0 [−48.6 to 293.7]%/m vs. 21.1 [-33.7-246.0]%/m), indicating the repeatability of the calculation of TGR. Taken together, these results imply that translation of TGR into clinical practice may allow earlier and more precise prediction of clinical outcomes in oncotherapy. Our study further and for the first time showed that the natural tumor growth kinetics, estimated as TGR_0, could predict the efficacy of ICI in NSCLC. This association was consistent across different subgroups and was maintained in multivariate regression analysis.

The TGR_0 could therefore have a potential in tailoring on-treatment imaging schemes and early prediction of risk of disease progression. Based on our findings, patients with high TGR_0 should undergo more frequent follow-up imaging because of their shorter PFS, namely higher risk of experiencing early disease progression; while patients with low TGR_0 are more likely to have durable clinical benefit and could receive follow-up imaging assessment of longer interval to cut down the radiation exposure and examination cost. TGR also played a role in examining anti-tumor drug activity and guiding "go/no go" decision making in the early drug

TABLE 3 | Univariate and multivariate analyses of progression-free survival.

	Univariate analysis		Multivariate analysis	
	HR (95% CI)	***P*-value**	**HR (95% CI)**	***P*-value**
Age, years				
< 55	1.40 (0.88-2.24)	0.156	1.46 (0.80-2.67)	0.212
≥ 55	1 [Reference]	NA	1 [Reference]	NA
Gender				
Male	1 [Reference]	NA	1 [Reference]	NA
Female	1.49 (0.91-2.45)	0.115	1.44 (0.74-2.79)	0.282
ECOG PS				
0	1 [Reference]	NA	1 [Reference]	NA
1	1.09 (0.67-1.78)	0.721	0.99 (0.56-1.75)	0.979
2-3	3.35 (1.14-9.80)	0.027	1.49 (0.39-5.79)	0.561
Smoking status				
Never smoker	1.16 (0.72-1.86)	0.545	1 [Reference]	NA
Current or former smoker	1 [Reference]	NA	1.18 (0.60-2.33)	0.637
Histology				
Squamous cell carcinoma	1 [Reference]	NA	1 [Reference]	NA
Nonsquamous cell carcinoma	1.14 (0.70-1.87)	0.590	1.11 (0.55-2.24)	0.780
No. of prior treatment lines				
0-1	1 [Reference]	NA	1 [Reference]	NA
≥2	2.98 (1.76-5.02)	<0.001	3.36 (1.58-7.15)	0.002
No. of metastatic sites				
1-2	1 [Reference]	NA	1 [Reference]	NA
≥3	2.52 (1.55-4.10)	<0.001	1.97 (1.00-3.88)	0.051
Prior radiotherapy				
Yes	1.10 (0.64-1.90)	0.736	1 [Reference]	NA
No	1 [Reference]	NA	1.92 (0.96-3.83)	0.066
EGFR mutation status				
Negative	1 [Reference]	NA	1 [Reference]	NA
Positive	2.00 (0.98-4.06)	0.056	1.00 (0.39-2.61)	0.917
Not available	1.41 (0.80-2.49)	0.233	2.80 (0.73-10.77)	0.135
ALK translocation				
Negative	1 [Reference]	NA	1 [Reference]	NA
Positive	4.69 (1.61-13.70)	0.005	2.43 (0.67-8.82)	0.177
Not available	1.24 (0.74-2.08)	0.424	0.59 (0.18-1.86)	0.365
SLD_0, mm				
≤ 130	1 [Reference]	NA	1 [Reference]	NA
> 130	5.79 (2.64-12.73)	<0.001	10.70 (4.20-27.23)	<0.001
TGR_0, %/m				
≤ 25.3	1 [Reference]	NA	1 [Reference]	NA
> 25.3	1.97 (1.21-3.21)	0.006	1.97 (1.08-3.60)	0.026

HR, hazard ratio; CI, confidence interval; NA, not applicable; ECOG PS, Eastern Cooperative Oncology Group performance status; EGFR, epidermal growth factor receptor; ALK, anaplastic lymphoma kinase; SLD_0, sum of the longest diameters of the target lesions at baseline; TGR_0, pre-treatment tumor growth rate.

development. Although the rationale behind the negative impact of TGR_0 on the efficacy of ICI is unclear, it could be hypothesized that the immune microenviroment of fast-growing tumor is unfavorable for the action of PD-1 axis inhibitors. Another possible explanation is that the time for the adaptive immune response and tumor killing after PD-1 axis inhibition is too long compare with the tumor growth rate. These results implied that fast-growing tumors should avoid being treated with single agent ICI. This could be viewed from the case of small cell lung cancer, which is a typical type of fast-growing tumor and have poor responsiveness to single agent ICI but demonstrates improved survival with chemoimmunotherapy combinations (30). Also, our results highlight the need for future exploration of combining TGR and RECIST criteria to refine the follow-up schemes as well as the role of ICI plus chemotherapy in tumors with high TGR_0.

Our study failed to observe significant difference in OS between TGR_0 strata, which might be due to the divergent sensitivity of subsequent treatment (chemotherapy as the mainstream one) in these two groups, the imbalance of subsequent treatment, and the relatively small sample size. Nevertheless, we also found that high TGR_0 was correlated with low DCB rate and a tendency towards lower ORR. Similar to our observation, Yvonne Purcell et al. elucidated that the mean pre-treatment TGR was not significant different between the objective response (OR) and non-OR group in hepatocellular carcinoma treated with transarterial chemoembolization (19). This is clinically relevant because it has been showed that ORR was poorly correlated with long-term survival for immunotherapy (12, 31), indicating the inadequacy of RECIST criteria which only capture tumor volume change but miss out temporal information. Taken together, these results indicate that TGR_0 is a predictive

Subgroup	$TGR_0 \leq 25.3\%/m$ Patients (%)	$TGR_0 \leq 25.3\%/m$ Median PFS (months)	$TGR_0 > 25.3\%/m$ Patients (%)	$TGR_0 > 25.3\%/m$ Median PFS (months)	Hazard ratio (95% CI)	*P*-value
All patients	46 (57.5)	2.7	34 (42.5)	1.8	1.97 (1.21–3.21)	0.006
Age,years						
< 55	21 (52.5)	2.1	19 (47.5)	1.6	1.92 (0.97–3.79)	0.061
≥ 55	25 (62.5)	4.2	15 (37.5)	2.1	1.91 (0.95–3.85)	0.072
Gender						
Female	11 (42.3)	2.7	15 (57.7)	1.5	1.78 (0.77–4.16)	0.180
Male	35 (64.8)	3.6	19 (35.2)	2.1	1.95 (1.06–3.60)	0.033
ECOG PS						
0	17 (54.8)	4.1	14 (45.2)	1.8	1.94 (0.89–4.26)	0.097
1	27 (60.0)	3.6	18 (40.0)	2.0	2.07 (1.06–4.04)	0.032
2–3	2 (50.0)	1.4	2 (50.0)	0.2	2.56 (0.23–29.12)	0.448
Smoking status						
Never smoker	23 (47.9)	2.7	25 (52.1)	1.8	2.19 (1.14–4.19)	0.018
Current or former smoker	23 (71.9)	3.6	9 (28.1)	1.8	1.58 (0.71–3.52)	0.261
Histology						
Squamous	18 (58.1)	3.6	13 (41.9)	1.8	2.16 (0.94–4.95)	0.068
Nonsquamous	28 (57.1)	2.5	21 (42.9)	2.1	1.76 (0.96–3.25)	0.068
No. of prior therapy lines						
0–1	28 (57.1)	8.3	21 (42.9)	2.1	2.12 (1.09–4.11)	0.026
≥ 2	18 (58.1)	2.1	13 (41.9)	1.6	3.17 (1.37–7.34)	0.007
No. of metastatic sites						
1–2	28 (63.6)	6.4	16 (36.4)	2.1	2.84 (1.40–5.78)	0.004
≥ 3	18 (50.0)	1.8	18 (50.0)	1.8	1.10 (0.56–2.16)	0.779
Prior radiotherapy						
Yes	10 (52.6)	2.0	9 (47.4)	2.2	1.01 (0.37–2.72)	0.987
No	36 (59.0)	3.6	25 (41.0)	1.8	2.46 (1.39–4.34)	0.002
SLD_0, mm						
≤ 130	43 (61.4)	4.1	27 (38.6)	2.1	1.92 (1.13–3.25)	0.015
> 130	3 (30.0)	1.2	7 (70.0)	1.4	0.78 (0.18–3.31)	0.733

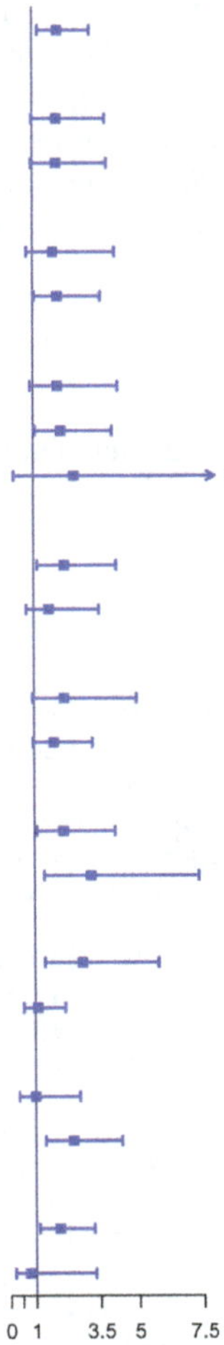

FIGURE 5 | Subgroup analysis of PFS according to TGR_0 stratification. Findings were examined by Cox proportional hazard regression analysis.

rather than a prognostic factor for aNSCLC patients undergoing ICI therapy. It is therefore more reliable to guide patients' management in clinical practice.

Our study has several limitations. First, the study was retrospectively conducted at a single institute with a moderate sample size. Statistical power was limited and could explain why the ORR and the OS between high and low TGR_0 groups did not reach statistical significance. Prospective or external validation of our work is required in another cohort with larger sample size. However, we think our finding is relatively reliable and reproducible since the predictive value of TGR is confirmed in various cancers undergoing different treatment therapies. Second, the strict inclusion criteria, especially the requirements of two consecutive imaging during wash-out period, may cause potential selection bias. Third, target lesions selected for calculation of TGR might not represent the whole tumor burden as new lesions and non-target lesions were not taken into account. Dissociated or mixed response phenomenon may confound the accurate tumor kinetics assessment after treatment initiation (32). Fourth, Limited to the retrospective nature of our work, we were unable to estimate predictive value of PD-L1 status and TMB level for only 3 patients had detected these two items. The main reason was that PD-L1 and TMB testing were not mandatory for using immunotherapy regimens since most patients in our study received ICIs in two or more lines of treatment. When we sought to re-evaluate PD-L1 and TMB status, the tissues were insufficient because all were from small biopsies. Last, the clinical application of TGR_0 may be limited by the economic and ethical consideration of additional imaging evaluation required during wash-out period. However, considering the risk of early disease progression and cost of ICI treatments, we think such procedure might still have clinical relevance. Despite these limitations, our findings suggested that TGR_0 has potential value for clinical utility by predicting risk of progression and providing complementary information to RECIST criteria.

CONCLUSIONS

Higher pre-treatment TGR was significantly associated with inferior PFS and less durable clinical benefit in aNSCLC patients undergoing anti-PD-1/PD-L1 monotherapy. TGR_0 could provide additional information for predicting the efficacy of immune checkpoint inhibition and facilitate tailoring patient's management. The potential role of TGR_0 in the treatment decision requires further validation in another cohort and future prospective studies.

AUTHOR CONTRIBUTIONS

SH and LZ put forward the study concept and design of the work. All authors contributed to the acquisition, analysis, or interpretation of data. L-NH, XZ, and HL drafted the manuscript. SH and LZ helped with funding acquisition. SH and YH edited the manuscript. LZ contributed to the study supervision. All authors contributed to the article and approved the submitted version.

ACKNOWLEDGMENTS

We sincerely appreciate all the patients and their family who were included in this retrospective study.

REFERENCES

1. Borghaei H, Paz-Ares L, Horn L, Spigel DR, Steins M, Ready NE, et al. Nivolumab versus Docetaxel in Advanced Nonsquamous Non-Small-Cell Lung Cancer. *N Engl J Med* (2015) 373:1627–39. doi: 10.1056/NEJMoa1507643
2. Brahmer J, Reckamp KL, Baas P, Crino L, Eberhardt WE, Poddubskaya E, et al. Nivolumab versus Docetaxel in Advanced Squamous-Cell Non-Small-Cell Lung Cancer. *N Engl J Med* (2015) 373:123–35. doi: 10.1056/NEJMoa1504627
3. Fehrenbacher L, Spira A, Ballinger M, Kowanetz M, Vansteenkiste J, Mazieres J, et al. Atezolizumab versus docetaxel for patients with previously treated non-small-cell lung cancer (POPLAR): a multicentre, open-label, phase 2 randomised controlled trial. *Lancet* (2016) 387:1837–46. doi: 10.1016/s0140-6736(16)00587-0
4. Gettinger S, Horn L, Jackman D, Spigel D, Antonia S, Hellmann M, et al. Five-Year Follow-Up of Nivolumab in Previously Treated Advanced Non-Small-Cell Lung Cancer: Results From the CA209-003 Study. *J Clin Oncol Off J Am Soc Clin Oncol* (2018) 36:1675–84. doi: 10.1200/jco.2017.77.0412
5. Mok TSK, Wu Y-L, Kudaba I, Kowalski DM, Cho BC, Turna HZ, et al. Pembrolizumab versus chemotherapy for previously untreated, PD-L1-expressing, locally advanced or metastatic non-small-cell lung cancer (KEYNOTE-042): a randomised, open-label, controlled, phase 3 trial. *Lancet* (2019) 393:1819–30. doi: 10.1016/s0140-6736(18)32409-7
6. Kim JY, Lee KH, Kang J, Borcoman E, Saada-Bouzid E, Kronbichler A, et al. Hyperprogressive Disease during Anti-PD-1 (PDCD1) / PD-L1 (CD274) Therapy: A Systematic Review and Meta-Analysis. *Cancers (Basel)* (2019) 11 (11):1699. doi: 10.3390/cancers11111699
7. Mushti SL, Mulkey F, Tang S, Singh H, Lemery SJ, Goldberg KB, et al. Immune Response Evaluation and Treatment with Immune Checkpoint Inhibitors Beyond Clinical Progression: Response Assessments for Cancer Immunotherapy. *Curr Oncol Rep* (2020) 22:116. doi: 10.1007/s11912-020-00974-z
8. Bodor JN, Boumber Y, Borghaei H. Biomarkers for immune checkpoint inhibition in non-small cell lung cancer (NSCLC). *Cancer* (2020) 126:260–70. doi: 10.1002/cncr.32468
9. Eisenhauer EA, Therasse P, Bogaerts J, Schwartz LH, Sargent D, Ford R, et al. New response evaluation criteria in solid tumours: revised RECIST guideline (version 1.1). *Eur J Cancer* (2009) 45:228–47. doi: 10.1016/j.ejca.2008.10.026
10. Maitland ML, Schwartz LH, Ratain MJ. Time to tumor growth: a model end point and new metric system for oncology clinical trials. *J Clin Oncol Off J Am Soc Clin Oncol* (2013) 31:2070–2. doi: 10.1200/jco.2013.49.3635
11. Nishino M, Dahlberg SE, Adeni AE, Lydon CA, Hatabu H, Janne PA, et al. Tumor Response Dynamics of Advanced Non-small Cell Lung Cancer Patients Treated with PD-1 Inhibitors: Imaging Markers for Treatment Outcome. *Clin Cancer Res* (2017) 23:5737–44. doi: 10.1158/1078-0432.CCR-17-1434
12. Ritchie G, Gasper H, Man J, Lord S, Marschner I, Friedlander M, et al. Defining the Most Appropriate Primary End Point in Phase 2 Trials of Immune Checkpoint Inhibitors for Advanced Solid Cancers: A Systematic Review and Meta-analysis. *JAMA Oncol* (2018) 4:522–8. doi: 10.1001/jamaoncol.2017.5236
13. Shukuya T, Mori K, Amann JM, Bertino EM, Otterson GA, Shields PG, et al. Relationship between Overall Survival and Response or Progression-Free Survival in Advanced Non-Small Cell Lung Cancer Patients Treated with Anti-PD-1/PD-L1 Antibodies. *J Thorac Oncol* (2016) 11:1927–39. doi: 10.1016/j.jtho.2016.07.017
14. Zhang J, Huang Y, Li X, Guo Y, Zhao Y, Xue C, et al. The impact of tumor size change after target therapy on survival: analysis of patients enrolled onto three clinical trials of advanced NSCLC from one institution. *Onco Targets Ther* (2012) 5:349–55. doi: 10.2147/OTT.S38441
15. Zhou T, Zheng L, Hu Z, Zhang Y, Fang W, Zhao Y, et al. The effectiveness of RECIST on survival in patients with NSCLC receiving chemotherapy with or without target agents as first-line treatment. *Sci Rep* (2015) 5:7683. doi: 10.1038/srep07683
16. Evan GI, Vousden KH. Proliferation, cell cycle and apoptosis in cancer. *Nature* (2001) 411:342–8. doi: 10.1038/35077213
17. Ferte C, Fernandez M, Hollebecque A, Koscielny S, Levy A, Massard C, et al. Tumor growth rate is an early indicator of antitumor drug activity in phase I clinical trials. *Clin Cancer Res* (2014) 20:246–52. doi: 10.1158/1078-0432.CCR-13-2098
18. Dromain C, Pavel ME, Ruszniewski P, Langley A, Massien C, Baudin E, et al. Tumor growth rate as a metric of progression, response, and prognosis in pancreatic and intestinal neuroendocrine tumors. *BMC Cancer* (2019) 19:66. doi: 10.1186/s12885-018-5257-x
19. Purcell Y, Sartoris R, Paradis V, Vilgrain V, Ronot M. Influence of pretreatment tumor growth rate on objective response of hepatocellular carcinoma treated with transarterial chemoembolization. *J Gastroenterol Hepatol* (2020) 35:305–13. doi: 10.1111/jgh.14816
20. Stein WD, Wilkerson J, Kim ST, Huang X, Motzer RJ, Fojo AT, et al. Analyzing the pivotal trial that compared sunitinib and IFN-alpha in renal cell carcinoma, using a method that assesses tumor regression and growth. *Clin Cancer Res* (2012) 18:2374–81. doi: 10.1158/1078-0432.CCR-11-2275
21. Lamarca A, Crona J, Ronot M, Opalinska M, Lopez Lopez C, Pezzutti D, et al. Value of Tumor Growth Rate (TGR) as an Early Biomarker Predictor of Patients' Outcome in Neuroendocrine Tumors (NET)-The GREPONET Study. *Oncologist* (2019) 24:e1082–e90. doi: 10.1634/theoncologist.2018-0672
22. Grande E, Martinez-Saez O, Gajate-Borau P, Alonso-Gordoa T. Translating new data to the daily practice in second line treatment of renal cell carcinoma: The role of tumor growth rate. *World J Clin Oncol* (2017) 8:100–5. doi: 10.5306/wjco.v8.i2.100
23. Ferte C, Koscielny S, Albiges L, Rocher L, Soria JC, Iacovelli R, et al. Tumor growth rate provides useful information to evaluate sorafenib and everolimus treatment in metastatic renal cell carcinoma patients: an integrated analysis of the TARGET and RECORD phase 3 trial data. *Eur Urol* (2014) 65:713–20. doi: 10.1016/j.eururo.2013.08.010

24. Champiat S, Dercle L, Ammari S, Massard C, Hollebecque A, Postel-Vinay S, et al. Hyperprogressive Disease Is a New Pattern of Progression in Cancer Patients Treated by Anti-PD-1/PD-L1. *Clin Cancer Res* (2017) 23:1920–8. doi: 10.1158/1078-0432.CCR-16-1741
25. von Elm E, Altman DG, Egger M, Pocock SJ, Gøtzsche PC, Vandenbroucke JP. The Strengthening the Reporting of Observational Studies in Epidemiology (STROBE) statement: guidelines for reporting observational studies. *Lancet (London England)* (2007) 370:1453–7. doi: 10.1016/s0140-6736(07)61602-x
26. Camp RL, Dolled-Filhart M, Rimm DL. X-tile: a new bio-informatics tool for biomarker assessment and outcome-based cut-point optimization. *Clin Cancer Res* (2004) 10:7252–9. doi: 10.1158/1078-0432.Ccr-04-0713
27. Ito T, Honma Y, Hijioka S, Kudo A, Fukutomi A, Nozaki A, et al. Phase II study of lanreotide autogel in Japanese patients with unresectable or metastatic well-differentiated neuroendocrine tumors. *Invest New Drugs* (2017) 35:499–508. doi: 10.1007/s10637-017-0466-8
28. Osorio B, Yegya-Raman N, Kim S, Simone CB 2nd, Theodorou RossC, Deek MP, et al. Clinical significance of pretreatment tumor growth rate for locally advanced non-small cell lung cancer. *Ann Transl Med* (2019) 7:95. doi: 10.21037/atm.2019.02.14
29. Ten Berge D, Hurkmans DP, den Besten I, Kloover JS, Mathijssen RHJ, Debets R, et al. Tumour growth rate as a tool for response evaluation during PD-1 treatment for non-small cell lung cancer: a retrospective analysis. *ERJ Open Res* (2019) 5(4):00179–2019. doi: 10.1183/23120541.00179-2019
30. Tay RY, Heigener D, Reck M, Califano R. Immune checkpoint blockade in small cell lung cancer. *Lung Cancer (Amsterdam Netherlands)* (2019) 137:31–7. doi: 10.1016/j.lungcan.2019.08.024
31. Zhang J, Liang W, Liang H, Wang X, He J. Endpoint surrogacy in oncological randomized controlled trials with immunotherapies: a systematic review of trial-level and arm-level meta-analyses. *Ann Transl Med* (2019) 7:244. doi: 10.21037/atm.2019.04.72
32. Tozuka T, Kitazono S, Sakamoto H, Yoshida H, Amino Y, Uematsu S, et al. Dissociated responses at initial computed tomography evaluation is a good prognostic factor in non-small cell lung cancer patients treated with anti-programmed cell death-1/ligand 1 inhibitors. *BMC Cancer* (2020) 20:207. doi: 10.1186/s12885-020-6704-z

12

Efficacy of Combination Chemo-Immunotherapy as a First-Line Treatment for Advanced Non-Small-Cell Lung Cancer Patients with HER2 Alterations

Shuang Zhao[1], Xinghong Xian[2], Panwen Tian[1], Weimin Li[1], Ke Wang[1] and Yalun Li[1*]*

[1] *Department of Respiratory and Critical Care Medicine, West China Hospital, Sichuan University, Chengdu, China,*
[2] *Clinical Medicine of West China Medical School/West China Hospital, Sichuan University, Chengdu, China*

Correspondence:
Ke Wang
wang2ke@126.com
Yalun Li
lunlunhx@qq.com

Objective: Although the treatment of non-small-cell lung cancer (NSCLC) patients with human epidermal growth factor receptor 2 (HER2) alterations has been studied for years, the overall response rate (ORR) of these patients is still unsatisfactory, and more therapeutic strategies are needed. Little is known about the combination of chemo- and immunotherapy in HER2-altered lung cancer treatment.

Materials and Methods: We report five cases of advanced NSCLC with HER2 insertion mutation or amplification treated with immunotherapy combined with chemotherapy as the first-line treatment. The HER2 alteration type, duration of treatment and survival were also analyzed.

Results: The five advanced NSCLC patients, three with HER2 mutations and two with HER2 amplifications, received chemo-immunotherapy as the first-line treatment. The average patient age was 54.6 years. Three patients were females, and two were males. Among all the patients, only one had a smoking history. The immunotherapies used were as follows: two patients were treated with sintilimab, and three patients were treated with pembrolizumab. Only one patient had squamous carcinoma, and she was also the only patient with a complete response (CR). The progression-free survival (PFS) ranged from 2-12 months, with a median PFS of 8.0 months.

Conclusions: Chemo-immunotherapy may be a promising first-line treatment option for NSCLC patients with HER2 alterations. Further clinical trials are required to confirm this therapeutic option.

Keywords: human epidermal growth factor receptor2, immunotherapy, chemotherapy, non-small-cell lung cancer, prognosis

INTRODUCTION

Lung cancer is known as one of the deadliest cancers worldwide and causes more deaths than prostate, breast, brain and colorectal cancers combined (1). Non-small-cell lung cancer (NSCLC) comprises approximately 85% of all lung cancer cases (2). Human epidermal growth factor 2 (HER2) is a rare oncogenic driver that is altered in 1% to 3% of NSCLC patients (3). The main types of HER2 alterations in lung cancer include gene insertion mutation, gene amplification and protein overexpression (4). Chemotherapy remains an important component of treatment for HER2-altered NSCLC patients, although HER2 positive tumors are relatively insensitive to chemoradiotherapy (5, 6). Several HER2-targeted tyrosine kinase inhibitors (TKIs) and antibodies have also been tested for the treatment of these patients. However, the overall response rate (ORR) was unsatisfactory, at only 7.4% for HER2-targeted TKIs such as neratinib, lapatinib and afatinib (7). More therapeutic strategies for NSCLC patients with HER2 alterations are needed. Little is known about the combination of immunotherapy and chemotherapy in the treatment of lung cancer with HER2 alterations. Therefore, we described five advanced NSCLC cases with HER2 mutation or amplification and immunotherapy combined with chemotherapy as the first-line treatment. We hope this case series will provide new clinical therapeutic insight for this class of patients.

CASE PRESENTATION

From January 2019 to June 2020, five patients with advanced NSCLC with HER2 alterations and chemo-immunotherapy as the first-line treatment were admitted to the Lung Cancer Center, West China Hospital, Sichuan University. High-throughput next-generation sequencing (NGS) technology was used to assess the presence and type of HER2 alterations in the biopsy specimens of all patients. The status of PD-L1 was also tested by immunohistochemistry. This retrospective study was approved by the Committee on Medical Ethics of West China Hospital, Sichuan University.

Patients With HER2 Mutation

Three patients harbored HER2 insertion mutations.

The first patient (Case 1) was a 37-year-old Asian female who was a never-smoker and had a symptom of severe headache. She was finally diagnosed with left lung adenocarcinoma with brain, bone, hilar and mediastinal lymph node metastases (cT2N2M1c, stage IVB). She harbored a HER2 insertion mutation in exon 20 (p. A775_G776insYVMA). EGFR, ALK, ROS-1 and PD-L1 testing was performed, and none of these targets were expressed. She received chemotherapy (carboplatin and pemetrexed) and sintilimab for 6 cycles with a partial response (PR) as her best response. Then, she experienced progressive disease (PD) with new brain metastases and was treated with pyrotinib, a pan-ErbB receptor TKI, for 2 months. However, she continued to progress with multiple new brain metastases and died because of a hemorrhagic cerebral hernia.

The second patient (Case 2) was a 65-year-old Asian man with a 10-pack-year smoking history who was diagnosed with cT4N3M1c stage IVB lung adenocarcinoma by pleural effusion smear and cytological examination. He complained of cough for 4 months. The NGS panel revealed a HER2 mutation (exon 20, p. A775_G776insYVMA) without concurrent alterations or PD-L1 expression. He was treated with carboplatin and pemetrexed combined with sintilimab for 4 cycles. His best response was stable disease (SD). Then, he experienced progressive malignant pleural effusion. One month after starting anlotinib, a chest CT scan showed a reduction in pleural effusion. The patient maintained SD until his last visit.

The third patient (Case 3) was a 52-year-old Asian man who was a never-smoker and developed cough and bloody sputum for 2 months. Chest CT showed a left lower lung mass with multiple bilateral pulmonary nodules. Brain MRI and bone single photon emission CT (SPECT) were all negative. Through percutaneous lung biopsy and left supraclavicular lymph node biopsy, he was finally diagnosed with cT4N3M1c stage IVB right lung adenocarcinoma. A HER2 mutation (exon 20, p. A775_G776insYVMA) was found from his initial molecular testing, but no other gene alterations were identified. He received carboplatin and pemetrexed chemotherapy and pembrolizumab for 2 cycles. Unfortunately, he experienced rapid progression within 2 months. He was then treated with docetaxel, carboplatin and bevacizumab for 1 month. He is currently enrolled in an EGFR/HER2-targeted TKI clinical trial (DZD9008).

Patients With HER2 Amplification

There were two patients with HER2 amplification.

The fourth patient (Case 4) was a 72-year-old Asian female never-smoker who complained of dorsalgia for 9 months. She was diagnosed with lung adenocarcinoma by percutaneous lung biopsy. CT showed metastatic mediastinal lymphadenopathy, SPECT scanning showed multiple bone metastases, and MRI showed evidence of brain metastases. The clinical stage was cT1N2M1c stage IVB. She was found to have HER2 amplification (copy number:2.6) without other gene alterations or PD-L1 expression. She was treated with carboplatin, pemetrexed, and pembrolizumab for 9 cycles. Then, she progressed with multiple new liver and bone metastases after 12 months and started on docetaxel and pembrolizumab with radiographic evidence of SD, which was sustained for 4.0 months up to the study endpoint.

The fifth patient (Case 5) was a 47-year-old Asian female never-smoker who had no symptoms. Her chest CT scan showed multiple pulmonary nodules. She was diagnosed with cT4N0M1a stage IVA lung squamous carcinoma by percutaneous lung biopsy. NGS testing of her lung biopsy specimen was performed, and it showed HER2 amplification (copy number:3.22). EGFR, ALK, ROS-1 and PD-L1 expression were all negative. She received chemotherapy (carboplatin and pemetrexed) and pembrolizumab for 4 cycles followed by pembrolizumab maintenance therapy, with a complete response (CR) as her best response. The patient was still in remission at the endpoint of this study.

Summary of Patients

The average patient age was 54.6 years. Three patients were females, and two were males. Among all the patients, only one had a smoking history (Case 2). The HER2 mutation type, treatments, responses and progression-free survival (PFS) for the above five patients are summarized in **Table 1**. The median PFS (mPFS) was 8 months, ranging from 2-12 months. The immunotherapies used were as follows: two patients were treated with sintilimab (Case 1 and Case 2), and three patients were treated with pembrolizumab (Case 3, Case 4 and Case 5). Only one patient (Case 5) had squamous carcinoma, and she was also the only patient with a CR. **Figure 1** displays the representative chest CT images of all the patients' best responses.

DISCUSSION

Five advanced NSCLC patients, three with HER2 mutations and two with HER2 amplifications, received chemoimmunotherapy as the first-line treatment. Among all the patients, the immunotherapies used were as follows: two patients were treated with sintilimab, and three patients were treated with pembrolizumab. Only one patient had squamous carcinoma, and she was also the only patient with a CR. The PFS ranged from 2-12 months, with a median PFS of 8.0 months.

HER2, also known as ERBB2, is a cell surface receptor tyrosine kinase of the ERBB family that is considered an oncogenic driver in many cancers, notably breast, ovarian and gastroesophageal cancers (8). The HER2 receptor is activated via heterodimerization or homodimerization with other ERBB family receptors, inducing activation of EGFR signaling (9). The main types of HER2 alterations in lung cancer include gene insertion mutation, gene amplification and protein overexpression. HER2 insertion mutations and amplifications have been reported in approximately 2-5% and 2-3% of lung adenocarcinomas, respectively (10–12).

Recently, many clinical trials have focused on HER2-targeted therapy for HER2-positive NSCLC. However, the results are ambiguous and insufficient. Trastuzumab, a monoclonal antibody for the HER2 receptor, did not show definite benefits for HER2-positive NSCLC patients (13). In contrast, TKIs targeting both HER2 and EGFR were shown to exhibit a therapeutic response. In the EUHER2 study, HER2-targeted drugs, including trastuzumab, lapatinib, neratinib and afatinib, did not show clear survival benefits compared with conventional therapy, including chemotherapy and reversible EGFR-TKIs (7). Among them, afatinib, an irreversible ERBB family blocker, might be a promising therapeutic choice for HER2-mutant NSCLC with progression after previous chemotherapy or reversible EGFR-TKI treatment (14). Afatinib showed a response rate of 18.2% and an mPFS of 3.9 months in the EUHER2 study (7), but recent phase II trials found that only

TABLE 1 | The characteristics, treatments, responses and progression free survival (PFS) for the patients.

Patient	Histopathological type	Gender	Age	Smoking	HER2	First-Line Treatment			Second -Line Treatment			OS
						Treatment	Best Disease Response	PFS1	Treatment	Best Disease Response	PFS2	
1#	ADC	female	37	Never	insertion mutation	AC+ sintilimab	PR	7m	pyrotinib	PD	4m	11m
2#	ADC	male	65	Current	insertion mutation	AC+ sintilimab	SD	8m	anlotinib	N/A	N/A	N/A >10m
3#	ADC	male	52	Never	insertion mutation	AC+ pembrolizumab	PD	2m	DC+ bevacizumab	SD	N/A	N/A >4m
4#	ADC	female	72	Never	amplification	AC+ pembrolizumab	SD	12m	D+ pembrolizumab/	SD	N/A	N/A >16m
5#	SCC	female	47	Never	amplification	AC +pembrolizumab; Pembrolizumab.	CR	N/A >12m			N/A	N/A >12m

A, pemetrexed; C, carboplatin; D, docetaxel; K, pembrolizumab; HER2, human epidermal growth factor receptor 2; ADC, adenocarcinoma; SCC, squamous carcinoma; OS, overall survival.

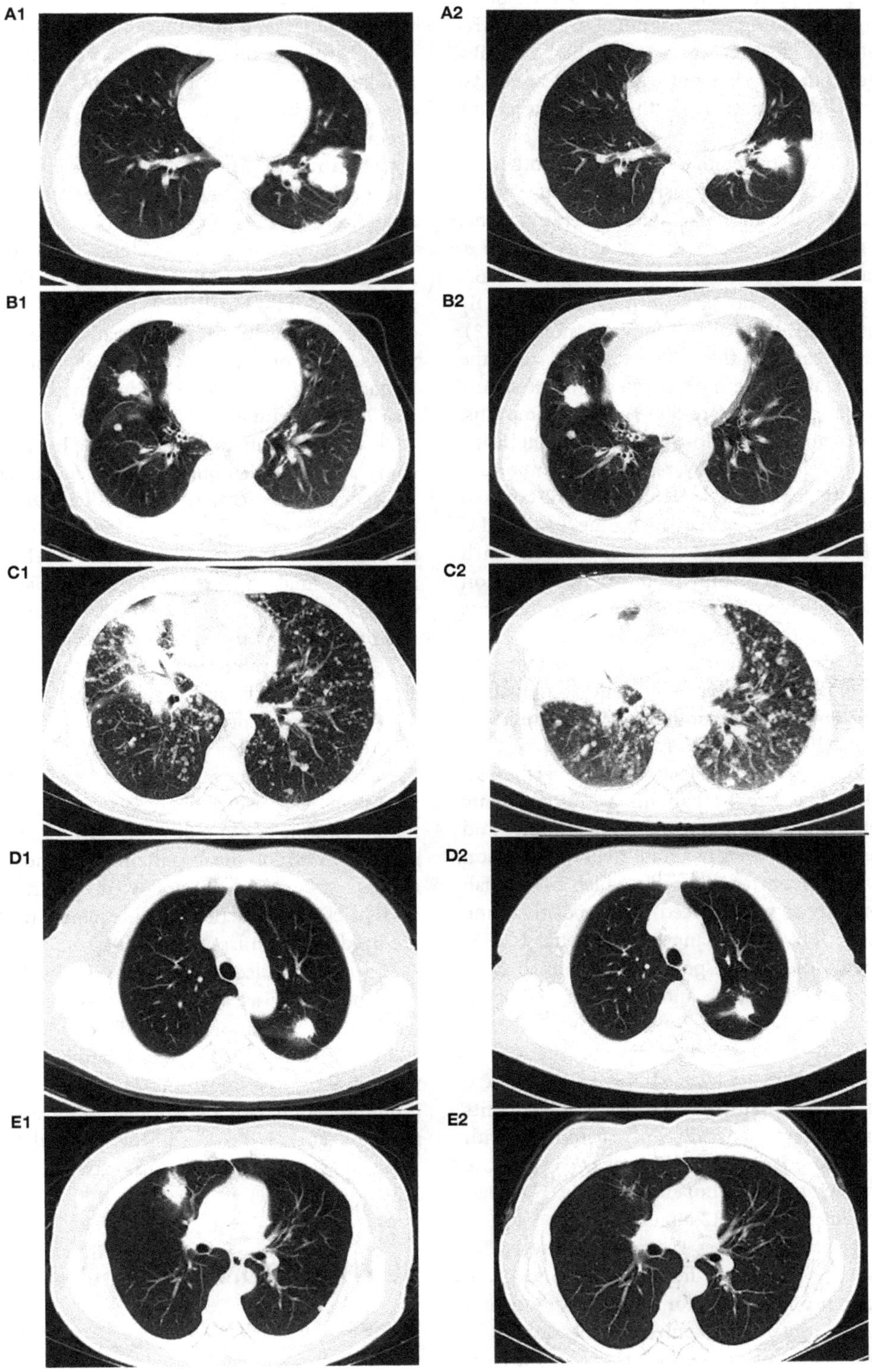

FIGURE 1 | CT imaging of best disease response of patients: Case 1 at beginning of therapy **(A1)** and 4 months after receiving carboplatin+pemetrexed chemotherapy and sintilimab **(A2)** Case 2 at beginning of therapy **(B1)** and 5 months after receiving carboplatin+pemetrexed chemotherapy and sintilimab **(B2)** Case 3 at beginning of therapy **(C1)** and 2 months after receiving carboplatin+pemetrexed chemotherapy and pembrolizumab**(C2)** Case 4 at beginning of therapy **(D1)** and 10 months after receiving carboplatin+pemetrexed chemotherapy and pembrolizumab **(D2)** Case 5 at beginning of therapy **(E1)** and 6 months after treatment with carboplatin, pemetrexed, and pembrolizumab for 4 cycles followed by pembrolizumab maintenance **(E2)**.

patients with specific HER2 mutations had durable responses to afatinib (15). Subsequently, preliminary results for several other HER2 kinase inhibitors, including temsirolimus (16) and TAK-788 (17), have indicated an effect on regression in these patients. Thus far, HER2-targeted therapy has not achieved ideal effects, and the treatment of NSCLC patients with HER2 alterations remains a major challenge.

The advantages of HER2-targeted therapy over chemotherapy in HER2-positive NSCLC are inconclusive. Previous studies suggested that the mPFS durations of chemotherapy alone, pemetrexed ± platinum/bevacizumab, gemcitabine, taxane ± platinum/bevacizumab, and vinorelbine were 4.3 months, 6.2 months, 2.6 months, 4 months and 3.5 months, respectively. By comparison, the mPFS of HER2 TKIs was only 2.2 months (18). For HER2-mutant lung cancers, the ORR was 36%, and the mPFS was 5.1 months with chemotherapy as the first-line therapy (6). The ORR and mPFS were 50.9% and 4.8 months, respectively, with trastuzumab or ado-trastuzumab emtansine (T-DM1) (7). Therefore, chemotherapy remains an important component of treatment, while the benefit of HER2-targeted therapy is inconclusive. However, the outcome of NSCLC patients with HER2 alterations who are treated with chemotherapy can be further improved by combination treatment, and thus, additional therapies for these patients are warranted.

Immunotherapies are also worth considering for the treatment of patients with HER2 alterations. The combination treatment of pembrolizumab and chemotherapy was included in the guidelines as a first-line treatment for advanced NSCLC based on the KEYNOTE-189 trial (19, 20). Nevertheless, immunotherapy is less effective in patients with oncogenic mutations than in patients without oncogenic mutations, and anti-PD-1/PD-L1 therapy may even facilitate hyperprogression (21). Chiara Catania et al. reported a case in which nivolumab had strong antitumor activity in advanced HER2-positive lung cancer (22). Conversely, Jody C. Chuang reported that HER2-mutated NSCLC patients did not respond to nivolumab (23). Mazieres et al. reported an ORR of 7% and a median PFS of 2.5 months amongst 29 patients with HER2 altered advanced lung cancer when treated with single agent immune checkpoint inhibitors (24). In our study, five advanced NSCLC cases were described. The results showed that the PFS times of the patients ranged from 2–12 months, with an mPFS of 8.0 months with chemoimmunotherapy. Based on our experience, we propose that chemoimmunotherapy may be a hopeful first-line treatment option for NSCLC patients with HER2 alterations.

NSCLC has distinct clinical features according to the HER2 alteration type; however, both amplification and oncogenic mutation in HER2 can promote receptor hyperactivation and tumor growth (25). HER2 mutations mainly occur at exon 20 in the protein kinase domain and are recognized as primary drivers in lung cancer, similar to other oncogenic drivers, such as EGFR, ROS, ALK, KRAS and BRAF (11). In NSCLC, it is controversial whether HER2 amplification is a driver gene. Some studies have suggested that amplification of ERBB2 is a driver event specifically in oncogene-negative lung adenocarcinoma (12). However, HER2 amplification may not be associated with HER2 mutation, and they may be involved in distinct clinical entities that need different therapeutic methods (26). Case reports have suggested that pyrotinib and afatinib may also be effective for lung adenocarcinoma patients with coexisting HER2 mutation and amplification (27, 28). The anti-HER2 antibody-drug conjugates (ADCs) have shown greater clinical benefit than TKIs in HER2-amplified cancers (29), specifically T-DM1 and deruxtecan-trastuzumab (T-DXd). T-DM1 was clinically effective in ERBB2-amplified/mutant lung cancer patients, and the ORR was 51%, with a mPFS of 5 months (30, 31). For heavily pretreated HER2-mutant NSCLC, a phase I study showed that the ORR of T-DXd was 72.7%, and the median PFS was 11.3 months (95% CI, 8.1–14.3) (32). Then in an ongoing phase II study (DESTINY-Lung01 study), T-DXd demonstrated an encouraging efficacy in this molecular subset of lung cancers. The ORR was 61.9%, and the median PFS was 14.0 months (95% CI, 6.4–14.0) (33). However, all of these studies are still in phase I or II, and the sample size is relatively small. Therefore, further exploration is required to identify specific types of HER2 alterations and assess their potential as novel therapeutic targets.

There are several limitations to this study. First, the sample size was too small, and the statistical results may have biased. Therefore, more prospective, larger sample size, randomized, controlled studies are needed. Second, the PD-L1 expression of these patients was negative, so the impact of PD-L1 status on the treatment response in these patients is unknown. Finally, the follow-up time of our study was only 12 months, and the overall survival (OS) of most patients was not reached. Thus, the patients still need to be followed up. Thus, the evidence from current clinical practice is inadequate, and further clinical data are needed to confirm our results.

To our knowledge, this study is the first to report chemo-immunotherapy as a first-line treatment for advanced NSCLC with HER2 alterations. Overall, our study aimed to provide additional data regarding the treatment of NSCLC with HER2 mutation or amplification. The results suggest that chemo-immunotherapy may be a hopeful first-line treatment option for these patients. However, further clinical trials are required to expand treatment options for NSCLC patients with HER2 alterations.

AUTHOR CONTRIBUTIONS

SZ wrote the manuscript. SZ and XX collected the data. SZ and PT analyzed the data. KW and YL revised the manuscript. KW and WL designed the manuscript. KW and YL reviewed the

REFERENCES

1. Siegel RL, Miller KD, Jemal A. Cancer statistics, 2020. *CA Cancer J Clin* (2020) 70:7–30. doi: 10.3322/caac.21590

2. Majem M, Juan O, Insa A, Reguart N, Trigo JM, Carcereny E, et al. SEOM clinical guidelines for the treatment of non-small cell lung cancer (2018). *Clin Transl Oncol* (2019) 21:3–17. doi: 10.1007/s12094-018-1978-1

3. Campbell JD, Alexandrov A, Kim J, Wala J, Berger AH, Pedamallu CS, et al. Distinct patterns of somatic genome alterations in lung adenocarcinomas and squamous cell carcinomas. *Nat Genet* (2016) 48:607–16. doi: 10.1038/ng.3564
4. Peters S, Zimmermann S. Targeted therapy in NSCLC driven by HER2 insertions. *Transl Lung Cancer Res* (2014) 3:84–8. doi: 10.3978/j.issn.2218-6751.2014.02.06
5. Kuyama S, Hotta K, Tabata M, Segawa Y, Fujiwara Y, Takigawa N, et al. Impact of HER2 gene and protein status on the treatment outcome of cisplatin-based chemoradiotherapy for locally advanced non-small cell lung cancer. *J Thorac Oncol* (2008) 3:477–82. doi: 10.1097/JTO.0b013e31816e2ea3
6. Wang Y, Zhang S, Wu F, Zhao J, Li X, Zhao C, et al. Outcomes of Pemetrexed-based chemotherapies in HER2-mutant lung cancers. *BMC Cancer* (2018) 18:326. doi: 10.1186/s12885-018-4277-x
7. Mazières J, Barlesi F, Filleron T, Besse B, Monnet I, Beau-Faller M, et al. Lung cancer patients with HER2 mutations treated with chemotherapy and HER2-targeted drugs: results from the European EUHER2 cohort. *Ann Oncol* (2016) 27:281–6. doi: 10.1093/annonc/mdv573
8. Baselga J, Swain SM. Novel anticancer targets: revisiting ERBB2 and discovering ERBB3. *Nat Rev Cancer* (2009) 9:463–75. doi: 10.1038/nrc2656
9. Oxnard GR, Binder A, Jänne PA. New targetable oncogenes in non-small-cell lung cancer. *J Clin Oncol* (2013) 31:1097–104. doi: 10.1200/JCO.2012.42.9829
10. Arcila ME, Chaft JE, Nafa K, Roy-Chowdhuri S, Lau C, Zaidinski M, et al. Prevalence, clinicopathologic associations, and molecular spectrum of ERBB2 (HER2) tyrosine kinase mutations in lung adenocarcinomas. *Clin Cancer Res* (2012) 18:4910–8. doi: 10.1158/1078-0432.CCR-12-0912
11. Kris MG, Johnson BE, Berry LD, Kwiatkowski DJ, Iafrate AJ, Wistuba II, et al. Using multiplexed assays of oncogenic drivers in lung cancers to select targeted drugs. *JAMA* (2014) 311:1998–2006. doi: 10.1001/jama.2014.3741
12. Cancer Genome Atlas Research Network. Comprehensive molecular profiling of lung adenocarcinoma. *Nature* (2014) 511:543–50. doi: 10.1038/nature13385
13. Mar N, Vredenburgh JJ, Wasser JS. Targeting HER2 in the treatment of non-small cell lung cancer. *Lung Cancer* (2015) 87:220–5. doi: 10.1016/j.lungcan.2014.12.018
14. Oh IJ, Hur JY, Park CK, Kim YC, Kim SJ, Lee MK, et al. Clinical Activity of Pan-HER Inhibitors Against HER2-Mutant Lung Adenocarcinoma. *Clin Lung Cancer* (2018) 19:e775–81. doi: 10.1016/j.cllc.2018.05.018
15. Kris MG, Camidge DR, Giaccone G, Hida T, Li BT, O'Connell J, et al. Targeting HER2 aberrations as actionable drivers in lung cancers: phase II trial of the pan-HER tyrosine kinase inhibitor dacomitinib in patients with HER2-mutant or amplified tumors. *Ann Oncol* (2015) 26(7):1421–7. doi: 10.1093/annonc/mdv186
16. Besse B, Soria J-C, Yao B, Kris M, Chao B, Cortot A, et al. Neratinib (N) with or Without Temsirolimus (Tem) in Patients (Pts) with Non-Small Cell Lung Cancer (Nsclc) Carrying Her2 Somatic Mutations: an International Randomized Phase II Study. *Ann Oncol* (2014) 25(suppl 4):v1–v41. doi: 10.1093/annonc/mdu438.47
17. Janne PA, Neal JW, Camidge DR, Spira AI, Piotrowska Z, Horn L, et al. Antitumor activity of TAK-788 in NSCLC with EGFR exon 20 insertions. *J Clin Oncol* (2019) 37 May (15_suppl):9007. doi: 10.1200/JCO.2019.37.15_suppl.9007
18. Eng J, Hsu M, Chaft JE, Kris MG, Arcila ME, Li BT. Outcomes of chemotherapies and HER2 directed therapies in advanced HER2-mutant lung cancers. *Lung Cancer* (2016) 99:53–6. doi: 10.1016/j.lungcan.2016.05.030
19. Gadgeel S, Rodríguez-Abreu D, Speranza G, Esteban E, Felip E, Dómine M, et al. Updated Analysis From KEYNOTE-189: Pembrolizumab or placebo plus pemetrexed and platinum for previously untreated metastatic nonsquamous non-small-cell lung cancer. *J Clin Oncol* (2020) 38:1505–17. doi: 10.1200/JCO.19.03136
20. Gandhi L, Rodríguez-Abreu D, Gadgeel S, Esteban E, Felip E, De Angelis F, et al. KEYNOTE-189 Investigators. Pembrolizumab plus Chemotherapy in Metastatic Non-Small-Cell Lung Cancer. *N Engl J Med* (2018) 37:2078–92. doi: 10.1056/NEJMoa1801005
21. Pardoll DM. The blockade of immune checkpoints in cancer immunotherapy. *Nat Rev Cancer* (2012) 12:252–64. doi: 10.1038/nrc3239
22. Catania C, Passaro A, Rocco EG, Spitaleri G, Barberis M, Noberasco C, et al. Dramatic Antitumor Activity of Nivolumab in Advanced HER2-Positive Lung Cancer. *Clin Lung Cancer* (2016) 17:e179–83. doi: 10.1016/j.cllc.2016.05.004
23. Chuang JC, Stehr H, Liang Y, Das M, Huang J, Diehn M, et al. ERBB2-Mutated Metastatic Non-Small Cell Lung Cancer: Response and Resistance to Targeted Therapies. *J Thorac Oncol* (2017) 12:833–42. doi: 10.1016/j.jtho.2017.01.023
24. Mazieres J, Drilon A, Lusque A, Mhanna L, Cortot AB, Mezquita L, et al. Immune checkpoint inhibitors for patients with advanced lung cancer and oncogenic driver alterations: results from the IMMUNOTARGET registry. *Ann Oncol* (2019) 30(8):1321–8. doi: 10.1093/annonc/mdz167
25. Yarden Y, Sliwkowski MX. Untangling the ErbB signalling network. *Nat Rev Mol Cell Biol* (2001) 2:127–37. doi: 10.1038/35052073
26. Li BT, Ross DS, Aisner DL, Chaft JE, Hsu M, Kako SL, et al. HER2 Amplification and HER2 Mutation Are Distinct Molecular Targets in Lung Cancers. *J Thorac Oncol* (2016) 1:414–9. doi: 10.1016/j.jtho.2015.10.025
27. Shan J, Ruan J, Tan Y, Yan L, Chen S, Du M, et al. Efficacy of Pyrotinib in a Heavily Pretreated Patient with Lung Adenocarcinoma Harboring HER2 Amplification and Exon 20 Insertions: A Case Report. *Oncol Targets Ther* (2020) 13:9849–56. doi: 10.2147/OTT.S271999
28. Liu X, Cao Y, Li Y, Duan X. Advanced lung adenocarcinoma with coexistent HER2 mutation and amplification and response to afatinib: a case report. *Ann Palliat Med* (2020) 9(2):483–7. doi: 10.21037/apm.2020.02.14
29. Moasser MM. Two dimensions in targeting HER2. *J Clin Oncol* (2014) 32:2074–7. doi: 10.1200/JCO.2014.55.7652
30. Li BT, Michelini F, Misale S, Cocco E, Baldino L, Cai Y, et al. HER2-Mediated Internalization of Cytotoxic Agents in ERBB2 Amplified or Mutant Lung Cancers. *Cancer Discovery* (2020) 10:674–87. doi: 10.1158/2159-8290.CD-20-0215
31. Li BT, Shen R, Buonocore D, Olah ZT, Ni A, Ginsberg MS, et al. Ado-trastuzumab emtansine for patients with HER2-mutant lung cancers: results from a phase II bsket trial. *J Clin Oncol* (2018) 36(24):2532–7. doi: 10.1200/JCO.2018.77.9777
32. Tsurutani J, Iwata H, Krop I, Jänne PA, Doi T, Takahashi S, et al. Targeting HER2 with Trastuzumab Deruxtecan: A Dose-Expansion, Phase I Study in Multiple Advanced Solid Tumors. *Cancer Discovery* (2020) 10(5):688–701. doi: 10.1158/2159-8290.CD-19-1014
33. Egbert FS, Kazuhiko N, Misako N, Enriqueta F, Yasushi G, Li BT, et al. Trastuzumab deruxtecan (T-DXd; DS-8201) in patients with HER2-mutated metastatic non-small cell lung cancer (NSCLC): Interim results of DESTINY-Lung01. *J Clin Oncol* (2020) 31(suppl 3):235. doi: 10.1200/jco.2020.38.15_suppl.9504

13

Development and Validation of a Nomogram for Predicting Prognosis to Immune Checkpoint Inhibitors Plus Chemotherapy in Patients with Non-Small Cell Lung Cancer

Hao Zeng[1†], *Wei-wei Huang*[2†], *Yu-jie Liu*[1], *Qin Huang*[3], *Sheng-min Zhao*[3], *Ya-lun Li*[3*], *Pan-wen Tian*[3*] *and Wei-min Li*[2]

[1] Department of Respiratory and Critical Care Medicine, West China Hospital, West China School of Medicine, Sichuan University, Chengdu, China, [2] Department of Respiratory and Critical Care Medicine, West China Hospital, Sichuan University, Chengdu, China, [3] Department of Respiratory and Critical Care Medicine, Lung Cancer Treatment Center, West China Hospital, Sichuan University, Chengdu, China

***Correspondence:**
Ya-lun Li
lunlunhx@qq.com
Pan-wen Tian
mrascend@163.com

†These authors have contributed equally to this work

Background: Immune checkpoint inhibitors (ICIs) plus chemotherapy improved the prognosis of patients with non-small cell lung cancer (NSCLC); however, reliable prognostic biomarkers are lacking. We explored factors associated with prognosis and developed a predictive model.

Methods: We retrospectively analyzed 130 consecutive stage IIIA–IVB NSCLC patients treated with ICIs combined with chemotherapy. Cox univariate and multivariate proportional hazards regression analyses were used to identify prognostic factors associated with progression-free survival (PFS). A nomogram was developed based on key factors in the training cohort (n = 86) and evaluated in the validation cohort (n = 44). According to the nomogram-based total point scores, we divided patients into low- and high-risk groups.

Results: In the training cohort, bone metastases (p = 0.017) and an increased derived neutrophil-to-lymphocyte ratio (p = 0.018) were significantly associated with poor PFS, while smoking (p = 0.007) and programmed death-ligand 1 (PD-L1) ≥50% (p = 0.001) were associated with improved PFS. A nomogram based on these factors was developed to predict PFS at 3, 6, and 12 months. The C-index of the nomogram to predict PFS was 0.725 (95% CI: 0.711–0.739) in the training cohort and 0.688 (95% CI: 0.665–0.711) in the validation cohort. The area under the curve (AUC) exhibited an acceptable discriminative ability, and calibration curves demonstrated a consistency between the actual results and predictions. In the training cohort, the median PFS (mPFS) was 12.3 and 5.7 months in the low- and high-risk groups, respectively (p < 0.001). In the validation cohort, the mPFS was 12.6 and 6.2 months in the low- and high-risk groups, respectively (p = 0.021).

Conclusions: A predictive nomogram was developed to help clinicians assess prognosis early for advanced NSCLC patients who received ICI plus chemotherapy.

Keywords: immune checkpoint inhibitors, chemotherapy, non-small cell lung cancer (NSCLC), nomogram, progression-free survival (PFS)

INTRODUCTION

According to Global Cancer Statistics in 2020, lung cancer is the second most commonly diagnosed malignant tumor and remains the leading cause of cancer death in the world (1). Non-small cell lung cancer (NSCLC) accounts for approximately 85% of all lung cancers (2). In advanced NSCLC lacking actionable oncogenic drivers, platinum-based chemotherapy has traditionally been used as a treatment. However, the median progression-free survival (mPFS) time in response to this therapy is only 5–6 months (3). In recent years, considerable successes have been achieved using novel therapeutic strategies, i.e., immune checkpoint inhibitors (ICIs), as first-line and second-line treatments in patients with NSCLC (4, 5). Unfortunately, nearly 60% of patients with advanced NSCLC do not benefit from ICIs (6). Remarkable heterogeneity regarding their objective response rate, survival, immune-related adverse events (irAEs) in individual NSCLC patients, and limits in current biomarkers have driven some studies to look for new prognostic markers or to develop a comprehensive model to optimize patient benefit (7, 8).

Based on KEYNOTE-189, KEYNOTE-021, and KEYNOTE-407, the National Comprehensive Cancer Network (NCCN) guidelines recommend platinum-based chemotherapy plus ICIs as category 1 agents for first-line therapy in advanced NSCLC patients without actionable oncogenic drivers (4, 9–12). In clinical practice, the Chinese Experts Consensus made the same recommendation (13). However, in a subgroup analysis of PFS, a programmed death-ligand 1 tumor proportion score (PD-L1 TPS) <1% was not associated with PFS, which means that the level of PD-L1 expression was not entirely associated with the prognosis. PD-L1 as a predictive biomarker for patients treated with PD-1 inhibitors unfortunately remains complex, with inconsistent data between studies (4, 12, 14, 15). Similarly, there is no association between tissue tumor mutation burden (TMB) and efficacy for pembrolizumab plus chemotherapy or chemotherapy alone based on KEYNOTE-189, KEYNOTE-021, and KEYNOTE-407 (4, 10, 12). Some clinical characteristics and peripheral blood markers have been found to be related to the prognosis of patients treated with immunotherapy alone, such as liver or lung metastases, neutrophil-to-lymphocyte ratio (NLR), and derived NLR (dNLR) (6, 15–17). Based on NLR, serum albumin concentration, and lactate dehydrogenase (LDH), Lenci et al. developed a Gustave Roussy Immune (GRIm) score for advanced NSCLC patients treated with first-line pembrolizumab and showed that the low GRImT1 group had significantly longer PFS than the high GRImT1 group (18). However, the GRIm score only includes peripheral blood markers, and the utility for patients who receive chemoimmunotherapy is unknown. More comprehensive prognostic factors are needed. For example, in the real-world context, Cantini et al. even reported that high-intensity statins are associated with better PFS in advanced NSCLC patients treated with PD-1 inhibitors (19). There are currently limited biomarkers and no predictive model for patients with advanced NSCLC treated with PD-1 inhibitors plus chemotherapy. Therefore, it is necessary to explore biomarkers that are prognostic factors of these populations to identify patients who would benefit from chemoimmunotherapy.

We therefore conducted a study to assess prognostic factors in advanced NSCLC patients treated with PD-1 inhibitor plus chemotherapy. Finally, we aimed to develop a nomogram that is a reliable and convenient prognostic tool to quantify risk of progression for cancer patients (14, 16, 20) to accurately predict PFS.

MATERIAL AND METHODS

Patients

We reviewed the electronic medical records of all patients with unresectable and metastatic (stage IIIA to IVB) NSCLC who received PD-1 inhibitor plus chemotherapy at West China Hospital between October 2017 and September 2020. A total of 158 consecutive patients were reviewed. The inclusion criteria were as follows: 1) pathologically confirmed NSCLC; 2) patients without actionable oncogenic drivers; and 3) patients with complete clinical data and follow-up information. Patients with other malignancies were excluded. Computer-generated random numbers were used to assign these patients into a training cohort and an internal validation cohort. The workflow of patient selection is shown in **Figure 1**. This study was approved by the Ethics Committee of West China Hospital (No. 2018-603), and the project was performed in accordance with the Declaration of Helsinki as revised in 2013.

Data Collection

Data on clinical characteristics, laboratory parameters, and treatment information were extracted from the electronic inpatient record system of each patient and were updated as of February 1, 2021. Clinicopathological characteristics included sex, age, height, weight, clinical stage, smoking history, histology, metastatic sites, and PD-L1 expression level. Baseline (before the first injection of PD-1 inhibitor plus chemotherapy) peripheral blood indicators included LDH, red blood cell (RBC) count, hemoglobin (HB) count, platelet count, white blood cell (WBC) count, absolute neutrophil count (ANC), absolute lymphocyte count (ALC), absolute monocyte count (AMC), absolute eosinophil count (AEC), and carcinoembryonic antigen (CEA). Treatment records included the number of treatment lines,

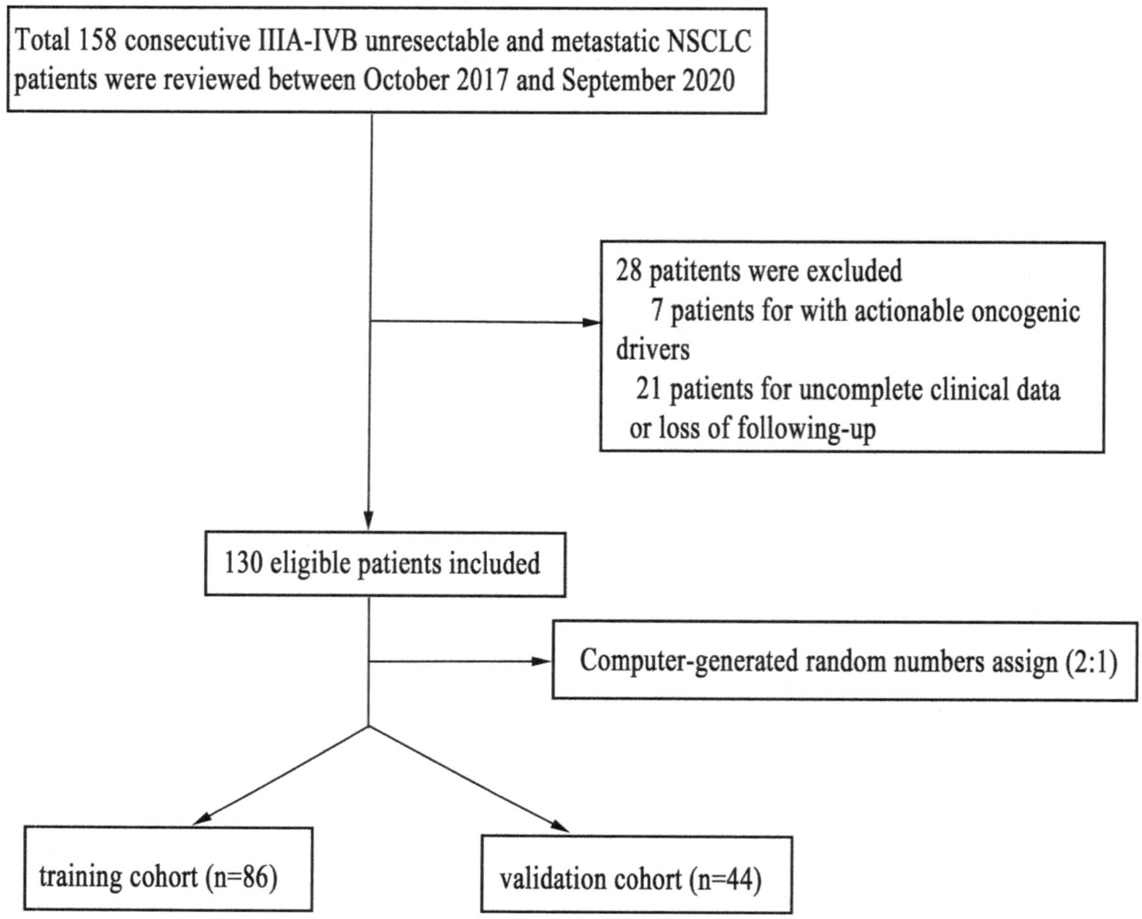

FIGURE 1 | The workflow of patient selection.

immunotherapy combined with chemotherapy regimens, and commencement/progression time of the treatment strategy. NLR = ANC/ALC, dNLR = ANC/(WBC − ANC) as defined previously (14).

Treatment and Efficiency Assessment

Among the 130 patients, 88 patients were treated with pembrolizumab plus chemotherapy, 19 patients were treated with nivolumab plus chemotherapy, 13 patients were treated with sintilimab plus chemotherapy, five patients were treated with camrelizumab plus chemotherapy, two patients were treated with tislelizumab plus chemotherapy, two patients were treated with penpulimab plus chemotherapy, and one patient was treated with durvalumab plus chemotherapy (details shown in **Table S1**). The radiological response of tumors was evaluated using computed tomography every 8–10 weeks, and the radiologist was independent and blinded. Disease progression was evaluated according to the immune-related Response Evaluation Criteria in Solid Tumors Criteria (i-RECIST) (21). PFS was defined as the time from the date of treatment initiation until radiographic progression or death from any cause, whichever occurred first. Patients without radiographic disease progression on the date of the last follow-up were classified as censored.

Statistical Analysis

The median and interquartile range (IQR) were used to describe continuous variables. Frequencies and percentages were used to describe categorical variables. Laboratory parameters were assessed as continuous variables. Age of 65 years was used as the cutoff point to convert age into a dichotomous variable. Body mass index (BMI) was divided into three groups according to Chinese standards (BMI < 18.5, underweight; 18.5 ≤ BMI < 24, normal; and BMI ≥ 24, overweight). Cox univariate and multivariate proportional hazards regression analyses were used to evaluate the impact of laboratory parameters and clinical characteristics on PFS. Variables with a p-value less than 0.1 in the univariate analysis were included in multivariate analysis. A two-tailed p-value of <0.05 was considered statistically significant.

In the training set, predictors derived from the multivariate Cox regression analysis were used to construct the nomogram and then validated in the validation cohort. Each nomogram was also validated internally by using bootstrap method with 1,000 resamples. The concordance index (C-index) and the area under the curve (AUC) were used to evaluate the discriminative ability of the nomogram. The first was computed in the Cox prediction models, while the second was obtained using receiver operating characteristic (ROC) curves with 3-, 6-, and 12-month PFS as binary outcomes. Calibration curves were used to compare the association between the actual outcomes and the predicted probabilities. Finally, we calculated the risk scores of all patients in the training set and validation set. We used X-tile software to select the cutoff point in the training set risk score, which was used to classify patients from the training set and validation set into two groups (low-risk group and high-risk group). The Cox proportional hazards regression model was used to compare whether the survival distributions differed between the two risk groups. Finally, we compared the current nomogram with Yuan's nomogram (14), which was developed to predict prognosis in NSCLC patients treated with anti–PD-1 antibody, to demonstrate the advantage of the current nomogram to guide treatment decisions for patients treated with ICIs combined with chemotherapy. All statistical analyses were performed using SPSS version 24.0 Statistical Software (SPSS Inc., Chicago, IL, USA) and the R program (version 4.2.0).

RESULTS

Patient Characteristics

We identified 158 consecutive IIIA–IVB unresectable and metastatic NSCLC patients who received PD-1 inhibitors plus chemotherapy. Of these, seven patients with actionable oncogenic drivers and 21 patients with incomplete clinical data or loss of follow-up were excluded, leaving 130 patients for analysis.

Among them, 86 patients were included in the model development cohort, and 44 were included in the validation cohort. Among 86 patients in the training cohort, the median age was 61.0 (53.0–68.0) years. Males accounted for 69 (80.23%), and smokers accounted for 67.44% of the subjects. Thirty (34.88%) patients had bone metastasis. Twenty (23.25%), 21 (24.42%), 23 (26.74%), and 22 (25.58%) patients had PD-L1 TPS <1%, ≥1%–49%, ≥50%, and unknown, respectively. The median dNLR was 2.19 (1.65, 3.30). Other clinical characteristics and laboratory parameters are shown in **Table 1**.

After a median follow-up period of 11.1 months (range 6.5–18.4 months), at the last date of follow-up, the mPFS of the 130 patients was 9.2 (7.9, 10.4) months, and 21 patients died. The PFS probability in the whole patient population was 90.7%, 69.1%, and 30.3% at 3, 6, and 12 months, respectively.

Independent Prognostic Factors in the Training Set

The results of univariate and multivariate survival analyses of PFS are listed in **Table 2**. Univariate analysis showed that sex, smoking status, PD-L1 expression, bone metastasis, ALC, dNLR, and CEA were related to PFS ($p < 0.1$). Next, all significant factors in the univariate analysis were entered into the multivariate analysis, which indicated that bone metastasis (HR = 2.071, 95% CI: 1.138–3.766, p = 0.017) and higher dNLR (HR = 1.142, 95% CI: 1.023–1.275, p = 0.018) were significantly associated with shortened PFS, while smoking (HR = 0.419, 95% CI: 0.223–0.789, p = 0.007) and PD-L1 ≥50% (HR = 0.211, 95% CI: 0.087–0.509, p = 0.001) were independent protective factors for PFS. The Kaplan–Meier survival curve analysis showed that patients who developed bone metastasis and never smoked had a shortened PFS, and PD-L1 ≥50% was related to a prolonged PFS (**Figure 2**).

Establishment of a Prognostic Nomogram for Progression-Free Survival

According to predictive factors identified in the training cohort, we developed a nomogram to predict the probability of PFS at 3, 6, and 12 months in NSCLC patients treated with ICIs plus chemotherapy (**Figure 3**). Each prognostic parameter was assigned a corresponding number of risk points on the points scale. We obtained a total score by delineating a vertical line and summing the corresponding risk points of each parameter. Finally, we drew a vertical line towards the PFS probability axis, which could help to estimate the specific probability of PFS at 3, 6, and 12 months for each specific NSCLC patient.

Evaluation and Validation of the Nomogram

The mPFS was 9.6 months (95% CI: 7.1, 12.1 months) in the validation set. The C-index of the nomogram to predict PFS was 0.725 (95% CI: 0.711–0.739) in the training cohort and 0.688 (95% CI: 0.665–0.711) in the validation cohort. In addition, the AUCs of the nomogram to predict PFS at 3, 6, and 12 months were 0.80 (95% CI: 0.66–0.91), 0.80 (95% CI: 0.69–0.89), and 0.84 (95% CI: 0.74–0.96) in the training cohort and 0.59 (95% CI: 0.41–0.75), 0.75 (95% CI: 0.57–0.93), and 0.85 (95% CI: 0.70–1.00) in the validation cohort, respectively (**Figure 4**). Additionally, there was good consistency between the actual outcomes and the predicted outcomes according to the calibration curves in the training cohort and validation cohort (**Figure 5**).

Furthermore, patients in the training set and validation set were divided into two subgroups according to the cutoff value of the nomogram-based total score: the low-risk group (0–100) and the high-risk group (>100). In the training set, 46 patients were assigned to the low-risk group, while 40 patients were assigned to the high-risk group. The Kaplan–Meier survival curve analysis showed that the mPFS was 12.3 (95% CI: 9.8, 14.9) months and 5.7 (95% CI: 1.7, 9.8) months in the low-risk group and high-risk group ($p < 0.001$), respectively. In the validation set, 20 patients were assigned to the low-risk group, while 24 patients were assigned to the high-risk group. The mPFS was 12.6 (95% CI: 9.2, 16.1) months and 6.2 (95% CI: 3.7, 8.7) months in the low-risk and high-risk groups (p = 0.021), respectively (**Figure 6**). Cox univariate regression analysis showed that patients in the high-risk group had a shortened PFS (HR = 4.726, 95% CI: 2.579–

TABLE 1 | Baseline clinical characteristics and laboratory parameters.

Variable	Training Set (*n* = 86)	Validation Set (*n* = 44)	Immunotherapy Combined With Chemotherapy Set (*n* = 130)
Characteristics			
Age, median, (25th, 75th)	61.0 (53.0, 68.0)	58.5 (51.2, 65.7)	61 (53.0, 67.0)
Gender, *n* (%)			
Male	69 (80.23)	33 (75.00)	102 (78.46)
Female	17 (19.77)	11 (25.00)	28 (21.54)
Smoking status, *n* (%)			
Never	28 (32.56)	17 (38.64)	45 (34.62)
Smoking	58 (67.44)	27 (61.36)	85 (65.38)
Diabetes or hypertension, *n* (%)			
No	59 (68.60)	32 (72.72)	91 (70.00)
Yes	27 (31.40)	12 (27.28)	39 (30.00)
BMI, *n* (%)			
<18.5	9 (10.47)	3 (6.81)	12 (9.23)
18.5-23.9	50 (58.14)	26 (59.09)	76 (58.46)
≥24	27 (31.39)	15 (34.10)	42 (32.31)
Histology, *n* (%)			
Squamous	34 (39.53)	21 (47.73)	55 (42.31)
Adenocarcinoma	50 (58.14)	19 (43.18)	69 (53.08)
Other NSCLC	2 (2.32)	4 (9.09)	6 (4.61)
Clinical stage, *n* (%)			
IIIA~IIIC	12 (13.95)	9 (20.45)	21 (16.15)
IV	74 (86.05)	35 (79.55)	109 (83.85)
N stage, *n* (%)			
N0~N1	19 (22.09)	6 (13.64)	25 (19.23)
N2~N3	67 (77.91)	38 (86.36)	105 (80.77)
Number of metastatic organs, *n* (%)			
≤1	49 (56.98)	27 (61.36)	76 (58.46)
>1	37 (43.02)	17 (38.64)	54 (41.54)
Metastatic, *n* (%)			
Brain	19 (22.09)	8 (18.18)	27 (20.77)
Liver	5 (5.81)	7 (15.91)	12 (9.23)
Bone	30 (34.88)	16 (36.36)	46 (35.38)
Adrenal	8 (9.30)	4 (9.09)	12 (9.23)
Pleural	20 (23.25)	15 (34.09)	35 (26.92)
Contralateral lung	33 (38.37)	13 (29.55)	46 (35.38)
Line of treatment, *n* (%)			
1	57 (66.28)	33 (75.00)	90 (69.23)
>1	29 (33.72)	11 (25.00)	40 (30.77)
Receipt of hormone treatment, *n* (%)			
No	26 (30.23)	18 (40.91)	44 (33.85)
Yes	60 (69.77)	26 (59.09)	86 (66.15)
PD-L1 TPS%, *n* (%)			
<1%	20 (23.25)	9 (20.46)	29 (22.30)
1%–49%	21 (24.42)	10 (22.73)	31 (23.85)
≥50%	23 (26.74)	8 (18.18)	31 (23.85)
Unknown	22 (25.58)	17 (38.64)	39 (30.00)
Laboratory parameters (25th, 75th)			
LDH (IU/L)	177 (150, 225)	172 (139, 226)	176 (146, 225)
RBC ($\times 10^{12}$/L)	4.32 (4.03, 4.76)	4.23 (3.88, 4.66)	4.29 (3.93, 4.71)
HB (g/L)	130 (119, 142)	126 (112, 136)	128 (116, 141)
Platelet ($\times 10^{9}$/L)	218 (166, 275)	245 (187, 314)	230 (171, 277)
WBC ($\times 10^{9}$/L)	7.39 (5.45, 8.80)	7.06 (5.05, 9.15)	7.22 (5.38, 8.92)
ANC ($\times 10^{9}$/L)	4.87 (3.60, 6.39)	5.12 (3.27, 6.80)	4.94 (3.50, 6.63)
AMC ($\times 10^{9}$/L)	0.49 (0.37, 0.67)	0.51 (0.34, 0.66)	0.50 (0.36, 0.67)
ALC ($\times 10^{9}$/L)	1.40 (0.91, 1.70)	1.50 (1.01, 2.00)	1.43 (0.96, 1.75)
AEC ($\times 10^{9}$/L)	0.13 (0.05, 0.23)	0.14 (0.08, 0.29)	0.14 (0.07, 0.25)
dNLR	2.19 (1.65, 3.30)	2.40 (1.62, 3.56)	2.20 (1.65, 3.31)
NLR	3.54 (2.37, 5.83)	3.76 (2.39, 5.96)	3.54 (2.39, 5.83)
CEA (ng/ml)	5.27 (1.81, 24.75)	3.39 (1.87, 8.35)	3.81 (1.81, 13.97)

BMI, body mass index; NSCLC, non-non-small cell lung cancer; LDH, lactate dehydrogenase; RBC, red blood cell count; HB, hemoglobin; WBC, white blood cell count; ANC, absolute neutrophil count; AMC, absolute monocyte count; ALC, absolute lymphocyte count; AEC, absolute eosinophil count; dNLR, derived neutrophil-to-lymphocyte ratio; NLR, neutrophil-to-lymphocyte ratio; CEA, carcinoembryonic antigen.

TABLE 2 | Univariate and multivariate Cox analyses of progression-free survival (PFS).

Variables	Univariate Analysis		Multivariate Analysis	
	HR (95% CI)	p	HR (95% CI)	p
Gender				
Male	1 [Reference]			
Female	1.927 (1.037, 3.582)	0.038		
Age years				
≤65	1 [Reference]			
>65	0.797 (0.444, 1.433)	0.449		
BMI (kg/m^2)		0.124		
<18.5	1 [Reference]			
18.5–23.9	0.659 (0.300, 1.446)	0.299		
≥24	0.417 (0.175, 0.996)	0.049		
Smoking status				
Never	1 [Reference]			
Smoking	0.397 (0.225, 0.700)	0.001	0.419 (0.223, 0.789)	0.007
Receipt of hormone treatment				
No	1 [Reference]			
Yes	0.946 (0.536, 1.670)	0.848		
Number of metastatic organs				
≤1	1 [Reference]			
>1	1.546 (0.904, 2.647)	0.112		
Clinical stage				
IIIA~IIIC	1 [Reference]			
IV	1.914 (0.817, 4.486)	0.135		
Histology		0.586		
Squamous	1 [Reference]			
Adenocarcinoma	1.345 (0.759, 2.386)	0.310		
Other NSCLC	1.398 (0.319, 6.123)	0.656		
Treatment lines				
1	1 [Reference]			
>1	0.856 (0.497, 1.475)	0.576		
PD-L1 TPS%		0.012		0.004
<1%	1 [Reference]			
Unknown	0.618 (0.296, 1.290)	0.200	0.543 (0.250, 1.178)	0.122
1%~49%	0.490 (0.229, 1.047)	0.065	0.473 (0.218, 1.023)	0.057
≥50%	0.271 (0.124, 0.593)	0.001	0.211 (0.087, 0.509)	0.001
Brain metastatic				
No	1 [Reference]			
Yes	1.578 (0.824, 3.022)	0.168		
Bone metastatic				
No	1 [Reference]			
Yes	1.955 (1.119, 3.417)	0.019	2.071 (1.138, 3.766)	0.017
Liver metastatic				
No	1 [Reference]			
Yes	1.624 (0.644, 4.094)	0.304		
Adrenal metastatic				
No	1 [Reference]			
Yes	0.822 (0.325, 2.077)	0.679		
Contralateral lung metastatic				
No	1 [Reference]			
Yes	0.707 (0.403, 1.240)	0.226		
Pleural metastatic				
No	1 [Reference]			
Yes	1.320 (0.704, 2.473)	0.387		
Diabetes or hypertension				
No	1 [Reference]			
Yes	0.680 (0.368, 1.258)	0.219		
N stage				
N0~N1	1 [Reference]			
N2~N3	0.956 (0.502, 1.820)	0.891		
LDH (IU/L)	1.001 (0.999, 1.003)	0.499		
RBC (×10^{12}/L)	0.885 (0.591, 1.324)	0.553		
HB (g/L)	0.994 (0.981, 1.007)	0.394		

(Continued)

TABLE 2 | Continued

Variables	Univariate Analysis		Multivariate Analysis	
	HR (95% CI)	p	HR (95% CI)	p
Platelet (×10^9/L)	0.999 (0.996, 1.002)	0.640		
WBC (×10^9/L)	1.022 (0.939, 1.113)	0.616		
ANC (×10^9/L)	1.047 (0.964, 1.137)	0.281		
AMC (×10^9/L)	0.335 (0.089, 1.258)	0.105		
ALC (×10^9/L)	0.678 (0.426, 1.077)	0.090		
AEC (×10^9/L)	0.822 (0.146, 4.622)	0.824		
dNLR	1.097 (0.999, 1.204)	0.053	1.142 (1.023, 1.275)	0.018
NLR	1.039 (0.983, 1.097)	0.176		
CEA (ng/ml)	1.002 (1.001, 1.004)	0.007		

BMI, body mass index; LDH, lactate dehydrogenase; RBC, red blood cell count; HB, hemoglobin; WBC, white blood cell count; ANC, absolute neutrophil count; AMC, absolute monocyte count; ALC, absolute lymphocyte count; AEC, absolute eosinophil count; dNLR, derived neutrophil-to-lymphocyte ratio; NLR, neutrophil-to-lymphocyte ratio; CEA, carcinoembryonic antigen.

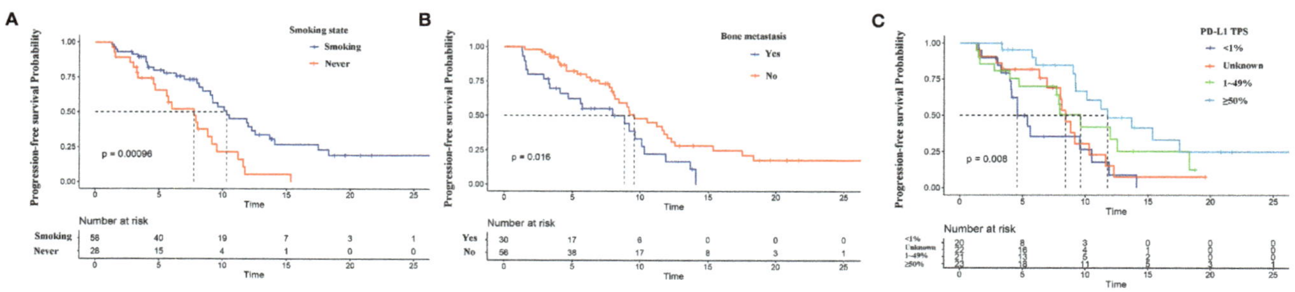

FIGURE 2 | Kaplan–Meier curves for progression-free survival (PFS) based on predictors from the nomogram. PFS according to **(A)** smoking, **(B)** bone metastasis status, and **(C)** programmed cell death ligand-1 (PD-L1) expression.

8.659, p < 0.001). Similarly, the high-risk group was linked to a shortened PFS in the validation set (HR = 2.422, 95% CI: 1.113–5.270, p = 0.026).

Comparison of Current Nomogram and Previous Nomogram

We compared the current nomogram model with Yuan's nomogram, which was developed to predict NSCLC patients treated with anti–PD–1 antibody. Decision curve analysis for 6- and 12-month PFS revealed that the current nomogram had a higher benefit (**Figure 7**).

DISCUSSION

Immunotherapy is widely used in the treatment of NSCLC patients who lack targetable aberrations and show improved efficacy over standard platinum-based doublet chemotherapy (22). Immunotherapy combined with chemotherapy has been recommended as category 1 for treating advanced NSCLC patients in the NCCN guidelines (9). Some studies have shown that pembrolizumab combined with chemotherapy has a better PFS than pembrolizumab alone for treating NSCLC patients (23, 24). However, studies about prognostic factors associated with shorter PFS for immunotherapy plus chemotherapy individuals are limited. This is the first study to develop a comprehensive model that incorporates PD-L1, easily accessible clinical characteristics, serum parameters, and imaging features to predict the probability of PFS at 3, 6, and 12 months for NSCLC patients treated with ICIs plus chemotherapy. Here, we identified four factors, including dNLR, smoking history, PD-L1 TPS, and bone metastasis, which were associated with PFS in this population.

Some recent papers about NLR, inflammation-related peripheral blood parameters, have been reported and have shown that increased NLR is associated with worsened prognosis in patients receiving immunotherapy (25). The lung immuno-oncology prognostic score (LIPS-3), which includes NLR, PD-L1 tumor cell expression level, and LDH, was developed to classify NSCLC patients with PD-L1 ≥50% who received first-line pembrolizumab and showed that NLR <4 was a significant prognostic factor (26). Similarly, some studies showed that a high dNLR was associated with poorer prognosis in patients treated with immunotherapy alone (27–29). Inflammation plays an important role in tumor development, affecting the survival of cancer patients. dNLR, a novel index derived from NLR, may reflect cancer-associated inflammation and determine disease progression (27). Mezquita et al. (27) showed that a baseline

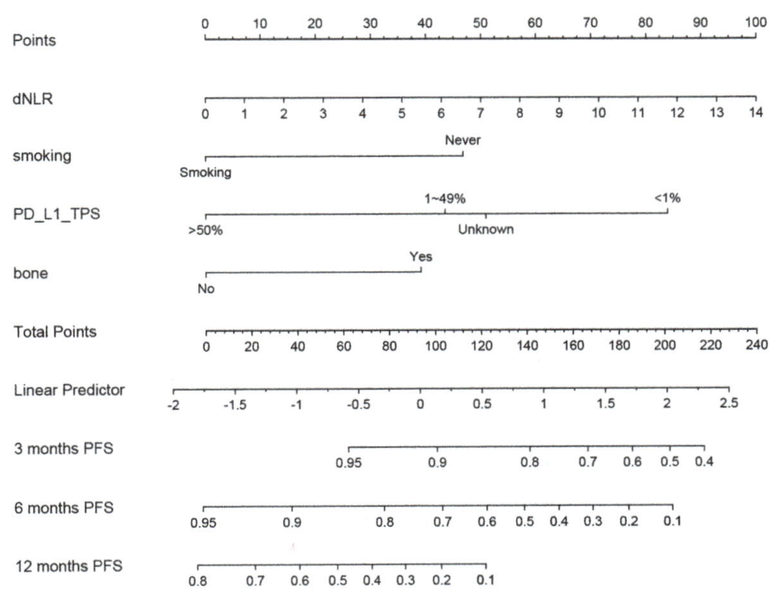

FIGURE 3 | Prognostic nomogram for non-small cell lung cancer (NSCLC) patients treating immune checkpoint inhibitors (ICIs) plus chemotherapy to assign their probability of progression-free survival (PFS) at 3, 6, and 12 months.

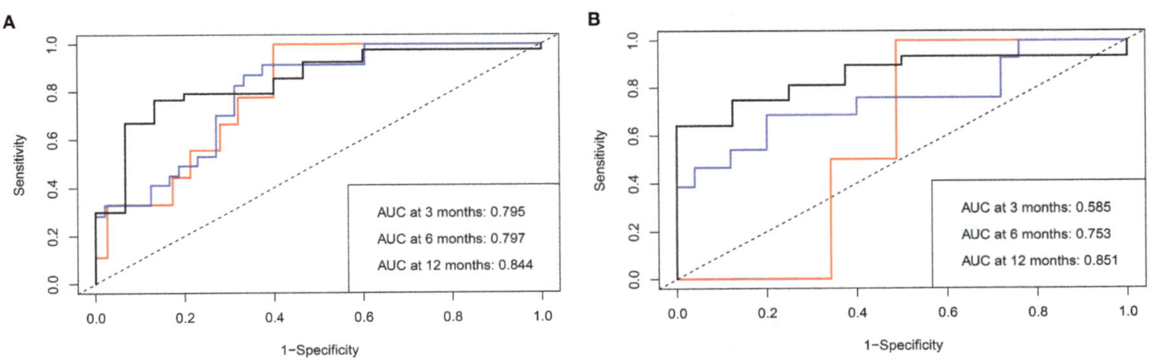

FIGURE 4 | Receiver operating characteristic (ROC) curves of the nomogram to predict progression-free survival (PFS) in both the training and validation cohorts. The area under the curve (AUC) of the probability of PFS at 3, 6, and 12 months in **(A)** the training and **(B)** validation cohorts, respectively.

dNLR >3 was independently associated with PFS in patients with advanced NSCLC treated with PD-1/PD-L1 inhibitors. Additionally, Yuan et al. (14) showed that a high dNLR was associated with a poorer OS and developed a nomogram that incorporated dNLR to predict prognosis of NSCLC patients treated with anti–PD–1 antibodies. In our present study, we found that increased dNLR was also correlated with poor outcomes with ICI plus chemotherapy.

Regarding clinical characteristics, our results showed that smoking was an independent protective factor for NSCLC patients treated with ICIs plus chemotherapy. Similarly, a previous study showed that current/former smokers experienced improved PFS and OS when PD-L1 expression ≥50% and first-line pembrolizumab was administered (30). Additionally, two studies aiming to develop nomograms to predict the prognosis of NSCLC patients treated with anti-PD-1 inhibitors both showed that smoking was associated with improved prognosis and incorporated it into the model (8, 14). Smokers were more likely to exhibit positive PD-L1 expression and higher TMB, which may improve the therapeutic efficacy of PD-1 inhibitors (31). The potential mechanism involved recruitment of tumor-infiltrating lymphocytes (TILs) and release of interferon-γ (IFN-γ) under a chronic inflammatory microenvironment caused by tobacco exposure, which induced PD-L1 expression and enhanced the stability of PD-L1 (8). Limited data from a meta-analysis indicated that both smokers and nonsmokers benefit from chemoimmunotherapy (32, 33), but our retrospective study yielded different PFS rates between smokers and never smokers.

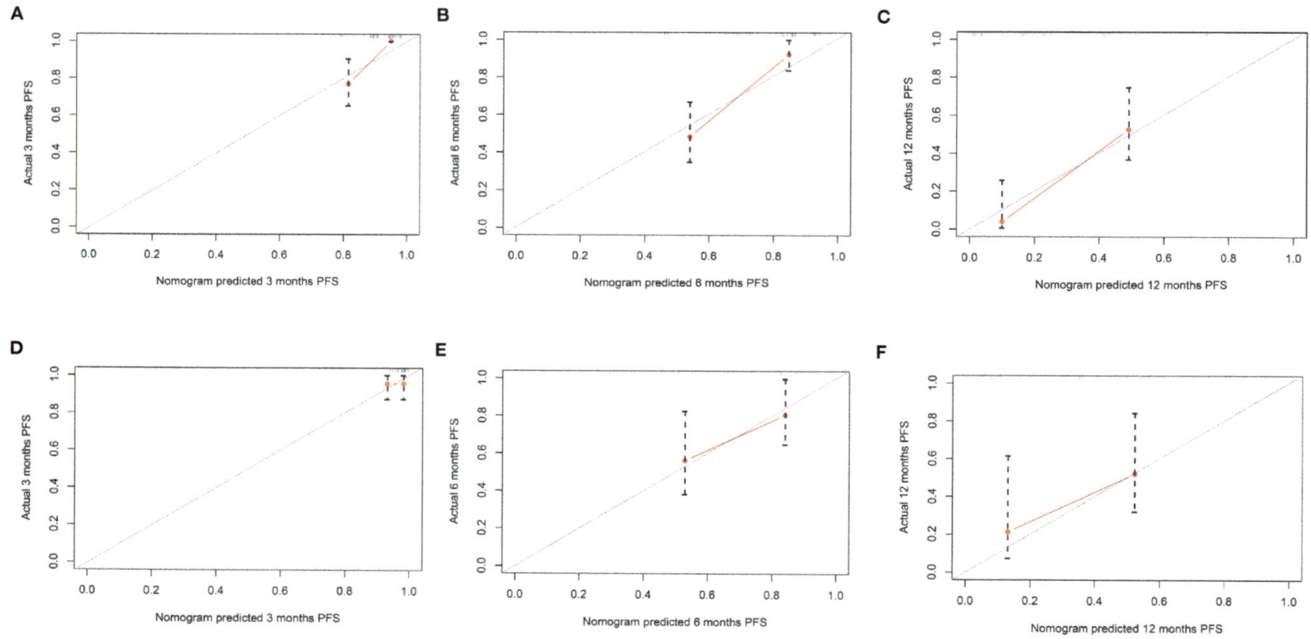

FIGURE 5 | The calibration curves of the nomogram for predicting progression-free survival (PFS) in both the training and validation cohorts. The x-axis represents the nomogram predicted probability, and the y-axis represents the actual probability of PFS. The red line indicates the performance of the nomogram, of which a closer fit to the gray line represents a better prediction. Calibration curves of the nomogram for predicting PFS at **(A)** 3, **(B)** 6, and **(C)** 12 months in the training cohort. Calibration curves of the nomogram to predict PFS at **(D)** 3, **(E)** 6, and **(F)** 12 months in the validation cohort.

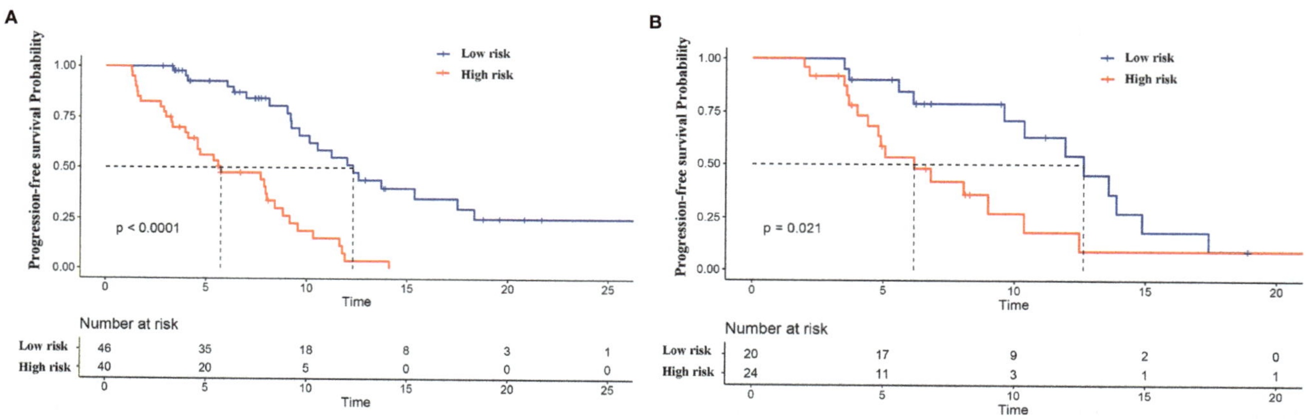

FIGURE 6 | Kaplan–Meier curves for two subgroups according to the cutoff value in the training cohort of the nomogram-based total score. The blue curve and red curve represent the low-risk (0–100) and high-risk (>100) groups, respectively. Kaplan–Meier curves for progression-free survival (PFS) in **(A)** the training cohort and **(B)** validation cohort.

To date, although its expression may vary over time and by site, PD-L1 expression is the only approved predictive biomarker for PD-(L)1 blockade in NSCLC. Not only the NCCN guidelines but also the American Society of Clinical Oncology (ASCO) and Ontario Health Cancer Care (CCO) NSCLC expert panels made recommendations for therapy for patients without driver alterations based on PD-L1 expression (9, 34). Our study demonstrates that high PD-L1 expression is related to prolonged PFS in NSCLC patients treated with ICIs plus chemotherapy.

A few studies have investigated the prognostic role of metastatic sites of disease in NSCLC patients treated with ICIs. Pantano et al. showed that the number of liver metastases is significantly correlated with time-to-treatment failure, while there was no statistically significant difference for bone

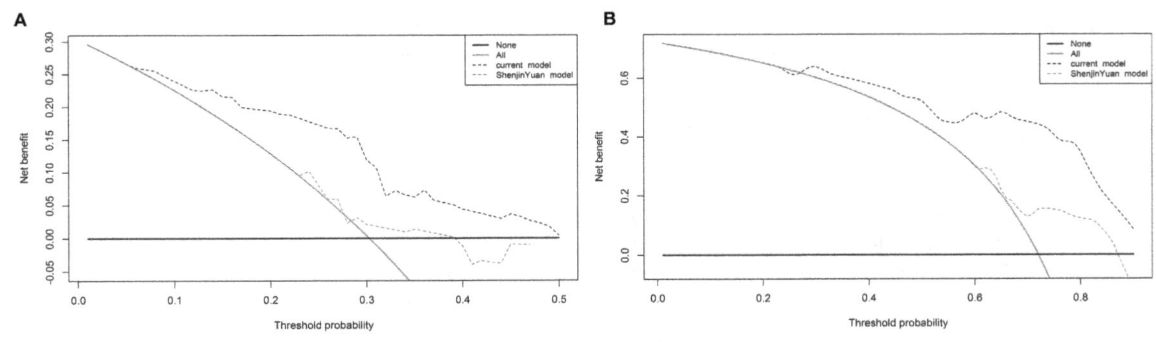

FIGURE 7 | Decision curve analysis for progression-free survival (PFS). The straight gray line represents the assumption that all patients will progress at **(A)** 6 and **(B)** 12 months, and the black horizontal line represents the assumption that no patients will progress at **(A)** 6 and **(B)** 12 months.

metastases (35). The incidence of bone metastases in NSCLC is 20%–40% (32). Bone marrow, a well-known secondary lymphatic organ, hosts several immune cells that are potentially able to affect systemic immunity and the therapeutic efficacy of immunotherapy (36, 37). In a retrospective study of NSCLC patients receiving nivolumab, patients with bone metastasis had significantly reduced PFS than patients without, which was similar to a study of patients receiving pembrolizumab showing that patients with bone metastasis exhibited significantly shorter PFS (37, 38). However, in another retrospective study of advanced NSCLC treated with pembrolizumab, bone metastasis did not affect PFS, which may be related to the relatively small sample size (39). In a real-life study, bone metastases were a general prognostic factor in NSCLC patients, regardless of the treatment; and most studies indicate that patients with bone metastases experience significantly shorter PFS (37, 40). For patients treated with ICIs plus chemotherapy, our study also demonstrated that bone metastasis was linked to a shortened PFS.

The C-index, AUC, and calibration curves implied the predictive accuracy of the current model as reported models, but the AUC of the nomogram to predict PFS at 3 months was relatively low in the validation cohort, which means that the model had a weak ability to predict PFS at 3 months but was better able to predict PFS at 6 and 12 months (14, 41). We attribute this to several causes. First, there was a relatively small sample size in the validation cohort. Second, as many studies have reported, the median time of irAEs is approximately 3 months, which may lead to changes in treatment regimens or even interruptions (42–44). The current nomogram model was compared with Yuan's model, which was developed to predict the prognosis of NSCLC patients treated with anti–PD–1 antibody (14). The current nomogram revealed an advantage in predicting the PFS of NSCLC patients treated with ICIs plus chemotherapy. To the best of our knowledge, this is the first nomogram based on PD-L1, clinical characteristics, laboratory parameters, and imaging features for predicting the prognosis of patients treated with ICI plus chemotherapy.

There are several limitations to our study. First, this was a retrospective study of a single center with a small population and lacks external validation. Larger-scale and multicenter prospective studies are needed to validate our findings. Second, this study only focused on PFS in NSCLC patients treated with PD-1 inhibitors plus chemotherapy due to the short follow-up time. Finally, this study lacks some other important predictive biomarkers, such as TILs, TMB, human leukocyte antigen (HLA), and broadly predictors, which should be explored in the future.

In conclusion, the novel nomogram model based on comprehensive factors has acceptable predictive accuracy and discriminative ability and could be applied to estimate the probability of PFS in advanced NSCLC patients treated with ICIs plus chemotherapy, especially for 6 and 12 months, and will assist clinicians in guiding treatment decisions in clinical practice. But larger samples, multicenter prospective studies, and external validation are still needed to develop a better nomogram for these populations.

AUTHOR CONTRIBUTIONS

HZ, W-wH, Y-jL, Y-lL, and P-wT contributed to the conception and design of the study. HZ, QH, S-mZ, Y-lL, and PT organized the database. HZ, W-wH, QH, and S-mZ performed the statistical analysis. HZ and W-wH wrote the first draft of the manuscript. HZ and W-wH contributed to this study equally. All authors contributed to the article and approved the submitted version.

012), the National Key Development Plan for Precision Medicine Research of China (2017YFC0910004), the Science and Technology Program of Sichuan, China (2020YFS0572), and the Major Science and Technology Innovation Project of Chengdu City, China (2020-YF08-00080-GX).

REFERENCES

1. Sung H, Ferlay J, Siegel RL, Laversanne M, Soerjomataram I, Jemal A, et al. Global Cancer Statistics 2020: GLOBOCAN Estimates of Incidence and Mortality Worldwide for 36 Cancers in 185 Countries. *CA Cancer J Clin* (2021) 71(3):209–49. doi: 10.3322/caac.21660
2. Rosell R, Karachaliou N. Large-Scale Screening for Somatic Mutations in Lung Cancer. *Lancet* (2016) 387(10026):1354–6. doi: 10.1016/s0140-6736(15)01125-3
3. Socinski MA, Bondarenko I, Karaseva NA, Makhson AM, Vynnychenko I, Okamoto I, et al. Weekly Nab-Paclitaxel in Combination With Carboplatin Versus Solvent-Based Paclitaxel Plus Carboplatin as First-Line Therapy in Patients With Advanced Non-Small-Cell Lung Cancer: Final Results of a Phase III Trial. *J Clin Oncol* (2012) 30(17):2055–62. doi: 10.1200/JCO.2011.39.5848
4. Gandhi L, Rodriguez-Abreu D, Gadgeel S, Esteban E, Felip E, De Angelis F, et al. Pembrolizumab Plus Chemotherapy in Metastatic Non-Small-Cell Lung Cancer. *N Engl J Med* (2018) 378(22):2078–92. doi: 10.1056/NEJMoa1801005
5. Morabito A. Second-Line Treatment for Advanced NSCLC Without Actionable Mutations: Is Immunotherapy the 'Panacea' for All Patients? *BMC Med* (2018) 16(1):24. doi: 10.1186/s12916-018-1011-0
6. Prelaj A, Tay R, Ferrara R, Chaput N, Besse B, Califano R. Predictive Biomarkers of Response for Immune Checkpoint Inhibitors in Non-Small-Cell Lung Cancer. *Eur J Cancer* (2019) 106:144–59. doi: 10.1016/j.ejca.2018.11.002
7. Tanizaki J, Haratani K, Hayashi H, Chiba Y, Nakamura Y, Yonesaka K, et al. Peripheral Blood Biomarkers Associated With Clinical Outcome in Non-Small Cell Lung Cancer Patients Treated With Nivolumab. *J Thoracic Oncol* (2018) 13(1):97–105. doi: 10.1016/j.jtho.2017.10.030
8. Chai R, Fan Y, Zhao J, He F, Li J, Han Y. Prognostic Nomogram on Clinicopathologic Features and Serum Indicators for Advanced Non-Small Cell Lung Cancer Patients Treated With Anti-PD-1 Inhibitors. *Ann Transl Med* (2020) 8(17):1078. doi: 10.21037/atm-20-4297
9. Ettinger DS, Wood DE, Aggarwal C, Aisner DL, Akerley W, Bauman JR, et al. NCCN Guidelines Insights: Non-Small Cell Lung Cancer, Version 1.2020. *J Natl Compr Canc Netw* (2019) 17(12):1464–72. doi: 10.6004/jnccn.2019.0059
10. Langer CJ, Gadgeel SM, Borghaei H, Papadimitrakopoulou VA, Patnaik A, Powell SF, et al. Carboplatin and Pemetrexed With or Without Pembrolizumab for Advanced, Non-Squamous Non-Small-Cell Lung Cancer: A Randomised, Phase 2 Cohort of the Open-Label KEYNOTE-021 Study. *Lancet Oncol* (2016) 17(11):1497–508. doi: 10.1016/s1470-2045(16)30498-3
11. Gadgeel S, Rodríguez-Abreu D, Speranza G, Esteban E, Felip E, Dómine M, et al. Updated Analysis From KEYNOTE-189: Pembrolizumab or Placebo Plus Pemetrexed and Platinum for Previously Untreated Metastatic Nonsquamous Non–Small-Cell Lung Cancer. *J Clin Oncol* (2020) 14:3814. doi: 10.1200/JCO.19.03136
12. Paz-Ares L, Luft A, Vicente D, Tafreshi A, Gumus M, Mazieres J, et al. Pembrolizumab Plus Chemotherapy for Squamous Non-Small-Cell Lung Cancer. *N Engl J Med* (2018) 379(21):2040–51. doi: 10.1056/NEJMoa1810865
13. Zhou C, Wang J, Bu H, Wang B, Han B, Lu Y, et al. Chinese Experts Consensus on Immune Checkpoint Inhibitors for Non-Small Cell Lung Cancer (2019 Version). *Zhongguo Fei Ai Za Zhi* (2020) 23(2):65–76. doi: 10.3779/j.issn.1009-3419.2020.02.01
14. Yuan S, Xia Y, Shen L, Ye L, Li L, Chen L, et al. Development of Nomograms to Predict Therapeutic Response and Prognosis of Non-Small Cell Lung Cancer Patients Treated With Anti-PD-1 Antibody. *Cancer Immunol Immunother* (2021) 70(2):533–46. doi: 10.1007/s00262-020-02710-9
15. Burdett N, Desai J. New Biomarkers for Checkpoint Inhibitor Therapy. *ESMO Open* (2020) 5(Suppl 1):e000597. doi: 10.1136/esmoopen-2019-000597
16. Botticelli A, Salati M, Di Pietro FR, Strigari L, Cerbelli B, Zizzari IG, et al. A Nomogram to Predict Survival in Non-Small Cell Lung Cancer Patients Treated With Nivolumab. *J Transl Med* (2019) 17(1):99. doi: 10.1186/s12967-019-1847-x
17. Garde-Noguera J, Martin-Martorell P, De Julian M, Perez-Altozano J, Salvador-Coloma C, Garcia-Sanchez J, et al. Predictive and Prognostic Clinical and Pathological Factors of Nivolumab Efficacy in Non-Small-Cell Lung Cancer Patients. *Clin Trans Oncol* (2018) 20(8):1072–9. doi: 10.1007/s12094-017-1829-5
18. Lenci E, Cantini L, Pecci F, Cognigni V, Agostinelli V, Mentrasti G, et al. The Gustave Roussy Immune (GRIm)-Score Variation Is an Early-On-Treatment Biomarker of Outcome in Advanced Non-Small Cell Lung Cancer (NSCLC) Patients Treated With First-Line Pembrolizumab. *J Clin Med* (2021) 10(5):1005. doi: 10.3390/jcm10051005
19. Cantini L, Pecci F, Hurkmans DP, Belderbos RA, Lanese A, Copparoni C, et al. High-Intensity Statins Are Associated With Improved Clinical Activity of PD-1 Inhibitors in Malignant Pleural Mesothelioma and Advanced Non-Small Cell Lung Cancer Patients. *Eur J Cancer* (2021) 144:41–8. doi: 10.1016/j.ejca.2020.10.031
20. Liang W, Zhang L, Jiang G, Wang Q, Liu L, Liu D, et al. Development and Validation of a Nomogram for Predicting Survival in Patients With Resected Non-Small-Cell Lung Cancer. *J Clin Oncol* (2015) 33(8):861–9. doi: 10.1200/JCO.2014.56.6661
21. Seymour L, Bogaerts J, Perrone A, Ford R, Schwartz LH, Mandrekar S, et al. iRECIST: Guidelines for Response Criteria for Use in Trials Testing Immunotherapeutics. *Lancet Oncol* (2017) 18(3):e143–52. doi: 10.1016/s1470-2045(17)30074-8
22. Carlisle JW, Steuer CE, Owonikoko TK, Saba NF. An Update on the Immune Landscape in Lung and Head and Neck Cancers. *CA: A Cancer J Clin* (2020) 70(6):505–17. doi: 10.3322/caac.21630
23. Kim R, Keam B, Hahn S, Ock CY, Kim M, Kim TM, et al. First-Line Pembrolizumab Versus Pembrolizumab Plus Chemotherapy Versus Chemotherapy Alone in Non-Small-Cell Lung Cancer: A Systematic Review and Network Meta-Analysis. *Clin Lung Cancer* (2019) 20(5):331–8.e4. doi: 10.1016/j.cllc.2019.05.009
24. Wang X, Niu X, An N, Sun Y, Chen Z. Comparative Efficacy and Safety of Immunotherapy Alone and in Combination With Chemotherapy for Advanced Non-Small Cell Lung Cancer. *Front Oncol* (2021) 11:611012. doi: 10.3389/fonc.2021.611012
25. Peng L, Wang Y, Liu F, Qiu X, Zhang X, Fang C, et al. Peripheral Blood Markers Predictive of Outcome and Immune-Related Adverse Events in Advanced Non-Small Cell Lung Cancer Treated With PD-1 Inhibitors. *Cancer Immunol Immunother* (2020) 69(9):1813–22. doi: 10.1007/s00262-020-02585-w
26. Banna GL, Cortellini A, Cortinovis DL, Tiseo M, Aerts J, Barbieri F, et al. The Lung Immuno-Oncology Prognostic Score (LIPS-3): A Prognostic Classification of Patients Receiving First-Line Pembrolizumab for PD-L1 >/= 50% Advanced Non-Small-Cell Lung Cancer. *ESMO Open* (2021) 6(2):100078. doi: 10.1016/j.esmoop.2021.100078
27. Mezquita L, Auclin E, Ferrara R, Charrier M, Remon J, Planchard D, et al. Association of the Lung Immune Prognostic Index With Immune Checkpoint Inhibitor Outcomes in Patients With Advanced Non-Small Cell Lung Cancer. *JAMA Oncol* (2018) 4(3):351–7. doi: 10.1001/jamaoncol.2017.4771
28. Li Y, Zhang Z, Hu Y, Yan X, Song Q, Wang G, et al. Pretreatment Neutrophil-To-Lymphocyte Ratio (NLR) May Predict the Outcomes of Advanced Non-Small-Cell Lung Cancer (NSCLC) Patients Treated With Immune Checkpoint Inhibitors (ICIs). *Front Oncol* (2020) 10:654. doi: 10.3389/fonc.2020.00654
29. Russo A, Franchina T, Ricciardi GRR, Battaglia A, Scimone A, Berenato R, et al. Baseline Neutrophilia, Derived Neutrophil-to-Lymphocyte Ratio (dNLR), Platelet-to-Lymphocyte Ratio (PLR), and Outcome in Non Small Cell Lung Cancer (NSCLC) Treated With Nivolumab or Docetaxel. *J Cell Physiol* (2018) 233(10):6337–43. doi: 10.1002/jcp.26609
30. Cortellini A, De Giglio A, Cannita K, Cortinovis DL, Cornelissen R, Baldessari C, et al. Smoking Status During First-Line Immunotherapy and Chemotherapy in NSCLC Patients: A Case-Control Matched Analysis From a Large Multicenter Study. *Thorac Cancer* (2021) 12(6):880–9. doi: 10.1111/1759-7714.13852
31. Xu Y, Li H, Huang Z, Chen K, Yu X, Sheng J, et al. Predictive Values of Genomic Variation, Tumor Mutational Burden, and PD-L1 Expression in Advanced Lung Squamous Cell Carcinoma Treated With Immunotherapy. *Transl Lung Cancer Res* (2020) 9(6):2367–79. doi: 10.21037/tlcr-20-1130
32. Passaro A, Attili I, Morganti S, Del Signore E, Gianoncelli L, Spitaleri G, et al. Clinical Features Affecting Survival in Metastatic NSCLC Treated With Immunotherapy: A Critical Review of Published Data. *Cancer Treat Rev* (2020) 89:102085. doi: 10.1016/j.ctrv.2020.102085

33. El-Osta HE, Mott FE, Burt BM, Wang DY, Sabichi AL. Predictors of Benefits From Frontline Chemoimmunotherapy in Stage IV Non-Small-Cell Lung Cancer: A Meta-Analysis. *Oncoimmunology* (2019) 8(12):e1665974. doi: 10.1080/2162402X.2019.1665974
34. Hanna NH, Schneider BJ, Temin S, Baker S, Brahmer J, Ellis PM, et al. Therapy for Stage IV Non-Small-Cell Lung Cancer Without Driver Alterations: ASCO and OH (CCO) Joint Guideline Update. *J Clin Oncol* (2020) 14:3814. doi: 10.1200/JCO.19.03022
35. Pantano F, Russano M, Berruti A, Mansueto G, Migliorino MR, Adamo V, et al. Prognostic Clinical Factors in Patients Affected by Non-Small-Cell Lung Cancer Receiving Nivolumab. *Expert Opin Biol Ther* (2020) 20(3):319–26. doi: 10.1080/14712598.2020.1724953
36. Xiang L, Gilkes DM. The Contribution of the Immune System in Bone Metastasis Pathogenesis. *Int J Mol Sci* (2019) 20(4):999. doi: 10.3390/ijms20040999
37. Landi L, D'Inca F, Gelibter A, Chiari R, Grossi F, Delmonte A, et al. Bone Metastases and Immunotherapy in Patients With Advanced Non-Small-Cell Lung Cancer. *J Immunother Cancer* (2019) 7(1):316. doi: 10.1186/s40425-019-0793-8
38. Hosoya K, Fujimoto D, Morimoto T, Kumagai T, Tamiya A, Taniguchi Y, et al. Clinical Factors Associated With Shorter Durable Response, and Patterns of Acquired Resistance to First-Line Pembrolizumab Monotherapy in PD-L1-Positive Non-Small-Cell Lung Cancer Patients: A Retrospective Multicenter Study. *BMC Cancer* (2021) 21(1):346. doi: 10.1186/s12885-021-08048-4
39. Kawachi H, Tamiya M, Tamiya A, Ishii S, Hirano K, Matsumoto H, et al. Association Between Metastatic Sites and First-Line Pembrolizumab Treatment Outcome for Advanced Non-Small Cell Lung Cancer With High PD-L1 Expression: A Retrospective Multicenter Cohort Study. *Invest New Drugs* (2020) 38(1):211–8. doi: 10.1007/s10637-019-00882-5
40. Cortellini A, Tiseo M, Banna GL, Cappuzzo F, Aerts JGJV, Barbieri F, et al. Clinicopathologic Correlates of First-Line Pembrolizumab Effectiveness in Patients With Advanced NSCLC and a PD-L1 Expression of ≥ 50. *Cancer Immunol Immunother* (2020) 69(11):2209–21. doi: 10.1101/2020.04.09.20047464
41. Cao X, Zheng YZ, Liao HY, Guo X, Li Y, Wang Z, et al. A Clinical Nomogram and Heat Map for Assessing Survival in Patients With Stage I Non-Small Cell Lung Cancer After Complete Resection. *Ther Adv Med Oncol* (2020) 12:1758835920970063. doi: 10.1177/1758835920970063
42. Delaunay M, Cadranel J, Lusque A, Meyer N, Gounant V, Moro-Sibilot D, et al. Immune-Checkpoint Inhibitors Associated With Interstitial Lung Disease in Cancer Patients. *Eur Respir J* (2017) 50(2):1700050. doi: 10.1183/13993003.00050-2017
43. Gkiozos I, Kopitopoulou A, Kalkanis A, Vamvakaris IN, Judson MA, Syrigos KN. Sarcoidosis-Like Reactions Induced by Checkpoint Inhibitors. *J Thorac Oncol* (2018) 13(8):1076–82. doi: 10.1016/j.jtho.2018.04.031
44. Suresh K, Voong KR, Shankar B, Forde PM, Ettinger DS, Marrone KA, et al. Pneumonitis in Non-Small Cell Lung Cancer Patients Receiving Immune Checkpoint Immunotherapy: Incidence and Risk Factors. *J Thorac Oncol* (2018) 13(12):1930–9. doi: 10.1016/j.jtho.2018.08.2035

14

Combination of Immune Checkpoint Inhibitors and Anti-Angiogenic Agents in Brain Metastases from Non-Small Cell Lung Cancer

Likui Fang, Wuchen Zhao, Bo Ye and Da Chen *

Department of Thoracic Surgery, Affiliated Hangzhou Chest Hospital, Zhejiang University School of Medicine, Hangzhou, China

***Correspondence:**
Da Chen
nuu2k@sina.com

Brain metastases remain a critical issue in the management of non-small cell lung cancer (NSCLC) because of the high frequency and poor prognosis, with survival rates often measured in just months. The local treatment approach remains the current standard of care, but management of multiple asymptomatic brain metastases always involves systemic therapy. Given that anti-angiogenic agents and immune checkpoint inhibitors (ICIs) both target the tumor microenvironment (TME), this combination therapy has become a promising strategy in clinical practice. Increasing number of preclinical and clinical studies have shown remarkable anti-tumor activity of the combination therapy, but the efficacy in brain metastases is unclear due to the strict selection criteria adopted in most clinical trials. This review briefly summarizes the potential synergistic anti-tumor effect and clinical development of the combination of anti-angiogenic agents and ICIs in NSCLC brain metastases, and discusses the existing challenges and problems.

Keywords: non-small cell lung cancer, brain metastases, immune checkpoint inhibitors, anti-angiogenesis, combination therapy

INTRODUCTION

Lung cancer is one of the most common malignant tumors and the leading cause of cancer-related mortality worldwide (1, 2). Non-small cell lung cancer (NSCLC) is the most frequent subtype of lung cancer and approximately 57% patients with NSCLC are in advanced stage including 20% presenting with brain metastases at the time of diagnosis (3). Brain metastases are also the common pattern of distant relapse after initial treatment (4, 5). Brain metastases are associated with poor prognosis and portend limited effective treatment options (6).

Current treatment strategies include local and systematic management. For the patients with symptomatic and immediately life-threatening brain metastases, surgical resection and radiotherapy are the major therapeutic approaches because of their relatively effective local control (7–9). However, surgery is typically reserved for intracranial hemorrhage, large lesions, and solitary brain metastases (10). Similarly, the use of stereotactic radiosurgery is limited by the number of metastatic lesions and is not suitable for the tumors which are larger than 4cm or located in critical structures (11, 12). Whole brain radiotherapy is still the main method for the patients with multiple brain metastases or when stereotactic radiosurgery is not feasible (13). Although local treatment has an irreplaceable status in brain metastases currently, its toxic effects should warrant enough attention, such as cognitive decline and symptomatic radiation necrosis (7, 14, 15). Moreover, local treatment could delay the initiation of systemic treatment, which would lead to the progression of primary tumors and compromise long-term outcomes.

Considering the limitations of local treatment, systematic therapy for NSCLC brain metastases has been explored due to its simultaneous treatment for both intracerebral and extracerebral diseases. Chemotherapy is not so often an effective approach for metastatic brain lesions, whereas tyrosine kinase inhibitors (TKIs) therapy such as Osimertinib in oncogene driven disease has shown a good activity also on brain metastases (16–18). In the era of immunotherapy, there is increasing evidence supporting the use of immune checkpoint inhibitors (ICIs) in the treatment of NSCLC brain metastases when no targetable driver mutation has been identified (19). Despite the encouraging data, only few patients respond to immunotherapy and additional combination treatment strategies are in urgent need. Given that both anti-angiogenesis and immune checkpoint blockade focus on targeting the tumor microenvironment (TME), the combination of ICIs and anti-angiogenic agents has become an attractive strategy. This review summarizes the potential synergistic anti-tumor effect and clinical development of this combination therapy strategy in NSCLC brain metastases.

POTENTIAL MECHANISMS

Tumorigenesis involves a succession of genetic alterations which have been classified into eight distinctive and complementary biologic capabilities, including sustaining proliferative signaling, evading growth suppressors, deregulating cellular energetics, enabling replicative immortality, resisting cell death, inducing angiogenesis, avoiding immune destruction and activating invasion and metastasis (20). Therefore, angiogenesis and immune escape are two critical processes of tumorigenesis. Moreover, TME is widely accepted as an important regulator of cancer formation and progression. The tumor vasculature is a key component of the microenvironment that can be targeted through the use of anti-angiogenic agents. Blood vascular and lymphatic endothelial cells have important roles in regulating the microenvironment and modulating the immune response. Improving access to the tumor through vascular normalization with anti-angiogenic agents may prove an effective combination strategy with immunotherapy approaches, and this combination therapy could have synergistic effects on TME to inhibit tumorigenesis. However, even though TME is a potentially rich source of therapeutic targets, our knowledge of the brain TME lacks comprehensive and integrative analysis.

The brain has long been regarded as immune privileged organ because blood brain barrier (BBB) and blood cerebrospinal fluid barrier (BCB) limit the entry of immune cells from the periphery. However, the immune privileged status of brain has been recently challenged by the discovery of lymphatic vessels that connect the central nervous system (CNS) with the periphery and are able to carry both fluid and immune cells (21, 22). This discovery leads to a reassessment of long-held assumptions in neuroimmunology and sheds new light on the application of immunotherapy in brain metastases. Several in-depth studies of immune microenvironmental landscape within CNS have revealed disease-specific enrichment of immune cells, including tissue-resident microglia, infiltrating monocyte-derived macrophages, neutrophils, and T cells (23, 24). Principal-component analysis has confirmed that monocyte-derived macrophages, neutrophils, and CD4+ and CD8+ T cells are the major immune cell determinants of the TME landscape of lung cancer brain metastases (24). In addition, brain metastases can disrupt the integrity of the BBB and BCB and recruit different immune cells from the myeloid and lymphoid lineage to the CNS (25). Angiogenesis is one of the specific hallmarks of NSCLC brain metastases and pivotal for the progression of metastasizing lesions, which have been proven by the observations of human autopsy specimens (26, 27). In addition, the tumor vasculature has important immunomodulatory roles including preventing the immune rejection of tumors (28). There have been several clinical studies suggesting that inclusion of anti-angiogenic therapies should be evaluated in selected patients with asymptomatic NSCLC brain metastases (29, 30). These findings provide theoretical supports for the use of ICIs and anti-angiogenic agents in NSCLC brain metastases. The development of this combination strategy is based on the understandings of the interaction between these two therapeutic interventions and their effects on the TME.

Anti-Angiogenic Agents Promote Anti-Tumor Immune Response

Angiogenesis involves many signaling pathways, such as vascular endothelial growth factor (VEGF)-VEGF receptor (VEGFR), platelet derived growth factor (PDGF)-PDGF receptor (PDGFR) and fibroblast growth factor (FGF)-FGF receptor (FGFR). These signaling pathways influence multiple steps of the cancer immune response (31, 32) (**Figure 1**). VEGF is one of the most studied factors triggering angiogenesis. In the circulation, the level of VEGF was found to be inversely correlated with the level of mature dendritic cell (DC) which is the main antigen-presenting cell (33). VEGF-VEGFR signaling pathway could inhibit the transcriptional activation of nuclear factor-κB to affect the differentiation and maturation of DCs (34, 35). Moreover, VEGF could also inhibit the antigen-presentation function of DCs by upregulating programmed cell death protein ligand-1 (PD-L1) expression on DCs (36). As a result, cancer antigens fail to be presented to T cells, leading to silence of cytotoxic T lymphocytes. In addition, PDGF could also restrain DC maturation (31). Anti-angiogenic agents could increase the level of mature DCs and enhance the uptake of antigen presentation, resulting in the promotion of anti-tumor immune response (37, 38).

T cell infiltration is widely accepted as a key component of adaptive cancer immune response. VEGF could inhibit the differentiation of CD8+ and CD4+ T cells from hematopoietic

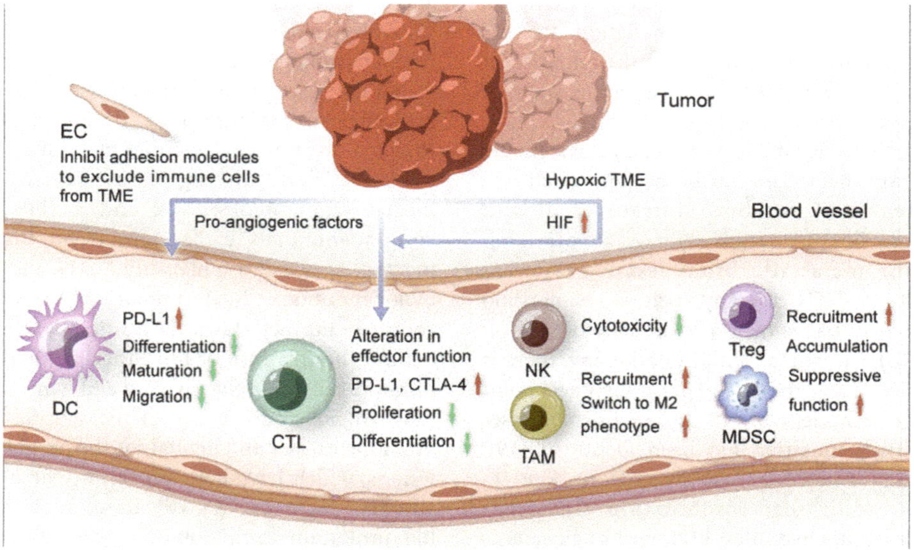

FIGURE 1 | The role of tumor angiogenesis in TME. Pro-angiogenic factors and hypoxia restrict the maturation and migration of dendritic cells, reduce the proliferation and differentiation of effector CTLs, and promote the recruitment of suppressive immune cells. TME, tumor microenvironment; DC, dendritic cell; CTL, cytotoxic T lymphocytes; NK, natural killer cell; TAM, tumor-associated macrophage; Treg, regulatory T cell; MDSC, myeloid-derived suppressor cell; EC, endothelial cell; HIF, hypoxia-inducible factor.

progenitor cells and lead to the occurrence of T-cell deficiency (39). Moreover, activation of VEGF-VEGFR signaling pathway on CD8+T cells could induce T cell exhaustion and reduce T cell cytotoxicity by increasing the expression of programmed cell death protein 1 (PD-1) and cytotoxic T-lymphocyte-associated protein 4 (CTLA-4) (40). Similarly, natural killer cells (NK) cytotoxicity could be impaired by VEGF-VEGFR signaling pathway (41). Overexpressed VEGF could also inhibit the recruitment of type 1 helper T cells (Th) at tumor site but enhance the recruitment and proliferation of immunosuppressive cells including regulatory T cells (Treg) and myeloid-derived suppressor cells (MDSC) to promote the formation of immunosuppressive microenvironment (31).

The steps of immune cells infiltrating into the TME include entering the tumor vessels, attaching to the endothelial cells and finally migrate to the TME through the vascular wall (42). Angiogenic molecules are capable to regulate the expression of different adhesion molecules such as intercellular adhesion molecule-1 (ICAM-1) and vascular cell adhesion molecule 1 (VCAM1) to inhibit the transfer of immune cells to TME (28). Moreover, tumor endothelial cells could not only form a specific selective barrier to inhibit the penetration of certain immune cells (31), but also modulate the activity and variability of immune cells to regulate immunosuppression (32).

Abnormal tumor vasculature could aggravate the hypoxia in TME, leading to immune suppression through multiple mechanisms including recruitment of MDSCs, accumulation of Tregs (43) and activation of hypoxia-inducible factor (HIF) which is a critical factor of regulating angiogenesis and immune response (44). HIF could participate in innate and adaptive immunity. For example, HIF could promote recruitment of monocytes and M2 tumor-associated macrophages (TAMs) by upregulating the expression of nuclear factor-κB (44). TAMs have emerged as prominent players in brain cancer (24). They are highly plastic cells that integrate input from cytokines, growth factors, and other stimuli, resulting in diverse activation states and cellular phenotypes, including promotion of invasion, angiogenesis, metastasis, and immune suppression (24). HIF could also inhibit DC maturation, inactivate cytotoxic T lymphocytes (CTLs) and target PD-L1 to evade anticancer immune responses (31).

Overall, the immunomodulatory effects of tumor vasculature are important targets in understanding and manipulating the TME. Anti-angiogenic therapy could not only normalize the tumor vasculature, but also transform the immunosuppressive TME to the immunosupportive one to improve anti-tumor immune response.

ICIs Enhance the Anti-Tumor Effects of Anti-Angiogenic Agents

Tumor immune response is closely influenced by angiogenesis. Meanwhile, tumor angiogenesis also highly depends on immunosuppressive microenvironment. ICIs could activate immune cells to secret immune-mediating cytokine with anti-angiogenesis effects to induce tumor vessel normalization (45). IFN-γ is one of the important mediums during the process (**Figure 2**). For example, the activation of IFN-γ signaling pathway on CD8+T cells might be one of the potential mechanisms of the vasculature-normalizing effect of ICIs (32). IFN-γ could inhibit some pathways inducing angiogenesis, such as Notch signaling pathway, to effectively retard tumor growth (31). IFN-γ could also reduce the VEGF secretion of tumor-

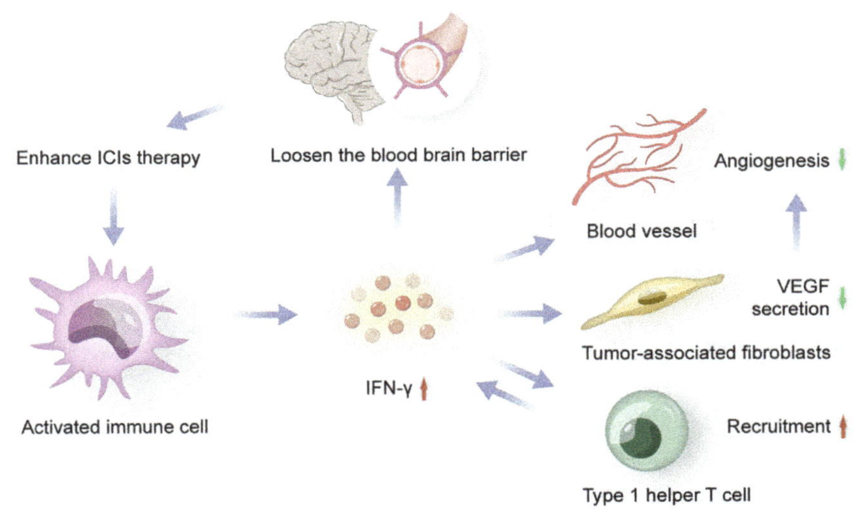

FIGURE 2 | Activated immune cell secretes IFN-γ to inhibit angiogenesis. ICIs, immune checkpoint inhibitors; VEGF, vascular endothelial growth factor.

associated fibroblasts to down-regulated angiogenesis (31). In addition, IFN-γ could increase expression of CXCL9, CXCL10, and CXCL1 which recruit Th1 cells (46), and Th1 cells could secrete IFN-γ in turn, which is significantly associated with vessel normalization (47). Besides, activated CD4+ T cells in the brain could loosen the BBB to circulating antibodies through local IFN-γ production, which is a mechanism that anti-PD-1/PD-L1 therapy could potentially enhance (48).

Immunosuppressive cells could also stimulate tumor angiogenesis by cooperating with pro-angiogenic factors. For instance, MDSCs could enhance the proliferation and migration of endothelial cells by secreting VEGF, and promote tumor angiogenesis by inducing the production of matrix metalloproteinase 9 to act on the extracellular matrix (31). DC precursors could induce tumor angiogenesis in cooperation with VEGF-VEGFR signaling pathway which could further induce DC precursor endothelial-like specialization and migration to blood vessels (31). Moreover, through the expression and secretion of pro-angiogenic factors, some other myeloid cell subgroups might be also equipped with the ability to promote angiogenesis, including TAMs, Tregs, B cells, monocytes and neutrophils (31). These basic researches have provided the evidence that anti-angiogenic therapy could be more effective following the generation of an immunosupportive microenvironment.

Basic researches have suggested that immune response and angiogenesis are mutually regulated, and alleviated immunosuppression coupled with normalization of the tumor vasculature could achieve a loop of positive feedback that promotes each other (32). Some preclinical studies indicated that the efficacy of ICIs combined with anti-angiogenesis was significantly superior to monotherapy in advanced NSCLC. Sha Zhao et al. demonstrated that based on syngeneic lung cancer mouse model, low-dose apatinib could result in alleviating hypoxia, increasing infiltration of CD8+ T cells, reducing recruitment of TAMs in tumor and decreasing TGF-β level both in tumor and serum (49). They also found that combining low-dose apatinib with anti-PD-L1 antibody could significantly retard tumor growth and metastases, and induce prolonged survival in mouse models (49). Additionally, apatinib could improve the anti-tumor efficacy of anti-PD-1 therapy *via* upregulating PD-L1 expression in a syngeneic mouse model (50), which might provide a rationale for this combination strategy in the clinic.

CLINICAL DATA

Based on the synergistic effect on TME, the combination of ICIs and anti-angiogenic agents has been performed in advanced NSCLC. Although data are still immature, clinical benefits have been obtained from this combination strategy. The results of clinical trials investigating the combination effect of anti-angiogenic agents and ICIs were presented in **Table 1**.

Herbst et al. designed a multi-cohort phase I trial (NCT02443324) to assess the effect of ramucirumab plus pembrolizumab in the patients with advanced NSCLC with prior progression on systemic therapy (51). This trial enrolled 27 patients with 77.8% adenocarcinoma and 14.8% squamous cell carcinoma. Median progression-free survival (PFS) was 9.7 months and overall survival (OS) rate at 6 month was 84.9%. Objective response rate (ORR) and disease control rate (DCR) were 30% and 85%, respectively. Treatment related adverse events (TRAEs) occurred in 25 (92.6%) patients with 18.5% grade 3 including adrenal insufficiency, delirium, hypertension, hyponatremia, infusion related reaction, proteinuria and respiratory failure. No grade 4-5 TRAEs occurred. In addition, Chu et al. conducted a phase Ib trial (NCT03628521) to evaluate

TABLE 1 | Clinical trials investigating the combination effect of anti-angiogenic agents and ICIs in NSCLC.

Clinical trial	Phase	Histology	Brain metastases	Treatment	Results	TRAEs
NCT02443324	I	Adenocarcinoma, 21/27 (77.8%) Squamous cell carcinoma, 4/27 (14.8%)	NA	Pembrolizumab plus ramucirumab	ORR, 30% DCR, 85% Median PFS, 9.7 m OS rate at 6 m, 84.9%	Total, 25/27 (92.6%) Grade 3, 5/27 (18.5%) Grade 4-5, 0/27 (0%)
NCT03628521	Ib	Squamous cell carcinoma, 12/22 (54.5%) Adenocarcinoma, 9/22 (40.9%)	4/22 (18.2%)	Sintilimab plus anlotinib	ORR, 72.7% DCR, 100% Median PFS, 15 m	Total, 22/22 (100%) Grade 3, 12/22 (54.5%) Grade 4-5, 1/22 (4.5%)
NCT01454102	I	Non-squamous cell carcinoma	NA	Nivolumab plus bevacizumab	ORR, 8% DCR, 58% Median PFS, 37.1 w OS rate at 1 y, 75%	Total, 11/12 (91.7%) Grade 3, 4/12 (33.3%) Grade 4-5, 0/12 (0%)
IMpower150	III	Non-squamous cell carcinoma	NA	Atezolizumab plus bevacizumab plus carboplatin plus paclitaxel	ORR, 63.5% DCR, 85.3% Median PFS, 8.3 m Median OS, 19.2 m	Total, 371/393 (94.4%) Grade 3-4, 219/393 (55.7%) Grade 5, 11/393 (2.8%)
NCT02039674	I	Non-squamous cell carcinoma	4/25 (16%)	Pembrolizumab plus bevacizumab plus carboplatin plus paclitaxel	ORR, 56% DCR, 76% Median PFS, 7.1 m Median OS, 16.7 m	Total, 23/24 (95.8%) Grade 3-4, 10/24 (41.7%) Grade 5, 0/24 (0%)

NSCLC, non-small cell lung cancer; m, month(s); w, weeks; y, year; NA, not applicable; ICIs, immune checkpoint inhibitors; ORR, objective response rate; DCR, disease control rate; PFS, progression-free survival; OS, overall survival; TRAEs, treatment related adverse events.

chemo-free first-line strategy of sintilimab combining anlotinib in treatment-naive and stage IIIB/IV NSCLC patients (52). Twenty-two patients were enrolled in the study and four had baseline brain metastases. The results showed high ORR (72.7%) and DCR (100%) with acceptable tolerability. The incidence rate of grade 3 TRAEs was 54.5%. No grade 4 TRAEs were observed, and one case of grade 5 immune-related pneumonitis occurred. The most common TRAEs were hemorrhage (59.1%), hypothyroidism (50.0%) and hyperuricemia (40.9%). Moreover, Rizvi et al. reported preliminary results from a phase I study (NCT01454102) evaluating the efficacy and safety of nivolumab plus bevacizumab as maintenance therapy in advanced NSCLC without progress on first-line platinum based chemotherapy (53). Median PFS was 37.1 weeks and 1-year OS rate was 75%. TRAEs occurred in 11/12 (91.7%) patients with 33.3% grade 3 and no grade 4 TRAEs. Grade 3 adverse events included pneumonitis, cough and tubulointerstitial nephritis.

IMpower150, a phase III randomized trial, showed a significant prognostic improvement with the addition of atezolizumab to bevacizumab and chemotherapy as first-line treatment for nonsquamous metastatic NSCLC (54). This clinical study enrolled a total of 1202 patients and randomly assigned them to three group, atezolizumab plus bevacizumab plus carboplatin plus paclitaxel (ABCP group, 400 patients), atezolizumab plus carboplatin plus paclitaxel (ACP group, 402 patients) and bevacizumab plus carboplatin plus paclitaxel (BCP group, 400 patients). The results indicated that ABCP group had higher rate of PFS at 12 months and objective response than BCP group, regardless of the PD-L1 expression status. It was worth mentioning that ABCP group also showed significant survival benefit in comparison to BCP group in the patients with sensitizing EGFR mutations and liver metastases (55). However, the frequency of TRAEs did not increase with the addition of atezolizumab and the safety profile was consistent with previously reported safety risks of the individual medicines (54). Although IMpower150 study confirmed successful combination of ICIs and anti-angiogenic agents in metastatic NSCLC, this study excluded patients if they had untreated metastases of the central nervous system. In contrast, a multi-cohort phase I study (NCT02039674) explored the anti-tumor activity and safety of pembrolizumab plus carboplatin-paclitaxel-bevacizumab in advanced non-squamous NSCLC without prior systemic therapy (56). This study randomly assigned patients into 3 cohorts (A, B and C) and the patients in cohort B received pembrolizumab plus carboplatin-paclitaxel-bevacizumab. Cohort B enrolled 25 patients with 4 (16%) brain metastases. ORR was 56% with 1 (4%) complete response and 13 (52%) partial response. Median PFS was 7.1 months and median OS was 16.7 months. TRAEs occurred in 95.8% patients and most events were of mild-to-moderate severity. It should be noted that TRAEs resulted in discontinuation of study treatment in 5 cases in cohort B, including neutropenia, autoimmune colitis, diarrhea, drug hypersensitivity, and pneumonitis.

A real-world retrospective study enrolled 69 patients with NSCLC to explore the efficacy of ICIs combining anti-angiogenesis therapy (57). Sixty-three (91.3%) patients were at stage IV and 16 (23.2%) had sensitizing EGFR mutations. Twenty-nine (42%) patients received nivolumab and 40 (58%) received pembrolizumab. Bevacizumab was used in 45 (65.2%) patients and the remaining patients received apatinib, anlotinib or endostar. ORR was 31.9% and DCR was 89.9%. Median PFS was 8.37 months, while median OS was not reached. It should be noted that the patients receiving combined therapy within 6 months after diagnosis had better ORR than those exceeding 6 months (59.1% *vs.* 19.1%, P = 0.001). These results suggested that it would be better to apply ICIs plus anti-angiogenic agents at the early stage after initial diagnosis. TRAEs appeared in 62% of patients. Most TRAEs were grade 1-2 with only 2 (2.9%) grade 3 (pneumonitis, diarrhea) and no grade 4-5 events. The most common adverse events were fatigue, decreased appetite and nausea.

The combination of ICIs and anti-angiogenic agents showed encouraging anti-tumor activity and tolerable safety profile. Due to the potential neurological sequelae, patients with brain metastases were often excluded from clinical trials. Major ongoing or planned trials investigating ICIs in combination with anti-angiogenic agents in patients with NSCLC (**Table 2**) include NCT03377023 (a trial of nivolumab plus ipilimumab plus nintedanib), NCT03689855 (a trial of atezolizumab plus ramucirumab), NCT03527108 (a trial of nivolumab plus ramucirumab) and NCT02681549 (a trial of pembrolizumab plus bevacizumab) (58). However, at the time of writing, there are no published trial data from prospective randomized controlled trials focusing on the effects of this combination strategy in NSCLC patients with brain metastases which warrant further studies.

PREDICTIVE INDICATORS

Despite the promising prospect of immunotherapy and anti-angiogenesis therapy in NSCLC brain metastases, this combination strategy still faces many challenges, one of which is identifying ideal predictive indicators to screen suitable populations. As for anti-angiogenesis therapy, circulating VEGF-A level was evaluated for the prognostic and predictive value in a retrospective analysis (59). This study included five trials involving three types of cancer, AVF2107 (colorectal cancer), E4599 (NSCLC), AVAiL (NSCLC), AVOREN (renal cell carcinoma) and AVF2938 (renal cell carcinoma). In E4599 trial, bevacizumab-based treatment was predictive for PFS benefit in high circulating VEGF-A group (>36 pg/mL) but not in low VEGF-A group. By contrast, circulating VEGF-A level (cutoff value, 45 pg/mL) was not prognostic for PFS and OS in AVAiL trial. Other biomarkers such as VEGFR-2, FGF-2 and IL-8 were proposed and investigated, but none could predict response to anti-angiogenesis therapy (60). Several studies indicated that anti-angiogenic TRAEs and the number of circulating endothelial cells were positively associated with the clinical benefit (60, 61), but none were validated for routine clinical use. Similarly, the use of ICIs for the treatment of intracranial metastatic tumors also requires effective predictive indicators. Previous studies have proven that the expression of PD-L1 and the presence of tumor-infiltrating lymphocytes (TILs) within TME are considered prognostic and predictive markers in patients treated with immunotherapy (62, 63). However, the PD-L1 expression and the presence of TILs might be different in CNS when compared with extracranial sites, with lower PD-L1 expression and less TILs infiltration in brain metastases compared with matched NSCLC primary tumors (64). Tumor mutational burden (TMB) was also a useful biomarker for response to ICIs in advanced NSCLC (65), but its value in brain metastases remains unclear. DNA mismatch repair-deficient (dMMR)/microsatellite instability-high (MSI-H) has also been reported to be able to predict the efficacy of ICIs, but the low frequency in NSCLC limits its clinical application (66).

As for the combination therapy, the phase Ib trial (NCT03628521) indicated that the patients with TMB ≥10 mutations per megabase showed higher ORR than those with TMB <10 mutations per megabase (85.7% *vs.* 63.6%) (52). It is worth mentioning that ORR in the patients with positive and negative PD-L1 expression was 69.2% and 75%, respectively (67). The phase I trial (NCT02039674) showed that patients with PD-L1 TPS ≥50% were seemed to have higher ORR than those with PD-L1 TPS <50% (75% *vs.* 47%) (56). IMpower150 also suggested that high expression of an effector T-cell (Teff) gene signature in the tumor was associated with survival benefit (54). However, in comparison to primary tumor of NSCLC, brain metastasis lesions displayed significant downregulation of genes related to immune response and immune cell activation (68). In addition, it is unclear whether aspects of the tumor vasculature are different in tumors that respond to immunotherapy and

TABLE 2 | Major ongoing or planned trials investigating ICIs in combination with anti-angiogenic agents in patients with NSCLC.

Clinical trial	Phase	Treatment (arm of combination therapy)	Planned patients	Primary objective
NCT03377023	I/II	Nivolumab plus ipilimumab plus nintedanib	Advanced or metastatic NSCLC	MTD, ORR
NCT03689855	II	Atezolizumab plus ramucirumab	Squamous or non-squamous NSCLC	ORR
NCT03527108	II	Nivolumab plus ramucirumab	Refractory or recurrent advanced NSCLC	DCR
NCT02681549	II	Pembrolizumab plus bevacizumab	Metastatic melanoma or NSCLC	BMRR

ICIs, immune checkpoint inhibitors; NSCLC, non-small cell lung cancer; MTD, maximum tolerated dose; ORR, objective response rate; DCR, disease control rate; BMRR, brain metastasis response rate.

those that do not, and if features such as hypoxia or production of pro-angiogenic factors may serve as predictive biomarkers. These problems suggest that it is unlikely to precisely predict the efficacy of immunotherapy and anti-angiogenesis combination in brain metastases through current biomarkers. The specific predictive indicators to distinguish appropriate population need further exploration.

DISCUSSION

Given recent advances in immunotherapy, emerging clinical evidence suggests that ICIs have anti-tumor effects in brain metastases from NSCLC. The OAK study showed that the hazard ratio (HR) for OS with atezolizumab *vs.* docetaxel was 0.73 for the overall population, 0.74 for patients without brain metastases, and 0.54 for patients with brain metastases (69). Similarly, the KEYNOTE-189 study comparing pembrolizumab plus chemotherapy with chemotherapy alone indicated that the HR for OS was 0.36 for patients with brain metastases, with 0.49 for the overall population and 0.53 for patients without brain metastases (70). A pooled analysis of CheckMate 063, 017 and 057 also demonstrated that nivolumab showed a survival advantage in second-line therapy for stable brain metastases when compared with docetaxel (71). Beyond oncogene-driven NSCLC, ICIs have recently shown promising activity in the CNS in patients with NSCLC brain metastases.

Despite the significant benefits of immunotherapy, there are still some problems such as limited patient response rates and drug resistance. Because of both targeting aspects of the TME, immunotherapy and anti-angiogenesis are expected to mutually enhance the anti-tumor effect through reprogramming the TME from immunosuppressive to immunosupportive, but whether this combination can improve response rate or delay drug resistance of monotherapy remains unclear and needs further clinical studies. Tumors can be categorized as inflamed and non-inflamed phenotypes based on the spatial localization of immune cells with respect to the tumor and stromal compartments (72). Almost all relevant therapeutic advances in the field of immunotherapy have been achieved in inflamed tumors, while non-inflamed tumors tend to respond poorly to ICIs (72). Whether anti-angiogenic therapy could expand the benefits of immune checkpoint inhibition to non-inflamed tumors requires additional researches. Clinically, steroids are frequently used in NSCLC patients with brain metastases with the aim of palliating cancer-related symptoms, but the use of steroids is associated with a lower efficacy of ICIs and a worse outcome (73). A retrospective study suggested that anlotinib could potentially replace glucocorticoids and effectively improve edema from brain metastases but this study only included 13 NSCLC patients with 23 brain metastases (74). Whether anti-angiogenesis can indeed counteract the negative effect of steroids needs further research. Hyperprogression is defined as rapid disease progression during immunotherapy, which is associated with poor survival outcome (75). In theory, rapidly proliferative cancer cells need an abundance of blood supply for nutrition, while bevacizumab could starve these cells of blood supply and nutrients and provide potential benefit (76). However, the clinical data is absent and needs further study.

Although the preliminary clinical results have suggested that immunotherapy and anti-angiogenesis combination could potentially provide significant activity against brain metastases, the field of this combination strategy faces many challenges in the pursuit of overcoming the defect of monotherapy and improving the outcome of patients. Firstly, there are various combination regimens involving ICIs (PD-1, PD-L1 and CTLA-4 inhibitors) and anti-angiogenic agents (anti-VEGF antibody, anti-VEGFR antibody and VEGFR TKIs). Which combination regimen is most effective for brain metastases remains to be answered by more data. Secondly, early phase clinical studies have reported the use time and the dosage of ICIs and anti-angiogenic agents (51–53), and the use of anti-angiogenic agents prior ICIs was seemed to be more beneficial *in vitro* and vivo experiments (77). However, no studies have analyzed the changes of pharmacokinetic and pharmacodynamic profiles of each agent after combinational use. The optimal time and sequence of each agent in the combination are currently unknown. The appropriate dosage of each agent also remains unclear. Thirdly, although preliminary studies have showed acceptable toxicities and tolerance of the combination therapy, those studies are at early phase and the samples are small. The toxicities still require close attention. Finally, lacking of efficient and sensitive predictive indicators for the combination therapy leads to difficult selection of optimal candidates.

In conclusion, although resolving the above problems requires a long distance, the combination of ICIs and anti-angiogenic agents has opened a new door for the treatment of NSCLC patients with brain metastases, and is expected to change the clinical management of those patients in the near future. Further studies are urgently needed to obtain the definitive data for the use of this combination strategy in clinic and facilitate the development of the optimal combination algorithm.

AUTHOR CONTRIBUTIONS

LF and DC performed a literature search, interpreted data, and wrote the manuscript. WZ and BY supervised and contributed to the writing process. All authors contributed to the article and approved the submitted version.

REFERENCES

1. Siegel RL, Miller KD, Jemal A. Cancer Statistics, 2020. *CA Cancer J Clin* (2020) 70(1):7–30. doi: 10.3322/caac.21590
2. Bray F, Ferlay J, Soerjomataram I, Siegel RL, Torre LA, Jemal A. Global Cancer Statistics 2018: GLOBOCAN Estimates of Incidence and Mortality Worldwide for 36 Cancers in 185 Countries. *CA Cancer J Clin* (2018) 68 (6):394–424. doi: 10.3322/caac.21492

3. Davis FG, Dolecek TA, McCarthy BJ, Villano JL. Toward Determining the Lifetime Occurrence of Metastatic Brain Tumors Estimated From 2007 United States Cancer Incidence Data. *Neuro-oncology* (2012) 14(9):1171–7. doi: 10.1093/neuonc/nos152
4. Churilla TM, Weiss SE. Emerging Trends in the Management of Brain Metastases From Non-small Cell Lung Cancer. *Curr Oncol Rep* (2018) 20 (7):54. doi: 10.1007/s11912-018-0695-9
5. Chen AM, Jahan TM, Jablons DM, Garcia J, Larson DA. Risk of Cerebral Metastases and Neurological Death After Pathological Complete Response to Neoadjuvant Therapy for Locally Advanced Nonsmall-Cell Lung Cancer: Clinical Implications for the Subsequent Management of the Brain. *Cancer* (2007) 109(8):1668–75. doi: 10.1002/cncr.22565
6. Sperduto PW, Kased N, Roberge D, Xu Z, Shanley R, Luo X, et al. Summary Report on the Graded Prognostic Assessment: An Accurate and Facile Diagnosis-Specific Tool to Estimate Survival for Patients With Brain Metastases. *J Clin Oncol* (2012) 30(4):419–25. doi: 10.1200/JCO.2011.38.0527
7. Alomari A, Rauch PJ, Orsaria M, Minja FJ, Chiang VL, Vortmeyer AO. Radiologic and Histologic Consequences of Radiosurgery for Brain Tumors. *J Neuro-oncol* (2014) 117(1):33–42. doi: 10.1007/s11060-014-1359-8
8. Redmond AJ, Diluna ML, Hebert R, Moliterno JA, Desai R, Knisely JP, et al. Gamma Knife Surgery for the Treatment of Melanoma Metastases: The Effect of Intratumoral Hemorrhage on Survival. *J Neurosurg* (2008) 109 Suppl:99–105. doi: 10.3171/JNS/2008/109/12/S16
9. Bansal P, Rusthoven C, Boumber Y, Gan GN. The Role of Local Ablative Therapy in Oligometastatic non-Small-Cell Lung Cancer: Hype or Hope. *Future Oncol (Lond Engl)* (2016) 12(23):2713–27. doi: 10.2217/fon-2016-0219
10. Flanigan JC, Jilaveanu LB, Chiang VL, Kluger HM. Advances in Therapy for Melanoma Brain Metastases. *Clin Dermatol* (2013) 31(3):264–81. doi: 10.1016/j.clindermatol.2012.08.008
11. Otake S, Goto T. Stereotactic Radiotherapy for Oligometastasis. *Cancers* (2019) 11(2):133–45. doi: 10.3390/cancers11020133
12. Collen C, Christian N, Schallier D, Meysman M, Duchateau M, Storme G, et al. Phase II Study of Stereotactic Body Radiotherapy to Primary Tumor and Metastatic Locations in Oligometastatic Nonsmall-Cell Lung Cancer Patients. *Ann Oncol* (2014) 25(10):1954–9. doi: 10.1093/annonc/mdu370
13. Li W, Yu H. Separating or Combining Immune Checkpoint Inhibitors (Icis) and Radiotherapy in the Treatment of NSCLC Brain Metastases. *J Cancer Res Clin Oncol* (2020) 146(1):137–52. doi: 10.1007/s00432-019-03094-9
14. Greene-Schloesser D, Robbins ME. Radiation-Induced Cognitive Impairment–From Bench to Bedside. *Neuro-oncology* (2012) 14(Suppl 4): iv37–44. doi: 10.1093/neuonc/nos196
15. Khan AJ, Dicker AP. On the Merits and Limitations of Whole-Brain Radiation Therapy. *J Clin Oncol* (2013) 31(1):11–3. doi: 10.1200/JCO.2012.46.0410
16. Reungwetwattana T, Nakagawa K, Cho BC, Cobo M, Cho EK, Bertolini A, et al. Cns Response to Osimertinib Versus Standard Epidermal Growth Factor Receptor Tyrosine Kinase Inhibitors in Patients With Untreated Egfr-Mutated Advanced non-Small-Cell Lung Cancer. *J Clin Oncol* (2018) 36(33):3290. doi: 10.1200/JCO.2018.78.3118
17. Gadgeel S, Peters S, Mok T, Shaw AT, Kim DW, Ou SI, et al. Alectinib Versus Crizotinib in Treatment-Naive Anaplastic Lymphoma Kinase-Positive (ALK +) non-Small-Cell Lung Cancer: CNS Efficacy Results From the ALEX Study. *Ann Oncol* (2018) 29(11):2214–22. doi: 10.1093/annonc/mdy405
18. Ernani V, Stinchcombe TE. Management of Brain Metastases in Non-Small-Cell Lung Cancer. *J Oncol Pract* (2019) 15(11):563–70. doi: 10.1200/JOP.19.00357
19. Wang S, Hu C, Xie F, Liu Y. Use of Programmed Death Receptor-1 and/or Programmed Death Ligand 1 Inhibitors for the Treatment of Brain Metastasis of Lung Cancer. *OncoTargets Ther* (2020) 13:667–83. doi: 10.2147/OTT.S235714
20. Hanahan D, Weinberg RA. Hallmarks of Cancer: The Next Generation. *Cell* (2011) 144(5):646–74. doi: 10.1016/j.cell.2011.02.013
21. Louveau A, Smirnov I, Keyes TJ, Eccles JD, Rouhani SJ, Peske JD, et al. Structural and Functional Features of Central Nervous System Lymphatic Vessels. *Nature* (2015) 523(7560):337–41. doi: 10.1038/nature14432
22. Raper D, Louveau A, Kipnis J. How Do Meningeal Lymphatic Vessels Drain the CNS? *Trends Neurosci* (2016) 39(9):581–6. doi: 10.1016/j.tins.2016.07.001
23. Quail DF, Joyce JA. The Microenvironmental Landscape of Brain Tumors. *Cancer Cell* (2017) 31(3):326–41. doi: 10.1016/j.ccell.2017.02.009
24. Klemm F, Maas RR, Bowman RL, Kornete M, Soukup K, Nassiri S, et al. Interrogation of the Microenvironmental Landscape in Brain Tumors Reveals Disease-Specific Alterations of Immune Cells. *Cell* (2020) 181(7):1643–60 e17. doi: 10.1016/j.cell.2020.05.007
25. Schulz M, Salamero-Boix A, Niesel K, Alekseeva T, Sevenich L. Microenvironmental Regulation of Tumor Progression and Therapeutic Response in Brain Metastasis. *Front Immunol* (2019) 10:1713. doi: 10.3389/fimmu.2019.01713
26. Berghoff AS, Rajky O, Winkler F, Bartsch R, Furtner J, Hainfellner JA, et al. Invasion Patterns in Brain Metastases of Solid Cancers. *Neuro-oncology* (2013) 15(12):1664–72. doi: 10.1093/neuonc/not112
27. Berghoff AS, Ilhan-Mutlu A, Dinhof C, Magerle M, Hackl M, Widhalm G, et al. Differential Role of Angiogenesis and Tumour Cell Proliferation in Brain Metastases According to Primary Tumour Type: Analysis of 639 Cases. *Neuropathol Appl Neurobiol* (2015) 41(2):e41–55. doi: 10.1111/nan.12185
28. Hendry SA, Farnsworth RH, Solomon B, Achen MG, Stacker SA, Fox SB. The Role of the Tumor Vasculature in the Host Immune Response: Implications for Therapeutic Strategies Targeting the Tumor Microenvironment. *Front Immunol* (2016) 7:621. doi: 10.3389/fimmu.2016.00621
29. Berghoff AS, Preusser M. Anti-Angiogenic Therapies in Brain Metastases. *Memo* (2018) 11(1):14–7. doi: 10.1007/s12254-018-0384-2
30. Shukla NA, Yan MN, Hanna N. The Story of Angiogenesis Inhibitors in Non-small-cell Lung Cancer: The Past, Present, and Future. *Clin Lung Cancer* (2020) 21(4):308–13. doi: 10.1016/j.cllc.2020.02.024
31. Guo F, Cui J. Anti-Angiogenesis: Opening a New Window for Immunotherapy. *Life Sci* (2020) 258:118163. doi: 10.1016/j.lfs.2020.118163
32. Song Y, Fu Y, Xie Q, Zhu B, Wang J, Zhang B. Anti-Angiogenic Agents in Combination With Immune Checkpoint Inhibitors: A Promising Strategy for Cancer Treatment. *Front Immunol* (2020) 11:1956. doi: 10.3389/fimmu.2020.01956
33. Galati D, Zanotta S, Canora A, Polistina GE, Nicoletta C, Ghinassi G, et al. Severe Depletion of Peripheral Blood Dendritic Cell Subsets in Obstructive Sleep Apnea Patients: A New Link With Cancer? *Cytokine* (2020) 125:154831. doi: 10.1016/j.cyto.2019.154831
34. Aggarwal V, Tuli HS, Varol A, Thakral F, Yerer MB, Sak K, et al. Role of Reactive Oxygen Species in Cancer Progression: Molecular Mechanisms and Recent Advancements. *Biomolecules* (2019) 9(11):735–60. doi: 10.3390/biom9110735
35. Alfaro C, Suarez N, Gonzalez A, Solano S, Erro L, Dubrot J, et al. Influence of Bevacizumab, Sunitinib and Sorafenib as Single Agents or in Combination on the Inhibitory Effects of VEGF on Human Dendritic Cell Differentiation From Monocytes. *Br J Cancer* (2009) 100(7):1111–9. doi: 10.1038/sj.bjc.6604965
36. Curiel TJ, Wei S, Dong H, Alvarez X, Cheng P, Mottram P, et al. Blockade of B7-H1 Improves Myeloid Dendritic Cell-Mediated Antitumor Immunity. *Nat Med* (2003) 9(5):562–7. doi: 10.1038/nm863
37. Long J, Hu Z, Xue H, Wang Y, Chen J, Tang F, et al. Vascular Endothelial Growth Factor (VEGF) Impairs the Motility and Immune Function of Human Mature Dendritic Cells Through the VEGF Receptor 2-RhoA-cofilin1 Pathway. *Cancer Sci* (2019) 110(8):2357–67. doi: 10.1111/cas.14091
38. Yang J, Yan J, Liu B. Targeting VEGF/VEGFR to Modulate Antitumor Immunity. *Front Immunol* (2018) 9:978. doi: 10.3389/fimmu.2018.00978
39. Ohm JE, Gabrilovich DI, Sempowski GD, Kisseleva E, Parman KS, Nadaf S, et al. VEGF Inhibits T-cell Development and may Contribute to Tumor-Induced Immune Suppression. *Blood* (2003) 101(12):4878–86. doi: 10.1182/blood-2002-07-1956
40. Voron T, Colussi O, Marcheteau E, Pernot S, Nizard M, Pointet AL, et al. VEGF-a Modulates Expression of Inhibitory Checkpoints on CD8+ T Cells in Tumors. *J Exp Med* (2015) 212(2):139–48. doi: 10.1084/jem.20140559
41. Lee JY, Park S, Min WS, Kim HJ. Restoration of Natural Killer Cell Cytotoxicity by VEGFR-3 Inhibition in Myelogenous Leukemia. *Cancer Lett* (2014) 354(2):281–9. doi: 10.1016/j.canlet.2014.08.027
42. Chen DS, Mellman I. Oncology Meets Immunology: The Cancer-Immunity Cycle. *Immunity* (2013) 39(1):1–10. doi: 10.1016/j.immuni.2013.07.012
43. Facciabene A, Peng X, Hagemann IS, Balint K, Barchetti A, Wang LP, et al. Tumour Hypoxia Promotes Tolerance and Angiogenesis Via CCL28 and T (reg) Cells. *Nature* (2011) 475(7355):226–30. doi: 10.1038/nature10169
44. Palazon A, Goldrath AW, Nizet V, Johnson RS. HIF Transcription Factors, Inflammation, and Immunity. *Immunity* (2014) 41(4):518–28. doi: 10.1016/j.immuni.2014.09.008
45. Yi M, Jiao D, Qin S, Chu Q, Wu K, Li A. Synergistic Effect of Immune Checkpoint Blockade and Anti-Angiogenesis in Cancer Treatment. *Mol Cancer* (2019) 18(1):60. doi: 10.1186/s12943-019-0974-6

46. Zheng X, Fang Z, Liu X, Deng S, Zhou P, Wang X, et al. Increased Vessel Perfusion Predicts the Efficacy of Immune Checkpoint Blockade. *J Clin Invest* (2018) 128(5):2104–15. doi: 10.1172/JCI96582
47. Tian L, Goldstein A, Wang H, Ching Lo H, Sun Kim I, Welte T, et al. Mutual Regulation of Tumour Vessel Normalization and Immunostimulatory Reprogramming. *Nature* (2017) 544(7649):250–4. doi: 10.1038/nature21724
48. Iwasaki A. Immune Regulation of Antibody Access to Neuronal Tissues. *Trends Mol Med* (2017) 23(3):227–45. doi: 10.1016/j.molmed.2017.01.004
49. Zhao S, Ren S, Jiang T, Zhu B, Li X, Zhao C, et al. Low-Dose Apatinib Optimizes Tumor Microenvironment and Potentiates Antitumor Effect of PD-1/PD-L1 Blockade in Lung Cancer. *Cancer Immunol Res* (2019) 7(4):630–43. doi: 10.1158/2326-6066.CIR-17-0640
50. Cai X, Wei B, Li L, Chen X, Liu W, Cui J, et al. Apatinib Enhanced anti-PD-1 Therapy for Colon Cancer in Mice Via Promoting PD-L1 Expression. *Int Immunopharmacol* (2020) 88:106858. doi: 10.1016/j.intimp.2020.106858
51. Herbst RS, Martin-Liberal J, Calvo E, Isambert N, Bendell J, Cassier P, et al. Previously Treated Advanced NSCLC Cohort From a Multi-Disease Phase 1 Study of Ramucirumab (R) Plus Pembrolizumab (P): Efficacy and Safety Data. *Ann Oncol* (2017) 28:ii32–ii3. doi: 10.1093/annonc/mdx091.010
52. Chu T, Zhong R, Zhong H, Zhang B, Zhang W, Shi C, et al. Phase Ib Study of Sintilimab Plus Anlotinib as First-line Therapy in Patients With Advanced non-Small Cell Lung Cancer. *J Thorac Oncol* (2020) 16(4):643–52. doi: 10.1016/j.jtho.2020.11.026
53. Rizvi NA, Antonia SJ, Shepherd FA, Chow LQ, Goldman J, Shen Y, et al. Nivolumab (Anti-Pd-1; BMS-936558, Ono-4538) Maintenance as Monotherapy or in Combination With Bevacizumab (BEV) for Non-Small Cell Lung Cancer (Nsclc) Previously Treated With Chemotherapy. *Int J Radiat OncologyBiologyPhysics* (2014) 90(5):S32. doi: 10.1016/j.ijrobp.2014.08.206
54. Socinski MA, Jotte RM, Cappuzzo F, Orlandi F, Stroyakovskiy D, Nogami N, et al. Atezolizumab for First-Line Treatment of Metastatic Nonsquamous Nsclc. *NEngl J Med* (2018) 378(24):2288–301. doi: 10.1056/NEJMoa1716948
55. Reck M, Mok TSK, Nishio M, Jotte RM, Cappuzzo F, Orlandi F, et al. Atezolizumab Plus Bevacizumab and Chemotherapy in non-Small-Cell Lung Cancer (Impower150): Key Subgroup Analyses of Patients With EGFR Mutations or Baseline Liver Metastases in a Randomised, Open-Label Phase 3 Trial. *Lancet Respir Med* (2019) 7(5):387–401. doi: 10.1016/S2213-2600(19)30084-0
56. Gadgeel SM, Stevenson JP, Langer CJ, Gandhi L, Borghaei H, Patnaik A, et al. Pembrolizumab and Platinum-Based Chemotherapy as First-Line Therapy for Advanced non-Small-Cell Lung Cancer: Phase 1 Cohorts From the KEYNOTE-021 Study. *Lung Cancer (Amsterdam Netherlands)* (2018) 125:273–81. doi: 10.1016/j.lungcan.2018.08.019
57. Qiu L, Zhao X, Shi W, Sun S, Zhang G, Sun Q, et al. Real-World Treatment Efficacy of Anti-Programmed Death-1 Combined With Anti-Angiogenesis Therapy in non-Small Cell Lung Cancer Patients. *Medicine* (2020) 99(24): e20545. doi: 10.1097/MD.0000000000020545
58. Popat S, Grohe C, Corral J, Reck M, Novello S, Gottfried M, et al. Anti-Angiogenic Agents in the Age of Resistance to Immune Checkpoint Inhibitors: Do They Have a Role in non-Oncogene-Addicted non-Small Cell Lung Cancer? *Lung Cancer (Amsterdam Netherlands)* (2020) 144:76–84. doi: 10.1016/j.lungcan.2020.04.009
59. Hegde PS, Jubb AM, Chen D, Li NF, Meng YG, Bernaards C, et al. Predictive Impact of Circulating Vascular Endothelial Growth Factor in Four Phase III Trials Evaluating Bevacizumab. *Clin Cancer Res* (2013) 19(4):929–37. doi: 10.1158/1078-0432.CCR-12-2535
60. Giuliano S, Pages G. Mechanisms of Resistance to Anti-Angiogenesis Therapies. *Biochimie* (2013) 95(6):1110–9. doi: 10.1016/j.biochi.2013.03.002
61. Liu X, Qin S, Wang Z, Xu J, Xiong J, Bai Y, et al. Early Presence of Anti-Angiogenesis-Related Adverse Events as a Potential Biomarker of Antitumor Efficacy in Metastatic Gastric Cancer Patients Treated With Apatinib: A Cohort Study. *J Hematol Oncol* (2017) 10(1):153. doi: 10.1186/s13045-017-0521-0
62. Mok TSK, Wu YL, Kudaba I, Kowalski DM, Cho BC, Turna HZ, et al. Pembrolizumab Versus Chemotherapy for Previously Untreated, PD-L1-expressing, Locally Advanced or Metastatic non-Small-Cell Lung Cancer (KEYNOTE-042): A Randomised, Open-Label, Controlled, Phase 3 Trial. *Lancet (Lond Engl)* (2019) 393(10183):1819–30. doi: 10.1016/S0140-6736(18)32409-7
63. Rossi S, Finocchiaro G, Marchetti S, Toschi L, Santoro A. Checkpoint Inhibitors: 'Raising the Bar' Also in Brain Metastases From non-Small-Cell Lung Cancer? *Immunotherapy* (2018) 10(5):403–10. doi: 10.2217/imt-2017-0151
64. Vilarino N, Bruna J, Bosch-Barrera J, Valiente M, Nadal E. Immunotherapy in NSCLC Patients With Brain Metastases. Understanding Brain Tumor Microenvironment and Dissecting Outcomes From Immune Checkpoint Blockade in the Clinic. *Cancer Treat Rev* (2020) 89:102067. doi: 10.1016/j.ctrv.2020.102067
65. Marabelle A, Fakih M, Lopez J, Shah M, Shapira-Frommer R, Nakagawa K, et al. Association of Tumour Mutational Burden With Outcomes in Patients With Advanced Solid Tumours Treated With Pembrolizumab: Prospective Biomarker Analysis of the Multicohort, Open-Label, Phase 2 KEYNOTE-158 Study. *Lancet Oncol* (2020) 21(10):1353–65. doi: 10.1016/S1470-2045(20)30445-9
66. Asaoka Y, Ijichi H, Koike K. Pd-1 Blockade in Tumors With Mismatch-Repair Deficiency. *N Engl J Med* (2015) 373(20):1979. doi: 10.1056/NEJMc1510353
67. Han B, Chu T, Zhong R, Zhong H, Zhang B, Zhang W, et al. Efficacy and Safety of Sintilimab With Anlotinib as First-Line Therapy for Advanced non-Small Cell Lung Cancer (Nsclc). *J Thoracic Oncol* (2019) 14(10):S129. doi: 10.1016/j.jtho.2019.08.269
68. Tsakonas G, Lewensohn R, Botling J, Ortiz-Villalon C, Micke P, Friesland S, et al. An Immune Gene Expression Signature Distinguishes Central Nervous System Metastases From Primary Tumours in non-Small-Cell Lung Cancer. *Eur J Cancer (Oxford Engl 1990)* (2020) 132:24–34. doi: 10.1016/j.ejca.2020.03.014
69. Rittmeyer A, Barlesi F, Waterkamp D, Park K, Ciardiello F, von Pawel J, et al. Atezolizumab Versus Docetaxel in Patients With Previously Treated non-Small-Cell Lung Cancer (OAK): A Phase 3, Open-Label, Multicentre Randomised Controlled Trial. *Lancet (London England)* (2017) 389(10066):255–65. doi: 10.1016/S0140-6736(16)32517-X
70. Gandhi L, Rodriguez-Abreu D, Gadgeel S, Esteban E, Felip E, De Angelis F, et al. Pembrolizumab Plus Chemotherapy in Metastatic non-Small-Cell Lung Cancer. *N Engl J Med* (2018) 378(22):2078–92. doi: 10.1056/NEJMoa1801005
71. Goldman JW, Crino L, Vokes EE, Holgado E, Reckamp K, Pluzanski A, et al. Nivolumab (Nivo) in Patients (Pts) With Advanced (Adv) NSCLC and Central Nervous System (Cns) Metastases (Mets). *J Thoracic Oncol* (2016) 11(10):S238–S9. doi: 10.1016/j.jtho.2016.08.107
72. Hegde PS, Chen DS. Top 10 Challenges in Cancer Immunotherapy. *Immunity* (2020) 52(1):17–35. doi: 10.1016/j.immuni.2019.12.011
73. Fuca G, Galli G, Poggi M, Lo Russo G, Proto C, Imbimbo M, et al. Modulation of Peripheral Blood Immune Cells by Early Use of Steroids and its Association With Clinical Outcomes in Patients With Metastatic non-Small Cell Lung Cancer Treated With Immune Checkpoint Inhibitors. *ESMO Open* (2019) 4(1):e000457. doi: 10.1136/esmoopen-2018-000457
74. Zhuang H, Wang Y, Cheng C, Shi S. The Efficacy of Anlotinib Instead of Glucocorticoids for Edema Induced by Brain Metastases in NSCLC Patients With anti-PD1/PDL-1 Immunotherapy. *Neuro-oncology* (2021) 23(1):169–71. doi: 10.1093/neuonc/noaa236
75. Billan S, Kaidar-Person O, Gil Z. Treatment After Progression in the Era of Immunotherapy. *Lancet Oncol* (2020) 21(10):e463–e76. doi: 10.1016/S1470-2045(20)30328-4
76. Venniyoor A. Synergism Between Anti-Angiogenic and Immune Checkpoint Inhibitor Drugs: A Hypothesis. *Med Hypotheses* (2021) 146:110399. doi: 10.1016/j.mehy.2020.110399
77. Yang Y, Li L, Jiang Z, Wang B, Pan Z. Anlotinib Optimizes Anti-Tumor Innate Immunity to Potentiate the Therapeutic Effect of PD-1 Blockade in Lung Cancer. *Cancer Immunol Immunother CII* (2020) 69(12):2523–32. doi: 10.1007/s00262-020-02641-5

15

A Computed Tomography-Derived Radiomics Approach for Predicting Uncommon EGFR Mutation in Patients with NSCLC

Wufei Chen, Yanqing Hua, Dingbiao Mao, Hao Wu, Mingyu Tan, Weiling Ma, Xuemei Huang, Jinjuan Lu, Cheng Li and Ming Li**

Department of Radiology, Huadong Hospital, Fudan University, Shanghai, China

Correspondence:
Yanqing Hua
huayqhd@163.com
Ming Li
minli77@163.com

Purpose: This study aims to develop a CT-based radiomics approach for identifying the uncommon epidermal growth factor receptor (EGFR) mutation in patients with non-small cell lung cancer (NSCLC).

Methods: This study involved 223 NSCLC patients (107 with uncommon EGFR mutation-positive and 116 with uncommon EGFR mutation-negative). A total of 1,269 radiomics features were extracted from the non-contrast-enhanced CT images after image segmentation and preprocessing. Support vector machine algorithm was used for feature selection and model construction. Receiver operating characteristic curve analysis was applied to evaluate the performance of the radiomics signature, the clinicopathological model, and the integrated model. A nomogram was developed and evaluated by using the calibration curve and decision curve analysis.

Results: The radiomics signature demonstrated a good performance for predicting the uncommon EGFR mutation in the training cohort (area under the curve, AUC = 0.802; 95% confidence interval, CI: 0.736–0.858) and was verified in the validation cohort (AUC = 0.791, 95% CI: 0.642–0.899). The integrated model combined radiomics signature with clinicopathological independent predictors exhibited an incremental performance compared with the radiomics signature or the clinicopathological model. A nomogram based on the integrated model was developed and showed good calibration (Hosmer–Lemeshow test, P = 0.92 in the training cohort and 0.608 in the validation cohort) and discrimination capacity (AUC of 0.816 in the training cohort and 0.795 in the validation cohort).

Conclusion: Radiomics signature combined with the clinicopathological features can predict uncommon EGFR mutation in NSCLC patients.

Keywords: NSCLC, computed tomography, uncommon EGFR, radiomics, nomogram

INTRODUCTION

Lung cancer is one of the leading causes of cancer-related deaths worldwide. Thereinto, non-small cell lung cancer (NSCLC) accounts for approximately 85% of all lung cancer cases (1). Over the past decade, the research of molecular targeted agents for NSCLC has made a great progress. The role of molecular targeted biomarkers in the process of oncotherapy has been further promoted (2). The epidermal growth factor receptor (EGFR) has been identified as the most common therapeutic biomarker for NSCLC. EGFR-TKI (tyrosine kinase inhibitor) treatment in EGFR mutation-activating patients has manifested superior progression-free survival benefits compared with standard chemotherapy (3). Of note is the fact that the therapeutic efficiency is closely related to the subtype of EGFR mutations. The mutation anchoring the uncommon site is thought to associate with poor outcomes, as it represents a higher heterogeneity (4, 5). Taking this into account, the accurate identification of uncommon EGFR mutation will play an essential role in the therapeutic decision-making of NSCLC patients.

At present, the acquisition of EGFR mutation status mainly depends on tissue biopsy. However, more than 50% of NSCLC patients get insufficient tissue in clinical practice (6). What is more, adverse events of percutaneous puncture, such as hemorrhage and pneumothorax, were reported in 17.1% among elderly patients (7). Thus, a non-invasive, convenient, and cost-effective alternative is desired (8).

Recently, radiomics is regarded to have a promising role for diagnostic support as it is non-invasive and has quantitative property to tumor heterogeneity. Previous studies demonstrated that radiomics signature could provide novel predictive indicators for the EGFR expression of NSCLC patients (9, 10). However, the study of predicting the subtype of EGFR mutation with radiomics analysis has been rarely reported.

This study aimed to evaluate the feasibility of radiomics approach to predict the uncommon EGFR mutation in NSCLC patients. We expect that this approach will become an alternative for optimizing the treatment for NSCLC patients.

MATERIALS AND METHODS

Data of Patients

This study was approved by our institutional review board, and the informed consent requirement for using desensitized data was waived. Consecutive patients with pathologically confirmed NSCLC from January 2016 to December 2020 were retrospectively analyzed. CT images and clinicopathological data were collected from the picture archiving and communication system (PACS) and the hospital information system in our institution. EGFR mutations of wild, common, and uncommon type were examined with human gene mutation detection kit (AmoyDx, China) *via* real-time polymerase chain reaction (PCR)-based assay and confirmed through direct sequencing.

The inclusion criteria were as follows: (a) no chemotherapy, radiotherapy, or targeted therapy before CT acquisition and PCR analysis; (b) cases with radiomics features that could be effectively extracted from the CT images; and (c) available clinicopathological data.

Finally, a total of 223 patients (107 with uncommon EGFR mutation, 73 with common EGFR mutation, and 43 with wild type) were enrolled in this study. The cases were randomly divided into the training cohort and the validation cohort at a ratio of 4:1.

Image Acquisition and Segmentation

All patients in this study underwent non-contrast-enhanced CT that covered the entire thorax. The scanning parameters are detailed in **Supplementary Table S2**. Images in DICOM format were derived from PACS in our institution. We used a commercially available segmentation software (Yizhun CIPS, version 4.0; http://www.yizhun-ai.com/Content/477572.html) and its lung tumor analysis tool as our image segmentation platform. The regions of interest (ROI) were delineated manually by two radiologists with more than 6 and 13 years of experience in chest CT interpretation with reference to the mediastinum and lung window, respectively. Both radiologists were blinded to the clinicopathological information and EGFR mutation status. Another radiologist with 7 years of experience independently segmented a random set of 20 nodules to assess the inter-observer reproducibility.

Radiomic Feature Extraction and Selection

The radiomics feature extraction in this study was performed with pyRadiomics (https://doi.org/10.1158/0008-5472.CAN-17-0339). Before the feature extraction, we used the nearest neighbor interpolation algorithm to resample the voxel into an isotropic distribution of 1 × 1 × 1 mm. Gaussian filter was used to modify the outlier value of voxel to reduce the photon noise influence on the radiomics features. A total of 1,269 radiomics features, which made up a mineable database for excavating the phenotype biomarker of the uncommon EGFR mutation, were extracted from the ROI. The definition of these radiomics features is available at http://pyradiomics.readthedocs.io/en/latest/features.html.

Inter-class correlation coefficient (ICC) was used to assess the inter-observer reproducibility of the extractive features. An ICC >0.75 was considered a good agreement. Stable and reproducible features were entered in the process of feature selection. Maximal relevance and minimal redundancy was used to reduce the redundant features.

Prediction Model Construction

The support vector machine (SVM), which is suitable for a small sample set, was adopted to construct the radiomics model in this study. The key features and their corresponding weight were calculated and screened out in the training cohort. Then, a radiomic score (Rad-score) was built by the weighted linear combination of all key features.

To explore the optimal model, another model based on clinicopathological features, including sex, age, smoking history, tumor grade, tumor biomarkers, stage, and Eastern Cooperative Oncology Group Performance Status (ECOG PS), was simultaneously built with multivariate logistic regression analysis. An integrated model, which included the Rad-score and the clinicopathological independent predictors, was also constructed.

Receiver operating characteristic (ROC) curve analysis was used to evaluate the predictive performance of each model. Then, the superior model was chosen to draw a nomogram for evaluating the clinical application. The calibration curve was plotted to explore the predictive accuracy of the nomogram. Decision curve analysis (DCA) was implemented to quantify the net benefits.

Statistical Analysis

Statistical analysis was performed using R software (version 3.6.2; R Foundation for Statistical Computing, Vienna, Austria; http://www.Rproject.org) and SPSS 21.0 (IBM, Chicago, IL, USA). R packages of "e1071", "rms", and "rmda" were implanted to execute the algorithm of SVM, nomogram, and DCA, respectively. Multivariate binary logistic regression was done with input parameter strategy. Independent *t*-test was used for the continuous variables, and chi-square test or Fisher's exact test was used for the categorical variables. All statistical tests were two-tailed, and P <0.05 indicated a significant difference.

RESULTS

Performance of the Clinicopathological Model

Among the full cohort, 107 patients were tested as uncommon EGFR mutation. The number of 20-INS, G719X, L861Q, S768I, and mixed was 23 (21.5), 33 (30.8), 26 (24.3), 11 (10.3), and 14 (13.1), respectively. No patients in this study had more than 2 exon mutations. Most patients exhibited a histological type of lung adenocarcinoma. According to disease-free survival (11), we incorporated the histological subtypes of non-mucinous lepidic predominant, acinar predominant, and papillary predominant adenocarcinoma into the low/intermediate-grade cohort and other subtypes, including solid predominant, micropapillary predominant invasive mucinous adenocarcinoma, and SCC, into the high-grade cohort. The EGFR mutation and histological subtype are detailed in **Supplementary Table S1**.

The clinicopathological features of the training and the validation cohorts are summarized in **Table 1**. Univariate analysis indicated that there was no significant difference in age, sex, smoking status, or tumor markers of NSE, CA125, SCC, CY21-1, stage, and ECOG PS between uncommon EGFR mutation-positive and uncommon EGFR mutation-negative (P > 0.05). Within the two cohorts, the uncommon EGFR mutation-positive showed a significant difference in serum

TABLE 1 | Clinicopathological data of patients in the training and validation cohorts.

Variable	Training cohort			Validation cohort			P
	Uncommon EGFR (+)	Uncommon EGFR (-)	P	Uncommon EGFR (+)	Uncommon EGFR (-)	P	
Age (mean ± SD)	64.93 ± 10.07	63.29 ± 9.89	0.273	65.47 ± 9.14	64.82 ± 13.7	0.856	0.543
Sex, *n* (%)			0.270			0.098	0.064
Male	45 (52.3)	41 (44.1)		16 (76.2)	12 (52.2)		
Female	41 (47.7)	52 (55.9)		5 (23.8)	11 (47.8)		
Smoking status, *n* (%)			0.879			0.063	0.822
Smoker	7 (8.1)	7 (7.5)		18 (85.7)	23 (100)		
Never smoker	79 (91.9)	86 (92.5)		3 (14.3)	0 (0)		
Grade, *n* (%)			**0.036**			**0.032**	0.137
Low/intermediate	62 (72.1)	79 (84.9)		11 (52.4)	19 (82.6)		
High	24 (27.9)	14 (15.1)		10 (47.6)	4 (17.4)		
Tumor marker (mean ± SD)							
CEA	7.63 ± 6.13	5.78 ± 5.49	**0.035**	8.53 ± 8.18	4.53 ± 4.20	**0.045**	0.823
NSE	2.87 ± 2.27	3.03 ± 2.99	0.695	2.46 ± 1.38	3.75 ± 3.11	0.087	0.686
CA125	9.49 ± 8.39	9.63 ± 6.18	0.898	8.67 ± 11.51	6.47 ± 13.48	0.567	0.157
SCC	0.69 ± 1.29	0.81 ± 1.23	0.506	0.92 ± 1.7	0.53 ± 0.28	0.294	0.848
CY21-1	3.61 ± 9.03	3.40 ± 3.65	0.834	3.52 ± 2.59	2.06 ± 2.34	0.056	0.475
Stage, *n* (%)			0.060			0.216	0.266
I	52 (60.5)	58 (62.4)		11 (52.4)	15 (65.2)		
II	9 (10.5)	11 (11.8)		1 (4.8)	1 (4.3)		
III	10 (11.6)	2 (2.2)		0 (0)	2 (8.7)		
IV	15 (17.4)	22 (23.7)		9 (42.9)	5 (21.7)		
ECOG PS, *n* (%)			0.368			0.594	0.580
0	29 (33.7)	34 (36.6)		6 (28.6)	6 (26.1)		
1	31 (36.0)	33 (35.5)		9 (42.9)	8 (34.8)		
2	18 (20.9)	23 (24.7)		5 (23.8)	5 (21.7)		
3	8 (9.3)	3 (3.2)		1 (4.8)	4 (17.4)		
Rad_score (mean ± SD)	0.55 ± 0.68	-0.29 ± 0.68	**0.001**	0.40 ± 0.84	-0.48 ± 0.68	**0.001**	0.970

Bold values: P < 0.05.

carcinoembryonic antigen (CEA) and tumor grade ($P < 0.05$). Accordingly, these two features were selected to establish a clinicopathological model with multivariate logistic regression analysis. The ROC curves for the clinicopathological model showed an acceptable performance (AUC of 0.665, 95% CI: 0.5995–0.727, sensitivity 63.55%, and specificity 62.93%).

Performance of the Radiomics Model

The workflow of radiomics analysis is indicated in **Figure 1**. A total of 1,018 features with ICCs >0.75 were reserved according to the re-segmentation data. After SVM analysis, 10 robust radiomics features, which were associated with an uncommon EGFR mutation, remained in the training cohort. The detailed formula of the Rad-score is shown in the **Supplementary Material**. The ROC curve for the radiomics signature showed a good performance in the training cohort (AUC = 0.802; 95% CI: 0.736–0.858; sensitivity, 82.56%; and specificity, 78.49%) and was then verified in the validation cohort (AUC = 0.791; 95% CI: 0.642–0.899; sensitivity, 61.90%; and specificity, 91.30%).

Performance of the Integrated Model

Subsequently, we established an integrated model with Rad-score, serum CEA, and the tumor grade. According to the multivariable logistic regression analysis, only Rad-score was independently associated with the uncommon EGFR mutation in the training cohort. The corresponding regression equation was as follows:

$$\text{logit}(p) = -0.417 + 1.601 \times \text{Rad} - \text{score} + 0.058 \times \text{CEA} - 0.334 \times \text{grade}.$$

The integrated model showed an incremental performance in the training cohort (AUC of 0.816; 95% CI: 0.751–0.870; sensitivity, 86.05%; and specificity, 70.97%) and AUC of 0.795 (95% CI: 0.646–0.902; sensitivity, 66.67%; and specificity, 91.3%) in the validation cohort.

The comparison of the three developed models is shown in **Figure 2**. According to the DeLong test, both the radiomics signature and the integrated model were superior to the clinicopathological model ($P < 0.05$). However, no statistical difference was found between the radiomics signature and the integrated model ($P > 0.05$).

Nomogram Construction

To visualize the potential application of the developed model, a nomogram based on the integrated model was delineated (seen

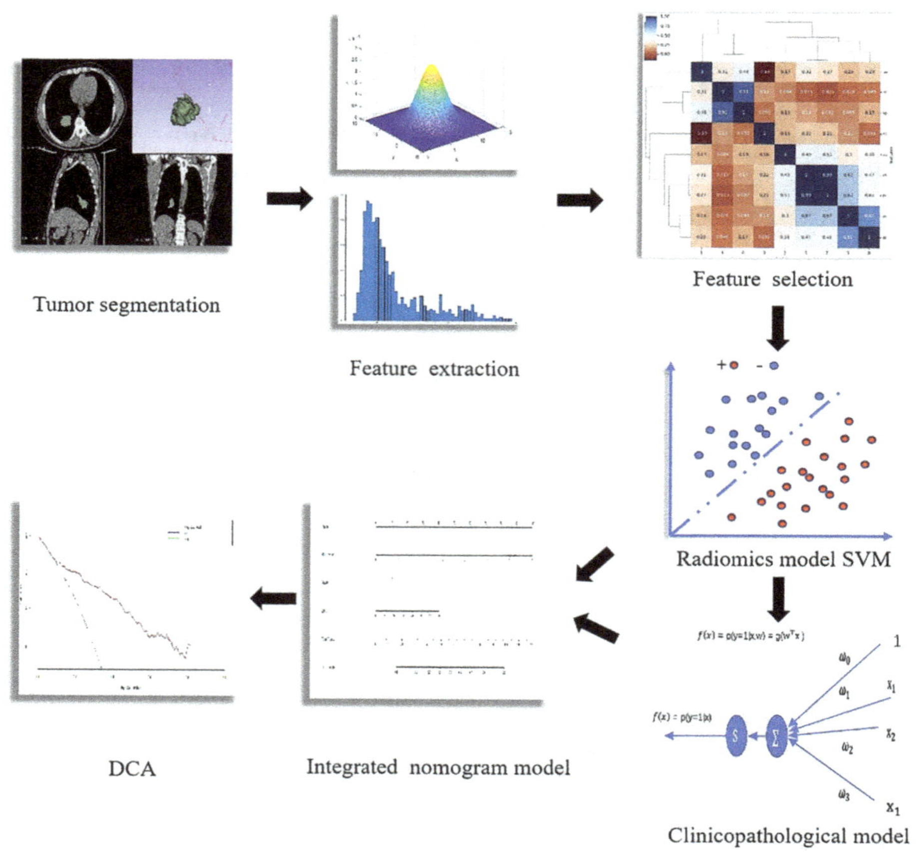

FIGURE 1 | Workflow of the radiomics analysis.

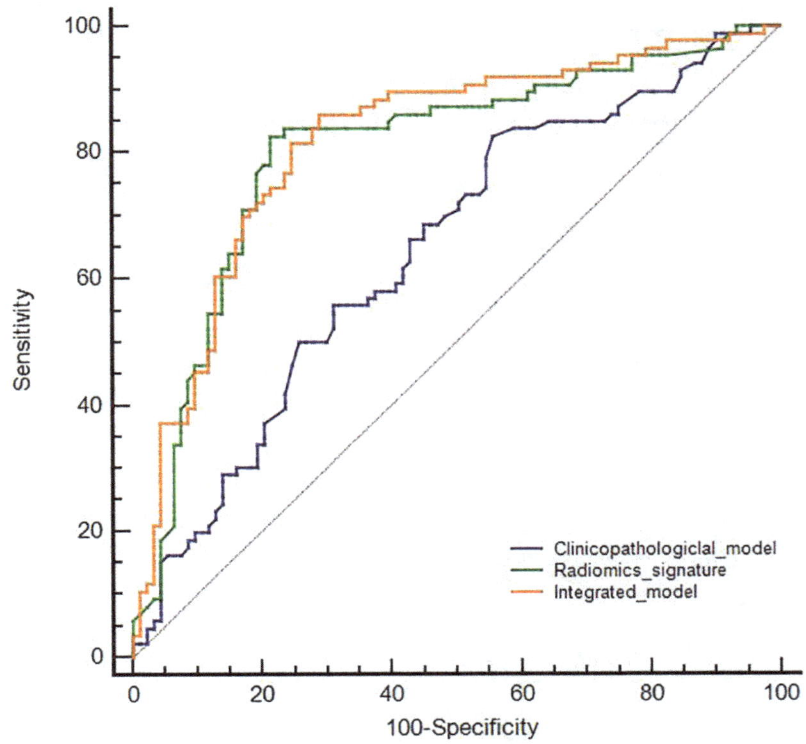

FIGURE 2 | Receiver operating characteristic curves of the developed models in the training cohort.

in **Figure 3**). The Hosmer–Lemeshow test showed no significant statistical difference between calibration curves and ideal curves both in the training cohort (P = 0.92) and in the validation cohort (P = 0.608). The calibration curve of the nomogram for the probability of the uncommon EGFR mutations demonstrated a good agreement (shown in **Figure 4**).

DCA was performed for the nomogram. As shown in **Figure 5** (red line), using the nomogram model to predict the uncommon

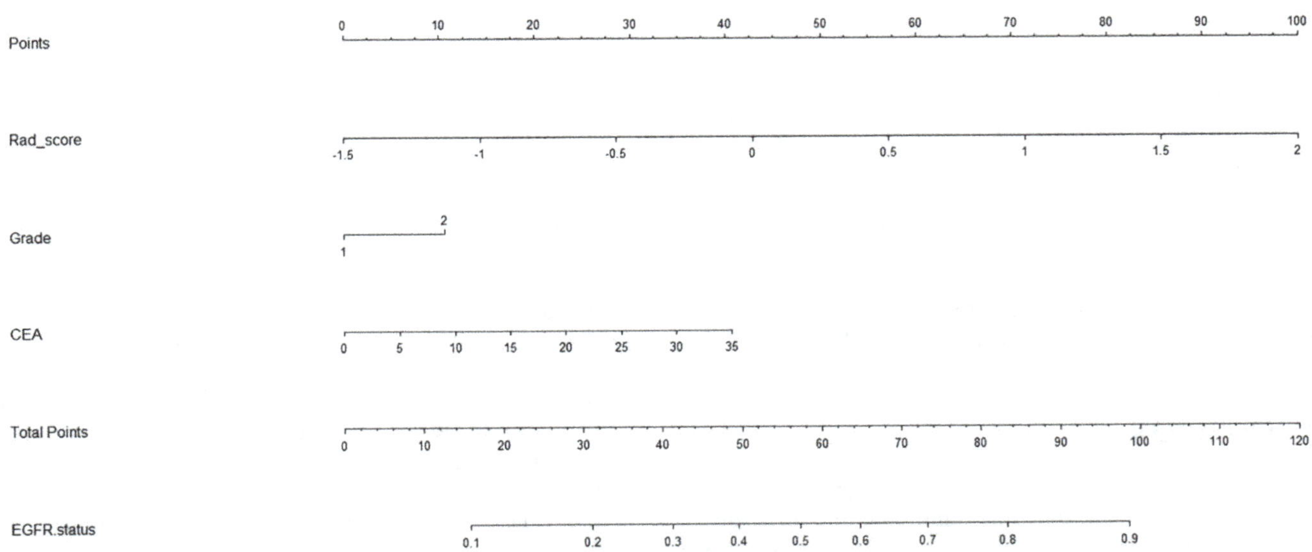

FIGURE 3 | Radiomics nomogram. The nomogram incorporated the radiomics signature with serum carcinoembryonic antigen and tumor grade.

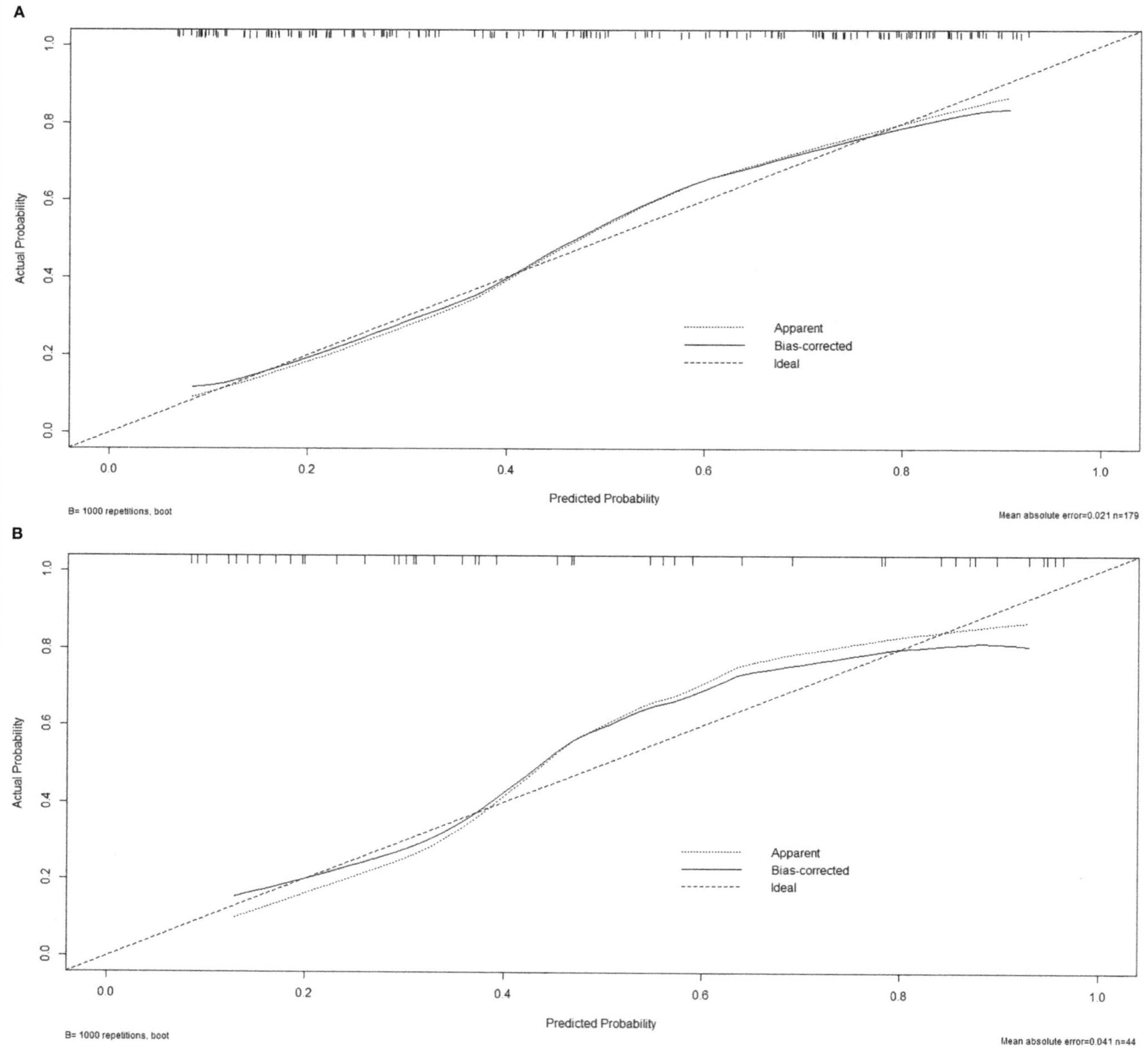

FIGURE 4 | Calibration curve. **(A)** Calibration curve of the nomogram in the training cohort. **(B)** Calibration curve in the validation cohort.

EGFR mutation added more benefit than using the treat-all scheme or the treat-none scheme with the threshold probabilities >10%.

DISCUSSION

In this study, we developed a radiomics signature for non-invasive predicting of the uncommon EGFR mutation in NSCLC patients. The radiomics signature demonstrated good performance both in the training cohort (AUC = 0.802) and in the validation cohort (AUC = 0.791). We subsequently combined the radiomics signature with the clinicopathological independent predictors to construct an integrated model. The integrated model achieved an incremental performance with an AUC of 0.816 in the training cohort and 0.795 in the validation cohort. The nomogram based on the integrated model demonstrated an easy-to-use value with a good agreement on the calibration curve. When the DCA threshold probabilities >10%, using the nomogram obtained more benefit than using the treat-all scheme or the treat-none scheme.

Our results are in line with previous studies. Yip et al. (12) demonstrated that radiomics signature could successfully

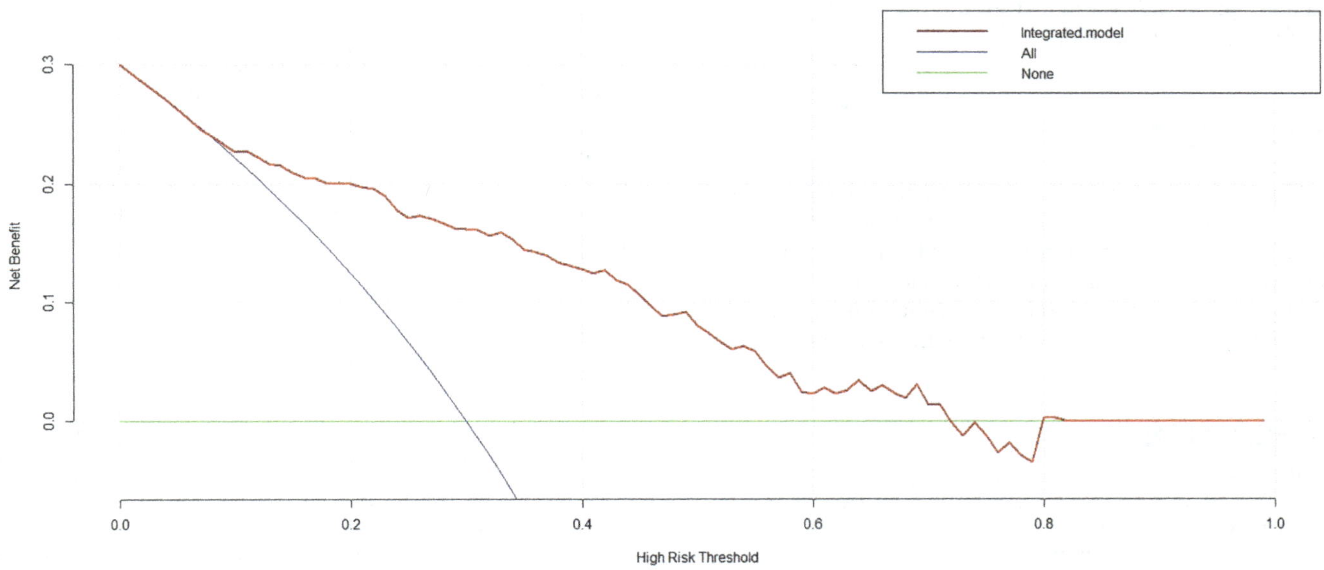

FIGURE 5 | Decision curve analysis for the nomogram. With the threshold probabilities >10%, using the nomogram to predict the uncommon epidermal growth factor receptor status added more benefit than using the treat-all scheme or the treat-none scheme.

identify the EGFR-activating mutation in lung adenocarcinoma patients. Mei et al. (13) obtained moderate diagnostic performance in assessing the correlation between the radiomics features and EGFR exon 19 or 21 mutations of lung adenocarcinoma. To the best of our knowledge, this study is one of the firsts to evaluate the feasibility of radiomics features in predicting the uncommon EGFR mutation of NSCLC. Our result is reasonable, such that NSCLC with uncommon EGFR mutation represents a higher heterogeneous subgroup (14, 15), in which the heterogeneity is closely associated with radiomics phenotypes. We believe that our radiomics signature could provide clinical feasibility for identifying the uncommon EGFR mutation. In consideration of the different mechanisms of resistance (16, 17), our future study will dedicate to investigating the radiomics changes correlating with the subtype of uncommon EGFR mutation such as C797S and T790M.

Clinicopathological factors have been recognized as an important indicator of EGFR mutation (18, 19). Previous researches (20) have demonstrated that the combination of clinicopathological factors and radiomics signature could complement the information and improve the model prediction ability for EGFR mutation. In this study, we found that serum CEA and tumor grade were potentially associated with uncommon EGFR mutation, whereas no significant correspondence was found in stage and ECOG PS, which had been proved to have independent prognostic value for NSCLC patients in previous studies. One explanation may be that both of these factors represent the general status of tumor and patients instead of intratumoral conditions. Our integrated model exhibited an incremental performance, but no significant difference was found between the integrated model and the radiomics signature, probably because the serum CEA and tumor grade are sensitive to the poor differentiation of tumor but insensitive to tumor heterogeneity.

We next constructed a radiomics nomogram based on the integrated model. As seen in **Figure 3**, the nomogram is expected to become a supporting tool for clinicians following their experience and judgment. It is worth noting that another minimally invasive approach of liquid biopsy has been receiving more and more attention in recent years (21, 22). Both radiomics and liquid biopsy could provide objective, comprehensive, and virtually real-time information for EGFR testing, but drawbacks in using them in isolation make them complementary. Firstly, ctDNA, as an example of liquid biopsy, is less sensitive and specific than ideal (23). It is unclear whether the sample could represent all genetic clones, such that ctDNA accounts for only 0.02 to 0.1% of the total DNA circulating. To make up for that, we can use radiomics to provide a full-field analysis and refine the liquid biopsy results. Besides this, no clear biological explanation has been made for radiomics. Liquid biopsy may help to decode the biological significance of tumor information. Lastly, both the radiomics and molecular protocols need to be standardized. Extremely sensitive analytical instruments are needed. In future articles, we plan to make a combination of these two data to improve the credibility of the results.

Nevertheless, there are remaining limitations to this study. Firstly, this was a retrospective study and performed in a single center. Selection bias in patients was inevitable. Secondly, the sample size of the entire cohort was relatively small. Larger-sample-size studies are needed to further validate the reliability of the model. Lastly, the reconstruction kernel and scanner parameters of different CT vendors may have affected the stability of the radiomics features. In future investigations, a multicenter and prospective study with standardized CT scanning protocol is warranted to improve the stratification of uncommon EGFR mutation.

CONCLUSION

NSCLC with uncommon EGFR mutation represents a highly heterogeneous entity, which exhibits resistant biological characteristics when treated with EGFR-TKI. The radiomics approach combined with clinicopathological information could effectively identify the uncommon EGFR mutation and help clinicians to optimize relevant therapeutic strategies.

AUTHOR CONTRIBUTIONS

YQH and ML designed the study, MYT, WLM, XMH, CL, and JJL collected the data, HW was added to assess the interobserver reproducibility of radiomics feature extraction, WFC performed the data analyses, DBM and WFC critically revised the manuscripts, YQH supervised the study, and WFC wrote the manuscript. YQH and ML made an equal contribution to this article. All authors contributed to the article and approved the submitted version.

REFERENCES

1. Hyuna S, Jacques F, Rebecca LS, Mathieu L, Isabelle S, Ahmedin J, et al. Global Cancer Statistics 2020: GLOBOCAN Estimates of Incidence and Mortality Worldwide for 36 Cancers in 185 Countries. *CA Cancer J Clin* (2020) 71(3):209–49. doi: 10.3322/caac.21660
2. Hong SJ, Kim TJ, Choi YW, Park JS, Chung JH, Lee KW. Radiogenomic Correlation in Lung Adenocarcinoma With Epidermal Growth Factor Receptor Mutations: Imaging Features and Histological Subtypes. *Eur Radiol* (2016) 26(10):3660–8.
3. Li S, Ding C, Zhang H, Song J, Wu L. Radiomics for the Prediction of EGFR Mutation Subtypes in Non-Small Cell Lung Cancer. *Med Phys* (2019) 46(10). doi: 10.1007/s00330-015-4196-z
4. Kuiper JL, Hashemi S, Thunnissen E, Snijders P, Nberg KG, Bloemena E, et al. Non-Classic EGFR Mutations in a Cohort of Dutch EGFR-Mutated NSCLC Patients and Outcomes Following EGFR-TKI Treatment. *Br J Cancer* (2016) 115(12):1504–12. doi: 10.1038/bjc.2016.372
5. Frega S, Lorenzi M, Fassan M, Indraccolo S, Pasello G. Clinical Features and Treatment Outcome of Non-Small Cell Lung Cancer (NSCLC) Patients With Uncommon or Complex Epidermal Growth Factor Receptor (EGFR) Mutations. *Oncotarget* (2017) 8(20):32626–38.
6. Shuo W, Jingyun S, Zhaoxiang Y, Di D, Dongdong Y, Mu Z, et al. Predicting EGFR Mutation Status in Lung Adenocarcinoma on Computed Tomography Image Using Deep Learning. *Eur Respir J* (2019) 53(3):1800986. doi: 10.1183/13993003.00986-2018
7. Overman MJ, Modak J, Kopetz S, Murthy R, Yao JC, Hicks ME, et al. Use of Research Biopsies in Clinical Trials: Are Risks and Benefits Adequately Discussed? *J Clin Oncol* (2013) 31(1):17–22. doi: 10.1200/JCO.2012.43.1718
8. Wu W, Chintan P, Patrick G, John Q, Philippe L, Johan B, et al. Exploratory Study to Identify Radiomics Classifiers for Lung Cancer Histology. *Front Oncol* (2016) 6(Suppl 2):71. doi: 10.3389/fonc.2016.00071
9. Emmanuel RV, Chintan P, Ying L, Thibaud PC, Gisele C, Olya S, et al. Somatic Mutations Drive Distinct Imaging Phenotypes in Lung Cancer. *Cancer Res: Off Organ Am Assoc Cancer Res Inc* (2017) 77(14):3922–30. doi: 10.3322/caac.21660
10. Zhang L, Chen B, Xia L, Song J, Jie T. Quantitative Biomarkers for Prediction of Epidermal Growth Factor Receptor Mutation in Non-Small Cell Lung Cancer. *Trans Oncol* (2017) 11(1):94. doi: 10.1016/j.tranon.2017.10.012
11. Akihiko Y, Noriko M, Gregory JR, Cami SS, William LG, Mark GK, et al. Impact of Proposed IASLC/ATS/ERS Classification of Lung Adenocarcinoma: Prognostic Subgroups and Implications for Further Revision of Staging Based on Analysis of 514 Stage I Cases. *Modern Pathol an Off J United States Can Acad Pathol Inc* (2011) 24(5):653–64. doi: 10.1038/modpathol.2010.232.
12. Yip SS, Kim J, Coroller T, Parmar C, Velazquez ER, Huynh E, et al. Associations Between Somatic Mutations and Metabolic Imaging Phenotypes in Non-Small Cell Lung Cancer. *J Nucl Med Off Publ Soc Nucl Med* (2016) 58(4):569–76. doi: 10.2967/jnumed.116.181826
13. Dongdong M, Yan L, Wang J, Yan W, Jingshan J. CT Texture Analysis of Lung Adenocarcinoma: Can Radiomic Features be Surrogate Biomarkers for EGFR Mutation Statuses. *Cancer Imaging Off Publ Int Cancer Imaging Soc* (2018) 18(1):52. doi: 10.1186/s40644-018-0184-2
14. Pilotto S, Rossi A, Vavalà T, Follador A, Tiseo M, Galetta D, et al. Outcomes of First-Generation EGFR-TKIs Against Non-Small-Cell Lung Cancer Harboring Uncommon EGFR Mutations: A Post-Hoc Analysis of the BE-POSITIVE Study. *Clin Lung Cancer* (2018) 19(1):93–104. doi: 10.1016/j.cllc.2017.05.016
15. Tu HY, Ke EE, Yang JJ, Sun YL, Yan HH, Zheng MY, et al. A Comprehensive Review of Uncommon EGFR Mutations in Patients With Non-Small Cell Lung Cancer. *Lung Cancer* (2017) 114:96–102. doi: 10.1016/j.lungcan.2017.11.005
16. Re MD, Cucchiara F, Petrini I, Fogli S, Passaro A, Crucitta S, et al. ErbB in NSCLC as a Molecular Target: Current Evidences and Future Directions. *ESMO Open* (2020) 5(4):e000724. doi: 10.1136/esmoopen-2020-000724
17. Mok TS, Wu YL, Ahn MJ, Garassino MC, Kim HR, Ramalingam SS, et al. Osimertinib or Platinum-Pemetrexed in EGFR T790M-Positive Lung Cancer. *N Engl J Med* (2017) 376(7):629–40. doi: 10.1056/NEJMoa1612674
18. Lohinai Z, Hoda MA, Fabian K, Ostoros G, Raso E, Barbai T, et al. Distinct Epidemiology and Clinical Consequence of Classic Versus Rare EGFR Mutations in Lung Adenocarcinoma. *J Thorac Oncol* (2015) 10(5):738–46. doi: 10.1097/JTO.0000000000000492
19. Tsai MJ, Hung JY, Lee MH, Kuo CY, Tsai YC, Tsai YM, et al. Better Progression-Free Survival in Elderly Patients With Stage IV Lung Adenocarcinoma Harboring Uncommon Epidermal Growth Factor Receptor Mutations Treated With the First-Line Tyrosine Kinase Inhibitors. *Cancers* (2018) 10(11):434. doi: 10.3390/cancers10110434
20. Liu Y, Kim J, Balagurunathan Y, Li Q, Garcia AL, Stringfield O, et al. Radiomic Features Are Associated With EGFR Mutation Status in Lung Adenocarcinomas. *Clin Lung Cancer* (2016) 17(5):441–8.e6. doi: 10.1016/j.cllc.2016.02.001
21. Saarenheimo J, Eigeliene N, Andersen H, Tiirola M, Jekunen A. The Value of Liquid Biopsies for Guiding Therapy Decisions in Non-Small Cell Lung Cancer. *Front Oncol* (2019) 9:129. doi: 10.3389/fonc.2019.00129
22. Russano M. Detection of Novel Driver Mutations in Liquid Biopsy: Case Report of a RET-Positive Lung Adenocarcinoma Treated With Pralsetinib. *Recenti Prog Med* (2021) 112(1):5e–9e. doi: 10.1701/3525.35131
23. Aggarwal C, Thompson JC, Black TA, Katz SI, Carpenter EL. Clinical Implications of Plasma-Based Genotyping With the Delivery of Personalized Therapy in Metastatic Non–Small Cell Lung Cancer. *JAMA Oncol* (2018) 5(2):173–80. doi: 10.1001/jamaoncol.2018.4305

16

Age-Associated Changes in Adverse Events Arising from Anti-PD-(L)1 Therapy

Xinyi Huang[1,2,3], *Tiantian Tian*[2,3], *Yan Zhang*[2,3], *Shengjian Zhou*[4], *Pingping Hu*[2,3*†] *and Jiandong Zhang*[2,3*†]

[1] Department of Oncology, Shandong Provincial Qianfoshan Hospital, Cheeloo College of Medicine, Shandong University, Jinan, China, [2] Department of Oncology, The First Affiliated Hospital of Shandong First Medical University & Shandong Provincial Qianfoshan Hospital, Jinan, China, [3] Shandong Lung Cancer Institute, Jinan, China, [4] Department of Oncology, Liangshan County People's Hospital, Jining, China

***Correspondence:**
Pingping Hu
hupingping0915@126.com
Jiandong Zhang
zhangjd2233@126.com

[†]These authors have contributed equally to this work

Background: Immune-related adverse events (irAEs) may complicate the immune checkpoint inhibition (ICI) therapy. The effect of age on these irAEs is not elucidated. The aim of the study was to compare the occurrence of irAEs in different age groups.

Methods: Patients with lung cancer receiving anti-programmed death- (ligand)1 (PD-(L)1) were selected from the US Food and Drug Administration Adverse Event Reporting System (FAERS) database. Immune cell infiltration data set was obtained from TIMER 2.0 web server. The patients were stratified for age as follows: <65 year-old (young patients, YP), 65 to 75 year-old (middle aged patients, MP), ≥75 year-old (old patients, OP). The severity of irAEs was compared using logistic binary regression model. The distribution differences of immune cell infiltration were estimated using non-parametric tests.

Results: Of all the 17,006 patients treated by anti-PD-(L)1, 7,355 were <65 (YP), 6,706 were 65–75 (MP), and 2,945 were ≥75 (OP). In general, we analyzed a total of 16 irAEs in this article and found that pulmonary toxicity was more frequent in OP (OP *vs.* YP: OR = 1.45, 95% CI: 1.28–1.64) and MP (MP *vs.* YP: OR = 1.38, 95% CI: 1.24–1.52), but hepatitis was less frequent in OP (OP *vs.* YP: OR = 0.56, 95% CI: 0.32–0.97) and MP (MP *vs.* YP: OR = 0.57, 95%CI: 0.38–0.85). Further analysis demonstrated that older patients showed less B cell, $CD8^+$ T cell and myeloid dendritic cell infiltration than younger patients.

Conclusions: Elderly patients exhibited higher incidences of pulmonary toxicity, while hepatitis was found at low incidence. Therefore, clinicians should carefully monitor comorbidities in elderly patients.

Keywords: aging, immune checkpoint inhibitors, immune-related adverse events, immune cell infiltration, lung cancer

INTRODUCTION

Programmed cell death protein-1 (PD-1) and programmed cell death protein- ligand 1 (PD-L1) are the two most intensively studied immune regulatory checkpoint pathways in cancer (1), which relies on the presence of ongoing antitumor immune response after blocking this pathway (2). Monoclonal antibody therapies at various clinical levels have now been developed to against these immune checkpoint proteins (3, 4). Immune checkpoint inhibitors (ICIs) against PD-(L)1 have changed the treatment landscape of many different cancers so far. Responses occur in a large proportion of patients and are often long-lasting and even curative (5, 6). PD-(L)1 inhibitors can reactivate previously activated T cells that have lost their effector and proliferative functions during the process of immune response. Potential host anti-tumor immune response is the basis for the clinical benefit of PD-(L)1 agents (7).

Although ICIs such as anti-PD-1 or anti-PD-L1 have been shown to be effective against many cancers, patients who receive ICIs may experience immune-related adverse events (irAEs). IrAEs are common side effects of checkpoint inhibition (CPI) therapy for PD-(L)1. It has been found that the toxic effects associated with ICIs may occur at any part of the body and result from the activation of autoreactive T cells, thereby destroying host tissues (8). The most representative irAEs are usually colitis, hepatitis, pneumonia, hypophysitis, thyroid toxicity, and skin toxicity, and adverse events involving the heart, nervous system, and other organs, though rare, can also occur. These rare, violent, and deadly toxic effects may complicate the transformative treatment of PD-(L)1. These toxic effects are a major clinical challenge and an obstacle to the development of more effective combinations (9).

ICIs has now showed noteworthy therapeutic advantages compared with traditional therapies. However, there is still relatively limited information on the use of ICIs and the irAEs generated by ICIs in older patients. Previous studies found that the body's immune system function declines with age, manifested by a higher tendency to respond to autoantigens, a decrease in the ability of host defenses against microbes and cancer, and disorders between different immune system components. These signs of a weakened immune system may be associated with "immunosenescence," which may reduce the efficacy and safety of immune-based therapies and may contribute to the increased incidence of irAEs and development of cancer (10, 11). As only a small part of the participants are 75 years or older, the representativeness of the elderly population in clinical trials is generally low. Research on the irAEs of elderly is sparse. In this study, we use two large real-world data sets to explore the differences of irAEs and determine the distribution differences of tumor-infiltrating immune cells among patients of different ages.

METHODS

Data Selection and Preprocessing

The US Food and Drug Administration Adverse Event Reporting System (FAERS) is a database designed to support the Food and Drug Administration (FDA)'s post-marketing monitoring program for drugs and therapeutic biological products. The database includes all adverse event information and medication error information. In this study, we extracted 17006 eligible lung cancer (LC) patients receiving PD-(L)1 inhibitor treatment registered as of December 31, 2019 from FAERS. The study was exempt from ethical review under the EKOS (Ethikkommission Ostschweiz, Switzerland) ethics committee policy because all of the analyzed data sets were identified and publicly available. Five reported PD-(L)1 monoclonal antibodies were searched from FAKERS public dashboard. Search terms included "nivolumab," "pembrolizumab," "atezolizumab," "avelumab," and "durvalumab." We also selected sixteen common irAEs, including pulmonary toxicity, radiation pneumonitis, myasthenia gravis, adrenal insufficiency, colitis, myocarditis, hepatitis, myositis, hypophysitis, encephalitis, skin reaction, diabetes, thyroid toxicity, hematologic toxicity, neurologic toxicity, and gastrointestinal reaction (9). Clinicopathological characteristics enrolled in the model were sex, serious, pathological type, and country. Serious means that one or more of the following outcomes were documented in the report: death, hospitalization, life-threatening, disability, congenital anomaly, and/or other serious outcome. Subsequently, the cohort was trichotomized into three (younger patients (YP) with age <65, middle aged patients (MP) with 65≤age<75, and elder patients with age≥75) subgroups using cut-off age of 65 and 75 years.

Tumor-Infiltrating Immune Cell Analysis

The data set of tumor-infiltrating immune cells was downloaded from TIMER 2.0 (http://timer.cistrome.org). TIMER 2.0 consists of three major components, including immune, exploration, and estimation. The estimation component was used to infer immune cell infiltration levels. The TIMER algorithm was chosen for our study. Then, the TIMER data set was matched with the lung cancer data set obtained from the Cancer Genome Atlas (TCGA) database (https://portal.gdc.cancer.gov) according to the TCGA ID number. Similarly, the immune infiltration data was stratified into three subgroups by age (<65 years, 65–75 years, and ≥75 years). A violin plot was constructed using Origin ver. 2019 to show the distribution of tumor-infiltrating immune cells.

Statistical Analysis

All data manipulation and statistical analyses were performed using IBM SPSS version 22 (IBM Corporation, Armonk, NY, USA) and Microsoft Excel (2016, Microsoft). The differences in irAEs of each age group were calculated using a crosstab. Univariate logistic binary regression analysis was applied to calculate the odds ratio (ORs) and 95% confidence intervals (CIs). Subsequently, multivariate logistic regression was used to estimate the odds ratios (ORs) and 95% CI for the association between age and different irAEs, while controlling for potential confounders, including sex, treatment modality, comorbidity (pre-existing autoimmune condition). A forest plot was generated using Stata ver.12.0 to summarize data for each group with ORs and 95% CIs to provide a visual analysis of studies evaluating fatal toxicity events. The distribution of immune cells among different age groups was analyzed using TIMER 2.0 web server. Statistically significant difference was defined as a P-value <0.05.

Ethical Statement

The authors are accountable for all aspects of the work in ensuring that questions related to the accuracy or integrity of any part of the work are appropriately investigated and resolved. Institutional review board approval was not required because FAERS is an unlinkable anonymized database open to the public. Informed consents from patients were waived due to the anonymity of individual patient data. The study was conducted in accordance with the Declaration of Helsinki (as revised in 2013).

RESULTS

Characteristics of the Study Population

In our study, we identified 17006 LC cases from FDA database. Among them, 7355 (43.2%) patients were in the YP (age <65) group, 6706 (39.4%) were in the MP (65≤age<75) group and 2945 (17.4%) were in the OP (age≥75) group. The median (range) age of YP, MP, and OP subgroups was respectively 58 (0–64), 69 (65–74), and 78 (75–101) years old. In total, 11335 (66.7%) of the patients were male, 10584 (62.2%) were non-small cell lung cancer, and 16351 (96.1%) had serious outcomes. The main countries were Japan (5826[34.3%]), United States (3506 [20.6%]), France (1881[11.1%]), and others (1562[9.2%]). The baseline characteristics in each subgroup are presented in **Table 1**.

We run an univariate and multivariate logistic regression analysis of the odds ratio for different irAEs (**Supplementary Table 1**). In the univariate analysis, the incidence of irAEs including pulmonary toxicity, radiation pneumonitis, hepatitis, hypophysitis, hematologic toxicity, and gastrointestinal reaction was significantly higher for OP than MP and YP, and subjects with pulmonary toxicity, radiation pneumonitis, adrenal insufficiency, encephalitis, skin reaction, hematologic toxicity were more likely to be males. Multivariate analysis, after controlling for the confounders, demonstrated an independent and significant association between demographic and clinical characteristics and the increased likelihood of irAEs (**Supplementary Table 1**). The risk of pulmonary toxicity was independently positively associated with older subjects [adjusted OR of 1.381 (95% CI 1.243–1.534, p<0.001) and being male [adjusted OR of 1.537 (95% CI 1.407–1.680, p<0.001); adjusted OR of 1.418 (95% CI 1.115–1.804, p=0.004)]. In addition, patients receiving combinational agent treatment [adjusted OR of 1.334 (95% CI 1.236–1.441, p<0.001)] were also observed with increased pulmonary toxicity. Independent negative associations were observed among the risk of combinational agent treatment [adjusted OR of 0.652 (95% CI 0.526–0.808, p<0.001] (**Supplementary Table 1**).

TABLE 1 | Characteristics of 17006 Patients.

Characteristics	All n=17006	age<65 n=7355	65≤age<75 n=6706	age≥75 n=2945	P-value
Sex, No. (%)					<0.001
Female	5414 (31.8)	2660 (36.2)	1895 (28.3)	859 (29.2)	
Male	11335 (66.7)	4582 (62.3)	4723 (70.4)	2030 (68.9)	
Not specified	257 (1.5)	113 (1.5)	88 (1.3)	56 (1.9)	
Serious, No. (%)					<0.001
Serious	16351 (96.1)	7074 (96.2)	6485 (96.7)	2792 (94.8)	
Non-serious	655 (3.9)	281 (3.8)	221 (3.3)	153 (5.2)	
Pathological type, No. (%)					<0.001
Non-small cell lung cancer	10584 (62.2)	4477 (60.9)	4151 (61.9)	1956 (66.4)	
Small cell lung cancer	631 (3.7)	316 (4.3)	219 (3.3)	96 (3.3)	
Not specified	5791 (34.1)	2562 (34.8)	2336 (34.8)	893 (30.3)	
Country, No. (%)					<0.001
Japan	5826 (34.3)	1906 (25.9)	2663 (39.7)	1257 (42.7)	
United States	3506 (20.6)	1598 (21.7)	1240 (18.5)	668 (22.7)	
France	1881 (11.1)	972 (13.2)	660 (9.8)	249 (8.5)	
Germany	963 (5.7)	504 (6.9)	340 (5.1)	119 (4.0)	
Italy	632 (3.7)	227 (3.1)	279 (4.2)	126 (4.3)	
Spain	414 (2.4)	220 (3.0)	144 (2.1)	50 (1.7)	
China	366 (2.2)	235 (3.2)	108 (1.6)	23 (0.8)	
United Kingdom	312 (1.8)	125 (1.7)	132 (2.0)	55 (1.9)	
Australia	300 (1.8)	120 (1.6)	121 (1.8)	59 (2.0)	
Canada	296 (1.7)	135 (1.8)	114 (1.7)	47 (1.6)	
Belgium	229 (1.3)	114 (1.5)	90 (1.3)	25 (0.8)	
Republic of Korea	142 (0.8)	66 (0.9)	62 (0.9)	14 (0.5)	
Netherlands	137 (0.8)	70 (1.0)	55 (0.8)	12 (0.4)	
Switzerland	117 (0.7)	55 (0.7)	42 (0.6)	20 (0.7)	
India	115 (0.7)	80 (1.1)	27 (0.4)	8 (0.3)	
Israel	108 (0.6)	46 (0.6)	37 (0.6)	25 (0.8)	
Brazil	100 (0.6)	49 (0.7)	41 (0.6)	10 (0.3)	
Others	1562 (9.2)	833 (11.3)	551 (8.2)	178 (6.0)	

Serious means that one or more of the following outcomes were documented in the report: death, hospitalization, life-threatening, disability, congenital anomaly, and/or other serious outcomes. Documenting one or more of these outcomes in a report does not necessarily mean that the suspect product(s) named in the report was the cause of the outcomes.

However, subjects who have hepatitis were younger [adjusted OR of 0.622 (95% CI 0.420–0.922, p=0.018)] and received combinational agents [adjusted OR of 2.924 (95% CI 1.966–4.349, p<0.001)].

Impact of Aging on Immune-Related Adverse Events

To confirm whether aging increases the risk of irAEs, we performed analyses of the association between age and irAEs using a crosstab. A total of 16 irAEs were included in our analysis (**Table 2, Supplementary Table 1**, P<0.05). Among 2137 (12.6%) patients with pulmonary toxicity, 772 (10.5%) were in the YP group, 939 (14%) were in the MP group, and 426 (14.5%) were in the OP group. Compared with YP, OP (OP vs. YP: adjusted OR = 1.381, 95% CI: 1.243–1.534; P<0.001) and MP (MP vs. YP: adjusted OR = 1.270, 95% CI: 1.163–1.388; P<0.001) had increased risks of developing pulmonary toxicity. We also found that OP group had a higher risk of developing pulmonary toxicity than MP group. Within 207 (1.2%) patients with adrenal insufficiency and 177 (1.0%) with hematologic toxicity, the risk of developing adrenal insufficiency (MP *vs.* YP: adjusted OR = 1.505, 95% CI: 1.092–2.074) in the MP group and hematologic toxicity (OP *vs.* YP: adjusted OR = 1.513, 95% CI: 1.024–2.236) in the OP group were higher than that in the YP group, while the risk of developing gastrointestinal reaction (OP *vs.* YP: adjusted OR=1.537, 95% CI: 1.041–2.268) in the OP group was higher than that in the YP group. However, in the 124 (0.7%) patients with hepatitis, both the OP (OP vs. YP: adjusted OR=0.504, 95% CI: 0.295–0.861) group and the MP (MP *vs.* YP: adjusted OR=0.614, 95%CI: 0.416–0.907) group reduced the risk of irAEs. Besides, the OP group had a lower risk of developing hepatitis than MP group. The risk of other irAEs did not differ among the YP, MP, and OP group (**Table 2**, P > 0.05).

In order to further explore the effect of irAEs on patients receiving anti-PD-(L)1 treatment in combination with anti-cytotoxic T lymphocyte-associated antigen-4 (CTLA-4) agents, we analyzed separately in OP, MP and YP subgroups. In YP subject treated with both anti-PD-(L)1 and anti-CTLA-4, 125 (4.0%) patients developed colitis, 49 (1.6%) developed hepatitis, 23 (0.7%) developed hypophysitis, 45 (1.4%) developed diabetes, implying an increased risk of irAEs with the combination treatment (**Table 3**, p<0.05). Among OP subjects, 29 (0.9%), 24 (0.7%), and 28 (0.8%) cases had an increased risk of developing hepatitis, hypophysitis, and encephalitis (**Table 3**, p<0.05). However, the risk of irAEs on patients aged 75 and older appeared to have no differences in treatment type.

The Distribution of Tumor-Infiltrating Immune Cells

To determine if aging affects tumor-associated immune cell infiltration as well as the number of immune cells primarily involved, split violin plots (**Figure 1**) were built, allowing a direct comparison between the two populations (OP and MP) and YP. As can be seen from **Figure 1A**, the immune cell infiltration level of B cell, CD8$^+$ T cell, and myeloid dendritic cell in the OP group was significantly reduced compared with YP group. These immune cells infiltrated exhibited similar distribution patterns between groups of MP and YP (**Figure 1B**, P<0.05). CD8$^+$ T cell, neutrophil, and macrophage infiltrated did not differ in the OP or MP group versus YP group. The statistical significance was lost in CD8$^+$ T cell, neutrophil and macrophage. Therefore, the OP and MP groups may have unique biological features that are different from YP group.

DISCUSSION

ICI therapy is now increasingly used to treat a variety of solid tumors, including LC. However, the use of PD-(L)1 pathway inhibitors, such as monoclonal antibodies against PD-1 or PD-L1, will inevitably generate a variety of adverse events. ICIs have their own idiosyncratic adverse events, collectively defined as irAEs. Although ICI has a safe toxicity profile in cancer treatment, the toxicity of these molecules may be more challenging in elderly patients due to reduced functional reserve, age-associated comorbidities and polypharmacy.

Some clinical trials have found the relationship between age and toxicities. A previous clinical trial analyzing pooled data from a Nivolumab Phase III registry of different cancer types found that patients aged 70 years and older had higher skin toxicities than those under 65 years old (12). There was also an increase rate of grade III to V toxicities in patients aged 70 years or over than those under 70 years of age (13). In addition, a research team from Sloan Kettering Cancer Center presented at the American Society of Clinical Oncology (ASCO) meeting the benefits and toxicity of ICIs in patients over 80 years of age for melanoma (14). They reported that older patients had slightly higher rates of irAEs and early discontinuation of treatment than younger people. Our comprehensive study that included 17006 patients from FDA database investigated the occurrence of irAEs in elderly patients with lung cancer as compared with younger patients and middle-aged patients. In our results, our analysis showed an increased level of toxicities in older patients than in their younger counterparts when treated with anti-PD-(L)1 agents. Besides, the OP subgroup was having a higher risk of irAEs than MP and YP subgroup. Toxicities were more frequent on lung and endocrine in OP and MP compared with YP (**Table 2**). These results showed strong evidence of the increasing toxicities of anti-PD-(L)1 for older patients.

In recent years, more and more researchers have reached a consensus that immunosenescence has become a vital intersection of the increasing frequency and severity of cancer, aging, and immunity (15). Immunosenescence refers to a phenomenon of decreased immune function as a result of age-associated declines and impairments of immune function, affecting the process of producing specific responses to foreign antigens and autoantigens (16). One of the major theories to explain immunosenescence is autoimmunity (17). With advancing age, the immune system's ability to distinguish between invaders and normal tissue diminishes and immune cells begin to attach normal body tissues. Similarly, irAEs are associated with infiltration of normal tissue by activated T cells responsible for autoimmunity. Autoimmune diseases caused by ICIs may be typical examples (18, 19).

TABLE 2 | Univariate and multivariate logistic regression analysis of the odds ratio for different irAEs, controlling for multiple conditions.

Variable	Category	Univariate			Multivariate			Univariate			Multivariate		
		Crude OR	95%CI	*p* value	Adjusted OR	95%CI	*p* value	Crude OR	95%CI	*p* value	Adjusted OR	95%CI	*p* value
		Pulmonary toxicity						Gastrointestinal reaction					
Age	65≤age<75	1.329	1.217–1.451	**<0.001**	1.270	1.163–1.388	**<0.001**	1.157	0.815–1.644	0.414	1.151	0.811–1.635	0.431
	≥75	1.414	1.274–1.570	**<0.001**	1.381	1.243–1.534	**<0.001**	1.527	1.035–2.253	**0.033**	1.537	1.041–2.268	**0.031**
Sex	Male	1.609	1.473–1.756	**<0.001**	1.537	1.407–1.680	**<0.001**	1.247	0.892–1.742	0.196			
Treatment modality	Combinational	1.334	1.236–1.441	**<0.001**	1.300	1.203–1.405	**<0.001**	1.503	1.110–2.035	**0.008**	1.509	1.114–2.044	**0.008**
Comorbidity	Yes	1.236	0.694–2.201	0.472				0.000	0.000	0.997			
		Myasthenia gravis						Adrenal insufficiency					
Age	65≤age<75	1.576	0.914–2.718	0.102				1.559	1.133–2.146	**0.006**	1.505	1.092–2.074	**0.012**
	≥75	3.031	1.751–5.246	**<0.001**				1.365	0.925–2.013	0.117	1.354	0.917–1.999	0.127
Sex	Male	0.795	0.516–1.226	0.299				1.411	1.028–1.936	**0.033**	1.341	0.976–1.843	0.070
Treatment modality	Combinational	0.768	0.502–1.177	0.226				1.481	1.123–1.953	**0.005**	1.432	1.084–1.892	**0.011**
Comorbidity	Yes	2.935	0.403–21.388	0.288				0.000	0.000	0.997			
		Colitis						Myocarditis					
Age	65≤age<75	1.103	0.920–1.323	0.289				1.248	0.898–1.733	0.187			
	≥75	1.079	0.865–1.345	0.501				1.018	0.670–1.547	0.933			
Sex	Male	1.011	0.851–1.202	0.897				0.886	0.651–1.205	0.441			
Treatment modality	Combinational	1.451	1.234–1.705	**<0.001**	1.433	1.219–1.684	**<0.001**	1.216	0.908–1.629	0.189			
Comorbidity	Yes	0.403	0.056–2.911	0.368				1.418	0.196–10.278	0.729			
		Hepatitis						Myositis					
Age	65≤age<75	0.610	0.412–0.904	**0.014**	0.614	0.416–0.907	**0.014**	1.230	0.857–1.767	0.262			
	≥75	0.499	0.292–0.852	**0.011**	0.504	0.295–0.861	**0.012**	1.488	0.988–2.242	0.057			
Sex	Male	0.921	0.633–1.338	0.665				1.450	1.012–2.076	0.043			
Treatment modality	Combinational	2.964	1.995–4.403	**<0.001**	2.924	1.966–4.349	**<0.001**	1.072	0.786–1.462	0.663			
Comorbidity	Yes	4.277	1.035–17.673	**0.045**	3.063	0.736–12.740	0.124	3.248	0.788–13.383	0.103			
		Hypophysitis						Encephalitis					
Age	65≤age<75	0.921	0.587–1.446	0.721				0.857	0.591–1.242	0.415			
	≥75	0.392	0.183–0.839	**0.016**				1.281	0.857–1.915	0.228			
Sex	Male	1.128	0.706–1.803	0.615				0.644	0.467–0.889	**0.007**	0.646	0.468–0.892	**0.008**
Treatment modality	Combinational	1.516	0.985–2.334	0.059				1.394	1.012–1.920	**0.042**	1.363	0.989–1.878	0.058
Comorbidity	Yes	0.000	0.000	0.997				0.000	0.000	0.997			
		Skin reaction						Diabetes					
Age	65≤age<75	1.092	0.847–1.409	0.496				1.226	0.942–1.595	0.130			
	≥75	0.957	0.695–1.319	0.790				1.121	0.811–1.550	0.488			
Sex	Male	0.708	0.560–0.894	**0.004**	0.721	0.571–0.911	**0.006**	1.219	0.941–1.579	0.135			
Treatment modality	Combinational	1.245	0.990–1.566	0.061				1.041	0.824–1.315	0.736			
Comorbidity	Yes	0.000	0.000	0.997				1.798	0.438–7.381	0.416			
		Thyroid toxicity						Hematologic toxicity					
Age	65≤age<75	0.848	0.723–0.994	**0.042**				0.802	0.650–0.991	**0.041**	1.130	0.795–1.607	0.496
	≥75	0.920	0.760–1.114	0.395				0.711	0.542–0.934	**0.014**	1.513	1.024–2.236	**0.037**
Sex	Male	0.877	0.756–1.017	0.083				0.818	0.670–0.998	**0.047**	1.228	0.878–1.719	0.231
Treatment modality	Combinational	0.996	0.864–1.148	0.955				1.503	1.110–2.035	**0.008**	1.511	1.115–2.047	**0.008**
Comorbidity	Yes	1.632	0.654–4.072	0.294				1.187	0.290–4.864	0.812			
		Neurologic toxicity											
Age	65≤age<75	0.795	0.329–1.919	0.609									
	≥75	0.174	0.022–1.348	0.094									
Sex	Male	1.194	0.463–3.080	0.713									
Treatment modality	Combinational	1.202	0.510–2.831	0.674									
Comorbidity	Yes	0.000	0.000	0.998									

irAEs, immune-related adverse events; Yes, with irAEs; No, without irAEs. Statistically significant values are in bold (p < 0.05).

TABLE 3 | The severity of irAEs in patients with/without anti-CTLA4 agents.

irAEs	Age<65		65≤age<75		Age≥75	
	Combinational agents		Combinational agents		Combinational agents	
	OR (95%CI)	P-value	OR (95%CI)	P-value	OR (95%CI)	P-value
Pulmonary toxicity	0.900 (0.701–1.155)	0.407	0.776 (0.596–1.011)	0.060	0.898 (0.597–1.351)	0.605
Myasthenia gravis	0.590 (0.079–4.407)	0.607	1.512 (0.460–4.967)	0.495	0.693 (0.094–5.109)	0.719
Adrenal insufficiency	1.731 (0.820–3.653)	0.150	1.176 (0.542–2.553)	0.681	1.060 (0.254–4.423)	0.936
Colitis	1.981 (1.348–2.910)	**<0.001**	1.530 (0.985–2.375)	0.058	1.712 (0.852–3.440)	0.131
Myocarditis	0.579 (0.181–1.851)	0.357	1.443 (0.661–3.150)	0.357	2.108 (0.638–6.965)	0.221
Hepatitis	3.307 (1.818–6.016)	**<0.001**	3.154 (1.392–7.145)	**0.006**	2.994 (0.678–13.211)	0.148
Myositis	0.226 (0.031–1.637)	0.141	0.477 (0.116–1.955)	0.304	1.143 (0.273–4.779)	0.855
Hypophysitis	5.354 (2.696–10.632)	**<0.001**	3.563 (1.560–8.142)	**0.003**	3.194 (0.390–26.125)	0.279
Encephalitis	1.831 (0.865–3.876)	0.114	2.396 (1.075–5.340)	**0.033**	1.821 (0.555–5.974)	0.323
Skin reaction	0.531 (0.216–1.307)	0.168	0.493 (0.181–1.342)	0.166	0.000 (0.000–0.000)	0.996
Diabetes	2.067 (1.186–3.604)	**0.010**	1.182 (0.596–2.345)	0.633	1.616 (0.578–4.520)	0.360
Thyroid toxicity	0.799 (0.514–1.243)	0.320	0.868 (0.519–1.451)	0.589	0.262 (0.064–1.065)	0.061
Hematologic toxicity	0.363 (0.160–0.823)	0.015	0.588 (0.259–1.337)	0.205	0.301 (0.042–2.179)	0.234
Neurologic toxicity	0.000 (0.000–0.000)	0.993	0.000 (0.000–0.000)	0.994	0.000 (0.000–0.000)	0.997
Gastrointestinal reaction	0.635 (0.198–2.036)	0.444	0.225 (0.031–1.626)	0.139	0.000 (0.000–0.000)	0.996

irAEs, Immune-related adverse events; CTLA-4, cytotoxic T lymphocyte-associated antigen-4. Statistically significant values are in bold (p<0.05).

T cells play an important role in anti-cancer immune defense mechanisms and they recognize tumor antigens, so they are activated and widely clear tumor cells. Studies have shown that diminished T-cell mediated immunity is the primary factor involved in the pathophysiology of immunosenescence (20). T cells undergo significant changes with aging: their absolute number, especially the naive $CD8^{+}$T cells, declines with aging, partly due to thymic retreat and lymphoid stem cell contraction (21–23), and thus resulting in a decreased T cell diversity, decreased T cell proliferation and survival after T cell receptor stimulation, altered cytokines, and decreased cytotoxicity of $CD8^{+}$T cells (24, 25). In this article, we explored the age-related immune cell alterations. Our results identified that older age is associated with less $CD8^{+}$ T cell. Therefore, the decrease in the number and function of $CD8^{+}$ T cells might lead to poor immunity in patients, which are more likely to have irAEs when using ICIs and thus have a direct impact on the efficacy and toxicity of ICIs in this population. Our current understanding of immunosenescence implicates changes in the adaptive immune system—particularly within T cell populations—as the primary determinants of declining immune function with age. On the other hand, with the increase of age, the infiltration of immune cells into normal tissues increases, which leads to immune hyperactivity and triggers autoimmunity, thereby potentially increasing the incidence of irAEs (17–19).

At the same time, irAEs may be more challenging in older patients due to reduced functional reserve and age-associated comorbidities. Therefore, early detection of irAEs should be strengthened for management of elderly patients, and the severity of irAEs should also be carefully monitored and evaluated as associated comorbidities may be more likely to be decompensated. Finally, it is well known that older patients have a higher prevalence of autoantibodies, and it is expected that ICIs may reveal subclinical autoimmune diseases. Therefore, it is

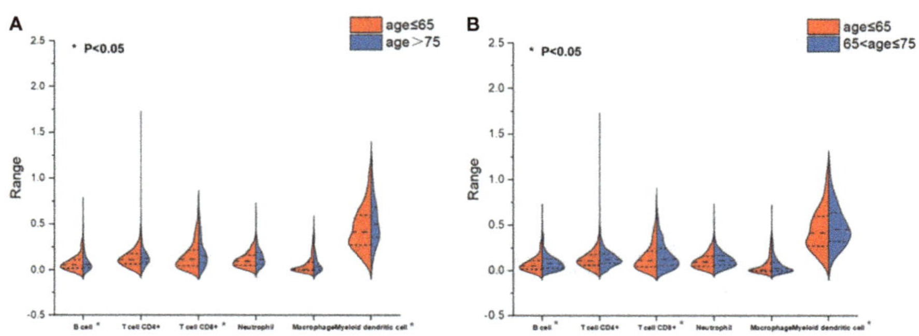

FIGURE 1 | Split violin plots estimating the distributions and levels of immune cell infiltration. **(A)** Infiltration differences of 6 immune cells between patients aged ≥75 (old patients) versus patients aged <65 (young patients). Red indicates the young patient subgroup and blue indicates the old patient subgroup. **(B)** Infiltration differences of six immune cells between patients aged 65 to <75 (middle-aged patients) versus patients aged <65 (young patients). Red indicates the young patient subgroup and blue indicates the middle-aged patient subgroup.

important to investigate individual or familial autoimmune diseases or viral infections before ICI treatment to prevent irAEs.

This study has some limitations that warrant mention. First, the present study was a retrospective study. Second, adverse events reported in the FAERS database cannot be identified whether they were caused by the drug. When submitting the reports, FDA does not require proof of a causal relationship between an adverse event and a drug, and reports typically do not include detailed information that evaluates an adverse event. Third, the information stored in the FAERS database is basically based on spontaneous reporting. Whether an event can be reported is influenced by a variety of factors, such as the time the product is on the market and the level of public awareness of adverse events. FDA is unable to collect all serious adverse events from patients, which leads to reporting bias.

In conclusion, our study compared the risks of irAEs and the distribution differences of tumor-infiltrating immune cells among different age groups based on real-world data analyses. Our analysis showed increased pulmonary toxicity and decreased hepatitis toxicity in the older group than younger group. Less B cell, $CD8^+$ T cell, and myeloid dendritic cell infiltration were observed in the patients aged ≥75 years. These trends often result in rapid clinical deterioration and poor outcomes. Therefore, clinicians should carefully assess and manage comorbidities in elderly patients, which is essential for better multidisciplinary cancer treatment.

Informed consents from patients were waived due to the anonymity of individual patient data. The study was conducted in accordance with the Declaration of Helsinki (as revised in 2013).

AUTHOR CONTRIBUTIONS

Conception and design: All authors. Administrative support: JZ. Provision of study materials or patients: All authors. Collection and assembly of data: PH, XH, TT, and YZ.Data analysis and interpretation: PH and XH. Manuscript writing: All authors. All authors contributed to the article and approved the submitted version.

ACKNOWLEDGMENTS

We gratefully acknowledge the US Food and Drug Administration Adverse Event Reporting System (FAERS) database and TIMER 2.0 web server for providing the primary data.

REFERENCES

1. Postow MA, Callahan MK, Wolchok JD. Immune Checkpoint Blockade in Cancer Therapy. *J Clin Oncol* (2015) 33(17):1974–82. doi: 10.1200/JCO.2014.59.4358
2. A R. Releasing the Brakes on Cancer Immunotherapy. *N Engl J Med* (2015) 373(16):1490–2. doi: 10.1056/NEJMp1510079
3. Mahoney KM, Freeman GJ, McDermott DF. The Next Immune-Checkpoint Inhibitors: PD-1/PD-L1 Blockade in Melanoma. *Clin Ther* (2015) 37(4):764–82. doi: 10.1016/j.clinthera.2015.02.018
4. Munoz-Unceta N, Burgueno I, Jimenez E, Paz-Ares L. Durvalumab in NSCLC: Latest Evidence and Clinical Potential. *Ther Adv Med Oncol* (2018) 10:1758835918804151. doi: 10.1177/1758835918804151
5. Xu Z, Yi FM, Yu DL, Xu JJ, Wei YP, Zhang WX. Nivolumab Provides Improved Effectiveness and Safety Compared With Docetaxel as a Second-Line Treatment for Advanced non-Small Cell Lung Cancer: A Systematic Review and Meta-Analysis. *Cancer Med-Us* (2019) 8(2):629–42. doi: 10.1002/cam4.1966
6. Shafique MR, Robinson LA, Antonia S. Durvalumab: A Potential Maintenance Therapy in Surgery-Ineligible non-Small-Cell Lung Cancer. *Cancer Manag Res* (2018) 10:931–40. doi: 10.2147/CMAR.S148009
7. Tumeh PC, Harview CL, Yearley JH, Shintaku IP, Taylor EJ, Robert L, et al. PD-1 Blockade Induces Responses by Inhibiting Adaptive Immune Resistance. *Nature* (2014) 515(7528):568–71. doi: 10.1038/nature13954
8. Baxi S, Yang A, Gennarelli RL, Khan N, Wang Z, Boyce L, et al. Immune-Related Adverse Events for Anti-PD-1 and Anti-PD-L1 Drugs: Systematic Review and Meta-Analysis. *BMJ* (2018) 360:k793. doi: 10.1136/bmj.k793
9. Wang DY, Salem JE, Cohen JV, Chandra S, Menzer C, Ye F, et al. Fatal Toxic Effects Associated With Immune Checkpoint Inhibitors: A Systematic Review and Meta-Analysis. *JAMA Oncol* (2018) 4(12):1721–8. doi: 10.1001/jamaoncol.2018.3923
10. Nishijima TF, Muss HB, Shachar SS, Moschos SJ. Comparison of Efficacy of Immune Checkpoint Inhibitors (Icis) Between Younger and Older Patients: A Systematic Review and Meta-Analysis. *Cancer Treat Rev* (2016) 45:30–7. doi: 10.1016/j.ctrv.2016.02.006
11. Pawelec G. Immunosenescence Comes of Age. Symposium on Aging Research in Immunology: The Impact of Genomics. *EMBO Rep* (2007) 8(3):220–3. doi: 10.1038/sj.embor.7400922
12. Spigel D, Schwartzberg L, Waterhouse D, Chandler J, Hussein M, Jotte R, et al. P3.02c-026 is Nivolumab Safe and Effective in Elderly and PS2 Patients With non-Small Cell Lung Cancer (NSCLC)? Results of Checkmate 153: Topic: it. *J Thorac Oncol* (2017) 12(1):S1287–8. doi: 10.1016/j.jtho.2016.11.1821
13. Singh H, Kim G, Maher VE, Beaver JA, Pai-Scherf LH, Balasubramaniam S, et al. FDA Subset Analysis of the Safety of Nivolumab in Elderly Patients With Advanced Cancers. *J Clin Oncol* (2016) 34(15_suppl):10010. doi: 10.1200/JCO.2016.34.15_suppl.10010
14. Friedman CF, Minehart J, Horvat TZ, Panageas K, Callahan MK, Chapman PB, et al. Efficacy and Safety of Checkpoint Blockade for Treatment of Advanced Melanoma (Mel) in Patients (Pts) Age 80 and Older (80+). *J Clin Oncol* (2016) 34(15_suppl):10009. doi: 10.1200/JCO.2016.34.15_suppl.10009
15. Hong H, Wang Q, Li J, Liu H, Meng X, Zhang HY, et al. Aging, Cancer and Immunity. *J Cancer* (2019) 10(13):3021–7. doi: 10.7150/jca.30723
16. Pawelec G DE, Larbi A. Immunosenescence and Cancer. *Crit Rev Oncol/Hematol* (2010) 75(2):165–72. doi: 10.1016/j.critrevonc.2010.06.012
17. Castelo-Branco C SI. The Immune System and Aging: A Review. *Gynecol Endocrinol* (2014) 30:16–22. doi: 10.3109/09513590.2013.852531
18. Dilas LT, Icin T, Paro JN, Bajkin I. Autoimmune Thyroid Disease and Other non-Endocrine Autoimmune Diseases. *Med Pregl* (2011) 64:183–7. doi: 10.2298/MPNS1104183T
19. Zgibor JC YL, Boudreau RM, et al. Community-Based Healthy Aging Interventions for Older Adults With Arthritis and Multimorbidity. *J Community Health* (2017) 42:390–9. doi: 10.1007/s10900-016-0268-5
20. Tomihara K CT, Zhang B. Optimization of Immunotherapy in Elderly Cancer Patients. *Crit Rev Oncogol* (2013) 18(6):573–83. doi: 10.1615/critrevoncog.2013010591
21. Britanova OV, Putintseva K, Shugay M, Merzlyak EM, Turchaninova MA, Staroverov DB, et al. Age-Related Decrease in TCR Repertoire Diversity Measured With Deep and Normalized Sequence Profiling. *J Immunol* (2014) 192(6):2689–98. doi: 10.4049/jimmunol.1302064

22. Ouyang Q, Wagner WM, Wikby A, Walter S, Aubert G, Dodi AI, et al. Large Numbers of Dysfunctional CD8+ T Lymphocytes Bearing Receptors for a Single Dominant CMV Epitope in the Very Old. *J Clin Immunol* (2003) 23 (4):247–57. doi: 10.1023/A:1024580531705
23. Quinn KM, Fox A, Harland KL, Russ BE, Li J, Nguyen THO, et al. Age-Related Decline in Primary CD8(+) T Cell Responses is Associated With the Development of Senescence in Virtual Memory CD8(+) T Cells. *Cell Rep* (2018) 23(12):3512–24. doi: 10.1016/j.celrep.2018.05.057
24. Mitchell WA LP, Aspinall R. Tracing Thymic Output in Older Individuals. *Clin Exp Immunol* (2010) 161(3):497–503. doi: 10.1111/j.1365-2249.2010.04209.x
25. Naylor K, Li G, Vallejo AN, Lee WW, Koetz K, Bryl E, et al. The Influence of Age on T Cell Generation and TCR Diversity. *J Immunol* (2005) 174 (11):7446–52. doi: 10.4049/jimmunol.174.11.7446

17

Blood Tumor Mutational Burden as a Predictive Biomarker in Patients with Advanced Non-Small Cell Lung Cancer (NSCLC)

Yuhui Ma[1], Quan Li[2], Yaxi Du[2], Jingjing Cai[3], Wanlin Chen[1], Guangqiang Zhao[1], Xing Liu[2], Hongsheng Li[3], Luyao Ma[2], Yunchao Huang[1,3] and Yongchun Zhou[3]**

[1] First Department of Thoracic Surgery, The Yunnan Cancer Hospital, Kunming, China, [2] Department of Key Laboratory of Lung Cancer, Key Laboratory of Lung Cancer Research of Kunming Medical University, Kunming, China, [3] Yunnan Cancer Hospital and The Third Affiliated Hospital of Kunming Medical University, Yunnan Cancer Center, Kunming, China

***Correspondence:**
Yongchun Zhou
chungui7625@163.com
Yunchao Huang
hycyn2008@163.com

This study was designed to investigate the impact of blood tumor mutational burden (bTMB) on advanced NSCLC in Southwest China. The relationship between the tTMB estimated by next-generation sequencing (NGS) and clinical outcome was retrospectively analyzed in tissue specimens from 21 patients with advanced NSCLC. Furthermore, the relationship between the bTMB estimated by NGS and clinical outcome was retrospectively assessed in blood specimens from 70 patients with advanced NSCLC. Finally, 13 advanced NSCLC patients were used to evaluate the utility of bTMB assessed by NGS in differentiating patients who would benefit from immunotherapy. In the tTMB group, tTMB ≥ 10 mutations/Mb was related to inferior progression-free survival (PFS) (hazard ratio [HR], 0.30; 95% CI, 0.08-1.17; log-rank $P = 0.03$) and overall survival (OS) (HR, 0.30; 95% CI, 0.08-1.16; log-rank $P = 0.03$). In the bTMB group, bTMB ≥ 6 mutations/Mb was associated with inferior PFS (HR, 0.32; 95% CI, 0.14-1.35; log-rank $P < 0.01$) and OS (HR, 0.31; 95% CI, 0.14-0.7; log-rank $P < 0.01$). In the immunotherapy section, bTMB ≥ 6 mutations/Mb was related to superior PFS (HR, 0.32; 95% CI, 0.14-1.35; log-rank $P < 0.01$) and objective response rates (ORRs) (bTMB < 6: 14.2%; 95% CI, 0.03-1.19; bTMB ≥ 6: 83.3%; 95% CI, 0.91-37.08; $P = 0.02$). These findings suggest that bTMB is a validated predictive biomarker for determining the clinical outcome of advanced NSCLC patients and may serve as a feasible predictor of the clinical benefit of immunotherapies (anti-PD-1 antibody) in the advanced NSCLC population in Yunnan Province.

Keywords: blood tumor mutational burden, next-generation sequencing, biomarker, immunotherapy, NSCLC

INTRODUCTION

Recently, immune checkpoint blockade (ICB) therapy has shown improved clinical benefits in patients with advanced non-small cell lung cancer (NSCLC) (1, 2). Tissue with high tumor mutational burden (tTMB-H), which is related to genomic instability and overall neoantigen load, is a new prognostic biomarker for clinical benefit to multiple ICB therapies (3–5). More recent studies have demonstrated a relationship between tTMB-H and superior clinical benefit in patients receiving anti-PD-1 (anti cognate ligand of programmed death 1) antibodies therapy (6–10). However, up to 30% to 50% of patients with advanced NSCLC cannot supply sufficient cancer tissue for TMB detection (9, 11). Therefore, there is an urgent need to create noninvasive methods that can differentiate patients who would benefit from ICB therapy.

More recent studies have demonstrated that blood tumor mutational burden (bTMB, measured by circulating tumor DNA [ctDNA]) may be a substitution for overall neoantigen production (12–14). Gandara et al. (12) found an association between high bTMB (≥ 16 mutations/Mb) and superior progression-free survival (PFS) with atezolizumab in NSCLC. Zhijie Wang et al. (13) reported that bTMB (≥ 6 mutations/Mb) is related to PFS and that objective response rates (ORRs) benefit from ICB therapy in NSCLC. However, most previous studies have shown that there is not a relationship between high bTMB and greater overall survival (OS) in NSCLC patients received ICB therapy (12, 13, 15). Moreover, whether bTMB can be estimated by ctDNA is still unclear (16). Therefore, further evidence of bTMB is needed to identify its utility value as a biomarker for immunotherapy.

bTMB testing facilities (by NGS) have been established in our cancer center since 2018. The bTMB status in advanced NSCLC patients in the Yunnan Province is not clear, so we first investigated advanced NSCLC with bTMB in Yunnan Province and further determined the feasibility of bTMB as a prognostic biomarker for ICB therapy.

MATERIALS AND METHODS

Patients

This research included 2 sections: we first recruited 21 advanced NSCLC patients (all of patients receiving platinum-based chemotherapy) and obtained tissue samples for retrospectively determining their tTMB status from the Yunnan Cancer hospital between February 2018 and August 2020. Second, we recruited 83 advanced NSCLC patients (70 patients receiving platinum-based chemotherapy and 13 patients receiving ICB therapy) with blood samples for retrospectively determining their bTMB status from the same center between January 2018 and August 2020. This work was performed in full accordance with the Declaration of Helsinki, and each patient provided informed consent. Protocol approval was acquired from the ethics committee of the Yunnan Cancer hospital. Advanced NSCLC patients from Yunnan Province with sufficient tissue or blood samples were considered eligible for this TMB analysis. Patients with known EGFR mutations or ALK translocations sensitive to targeted therapy or with an autoimmune disease were excluded. Twenty-one tissue samples underwent tTMB analysis, and 83 blood samples underwent bTMB analysis to obtain PFS and OS data. Finally, we collected other information, including clinical and molecular parameters.

DNA Extraction and NGS Library Construction

Plasma ctDNA extraction and purification [Thermo (k0782)], leukocyte enrichment from whole blood, and low-speed centrifugation for DNA extraction and quality identification (Qubit dsDNA HS Assay Kit) were performed before library construction. The ctDNA libraries were prepared by the Vazyme ND607 DNA Library Kit with unique identifiers (UIDs, also called barcodes) to tag individual DNA molecules. The extracted DNA was used for end repair and poly(A)-tail addition by KAPA enzymatic digestion. Target fragments were captured by magnetic beads, and PCR enrichment amplification was performed after hybridization.

The tumor tissue DNA extraction and NGS library construction were performed following the methods described in our previous study (17).

Sequencing and Data Processing

Captured probes were supplied by Integrated DNA Technologies (IDT) xGen Lockdown Probes (including 547 cancer-relevant genes) to evaluate the TMB, and then the probes were separately used to capture tissue gDNA and plasma ctDNA following standard protocols. Both captured libraries for tissue gDNA and plasma ctDNA were processed into the Illumina® HiSeq X-TEN for sequencing according to the manufacturer's instructions. Both raw parameters were processed by using Illumina® HiSeq X-TEN, and error reads were corrected by using the hg19 reference genome. Our program KEYseq V2.0 was used to analyze these data.

bTMB Detection

The TMB was calculated by summing all synonymous and nonsynonymous variants with ≥ 5% (0.5% in blood) frequency, which was demonstrated with the mutations per megabase (mut/Mb) unit, and germline variants and driver gene mutations were removed. Our bTMB algorithm contains single nucleotide polymorphism (SNP) sites and driver gene mutations filtering common untrue mutations, while synonymous mutations, small fragments and single base insertion-deletion mutations were not filtered. Our bTMB algorithm is based on the latest official standards of Foundation Medicine, a leading provider of genome sequencing analysis services. The tTMB cutoff point was 10 mutations/Mb, and the bTMB cutoff points were 6, 10, and 16 mutations/Mb based on recent studies (12, 13, 17).

Outcomes Assessment

In the group of patients who did not receive ICB therapy, PFS was defined as the time from the start of TMB detection to objective disease progression or death, and this was evaluated with the Response Evaluation Criteria In Solid Tumors (RECIST) v 1.1 or death. OS was defined as the time from the start of TMB detection until death due to any cause. In the group of patients who received ICB therapy, PFS was defined as the time from the start of ICB treatment to objective disease progression or death. OS was defined as the time from the start of ICB treatment to death due to any cause. The ORR is measured as the percentage of patients with a complete response (CR) or a partial response (PR) (as defined by RECIST v1.1). Tumor assessments were performed every 3 months after the first TMB detection, and the last follow-up was on August 8, 2020.

Statistical Analysis

Chi-square or Fisher's exact test was used to analyze the correlation between TMB and clinical data. For survival analysis, Kaplan-Meier curves (*P* values determined with log-rank test) were performed, and the hazard ratios (HRs) were calculated by using a Cox proportional hazards regression model. *P* levels < 0.05 (two-sided) were considered statistically significant. All statistical analyses were performed by SPSS 22.0 (SPSS, Inc., Chicago, IL, USA) and Graph-Pad Prism version 8.0 (San Diego, CA, USA).

RESULTS

Patient Characteristics

This study included 2 independent cohorts. Cohort 1 consisted of 21 patients with tissue samples; median age, 53 (range 36-75) years; 7 (33.3%) females. Cohort 2 consisted of 83 patients with blood samples; median age, 56 (range 31-82) years; 30 (36.1%) females. Thirteen patients received anti-PD-1 antibodies therapy as a second-line treatment. No evident differences were found in the patient characteristics (**eTables 1–3** in the **Supplement**).

tTMB Estimated by NGS and Clinical Outcomes of NSCLC Patients

In cohort 1, the cutoff level of bTMB was 10 mutations/Mb based on previous studies and FDA guidelines (4, 9). PFS and OS were evidently shorter in patients with tTMB-high (≥ 10 mutations/Mb) than in patients with tTMB-low (< 10 mutations/Mb). The median PFS was 8.5 months and 19.0 months, respectively (hazard ratio = 0.30, 95% CI 0.08 to 1.17, *p* = 0.03, **Figure 1A**). The median OS was 10.0 months and 21.0 months, respectively (hazard ratio = 0.30, 95% CI 0.08 to 1.16, *p* = 0.03, **Figure 1B**). In the univariable Cox proportional hazards regression model, the bTMB status was related to PFS and OS (HR, 3.87; 95% CI, 1.14-13.12; *p* = 0.03) (HR, 3.92; 95% CI, 1.15-13.35; *p* = 0.02) (**Tables 1, 2**). In the multivariable Cox proportional hazards regression model, the bTMB status was also associated with PFS and OS (HR, 4.20; 95% CI, 1.02-17.20; *p* = 0.04) (HR, 4.20; 95% CI, 1.01-17.49; *p* = 0.04) (**Tables 1, 2**).

bTMB Estimated by NGS and Clinical Outcomes of NSCLC Patient Who Did Not Receive ICB Therapy

In cohort 2, when the cutoff level of bTMB was 6, both HR and *P* levels were minimum values (**Figures 2A, B**). PFS and OS were evidently shorter in patients with bTMB-high (≥ 6 mutations/Mb) than in patient with bTMB-low (< 6 mutations/Mb). The median PFS was 10.0 months and 18.0 months, respectively (hazard ratio = 0.32, 95% CI 0.14 to 1.35, *p* < 0.01, **Figure 3A**). The median OS was 11.0 months and 25.0 months, respectively (hazard ratio = 0.31, 95% CI 0.14 to 0.7, *p* < 0.01, **Figure 3B**). In the univariable Cox proportional hazards regression model, bTMB status was related to PFS and OS (HR, 3.74; 95% CI, 1.85-7.54; *p* < 0.01) (HR, 4.48; 95% CI, 2.14-9.37; *p* < 0.01) (**Tables 3, 4**). In the multivariable Cox proportional hazards regression model, bTMB status was also related to PFS and OS (HR, 4.20; 95% CI, 1.02-17.20; *p* = 0.04) (HR, 4.20; 95% CI, 1.01-17.49; *p* = 0.04) (**Tables 3, 4**).

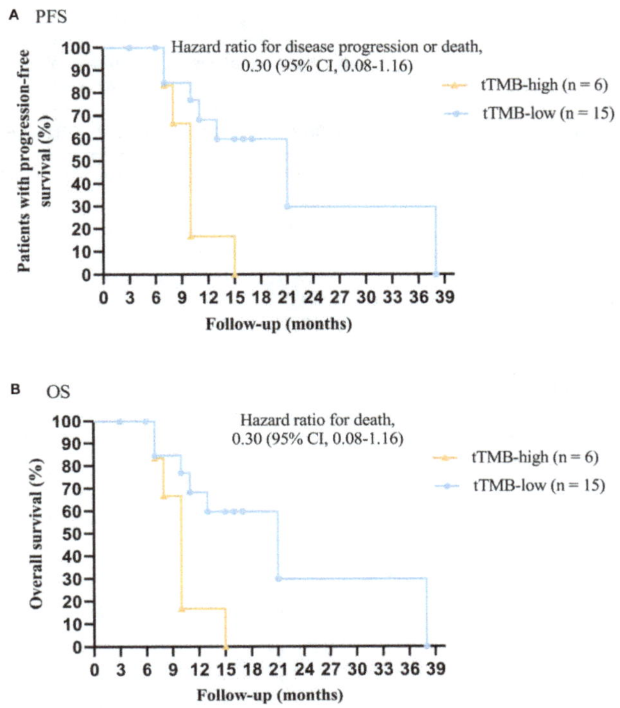

FIGURE 1 | Kaplan-Meier plots of PFS and OS of patients by tTMB status: **(A)** PFS by tTMB status. **(B)** OS by tTMB status.

TABLE 1 | Univariable and multivariable analysis of PFS.

	Progression-Free Survival			
	Univariable Analysis		Multivariable Analysis	
Characteristic	**HR (95% CI)**	***P***	**HR (95% CI)**	***P***
Age < 65 *vs* ≥ 65 y	0.94 (1.19-4.50)	*0.94*	NA	*NA*
Male *vs* female	1.56 (0.46-5.25)	*0.46*	NA	*NA*
Current or former *vs* never smoker	3.57 (0.98-12.91)	*0.05*	NA	*NA*
tTMB ≥ 10 *vs* < 10	3.87 (1.14-13.12)	*0.03a*	4.20 (1.02-17.20)	*0.04*[a]

[a]This p value indicates a statistically significant difference. NA, not applicable.

TABLE 2 | Univariable and multivariable analysis of OS.

	Overall survival			
	Univariable Analysis		Multivariable Analysis	
Characteristic	**HR (95% CI)**	***P***	**HR (95% CI)**	***P***
Age < 65 *vs* ≥ 65 y	0.99 (0.21-4.65)	*0.99*	NA	*NA*
Male *vs* female	1.53 (0.45-5.15)	*0.48*	NA	*NA*
Current or former *vs* never smoker	3.19 (0.89-11.42)	*0.07*	NA	*NA*
tTMB ≥ 10 *vs* < 10	3.92 (1.15-13.35)	*0.02[a]*	4.20 (1.01-17.49)	*0.04[a]*

[a]This p value indicates a statistically significant difference. NA, not applicable.

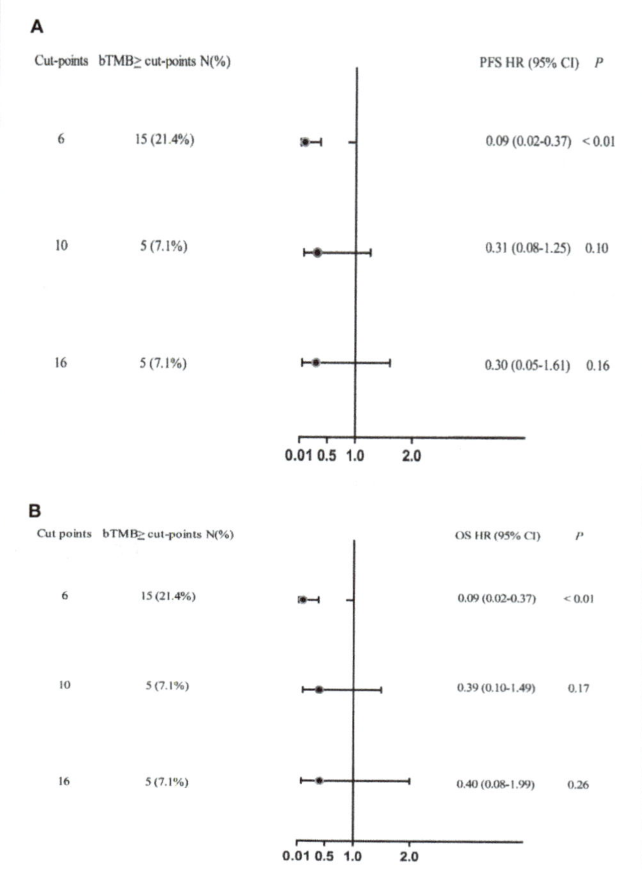

FIGURE 2 | Forest plots of HRs for the relationship between bTMB cutoff values and PFS and OS. **(A)** PFS and **(B)** OS in the bTMB cohort (excluding patients who treated with ICB therapy), bTMB cutoff values of ≥6, ≥10 and ≥16.

bTMB Estimated by NGS and Clinical Outcomes of NSCLC Patients Who Treated With ICB Therapy

In this work, we further investigated the relationship between bTMB status and clinical benefit in advanced NSCLC patients who treated with ICB (anti-PD-1 antibody) therapy. The PFS was significantly shorter in patients with bTMB-low (< 6 mutations/Mb) than in patients with bTMB-high (< 6 mutations/Mb). The median PFS was 4.0 months and 10.0 months, respectively (hazard ratio = 3.96, 95% CI 1.083 to 14.48, $p < 0.01$, **Figure 4A**). Furthermore, bTMB-high was related to a higher ORR than bTMB-low (83.3%; 95% CI, 0.91-37.08 *vs.* 14.2%; 95% CI, 0.03-1.19; $P = 0.02$, **Figure 4B**). Eventually, nonresponders had significantly lower bTMB levels than responders (median, 4; interquartile range, 1-8 *vs.* median, 11.5; interquartile range, 5.7-15, $P < 0.01$, **Figure 4C**).

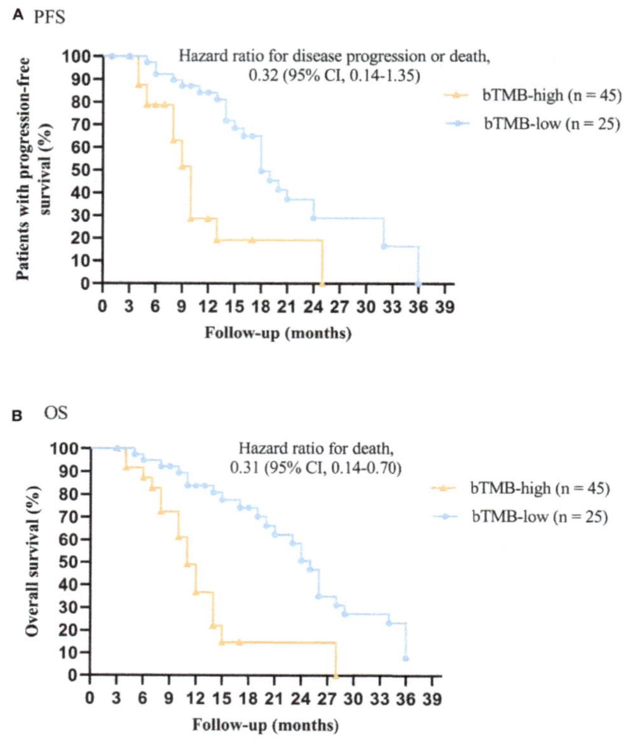

FIGURE 3 | Kaplan-Meier plots of PFS and OS of patients (excluding patients who received ICB therapy) by bTMB status. **(A)** PFS by bTMB status. **(B)** OS by bTMB status.

TABLE 3 | Univariable and multivariable analysis of PFS.

	Progression-Free Survival			
	Univariable Analysis		Multivariable Analysis	
Characteristic	**HR (95% CI)**	***P***	**HR (95% CI)**	***P***
Age < 65 *vs* ≥ 65 y	1.62 (0.77-3.44)	*0.20*	NA	*NA*
Male *vs* female	1.67 (0.86-3.23)	*0.12*	NA	*NA*
Current or former *vs* never smoker	1.31 (0.70-2.46)	*0.39*	NA	*NA*
bTMB ≥ 6 *vs* < 6	3.74 (1.85-7.54)	*<0.01[a]*	5.35 (2.39-11.97)	*<0.01[a]*

[a]This p value indicates a statistically significant difference. NA, not applicable.

TABLE 4 | Univariable and multivariable analysis of OS.

	Overall survival			
	Univariable Analysis		Multivariable Analysis	
Characteristic	**HR (95% CI)**	***P***	**HR (95% CI)**	***P***
Age < 65 *vs* ≥ 65 y	1.57 (0.74-3.31)	*0.23*	NA	*NA*
Male *vs* female	1.60 (0.85-3.00)	*0.14*	NA	*NA*
Current or former *vs* never smoker	1.46 (0.79-2.72)	*0.22*	NA	*NA*
bTMB ≥ 6 *vs* < 6	4.48 (2.14-9.37)	*<0.01*[a]	6.26 (2.71-14.46)	*<0.01*[a]

[a]*This p value indicates a statistically significant difference. NA, not applicable.*

Prevalence of Genetic Alterations in Patients

We found a wide range of cancer-related genetic alterations depended on tissue NGS genotyping. The landscape of genetic alterations had been shown in **Figure 5A**. The most frequently mutated genes were *TP53* (8 of 21, 38.1%) and *KRAS* (4 of 21, 19.0%). In addition, through plasma NGS genotyping, we also identified a wide range of cancer-related genetic alterations. The landscape of genetic alterations had been shown in **Figure 5B**. The most frequently mutated genes were *TP53* (29 of 83, 34.9%), *KRAS* (16 of 83, 19.3%) and *PIK3A* (12 of 83, 14.5%).

Mutation Variant Allele Frequency (VAF) Distribution of All Patients

In the tissue VAF subgroup, we found that the median TP53 VAF was 35.77% (range 5.06% to 42.20%) in patients with tTMB-low, while it was 28.93% (range 13.12% to 57.85%) in patients with tTMB-high. The median TP53 VAF was 14.50% (5.06% to 57.85%) in patients with adenocarcinoma and 38.27% (21.33% to 51.70%) in patients with squamous cell carcinoma. However, there were no significant differences in the tumor type and TMB level (**eTable 4**). In the blood VAF subgroup, we found that the median TP53 VAF was 7.76% (range 1.62% to 73.16%) in patients with bTMB-low and 17.18% (range 0.97% to 79.10%) in patients with bTMB-high. The median TP53 VAF was 12.18% (1.27% to 79.10%) in patients with adenocarcinoma and 11.92% (4.24% to 62.12%) in patients with squamous cell carcinoma. The median KRAS VAF was 13.13% (range 2.57% to 59.07%) in patients with bTMB-low and 28.71% (range 5.05% to 61.21%) in patients with bTMB-high. Similarly, there were no significant differences in the tumor type and TMB level (**eTable 5**).

DISCUSSION

In this work, we first examined the association between the tTMB values and advanced NSCLC patients' clinical outcomes who did not receive ICB therapy in Southwest China. Our findings were consistent with our previous study (17), and tTMB (cutoff value = 10 mutations/Mb) is a vital and independent predictive biomarker in advanced NSCLC. Many recent studies demonstrated that 30% to 50% of advanced NSCLC patients could not provide sufficient cancer tissue for tTMB detection (9, 12, 13). Therefore, whether bTMB could be a reliable biomarker to guide immunotherapies has attracted extensive attention from scientists. However, most of the research has focused on the relationship between bTMB values and advanced NSCLC

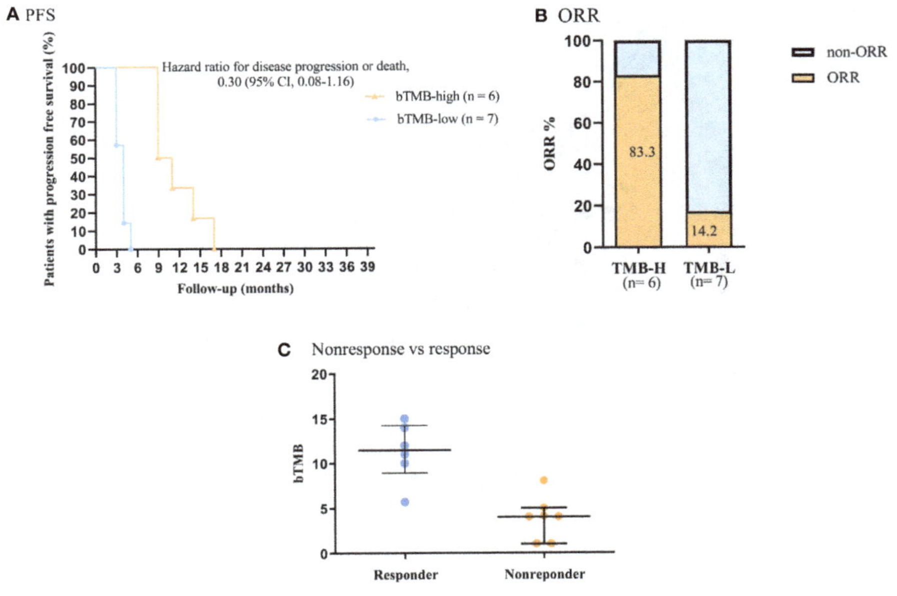

FIGURE 4 | Association of clinical outcome and bTMB in NSCLC patients received ICB therapy. **(A)** PFS by bTMB status. **(B)** Comparison of ORRs in the two bTMB groups (*P* =0.02). **(C)** Comparison of bTMB values between the nonresponse and response groups (*P* < 0.01).

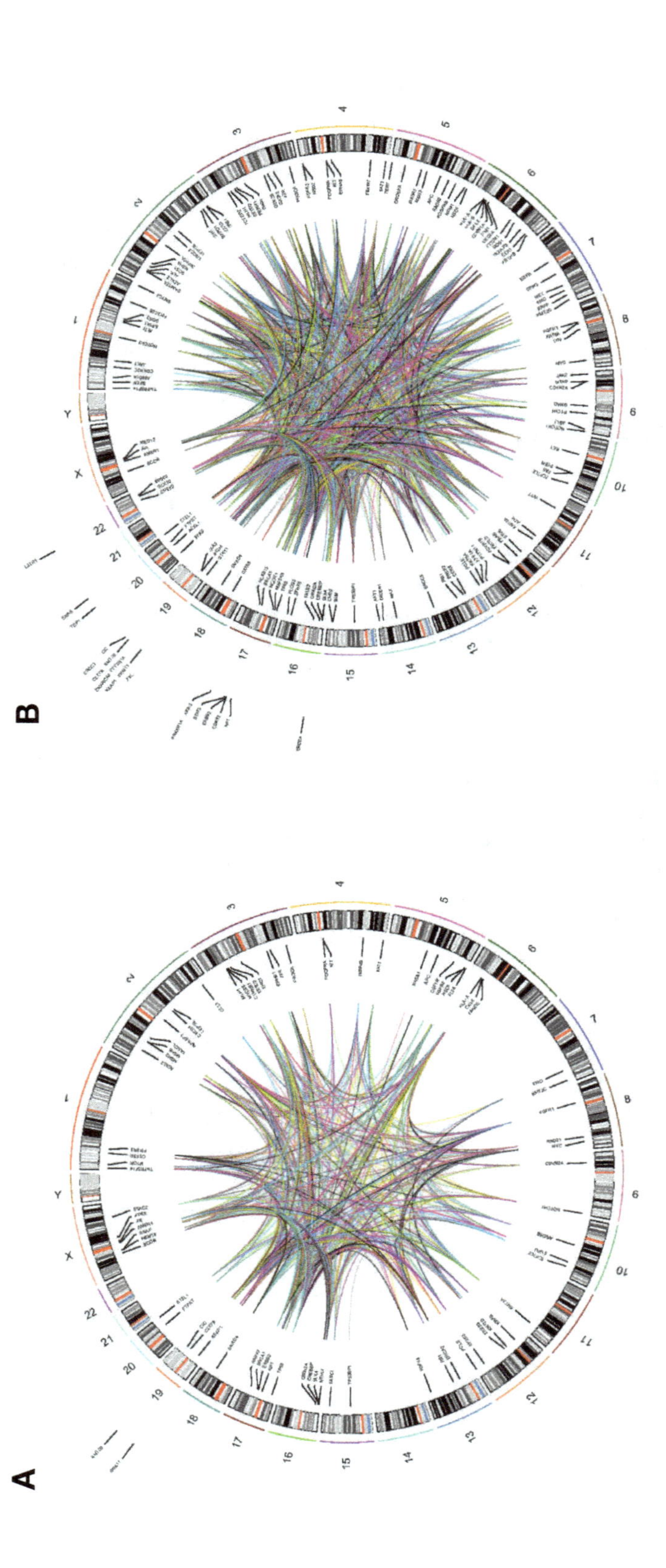

FIGURE 5 | Circos plot describing whole-genome DNA-seq data. *Track 1*: cytoband, chromosomes are depicted qter to pter. *Track 2*: Genomic location of mutant genes in tissues **(A)** or blood **(B)** of detected patients is located inside or outside cytoband of related genome. Gene name is in black represent. *Track 3*: Each line represent mutant genes existing in a patient.

patients' clinical benefits from ICB therapy. The relationship between bTMB values and clinical outcomes in patients who did not receive ICB therapy is still not clear. Herein, this is the study that demonstrates that advanced NSCLC patients (receiving platinum-based chemotherapy) with bTMB-low (cutoff value < 6 mutations/Mb) were associated with better outcomes in Yunnan Province (**Figures 3A, B**). These findings are similar to our previous tTMB study (17). It may be inferred that bTMB values are important for estimating advanced NSCLC patients' clinical outcomes and are similar to the outcomes estimated by tTMB levels.

This study also demonstrated that advanced NSCLC patients with bTMB-H (≥ 6 mutations/Mb) would benefit from ICB (anti-PD-1 antibody) therapy. These findings are also similar to those from previous studies (13). However, we also found that unlike tTMB, the OS benefit did not occur in advanced NSCLC patients with bTMB-H during ICB (anti-PD-1 antibody) therapy (1, 2). Therefore, more studies on bTMB are needed to investigate its intrinsic nature and reveal the potential mechanism.

The selection of bTMB cutoff points is still controversial (12, 13). Gandara et al. (12) and the phase III IMpower 110 study (18, 19) reported that advanced NSCLC patients with bTMB-H (≥ 16 mutations/Mb) would benefit from ICB therapy. More recently, MYSTIC study reported that advanced NSCLC patients with bTMB cutoff points (≥ 20 mutations/Mb) would benefit from ICB therapy (20). Subsequently, Zhijie Wang et al. (13) reported that advanced NSCLC patients with bTMB-H (≥ 6 mutations/Mb) would benefit from ICB therapy. In our study, we confirmed that the cutoff level of bTMB was 6 mutations/Mb, which is a suitable cutoff point that can differentiate advanced NSCLC patients from Yunnan Province who would benefit from ICB (anti-PD-1 antibody) therapy. The difference in the bTMB cutoff point between our findings and the other previous studies may result from five factors (12, 13, 18–20). First, the difference in the gene panel size between our research (547 cancer-relevant genes) and the study by Gandara et al. (394 cancer-relevant genes) may contribute to a discrepancy in the selection of the bTMB cutoff point. Second, the difference in patients' race between our research (all patients were Chinese) and Gandara et al.'s study (most patients were White) may contribute to a bias in the selection of the bTMB cutoff point. Third, the limited sample size in our study (only 13 patients received anti-PD-1 antibody therapy) may lead to a bias in the selection of the bTMB cutoff point. Fourth, the difference in the calculation of bTMB between our research (summing all synonymous and nonsynonymous variants) and other studies (summing all nonsynonymous variants) may contribute to a bias in the selection of the bTMB cutoff point (20, 21). Finally, our study was a retrospective analysis that may contribute to a statistical discrepancy. Therefore, further prospective studies with large sample sizes are needed.

In our study, a comprehensive analysis of genetic alterations in NSCLC patients demonstrated that the majority of mutations appeared in TP53 and KRAS (**Figure 5**). These findings are similar to our previous study (17).

In summary, our findings suggest that bTMB (cutoff point was 6 mutations per megabase) is a validated predictive biomarker for determining the clinical outcome of advanced NSCLC patients with chemotherapy. Using a bTMB cutoff point ≥ 6 mutations per megabase, we found that Yunnan advanced NSCLC patients who obtained an increased PFS benefit from anti-PD-1 antibody therapy. Further prospectively validated studies with large sample sizes are needed.

There are three limitations to our study. Firstly, our study was retrospective research, which may limit the interpretation of the clinical results. Secondly, the small sample size may cause unavoidable selection bias and measurement bias, relatively weakening the reliability of our conclusions. Thirdly, in our study, there were no matched blood and clinical tissue samples from the same patient for TMB detection. Therefore, it may lead to a bias between tTMB and bTMB in diagnostic concordance assessment. Further prospective researches are expected.

AUTHOR CONTRIBUTIONS

YZ, YH, and YM designed the study. YM, QL, YD, JC, WC, GZ, XL, HL, and LM finished the experiments. YM and YZ analyzed the parameters and wrote the research. All authors contributed to the research. All authors contributed to the article and approved the submitted version.

REFERENCES

1. Rittmeyer A, Barlesi F, Waterkamp D, Park K, Ciardiello F, Pawel J, et al. Atezolizumab Versus Docetaxel in Patients With Previously Treated non-Small-Cell Lung Cancer (OAK): A Phase 3, Open-Label, Multicentre Randomised Controlled Trial. *Lancet* (2017) 389:255–65. doi: 10.1016/S0140-6736(16)32517-X
2. Fehrenbacher L, Spira A, Ballinger M, Kowanetz M, Vansteenkiste J, Mazieres J, et al. Atezolizumab Versus Docetaxel for Patients With Previously Treated Non-Small-Cell Lung Cancer (POPLAR): A Multicentre, Open-Label, Phase 2 Randomised Controlled Trial. *Lancet* (2016) 387:1837–46. doi: 10.1016/S0140-6736(16)00587-0
3. Schumacher TN, Schreiber RD. Neoantigens in Cancer Immunotherapy. *Science* (2015) 348(6230):69–74. doi: 10.1126/science.aaa4971
4. Samstein RM, Lee CH, Shoushtari AN, Shoushtari AN, Hellmann MD, Shen R, et al. Tumor Mutational Load Predicts Survival After Immunotherapy Across Multiple Cancer Types. *Nat Genet* (2019) 51:202–6. doi: 10.1038/s41588-018-0312-8
5. Singal G, Miller PG, Agarwala V, Li G, Kaushik G, Backenroth D, et al. Association of Patient Characteristics and Tumor Genomics With Clinical Outcomes Among Patients With Non-Small Cell Lung Cancer Using a Clinicogenomic Database. *Jama* (2019) 321:1391–9. doi: 10.1001/jama.2019.3241
6. Carbone DP, Reck M, Paz-Ares L, Creelan B, Horn L, Steins M, et al. First-line Nivolumab in Stage IV or Recurrent non-Small-Cell Lung Cancer. *N Engl J Med* (2017) 376:2415–26. doi: 10.1056/NEJMoa1613493
7. Reck M, Schenker M, Lee KH, Provencio M, Nishio M, Lesniewski K, et al. Nivolumab Plus Ipilimumab Versus Chemotherapy as First-Line Treatment in Advanced Non-Small-Cell Lung Cancer With High Tumour Mutational Burden: Patient-Reported Outcomes Results From the Randomised, Open-Label, Phase III CheckMate 227 Trial. *Eur J Cancer* (2019) 116:137–47. doi: 10.1016/j.ejca.2019.05.008
8. Kowanetz M, Zou W, Shames D, Cummings C, Rizvi N, Spira A, et al. Tumor Mutation Burden (TMB) is Associated With Improved Efficacy of

Atezolizumab in 1L and 2L+ NSCLC Patients. *J Thorac Oncol* (2017) 12: S321–2. doi: 10.1016/j.jtho.2016.11.343

9. Hellmann MD, Ciuleanu TE, Pluzanski A, Lee JS, Otterson GA, Audigier-Valette C, et al. Nivolumab Plus Ipilimumab in Lung Cancer With a High Tumor Mutational Burden. *N Engl J Med* (2018) 378(22):2093–104. doi: 10.1056/NEJMoa1801946
10. Hellmann MD, Callahan MK, Awad MM, Calvo E, Ascierto PA, Atmaca A, et al. Tumor Mutational Burden and Efficacy of Nivolumab Monotherapy and in Combination With Ipilimumab in Small-Cell Lung Cancer. *Cancer Cell* (2018) 33(5):853–61, e854. doi: 10.1016/j.ccell.2018.04.001
11. Lim C, Tsao MS, Le LW, Shepherd FA, Feld R, Burkes RL, et al. Biomarker Testing and Time to Treatment Decision in Patients With Advanced Nonsmall-Cell Lung Cancer. *Ann Oncol* (2015) 26:1415–21. doi: 10.1093/annonc/mdv208
12. Gandara DR, Paul SM, Kowanetz M, Schleifman E, Zou W, Li Y, et al. Blood-Based Tumor Mutational Burden as a Predictor of Clinical Benefit in non-Small-Cell Lung Cancer Patients Treated With Atezolizumab. *Nat Med* (2018) 24(9):1441–8. doi: 10.1038/s41591-018-0134-3
13. Wang Z, Duan J, Cai S, Han M, Dong H, Zhao J, et al. Assessment of Blood Tumor Mutational Burden as a Potential Biomarker for Immunotherapy in Patients With Non-Small Cell Lung Cancer With Use of a Next-Generation Sequencing Cancer Gene Panel. *JAMA Oncol* (2019) 5(5):696–702. doi: 10.1001/jamaoncol.2018.7098
14. Wang Z, Duan J, Wang G, Zhao J, Xu JC, Han JF, et al. Allele Frequency-Adjusted Blood-Based Tumor Mutational Burden as a Predictor of Overall Survival for Patients With NSCLC Treated With Pd-(L)1 Inhibitors. *J Thorac Oncol* (2020) 15(4):556–67. doi: 10.1016/j.jtho.2019.12.001
15. Kim ES, Velcheti V, Mekhail T, Leal TA, Dowell JE, Tsai ML, et al. Lba55 Primary Efficacy Results From B-F1RST, a Prospective Phase II Trial Evaluating Blood-Based Tumour Mutational Burden (bTMB) as a Predictive Biomarker for Atezolizumab (Atezo) in 1L non-Small Cell Lung Cancer (NSCLC). *Ann Oncol* (2018) 29:mdy424.067. doi: 10.1093/annonc/mdy424.067
16. Torga G, Pienta KJ. Patient-Paired Sample Congruence Between 2 Commercial Liquid Biopsy Tests. *JAMA Oncol* (2018) 4(6):868–70. doi: 10.1001/jamaoncol.2017.4027
17. Ma Y, Li Q, Du Y, Chen WL, Zhao GQ, Liu X, et al. Tumor Mutational Burden and PD-L1 Expression in Non-Small-Cell Lung Cancer (NSCLC) in Southwestern China. *Onco Targets Ther* (2020) 13:5191–8. doi: 10.2147/OTT.S255947
18. Jassem J, Herbst RS, de Marinis F, Cadranel J, Csőszi T, Isla D, et al. *Impower110: Clinical Safety in a Phase Iii Study of Atezolizumab (Atezo) Monotherapy (Mono) vs Platinum-Based Chemotherapy (Chemo) in First-Line non-Small Cell Lung Cancer (Nsclc).* Alexandria, VA, USA: American Society of Clinical Oncology (2020). doi: 10.1200/JCO.2020.38.15_suppl.e21623
19. Herbst RS, Giaccone G, de Marinis F, Reinmuth N, Vergnenegre A, Barrios CN, et al. Atezolizumab for First-Line Treatment of PD-L1-Selected Patients With NSCLC. *N Engl J Med* (2020) 383(14):1328–39. doi: 10.1056/NEJMoa1917346
20. Si H, Kuziora M, Quinn KJ, Helman E, Ye JB, Liu F, et al. A Blood-based Assay for Assessment of Tumor Mutational Burden in First-line Metastatic NSCLC Treatment: Results From the MYSTIC Study. *Clin Cancer Res* (2020) 27 (6):1631–40. doi: 10.1158/1078-0432.CCR-20-3771
21. Litchfield K, Reading JL, Puttick C, Thakkar K, Abbosh C, Bentham R, et al. Meta-analysis of Tumor- and T Cell-Intrinsic Mechanisms of Sensitization to Checkpoint Inhibition. *Cell* (2021) 184(3):596–614.e14. doi: 10.1016/j.cell.2021.01.002

18

Pembrolizumab Alone or Combined with Chemotherapy in Advanced NSCLC with PD-L1 ≥ 50%: Results of a Retrospective Study

Ya Chen[†], Yanan Wang[†], Zhengyu Yang[†], Minjuan Hu, Yanwei Zhang, Fangfei Qian, Wei Zhang[*], Bo Zhang[*] and Baohui Han[*]

Department of Pulmonary, Shanghai Chest Hospital, Shanghai Jiao Tong University, Shanghai, China

***Correspondence:**
Baohui Han
18930858216@163.com
Bo Zhang
zb1063253078@163.com
Wei Zhang
18930858216@163.com

[†]*These authors share first authorship*

Objectives: Pembrolizumab plus platinum-based chemotherapy and pembrolizumab monotherapy (PM) both become standard of care in patients with advanced non-small-cell lung cancer (NSCLC) and a programmed death ligand 1 (PD-L1) tumor proportion score (TPS) greater than 50%. This study aimed to figure out the better treatment choice.

Method: In this retrospective analysis, we compared the clinical efficacy of PM and PC as first-line treatment in NSCLC patients with a PD-L1 ≥50% and negative for genomic alterations in the EGFR and ALK genes.

Result: Among the population, 115 patients received PC, and 91 patients received PM. Up to Dec 30, 2020, median follow-up was 17.13 months. The median progression-free survival (PFS) rates of PC and PM were 12.37 and 9.60 months (HR: 0.44, $p < 0.001$), respectively. The median overall survival (OS) rates were NE and 28.91 months (HR: 0.40, $p = 0.005$), respectively. Subgroup analysis found that the PFS benefit of PC was evident in most subgroups excepting patients with brain metastasis. The 1-year overall survival rates of PC and PM were 89.3% and 76.1%, respectively. The ORR was 61.7 and 46.9% ($p = 0.004$), respectively.

Conclusion: In patients with previously untreated, PD-L1 ≥50%, advanced NSCLC without EGFR or ALK mutations, the addition of pembrolizumab to standard platinum-based chemotherapy seems to be the preferred treatment, which needs to be validated by further prospective trials.

Keywords: non small cell lung cancer, pembrolizumab, chemotherapy, immunotherapy, programed cell death protein 1 (PD-1)

INTRODUCTION

The use of immune checkpoint inhibitors has greatly altered the standard of care in patients with advanced NSCLC. Pembrolizumab, an IgG4 monoclonal antibody against programmed cell death protein 1 (PD-1) has become a powerful treatment option in clinical practice nowadays.

The KEYNOTE-024 study compared pembrolizumab monotherapy (PM) *versus* chemotherapy in treatment-naïve patients with advanced non-small-cell lung cancer (NSCLC) with programmed death ligand 1 (PD-L1) tumor proportion score (TPS) of 50% or greater. PM achieved a remarkable improvement in terms of progression-free survival [PFS; hazard ratio (HR), 0.50; 95% CI, 0.37 to 0.68] and overall survival (OS; HR, 0.63; 95% CI, 0.47 to 0.86) (1, 2). Single-agent pembrolizumab becomes the standard of care in treatment-naïve NSCLC patients with a PD-L1 TPS ≥50% building on the results of KEYNOTE-024 study. Meanwhile, KEYNOTE-189 and KEYNOTE-407 revealed that pembrolizumab plus platinum-based chemotherapy (PC) significantly improved survival outcomes compared with chemotherapy in patients with metastatic non-squamous and squamous non-small-cell lung cancer (NSCLC), respectively.

Recently, updated analysis of KEYNOTE-024 showed that PM continued to provide remarkable clinical outcomes. The median PFS and OS of the PM group were 10.0 and 30.0 months, respectively. The 2-year overall survival rate was 51.5%, which was a breakthrough for NSCLC patients without EGFR/ALK mutation (1). Meanwhile, updated analysis of KEYNOTE-189 demonstrated that the PFS and OS of patients with PD-L1 ≥50% in the PC group were 11.1 and were not reached. The 2-year overall survival rate was 51.9% (3). Of interest, in patients with PD-L1 ≥50%, there seemed to be not much difference of the median PFS and the 2-year overall survival rate between the PM group in KEYNOTE-024 and the PC group in KEYNOTE-189. Recently, Liang et al. conducted an indirect comparison of clinical outcomes between immunotherapy plus chemotherapy (I + C) and immunotherapy alone. They found that I + C was superior to immunotherapy alone in terms of PFS (HR 0.54, 0.35–0.82) in patients with PD-L1 ≥50%. But the PFS benefit did not translate into an OS benefit (HR 0.75, 95% CI 0.51–1.10) (4). Kim et al. also compared the efficacy of I + C treatment and immunotherapy alone indirectly but reported different results. They found that pembrolizumab plus chemotherapy was superior to pembrolizumab alone in terms of PFS and OS in patients with PD-L1 ≥50% (5).

At present, PC and PM are both recommended with high evidence quality in NSCLC patients with PD-L1 TPS ≥50% without EGFR/ALK alterations according to NCCN and ASCO guideline (6). Of note, PM has been given a high-priority rating though it is difficult to figure out which one was the best option due to the absence of direct comparison. Several meta-analyses compared the efficacy of PC and PM indirectly but presented paradoxical result, which might be due to the inherent limitation such as the risk of systematic bias and confounding factors (5, 7–9). In this context, the present study aimed to figure out which therapy was the priority in this specific population by head-to-head comparison.

MATERIAL AND METHODS

Patients

The medical records of advanced NSCLC patients who received immunotherapy at the Shanghai Chest Hospital between Dec 1, 2017 and Oct 30, 2020 were screened. Two hundred and six patients met the following eligibility criteria: (1) advanced NSCLC (IIIB–IV); (2) histologically or cytologically proven NSCLC; (3) PD-L1 TPS ≥50% without sensitizing EGFR or ALK mutations; (4) pembrolizumab monotherapy or combined with chemotherapy as first-line treatment (chemotherapy agents were mainly pemetrexed, paclitaxel, or gemcitabine in combination with platinum) following standard medical instructions; (5) Eastern Cooperative Oncology Group performance status (ECOG PS) 0–1. Therapeutic schedule was decided by a physician under the principle that PC was priority, provided that patients has a high symptom and/or disease burden and/or large-volume visceral tumor and/or symptomatic brain metastasis (6). This study was approved by the Institutional Review Board of Shanghai Chest Hospital and carried out in accordance with the declaration of Helsinki.

Programmed Death Ligand 1 Tumor Proportion Score and Gene Detection

Tumor samples were obtained by tissue biopsy at the time that disease was diagnosed. PD-L1 expression was assessed before treatment detected by the PD-L1 IHC 22C3 pharmDx assay. Expression was classified to several types according to the tumor proportion score, TPS <0, 1–49 and ≥50%. The amplification refractory mutation system (ARMS) was used as the routine molecular technique for EGFR detection following the protocol of the DxS EGFR mutation test kit. The immunohistochemistry (IHC) and break-apart fluorescence *in situ* hybridization (FISH) were used as the routine molecular technique for ALK rearrangement detection.

Treatment and Clinical Response Evaluation

Therapeutic response evaluation, including enhanced chest computed tomography (CT) scan, and abdominal ultrasound scan, was performed every 4–6 weeks, while enhanced brain magnetic resonance imaging (MRI) was performed every half year if no lesion at baseline and no symptoms thereafter. If patients developed symptom during the treatment, the corresponding examination and evaluation were performed immediately. Clinical stage was determined by the 8th edition of the International Association for the Study of Lung Cancer (IASLC) tumor-node-metastasis (TNM) classification. The response was evaluated according to the Response Evaluation Criteria in Solid Tumors (RECIST) version 1.1.

Statistical Analysis

The characteristics of patients were compared using the $\chi 2$ test for categorical variables. The primary endpoints were PFS (calculated from disease diagnosis to disease progression or the last follow-up), OS (calculated from disease diagnosis to death or the last follow-up), and ORR. The median PFS and OS were estimated using the Kaplan–Meier method and compared by the log-rank test. Hazard ratios and associated 95% confidence intervals were calculated with the use of a stratified Cox proportional-hazards model. All p values were two-sided, and a P value <0.05 was considered statistically significant. All statistical analyses were performed using SPSS version 22.0 (IBM Corporation, Armonk, NY, USA).

RESULTS

Clinical Features

Two hundred and six patients met the eligibility criteria were included in this study. The patient selection procedure is shown in **Figure 1**. Among the 206 patients, 115 (55.8%) received PC and 91 (44.2%) received PM. The median follow-up time was 17.13 months. The median age was 65 (range 37–76) years and 67 (range 29–87) years in the PC and PM groups, respectively. Most patients were male (88.7% in PC and 87.9% in PM), current or former smoker (74.8% in PC and 79.1% in PM), stage IV (63.5% in PC and 64.8% in PM), adenocarcinoma (64.3% in PC and 53.8% in PM) and without brain metastasis (80.0% in PC and 90.1% in PM). The patients' baseline demographic and disease characteristics were generally well balanced between PC and PM groups except more patients with brain metastasis (BM) were in the PC group (p = 0.047) (**Table 1**).

Survival Analysis of PC and PM as First-Line Treatment in Patients With Advanced NSCLC

Up to Dec 30, 2020, 69 of 115 patients (60.0%) in the PC group and 57 of 91 patients (56.0%) in PM group had disease progression on first-line treatment. One hundred of 115 patients (87.0%) in the PC group and 69 of 91 patients (75.8%) in the PM group were still alive. The median PFS of PC and PM groups was 12.37 months (95% CI: 10.97–13.77) and 9.60 months (95% CI: 8.40–10.80), respectively (HR:0.44, $p < 0.001$) (**Figure 2A**). Median overall survival of PC and PM groups was not reached and 28.91 months (HR: 0.40, $p = 0.005$, **Figure 2B**), respectively. The 1-year overall survival rates of PC and PM were 89.3% and 76.1%, respectively.

Subgroup Analysis of PFS

A PFS benefit with PC was evident in most subgroups assessed (**Figure 3**), except for patients with brain metastasis (could not be calculated due to small sample in the PM group) and patients with previous adjuvant therapy (could not be calculated due to small sample).

Tumor Response of PC and PM as First-Line Treatment in Patients With Advanced NSCLC

The ORR (the proportion of patients with a confirmed complete or partial response) of PC and PM was 61.7 and 46.9%

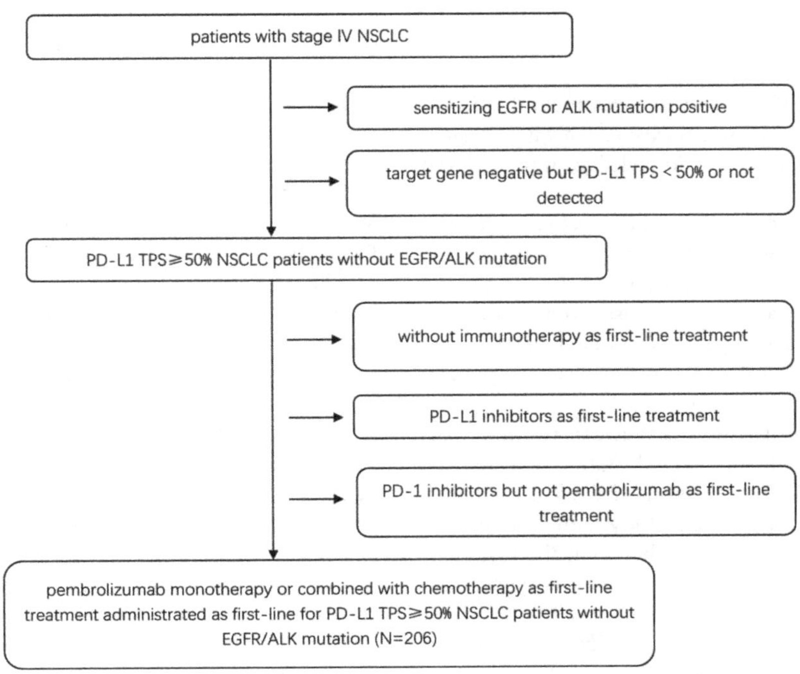

FIGURE 1 | Patient selection flow-chart.

TABLE 1 | Clinical characteristic of 206 patients of advanced NSCLC.

Variable	Pembrolizumab plus chemotherapy (N = 115)	Pembrolizumab (N = 91)	P value
Age			
Median (range)—year	65 (37–76)	67 (29–87)	
<65years—no. (%)	53 (46.1)	32 (35.2)	0.465
Sex—no. (%)			0.489
Male	102 (88.7)	80 (87.9)	
Female	13 (11.3)	11 (12.1)	
Smoking			0.529
Current or former smoker	86 (74.8)	72 (79.1)	
Never smoker	29 (25.2)	19 (20.9)	
Stage			0.840
IIIB–IIIC	42 (36.5)	32 (35.2)	
IV	73 (63.5)	59 (64.8)	
Histology			0.127
Squamous	41 (35.7)	42 (46.2)	
Adenocarcinoma	74 (64.3)	49 (53.8)	
Extrapulmonary metastasis			0.717
NO	59 (51.3)	49 (53.8)	
YES	56 (48.7)	42 (46.2)	
Central nervous system metastasis			0.047
NO	92 (80.0)	82 (90.1)	
YES	23 (20.0)	9 (9.9)	
Previous therapy for non-metastatic disease, n (%)			
Thoracic radiotherapy	19 (16.5)	13 (14.3)	0.660
Adjuvant therapy	9 (7.8)	9 (9.9)	0.602

Data are median (range) or n (%). NSCLC, non-small-cell lung cancer.

(p = 0.004), respectively. The disease control rates (the proportion of patients with a confirmed complete or partial response or stable disease) were 94.8 and 87.7%, respectively (p = 0.292). The change from baseline in the sum of the longest diameters of target lesions is shown in **Figures 4A, B**.

DISCUSSION

Survival analysis of PC and PM as first-line treatment in NSCLC patients with a PD-L1 TPS ≥50% was retrospectively investigated in the present study, which, to our knowledge, was analyzed directly for the first time.

Baseline characteristics were well balanced between PC and PM groups except more patients with brain metastasis were in the PC group. We found that adding chemotherapy to pembrolizumab resulted in a risk of disease progression that was 50% lower than the risks with pembrolizumab alone. Clinical outcomes, including PFS, OS, and ORR were improved significantly in the PC treatment arm.

KEYNOTE-189 (patients with adenocarcinoma) and KEYNOTE-407 (patients with squamous NSCLC) reported the median PFS as 11.1 and 8.00 months in patients with PD-L1 ≥50%, respectively (10, 11). The present study found the median PFS of PC group was 12.37 months, higher than the results of KEYNOTE-189 and KEYNOTE-407. The 1-year overall survival rate and ORR of PC in our study were 89.3% and 61.7%, which was comparable with the results of KEYNOTE-189 and KEYNOTE-407 in patients with PD-L1 ≥50% (11). Subgroup analysis of East Asia population and the rest of world population found that East Asia population had more reduced risk of disease progression and death than others in KEYNOTE-407. The HR of PFS was 0.49 and 0.58 in East Asia population and others, respectively. The HR of OS was 0.44 and 0.69, respectively. This racial difference might explain the greater survival benefit of PC in our study (11, 12). The median PFS of PM in our study was 9.60 months, which was between the values of 10.3 and 7.1 months of the patients with PD-L1 ≥50% in the KEYNOTE-024 and KEYNOTE-042 studies, respectively (2, 13). The median OS was 28.91 months in our study, slightly lower than 30.0 months of KEYNOTE-024 (1). ORR was 46.9% in our study, which was similar with the values of 44.8 and 39% in the KEYNOTE-024 and KEYNOTE-042 studies (2, 13). Those comparable results indicated the validity and reliability of our data. Recently, Wu et al. showed that Chinese patients from the KEYNOTE-042 global and China extension (NCT03850444) study could also obtain significant OS benefit from pembrolizumab treatment compared with standard chemotherapy (14). But details are not yet available. Thus, we look forward to explore whether efficacy of PM was comparable between our study and Wu's study.

Current treatment choice in the first-line setting in patients with NSCLC without targetable gene alterations depends on the PD-L1 expression levels. PC is the only alternative treatment of patients with low PD-L1 TPS (<50%) while PC and PM are both standard of care of patients with high PD-L1 TPS ≥50%). Deciding the optimal treatment in patients with a PD-L1 level ≥50% remains a challenge nowadays due to no direct comparison between PC and PM. Patients with a PD-L1 TPS ≥50% in KEYNOTE-042 did not replicate the remarkable result of KEYNOTE-024 because PFS was not superior in the pembrolizumab group and, in fact, was below that seen with chemotherapy for the first 6 months of treatment (15). And the

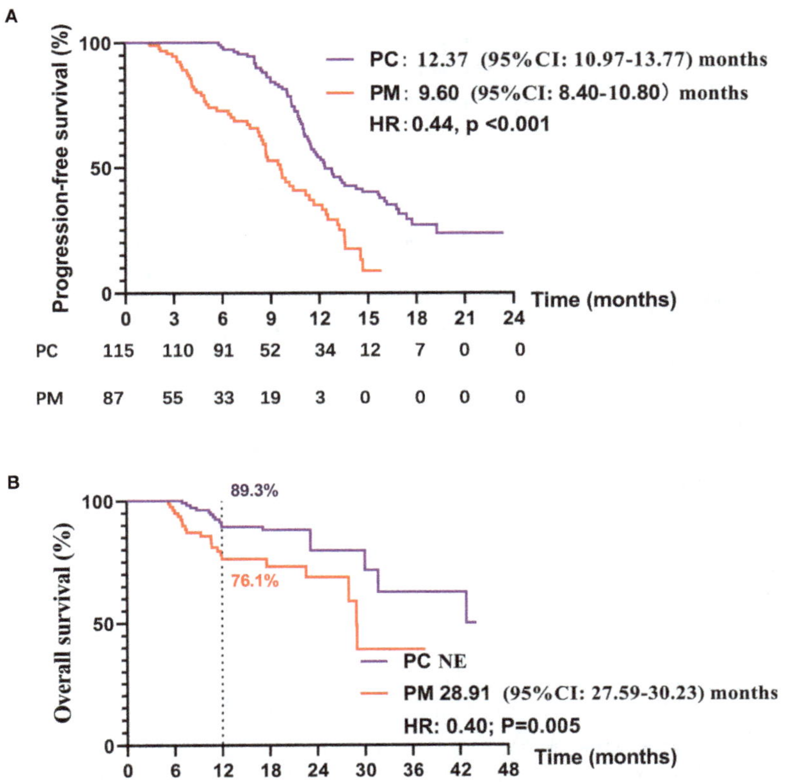

FIGURE 2 | Kaplan–Meier curves for **(A)** progression-free survival (PFS) and **(B)** overall survival (OS) in PC and PM groups.

difference was not explained convincingly. Thus, whether chemotherapy is indispensable for NSCLC patients with PD-L1 TPS ≥50% needs to be explored (15).

Several meta-analyses focused on the comparison of PC and PM but presented paradoxical result. A meta-analysis compared the OS between PM and PC in RCT trials and found that PC showed significant superiority to PM (HR: 0.87; 95% CI: 0.79–0.95) in general patients (6). Liu et al. focused on patients with PD-L1 TPS ≥50% and found that PC was superior to PM in terms of OS (HR =0.74, 95% CI: 0.56–0.98) but there was no difference on PFS (HR =0.83, 95% CI: 0.53–1.3) (9). Nevertheless, another analysis revealed a result that was almost converse to Liu's. PC performed significantly better than PM in terms of ORR (OR 1.60, 95% CI 1.20–2.20), PFS (HR 0.52, 95% CI 0.37–0.71) but not for OS (HR 0.75, 95% CI 0.51–1.10) in patients with PD-L1 high expression (10). In addition, Liang et al. found that PC was comparable to PM in terms of OS and PFS (HR = 1.01, 95% CI: 0.63 to 1.57 and HR = 0.59, 95% CI: 0.35 to 1.06) in patients with PD-L1 high expression by meta-analysis (7). Those results of meta-analysis were different or even opposite, which might be due to the inherent limitation such as the risk of systematic bias and confounding factors. Different search strategy, data extraction and statistical analysis also contributed to the huge difference. Thus, head-to-head comparison is needed to disperse the fog. Our study indicated that PC significantly improved PFS, OS, and ORR compared with PM. However, further clinical trials are needed to validate this benefit. INSIGNA (NCT 03793179), an ongoing randomized phase III study, compares the clinical outcomes of the pembrolizumab in combination with chemotherapy and pembrolizumab alone in treatment-naïve advanced non-squamous NSCLC with PD-L1 expression ≥1%. PERSEE (NCT 04547504), another ongoing phase III study, compares the pembrolizumab-chemotherapy combination and pembrolizumab alone as first-line treatment for advanced NSCLC with a PD-L1 expression ≥50%. These two ongoing trials focus on the same subject but target different populations, and we look forward to their clinical outcomes.

Subgroup analysis in our study found that the PFS benefit of PC was evident in most subgroups excepting for patients with brain metastasis and patients with previous adjuvant therapy because HR and 95% CI could not be calculated due to the small sample. Subgroup analysis may indicate that the benefit of PC over PM was universal across almost all population. Aguilar EJ et al. found that patients with NSCLC and PD-L1 TPS ≥90% treated with first-line pembrolizumab significantly improved clinical outcomes among patients with a PD-L1 TPS ≥50%, which indicated that PD-L1 expression can be divided more exquisitely according to prognosis (16). The subgroup of PD-L1 should also be further analyzed in our study but most PD-L1 expressions were labeled undefined, only

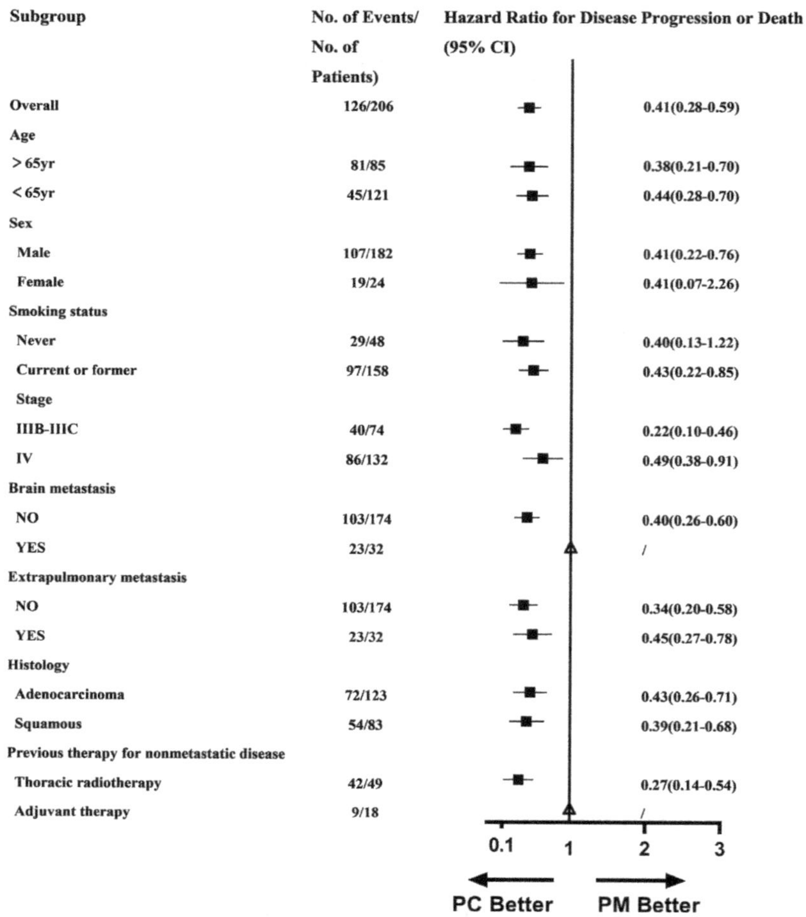

FIGURE 3 | Subgroup analysis of PFS in PC and PM groups.

with records of PD-L1 ≥50%. Aguilar EJ's study reminded us that the refinement of PD-L1 expression level was needed.

Apart from PD-L1 expression, more predictive biomarkers or prognostic factors, including but not limited to blood-based tumor mutational burden (bTMB), high body mass index (BMI), lactate dehydrogenase level (LDH), lung immune prognostic index (LIPI), serine/threonine kinase 11 gene (STK11) mutation, STING pathway, should be further analyzed to help identify the most effective treatment regimens for this specific population (17–21).

Ferrara R et al. proposed that PD-1/PD-L1 inhibitors or single-agent chemotherapy might be associated with hyperprogressive disease (22). In our study, every patient in the PC group received platinum-based chemotherapy instead of single-agent chemotherapy. Further study needs to be conducted to explore whether platinum is indispensable for NSCLC patients receiving immunotherapy plus chemotherapy. The mechanism of chemotherapy plus immunotherapy is not fully understood. However, there was evidence suggesting that chemotherapy can stimulate the antigenicity and immunogenicity of the host by enhancing antigen processing and presentation and by eliminating immune-suppressive myeloid derived suppressor cells (MDSC) and regulatory T cells (Tregs) (7, 23–26). Meanwhile, Ramakrishnan et al. proposed that chemotherapy may stimulate tumor cells to CTLs *via* the upregulation of mannose-6-phosphate receptors (MPRs), and autophagy may exert a tremendous influence in the immunogenic signaling during chemotherapy, which might contribute to the synergistic effect of chemotherapy and immunotherapy (23). Further exploration of the mechanism is needed.

Our study is limited by its retrospective nature. First, the sample size was relatively small and was collected from one center. Second, selection bias existed inevitably because of the missing data. Though the baseline clinical characteristics of patients in PC and PM groups were balanced well, we recognized the existence of selection bias that patients with no significant medical comorbidities were more likely to receive PC while patients with no significant medical comorbidities were more likely to receive PM. Also, the follow-up time was relatively short so that the median OS of PC was not mature, but to some extent K–M curve had showed significant difference between the two groups. Further follow-up should be conducted to confirm the OS benefit. Finally, though our study

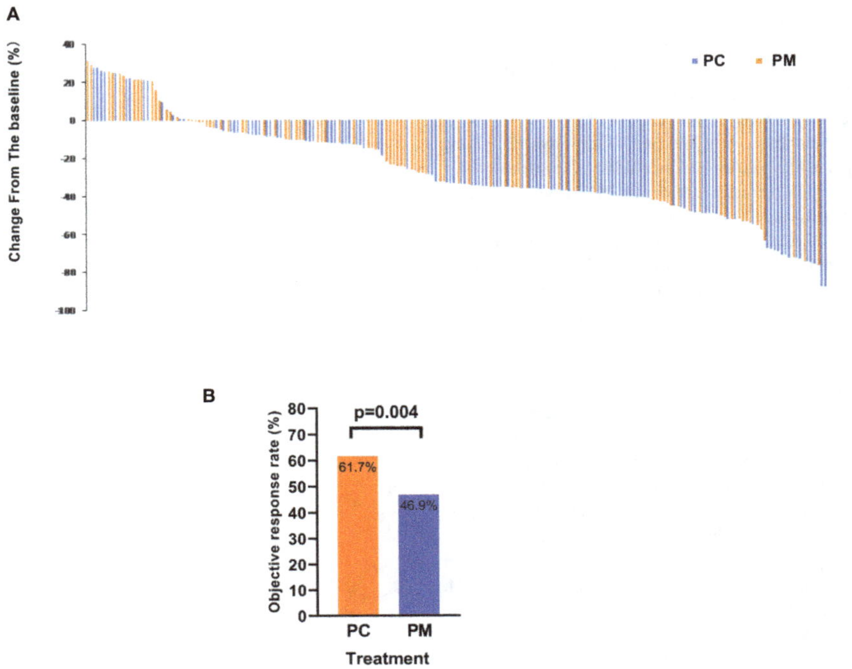

FIGURE 4 | The objective response rate is shown as a percent change of target lesions from baseline in PC and PM groups **(A)** and histograms showing the response rate **(B)**.

found that the clinical efficacy of the combination group was better than monotherapy, adverse events were not compared because of the incomplete records. Thus, prospective trials (INSIGNA and PERSEE) are indispensable for validating both efficacy and adverse events of these two treatments.

CONCLUSIONS

Direct comparison of clinical outcome between PC and PM in NSCLC patients with PD-L1 TPS ≥50% without driver alterations was reported for the first time. We found that PC improved PFS, OS, and ORR benefit over PM.

hospital. Requests to access the datasets should be directed to 18930858216@163.com.

AUTHOR CONTRIBUTIONS

YC, YW, and ZY have substantial contributions to the conception or design of the work, the collection and analysis of data, the writing and editing of the article. The rest authors have given substantial contributions to the work by providing editing and writing assistance. All authors contributed to the article and approved the submitted version.

REFERENCES

1. Reck M, Rodriguez-Abreu D, Robinson AG, Hui R, Csoszi T, Fulop A, et al. Updated Analysis of KEYNOTE-024: Pembrolizumab Versus Platinum-Based Chemotherapy for Advanced Non-Small-Cell Lung Cancer With PD-L1 Tumor Proportion Score of 50% or Greater. *J Clin Oncol* (2019) 37 (7):537–46. doi: 10.1200/JCO.18.00149
2. Herbst RS, Baas P, Kim DW, Felip E, Perez-Gracia JL, Han JY, et al. Pembrolizumab Versus Docetaxel for Previously Treated, PD-L1-Positive, Advanced Non-Small-Cell Lung Cancer (KEYNOTE-010): A Randomised Controlled Trial. *Lancet* (2016) 387(10027):1540–50. doi: 10.1016/S0140-6736(15)01281-7
3. Gadgeel S, Rodriguez-Abreu D, Speranza G, Esteban E, Felip E, Domine M, et al. Updated Analysis From KEYNOTE-189: Pembrolizumab or Placebo Plus Pemetrexed and Platinum for Previously Untreated Metastatic Nonsquamous Non-Small-Cell Lung Cancer. *J Clin Oncol* (2020) 38 (14):1505–17. doi: 10.1200/JCO.19.03136
4. Liang H, Liu Z, Cai X, Pan Z, Chen D, Li C, et al. PD-(L)1 Inhibitors vs. Chemotherapy vs. Their Combination in Front-Line Treatment for NSCLC: An Indirect Comparison. *Int J Cancer* (2019) 145(11):3011–21. doi: 10.1002/ijc.32366
5. Kim R, Keam B, Hahn S, Ock CY, Kim M, Kim TM, et al. First-Line Pembrolizumab Versus Pembrolizumab Plus Chemotherapy Versus Chemotherapy Alone in Non-Small-Cell Lung Cancer: A Systematic Review and Network Meta-Analysis. *Clin Lung Cancer* (2019) 20(5):331–8.e4. doi: 10.1016/j.cllc.2019.05.009
6. Hanna NH, Schneider BJ, Temin S, Baker S Jr., Brahmer J, Ellis PM, et al. Therapy for Stage IV Non-Small-Cell Lung Cancer Without Driver Alterations: ASCO and OH (Cco) Joint Guideline Update. *J Clin Oncol* (2020) 38(14):1608–32. doi: 10.1200/JCO.19.03022
7. Liang H, Lin G, Wang W, Huang J, Yang Y, Lan Y, et al. Feasibility and Safety of PD-1/L1 Inhibitors for Non-Small Cell Lung Cancer in Front-Line Treatment: A Bayesian Network Meta-Analysis. *Trans Lung Cancer Res* (2020) 9(2):188–203. doi: 10.21037/tlcr.2020.02.14
8. Liu T, Ding S, Dang J, Wang H, Chen J, Li G. First-Line Immune Checkpoint Inhibitors for Advanced Non-Small Cell Lung Cancer With Wild-Type Epidermal Growth Factor Receptor (EGFR) or Anaplastic Lymphoma

Kinase (ALK): A Systematic Review and Network Meta-Analysis. *J Thorac Dis* (2019) 11(7):2899–912. doi: 10.21037/jtd.2019.07.45
9. Liu J, Li C, Seery S, Yu J, Meng X. Identifying Optimal First-Line Interventions for Advanced Non-Small Cell Lung Carcinoma According to PD-L1 Expression: A Systematic Review and Network Meta-Analysis. *Oncoimmunology* (2020) 9(1):1746112. doi: 10.1080/2162402X.2020.1746112
10. Gandhi L, Rodriguez-Abreu D, Gadgeel S, Esteban E, Felip E, De Angelis F, et al. Pembrolizumab Plus Chemotherapy in Metastatic Non-Small-Cell Lung Cancer. *N Engl J Med* (2018) 378(22):2078–92. doi: 10.1056/NEJMoa1801005
11. Paz-Ares L, Luft A, Vicente D, Tafreshi A, Gümüş M, Mazières J, et al. Pembrolizumab Plus Chemotherapy for Squamous Non-Small-Cell Lung Cancer. *N Engl J Med* (2018) 379(21):2040–51. doi: 10.1056/NEJMoa1810865
12. Paz-Ares L, Vicente D, Tafreshi A, Robinson A, Soto Parra H, Mazieres J, et al. A Randomized, Placebo-Controlled Trial of Pembrolizumab Plus Chemotherapy in Patients With Metastatic Squamous NSCLC: Protocol-Specified Final Analysis of KEYNOTE-407. *J Thorac Oncol* (2020) 15 (10):1657–69. doi: 10.1016/j.jtho.2020.06.015
13. Mok TSK, Wu YL, Kudaba I, Kowalski DM, Cho BC, Turna HZ, et al. Pembrolizumab Versus Chemotherapy for Previously Untreated, PD-L1-Expressing, Locally Advanced or Metastatic Non-Small-Cell Lung Cancer (KEYNOTE-042): A Randomised, Open-Label, Controlled, Phase 3 Trial. *Lancet* (2019) 393(10183):1819–30. doi: 10.1016/s0140-6736(18)32409-7
14. Wu YL, Zhang L, Fan Y, Zhou J, Zhang L, Zhou Q, et al. 389p Updated Analysis From the KEYNOTE-042 China Study: 1L Pembrolizumab (Pembro) vs Chemotherapy (Chemo) in Chinese Patients (Pts) With Advanced NSCLC With PD-L1 Tps ≥1%. *Ann Oncol* (2020) 31:S1394. doi: 10.1016/j.annonc.2020.10.383
15. Smit EF, de Langen AJ. Pembrolizumab for All PD-L1-Positive NSCLC. *Lancet* (2019) 393(10183):1776–8. doi: 10.1016/s0140-6736(18)32559-5
16. Aguilar EJ, Ricciuti B, Gainor JF, Kehl KL, Kravets S, Dahlberg S, et al. Outcomes to First-Line Pembrolizumab in Patients With Non-Small-Cell Lung Cancer and Very High PD-L1 Expression. *Ann Oncol* (2019) 30 (10):1653–9. doi: 10.1093/annonc/mdz288
17. Chae YK, Davis AA, Raparia K, Agte S, Pan A, Mohindra N, et al. Association of Tumor Mutational Burden With DNA Repair Mutations and Response to Anti-PD-1/PD-L1 Therapy in Non-Small-Cell Lung Cancer. *Clin Lung Cancer* (2019) 20(2):88–96.e6. doi: 10.1016/j.cllc.2018.09.008
18. Agullo-Ortuno MT, Gomez-Martin O, Ponce S, Iglesias L, Ojeda L, Ferrer I, et al. Blood Predictive Biomarkers for Patients With Non-Small-Cell Lung Cancer Associated With Clinical Response to Nivolumab. *Clin Lung Cancer* (2020) 21(1):75–85. doi: 10.1016/j.cllc.2019.08.006
19. Jiang T, Bai Y, Zhou F, Li W, Gao G, Su C, et al. Clinical Value of Neutrophil-to-Lymphocyte Ratio in Patients With Non-Small-Cell Lung Cancer Treated With PD-1/PD-L1 Inhibitors. *Lung Cancer* (2019) 130:76–83. doi: 10.1016/j.lungcan.2019.02.009
20. Xu Z, Yan Y, Wang X, Zeng S, Gong Z. Lung Immune Prognostic Index for Outcome Prediction to Immunotherapy in Patients With NSCLC. *J Thorac Oncol* (2019) 14(9):e207–e8. doi: 10.1016/j.jtho.2019.04.027
21. Della Corte CM, Sen T, Gay CM, Ramkumar K, Diao L, Cardnell RJ, et al. STING Pathway Expression Identifies Non-Small Cell Lung Cancers With An Immune-Responsive Phenotype. *J Thorac Oncol* (2020) 15(5):777–91. doi: 10.1016/j.jtho.2020.01.009
22. Ferrara R, Mezquita L, Texier M, Lahmar J, Audigier-Valette C, Tessonnier L, et al. Hyperprogressive Disease in Patients With Advanced Non-Small Cell Lung Cancer Treated With PD-1/PD-L1 Inhibitors or With Single-Agent Chemotherapy. *JAMA Oncol* (2018) 4(11):1543–52. doi: 10.1001/jamaoncol.2018.3676
23. Ramakrishnan R, Gabrilovich DI. Novel Mechanism of Synergistic Effects of Conventional Chemotherapy and Immune Therapy of Cancer. *Cancer Immunol Immunother* (2013) 62(3):405–10. doi: 10.1007/s00262-012-1390-6
24. Ramakrishnan R, Huang C, Cho HI, Lloyd M, Johnson J, Ren X, et al. Autophagy Induced By Conventional Chemotherapy Mediates Tumor Cell Sensitivity to Immunotherapy. *Cancer Res* (2012) 72(21):5483–93. doi: 10.1158/0008-5472.CAN-12-2236
25. Ramakrishnan R, Assudani D, Nagaraj S, Hunter T, Cho HI, Antonia S, et al. Chemotherapy Enhances Tumor Cell Susceptibility to CTL-Mediated Killing During Cancer Immunotherapy in Mice. *J Clin Invest* (2010) 120(4):1111–24. doi: 10.1172/JCI40269
26. Pol J, Vacchelli E, Aranda F, Castoldi F, Eggermont A, Cremer I, et al. Trial Watch: Immunogenic Cell Death Inducers for Anticancer Chemotherapy. *Oncoimmunology* (2015) 4(4):e1008866. doi: 10.1080/2162402X.2015.1008866

19

Efficacy and Safety of Anlotinib in the Treatment of Small Cell Lung Cancer

Jing Yuan[†]*, Feng Cheng*[†]*, Guodong Xiao, Xiaofeng Wang and Huijie Fan*[*]

Department of Oncology, The First Affiliated Hospital of Zhengzhou University, Zhengzhou, China

***Correspondence:**
Huijie Fan
fanhuijie5542@163.com

[†]*These authors share first authorship.*

Aims: This study aimed to observe the efficacy and safety of anlotinib in the treatment of small cell lung cancer (SCLC) in the real world, as first-line maintenance therapy, second-line, and above.

Methods: Clinical data of 109 patients with SCLC treated with anlotinib and hospitalized at The First Affiliated Hospital of Zhengzhou University from June 2018 to June 2020 were retrospectively analyzed. Analysis of short-term efficacy and survival was performed, with $p<0.05$ being considered statistically significant.

Results: The median progression-free survival (mPFS) of anlotinib monotherapy used as first-line maintenance treatment of SCLC was 6.3 months (11.7 months in the limited phase and 5.8 months in the extensive phase) and median overall survival (mOS) was 16.7 months (not reached in limited phase, 12.6 months in extensive phase). In second-line treatment, anlotinib with chemotherapy prolonged PFS and OS as compared to anlotinib monotherapy ($p<0.05$). In third-line and above treatment, there was no improvement in mPFS with the chemotherapy combination regimen compared to anlotinib monotherapy (3.6 months vs. 3.8 months, $p=0.398$), with a trend toward impaired mOS (8.5 months vs. not achieved, $p=0.060$). Univariate analyses and multivariate analyses revealed that Eastern Cooperative Oncology Group performance status and liver metastases were independent prognostic factors affecting PFS and OS. No new anlotinib-related adverse reactions were identified.

Conclusion: Anlotinib was effective for first-line maintenance and second-line treatment, and the chemotherapy combination regimen was superior to monotherapy when applied as second-line treatment. However, this trend was not observed in third-line and above therapy.

Keywords: small cell lung cancer, anlotinib, maintenance therapy, second-line treatment, third-line treatment

INTRODUCTION

In recent years, among all cancers, lung cancer has the highest incidence and mortality rate worldwide (1). Small cell lung cancer (SCLC) is an aggressive neuroendocrine tumor, which accounts for approximately 15% of all lung cancers, and its biological and clinical characteristics are completely different from other types of lung cancers. SCLC is more sensitive to chemotherapy, but it easily develops resistance to chemotherapeutic drugs due to the rapid proliferation rate of the tumor. As a result, most patients experience disease progression soon after first-line treatment, and the efficacy of subsequent treatments is low. While the survival of patients with SCLC has improved over the years (2, 3), more safe and efficacious drugs are still urgently needed.

Anlotinib is a multi-targeted small molecule tyrosine kinase inhibitor (TKI) developed independently in China. In its phase II clinical trial ALTER1202, anlotinib was found to significantly prolong progression-free survival (PFS) and overall survival (OS) in third-line and above treatment of SCLC compared with a placebo. The Chinese treatment guidelines for SCLC have since been revised to reflect this new treatment (4). However, in practice, anlotinib is used not only in third-line and above therapies in the treatment of SCLC, but also in first-line maintenance therapy and second-line treatment. In terms of usage, it is rather common to combine chemotherapy, immunotherapy, or other treatments. However, there are few studies on the application of anlotinib in SCLC at the frontline. Therefore, this study aimed to analyze real-world data on anlotinib to evaluate whether anlotinib could provide additional benefits to SCLC patients as first-line maintenance therapy and second-line treatments, as well as whether combination therapy with chemotherapy or immune checkpoint inhibitors (ICIs) could further improve its efficacy.

MATERIALS AND METHODS

Clinical Data

Clinical data of patients with SCLC, treated with anlotinib hospitalized at The First Affiliated Hospital of Zhengzhou University from June 2018 to June 2020, were collected. The main inclusion criteria included: (1) pathologically confirmed SCLC; (2) patients with SCLC receiving first-line maintenance therapy with anlotinib or as second- or third-line after progression on prior therapies and subsequent treatments; (3) at least one observable or measurable lesion according to the Response Evaluation Criteria in Solid Tumors (RECIST) guidelines version 1.1. Those cases with no follow-up data after treatment with anlotinib were excluded. Based on the above criteria, 109 patients with SCLC were included. The study workflow is outlined in **Figure 1**.

Treatment Methods

Anlotinib capsules (Chia Tai Tianqing Pharmaceutical Group Co., Ltd., Approval No.: National Drug Code H20180002) were prescribed in an 8–12 mg dose and taken orally once a day for 2 weeks with a 1-week break. The dose prescribed depended on the patient's age, ECOG PS, and body surface area. The dose could be titrated downwards according to the patient's tolerance post-administration.

Evaluation of Efficacy and Observation Metrics

RECIST version 1.1 was used to evaluate the efficacy of the treatment. Responses were classified as complete response (CR), partial response (PR), stable disease (SD), and progressive disease (PD). The objective response rate (ORR) was calculated as the proportion of patients achieving CR or PR. The disease control rate (DCR) is the proportion of patients who achieved CR, PR, or SD. PFS is defined as the period from when a patient starts oral anlotinib until disease progression or death from any cause. OS is defined as the time from the start of patients receiving anlotinib until death due to any cause. For subjects who were lost to follow-up prior to death, the time of the last follow-up visit was recorded as the time of death.

The classification of drug-related adverse reactions was evaluated and recorded according to the Common Terminology Criteria for Adverse Events (CTCAE) version 4.03.

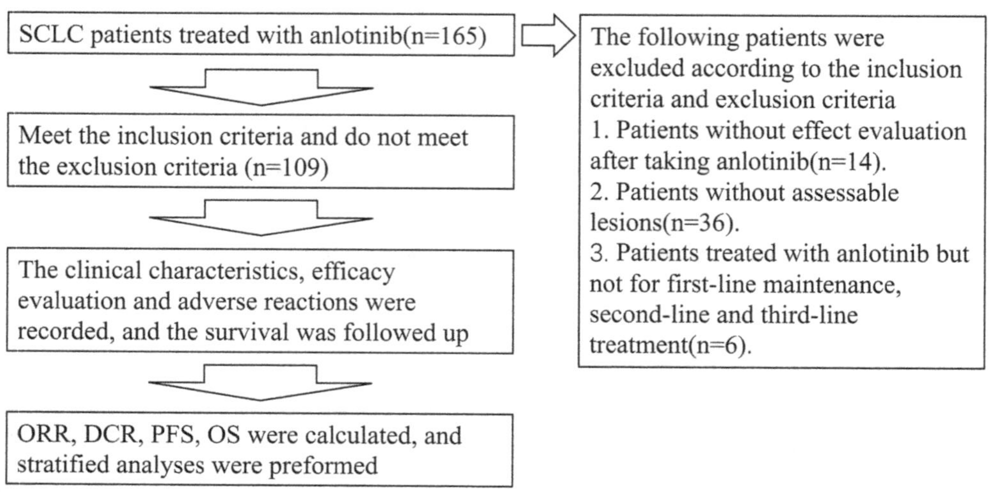

FIGURE 1 | Flow chart.

Follow-Up Visits

The final follow-up visit was conducted up to December 19, 2020, mainly by telephone and outpatient follow-up appointments. The time to disease progression or death was recorded. For the end of follow-up, cases with a follow-up outcome of "loss to follow-up" were considered as censored cases. There were 15 cases lost to follow-up in this study, with a 13.8% loss to follow-up rate and a median follow-up time of 16.7 months (95% CI: 10.3 months to 23.1 months).

Statistical Methods

SPSS version 18.0 was used for statistical analysis. The chi-square test was used for rate comparison, the Kaplan–Meier method was used for survival analysis, log-rank test was used to compare survival time between different groups, and the Cox regression method was used for multivariate analysis. A p-value of <0.05 was considered statistically significant.

RESULTS

Basic Patient Information

Clinical data were collected from 109 patients with SCLC treated with anlotinib. Information on age, sex, smoking history, ECOG PS, clinical staging, metastatic site, combination therapy with anlotinib, therapeutic drugs before and after anlotinib administration, and whether radiotherapy was done was collected. Detailed information is shown in **Table 1**.

TABLE 1 | Patient characteristics at baseline (n=109 cases).

Characteristic	Groups	Value (%)
Gender	Male	79 (72.5%)
	Female	30 (27.5%)
Age	≤65 years	74 (67.9%)
	>65 years	35 (32.1%)
Smoking history	Yes	56 (51.4%)
	No	53 (48.6%)
ECOG PS	0-1	94 (86.2%)
	≥2	15 (13.8%)
Disease extent	Limited	38 (34.9%)
	Extensive	71 (65.1%)
Brain metastases	Yes	31 (28.4%)
	No	78 (71.6%)
Liver metastases	Yes	11 (10.1%)
	No	98 (90.0%)
Treatment lines	Maintenance therapy after 1st line	35 (32.1%)
	2nd line	39 (35.8%)
	≥3rd line	35 (32.1%)
Ki67 index	≥90%	58 (53.2%)
	<90%	42 (38.5%)
	unknown	9 (8.3%)
PFS of 1st-line therapy	≤3 months	8 (7.3%)
	>3 months	101 (92.7%)
ICIs treatment	Yes	35 (32.1%)
	No	74 (67.9%)
Previous radiation therapy	Yes	59 (54.1%)
	No	50 (45.9%)
Previous antiangiogenic treatment	Yes	16 (14.7%)
	No	93 (85.3%)

Short-Term Efficacy

Treatment efficacy was evaluated for all 109 patients enrolled in this study. A total of 35 patients received anlotinib monotherapy as first-line maintenance. A total of 39 patients received anlotinib as second-line treatment with an overall ORR of 17.9% and DCR of 76.9%. Sixteen out of 39 patients received anlotinib monotherapy and 23 were treated with other drugs in combination (including chemotherapy, ICIs, and chemotherapy with ICIs). The ORR and DCR of combination therapy (ORR, 26.1%; DCR, 87%) were improved in comparison with monotherapy (ORR, 6.25%; DCR, 62.5%). However, there was no statistically significant difference (χ^2 value = 4.273, p=0.119). A total of 35 patients received anlotinib as third- and further-line treatment, with an overall ORR of 17.1% and an overall DCR of 85.7%. Twelve of the patients received anlotinib monotherapy, and 23 patients were treated in combination with other treatments (including chemotherapy, ICIs, and local treatment). The ORR and DCR of the combination therapy (ORR, 21.7%; DCR, 87%) were not statistically significant (χ^2 value = 1.010, p=0.750), as detailed in **Table 2**.

Survival Analysis

At the end of follow-up, 78 (71.6%) patients reached disease progression on anlotinib at their last follow-up, with an overall median PFS (mPFS) of 6.3 months. Forty-three patients reached the endpoint of death at their last follow-up, accounting for 39.4% of the total. The overall median OS (mOS) was 10.3 months.

Thirty-five patients with SCLC receiving anlotinib as first-line maintenance therapy (17 patients in the limited phase and 18 patients in the extensive phase) had an mPFS of 6.3 months (11.7 months in the limited phase and 5.8 months in the extensive phase) and an mOS of 16.7 months (not reached in the limited phase and 12.6 months in the extensive phase), as shown in **Figures 2A, B** and **Supplemental Figure 1A, B**.

The mPFS was 7.9 months for second-line treatment with anlotinib and 3.6 months for third-line and above therapy, as shown in **Table 3** and **Figure 2A**. In second-line treatment, mPFS was 5.7 months for the anlotinib monotherapy group (Group A) and 16.5 months for the anlotinib-chemotherapy combination group (Group A+C), with statistically significant difference (χ^2 = 4.208, p=0.04). In third-line and above therapy, mPFS for Group A and Group A+C were 3.8 months and 3.6 months, respectively, with no statistically significant difference (χ^2 = 0.138, p=0.711), as shown in **Figures 3A, C**.

The mOS of anlotinib, when administered in second-line treatment, was better than that of third-line and above therapy (p=0.037), as shown in **Table 3** and **Figure 2B**. In second-line treatment, mOS was not achieved in both the monotherapy and combination groups. The mOS was better in Group A+C than in Group A (χ^2 = 4.214, p=0.040). In third-line and above therapy, mOS was not achieved in Group A, and was 8.5 months in Group A+C (χ^2 = 3.027, p=0.082), as shown in **Figures 3B–D**.

TABLE 2 | Observation of short-term efficacy.

Treatment lines	Cases(n)	Combination therapy	PR	SD	PD	ORR	DCR	Total ORR	Total DCR
2st line	16	None	1	9	6	6.25%	62.5%	17.9%	76.9%
	16	Chemotherapy	2	12	2	12.5%	87.5%		
	5	ICIs	3	1	1	60%	80%		
	2	Chemothrapy & ICIs	1	1	0	50%	100%		
≥3rd line	12	None	1	9	2	8.3%	83.3%	17.1%	85.7%
	14	Chemotherapy	2	11	1	14.3%	92.9%		
	8	ICIs	3	3	2	37.5%	75%		
	1	Interventional therapy	0	1	0		100%		

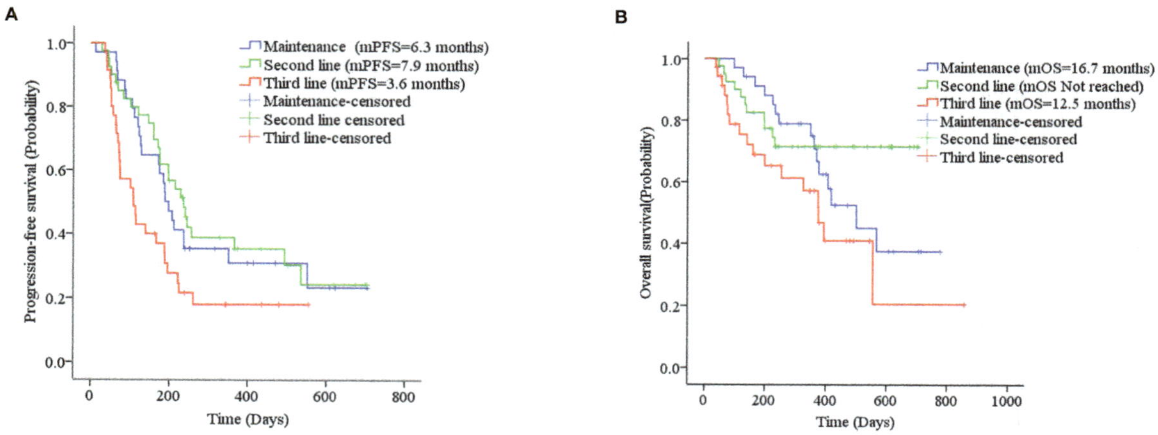

FIGURE 2 | **(A)** Kaplan–Meier plot of PFS among different treatment lines; **(B)** Kaplan–Meier plot of OS among different treatment lines.

TABLE 3 | Univariate survival analysis.

Characteristic	Groups	mPFS (m)	95%CI	χ^2 value	*P value*	mOS (m)	95%CI	χ^2value	*P value*
Gender	Male	6.3	5.6-7.0	0.002	0.969	16.7	3.8-24.1	0.771	0.38
	Female	5.6	2.3-8.9			18.5	NR		
Age	≤65	6.2	5.3-7.1	0.411	0.522	18.9	NR	0.011	0.918
	>65	6.6	4.8-8.5			18.5	9.9-27.1		
Smoking history	Yes	6.2	5.2-7.1	0.085	0.77	18.9	NR	0.029	0.864
	No	6.6	4.9-8.3			16.7	9.8-23.6		
ECOG PS	0-1	6.9	5.8-8.0	22.825	**<0.001**	NR	NR	36.972	**<0.001**
	≥2	2.3	1.8-2.7			4.6	2.4-6.8		
Disease extent	Limited	7.6	4.5-10.7	1.921	0.166	18.9	NR	0.877	0.349
	Extensive	6.2	5.3-7.1			16.7			
Brain metastases	Yes	6.3	4.0-8.5	0.049	0.824	NR	NR	2.053	1.052
	No	6.2	5.0-7.3			16.7	10.1-23.3		
Liver metastases	Yes	3.6	1.7-5.5	13.325	**<0.001**	6.6	3.8-9.4	27.415	**<0.001**
	No	6.6	5.5-7.7			NR	NR		
Treatment lines	Post 1st line maintenance	6.3	5.3-7.3	7.43	**0.024**	16.7	11.3-22.1	5.88	0.053
	2nd line	7.9	6.2-9.6	5.377		NR	NR	4.329	
	≥3 line	3.6	2.1-5.2			12.5	9.8-15.3		
Ki67 index	≥90%	5.9	4.8-6.9	0.19	0.663	16.7	9.6-23.8	0.768	0.381
	<90%	6.3	4.9-7.6			NR	NR		
PFS of 1st-line therapy	≤3 months	6.3	4.0-8.6	0.523	0.47	12.5	NR	0.014	0.906
	>3 months	6.3	5.5-7.1			18.5	NR		
ICIs treatment	Yes	5.9	2.7-9.1	1.659	0.198	12.5	3.8-21.2	2.373	0.123
	No	6.3	5.1-7.5			18.9	NR		
Previous radiation therapy	Yes	6.3	5.8-6.8	0.137	0.712	NR	NR	1.019	0.313
	No	5.7	2.7-8.7			13.9	8.6-19.3		
Previous antiangiogenic treatment	Yes	3.8	0.0-10.0	3.766	0.052	10.9	4.7-17.1	3.821	0.051
	No	6.3	5.3-7.3			18.9	NR		

CI, Confidence Interval; NR, Not Reached. P value less than 0.05 were shown in bold.

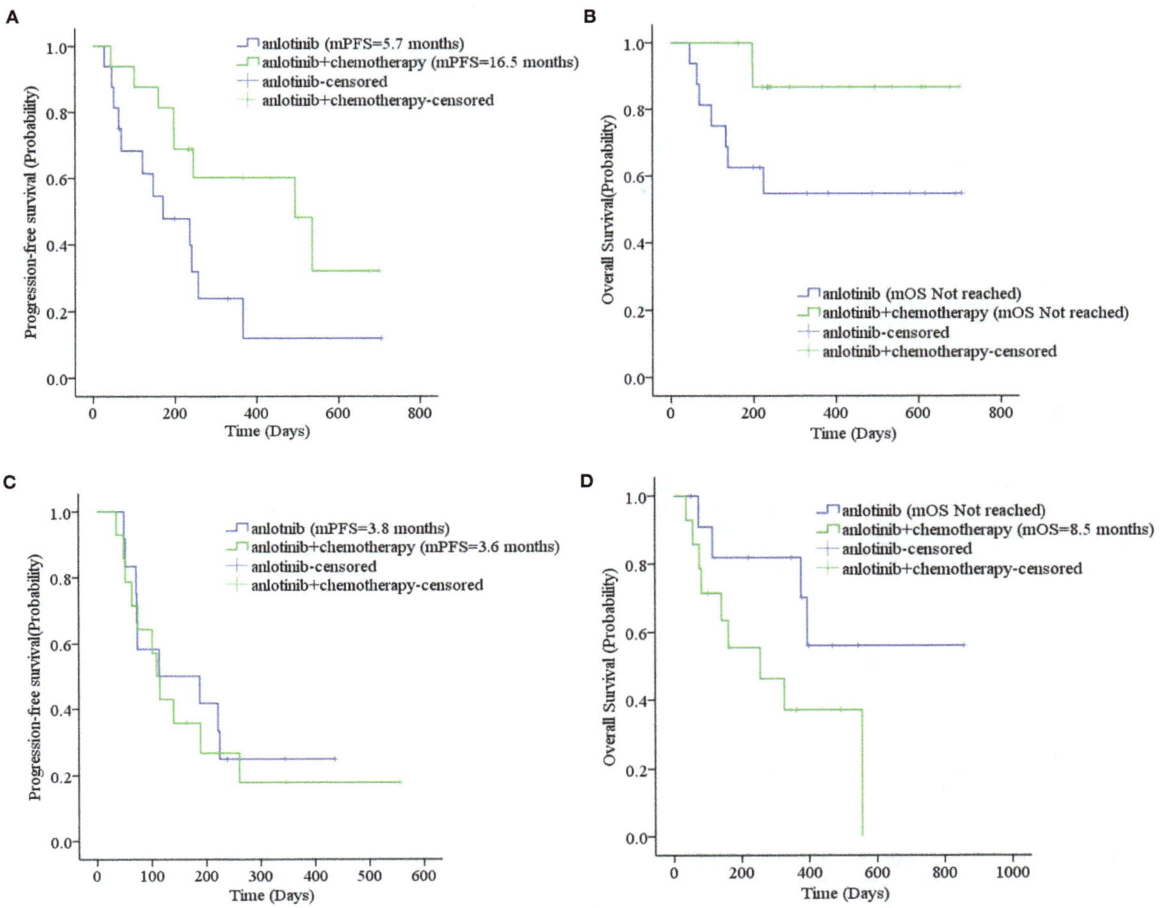

FIGURE 3 | **(A)** Progression-free survival stratified by treatment regimen in second-line therapy; **(B)** Overall survival stratified by treatment regimen in second-line therapy; **(C)** Progression-free survival stratified by treatment regimen in third- and further-line therapy; **(D)** Overall survival stratified by treatment regimen in third- and further-line therapy.

Sixteen patients who had received other anti-angiogenic treatments (including endostatin, bevacizumab, and apatinib) showed some difference in mPFS from those who had not received anti-angiogenic treatment (3.8 months vs. 6.3 months, p=0.052), as shown in **Table 3**. Considering that only one patient had received anti-angiogenic treatment (apatinib) with first-line therapy, we excluded the 35 patients in the first-line maintenance portion when evaluating the effect of anti-angiogenic agents on the efficacy of anlotinib. The PFS was 5.6 months for other patients who had previously used anti-angiogenic therapy compared to 6.3 months for those who had not, with no statistically significant difference (χ^2 = 1.936, p=0.164). There was also no statistically significant difference in mOS (χ^2 = 2.215, p=0.137), as shown in **Supplemental Figures 2A, B**. Eighteen patients were treated by ICIs previously or concomitantly with anlotinib. However, there were no significant differences in PFS (χ^2 = 1.659, p=0.198) and OS (χ^2 = 2.373, p=0.123) according to ICI treatment, as shown in **Table 3** and **Supplemental Figures 2C, D**. Patients with liver metastases and an ECOG PS score ≥2 had worse PFS and OS than the corresponding control group (p<0.001), as shown in **Table 3** and **Figure 4**. Cox regression analysis indicated that patients with ECOG PS ≥2 or liver metastases had a shorter PFS and OS (p<0.001), as shown in **Table 4**.

Evaluation of Drug Safety

Incidences of adverse reactions, such as fatigue, hand and feet reactions, hypertension, elevated ALT/AST, loss of appetite, and proteinuria, during the use of anlotinib were greater than 20%, regardless of severity grade. The incidence of grade 3 and above adverse reactions was 20.2%, and a total of four patients discontinued anlotinib due to intolerable adverse reactions (hemoptysis, elevated ALT/AST, severe thrombocytopenia, and joint pain), as shown in **Table 5**.

DISCUSSION

Angiogenesis is a key component of tumor proliferation and metastasis (5). It was found that vascular endothelial growth

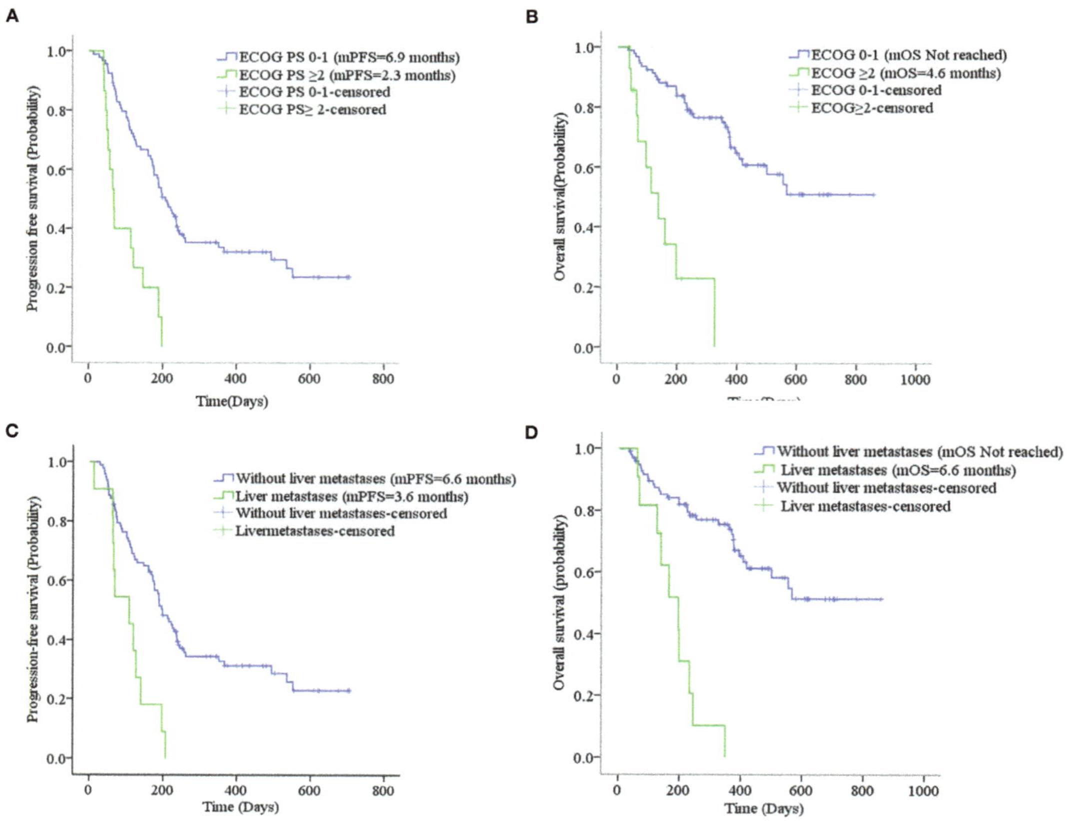

FIGURE 4 | **(A)** Progression-free survival stratified by ECOG PS; **(B)** Overall survival stratified by ECOG PS; **(C)** Progression-free survival stratified by liver metastases; **(D)** Overall survival stratified by liver metastases.

TABLE 4 | Cox regression analysis of PFS and OS.

Groups	PFS			OS		
	p value	HR	95%CI	*p* value	HR	95%CI
Liver metastases: Yes vs No	<0.001	3.769	1.921-7.391	<0.001	9.622	4.203-22.024
ECOG PS: ≥2 vs 0-1	<0.001	3.823	2.027-7.208	<0.001	9.968	4.232-23.479
Treatment lines: ≥3rd line vs 2nd line vs Post 1st line maintenance	0.145	1.258	0.924-1.713	0.225	1.288	0.856-1.936

factor (VEGF) levels were significantly higher in patients with SCLC than in the healthy population (6), suggesting that anti-angiogenic therapy may be effective in SCLC.

Anlotinib is a small molecule anti-angiogenic drug developed independently in China that inhibits tumor neovascularization by regulating VEGF, fibroblast growth factor, and platelet-derived growth factor receptors. It inhibits tumor growth by inhibiting c-Kit, a target related to tumor proliferation, invasion, and migration. Anlotinib has shown good efficacy and safety in lung cancer, soft tissue sarcoma, kidney cancer, and other cancer types (7–9). In the field of SCLC, the ALTER1202 study comparing the efficacy and safety of anlotinib against placebo for third-line and above treatment of SCLC showed that the anlotinib group had significantly better PFS and OS than the placebo group with a favorable safety profile (4, 10).

Maintenance therapy for SCLC is not as well reported. Trials on bevacizumab as first-line and first-line maintenance therapy for SCLC have been conducted; however, bevacizumab only improved PFS and did not prolong OS (11, 12). Sunitinib, a multi-targeted small molecule TKI, prolonged PFS (mPFS 3.7 months vs. 2.1 months, $p=0.02$), but was poorly tolerated and did not exhibit a significant difference in OS (9.0 months vs. 6.9 months, $p=0.16$) when compared to placebo as maintenance therapy after first-line chemotherapy for extensive stage SCLC (13). Studies have also attempted the use of a single chemotherapeutic agent as a first-line maintenance regimen for

TABLE 5 | Incidence of adverse reactions.

Adverse reaction	Any grade (%)	Grade 3/4 (%)
Fatigue	51 (46.8%)	6 (5.5%)
Hand-foot syndrome	41 (37.6%)	2 (1.83%)
Hypertension	35 (32.1%)	2 (1.83%)
ALT/AST elevation	28 (25.7%)	3 (2.8%)
Loss of appetite	26 (23.9%)	3 (2.8%)
Proteinuria	23 (21.1%)	1 (0.9%)
Hemoptysis	17 (15.6%)	3 (2.8%)
Oral mucositis	12 (11.0%)	0 (0%)
Thrombocytopenia	10 (9.2%)	1 (0.9%)
Thrombotic events	3 (2.8%)	1 (0.9%)
Joint pain	2 (1.83%)	0 (0%)
Prolonged Q-T interval	1 (0.9%)	0 (0%)

treatment, but the choice of irinotecan, topotecan, or etoposide did not significantly improve OS (14–16). In this study, 35 patients receiving anlotinib as first-line maintenance therapy were enrolled and all were treated with etoposide in combination with platinum as first-line chemotherapy. The mPFS for maintenance therapy with anlotinib in extensive stage SCLC was 5.8 months, and the mOS exceeded 1 year at 12.6 months.

Second-line treatment options are relatively limited for SCLC. Topotecan monotherapy is the standard second-line treatment regimen of SCLC (17). The PFS of relapsed SCLC treated with amrubicin or EP regimen rechallenge were 3.5 and 4.7 months respectively, which were better than that of the topotecan control groups (2.2 and 2.7 months respectively) (18, 19). ICIs such as nivolumab did not improve survival when compared with chemotherapy in relapsed SCLC (20, 21). In this study, the mPFS for second-line treatment with an anlotinib-containing regimen was 7.9 months. The PFS and OS of anlotinib-chemotherapy combination were significantly prolonged compared with anlotinib monotherapy. In third-line and above treatment, there was no benefit to PFS and even an impaired OS for the anlotinib-chemotherapy combination as compared to anlotinib monotherapy. Anlotinib-containing regimens may be an alternative for relapsed SCLC. However, the benefit of chemotherapy combination was greater in the second-line application of anlotinib, not in third-line and above applications. Therefore, it appears that different regimen designs should be chosen at different treatment times.

In a univariate analysis, liver metastasis and ECOG PS score were found to be prognostic factors for PFS and OS, which was consistent with previous studies (22). We also found that prior anti-angiogenic therapy did not affect the efficacy of anlotinib. Unfortunately, no synergistic effect of ICIs on anlotinib was observed in the study.

The incidence of common adverse effects and adverse reactions to anlotinib in this study were similar to those reported previously (4), suggesting that although anlotinib was often combined with other therapeutic agents in actual clinical application, there was no significant increase in the incidence of anlotinib-related adverse reactions.

In summary, we found further evidence for the use of anlotinib in first-line maintenance and second-line therapy, providing a new option for relapsed SCLC. In addition, we found that anlotinib had added benefit in combination with chemotherapy in second-line therapy; this was not observed in third-line therapy. This suggests that the formulation of individualized treatment plans will be of great help in improving the efficacy of SCLC treatment. However, the results should be validated by a randomized controlled prospective study.

AUTHOR CONTRIBUTIONS

This study was conceived, designed, and interpreted by HF and JY. JY performed the data analyses and drafted the manuscript; FC contributed significantly to analysis and manuscript preparation; GX and XW helped perform the analysis with constructive discussions. All authors read and approved the final manuscript.

ACKNOWLEDGMENTS

We would like to thank Editage (www.editage.cn) for English language editing.

SUPPLEMENTARY MATERIAL

Supplementary Figure 1 | (A) Progression-free survival stratified by clinical stage of SCLC when anlotinib was used as first-line maintenance regimen. **(B)** Overall survival stratified by clinical stage of SCLC when anlotinib was used as first-line maintenance regimen.

Supplementary Figure 2 | (A) Progression-free survival stratified by previous antiangiogenic treatment; **(B)** Overall survival stratified by previous antiangiogenic treatment; **(C)** Progression-free survival stratified by ICIs treatment; **(D)** Overall survival stratified by ICIs treatment.

REFERENCES

1. Bray F, Ferlay J, Soerjomataram I, Siegel RL, Torre LA, Jemal A. Global Cancer Statistics 2018: GLOBOCAN Estimates of Incidence and Mortality Worldwide for 36 Cancers in 185 Countries. *CA: Cancer J Clin* (2018) 68 (6):394–424. doi: 10.3322/caac.21492
2. Rudin CM, Poirier JT. Small-Cell Lung Cancer in 2016: Shining Light on Novel Targets and Therapies. *Nat Rev Clin Oncol* (2017) 14(2):75–6. doi: 10.1038/nrclinonc.2016.203
3. Gazdar AF, Bunn PA, Minna JD. Small-Cell Lung Cancer: What We Know, What We Need to Know and the Path Forward. *Nat Rev Cancer* (2017) 17(12):725–37.
4. Cheng Y, Wang Q, Li K, Shi J, Wu L, Han B, et al. OA13.03 Anlotinib as Third-Line or Further-Line Treatment in Relapsed SCLC: A Multicentre, Randomized, Double-Blind Phase 2 Trial. *J Thorac Oncol* (2018) 13(10):S351–2. doi: 10.1016/j.jtho.2018.08.308
5. Folkman J. Role of Angiogenesis in Tumor Growth and Metastasis. *Semin Oncol* (2002) 29(6 Suppl 16):15–8. doi: 10.1053/sonc.2002.37263
6. Tas F, Duranyildiz D, Oguz H, Camlica H, Yasasever V, Topuz E. Serum Vascular Endothelial Growth Factor (VEGF) and Interleukin-8 (IL-8) Levels in Small Cell Lung Cancer. *Cancer Invest* (2006) 24(5):492–6. doi: 10.1080/07357900600814771

7. Han B, Li K, Zhao Y, Li B, Cheng Y, Zhou J, et al. Anlotinib as a Third-Line Therapy in Patients With Refractory Advanced non-Small-Cell Lung Cancer: A Multicentre, Randomised Phase II Trial (ALTER0302). *Br J Cancer* (2018) 118(5):654–61. doi: 10.1038/bjc.2017.478
8. Chi Y, Fang Z, Hong X, Yao Y, Sun P, Wang G, et al. Safety and Efficacy of Anlotinib, a Multikinase Angiogenesis Inhibitor, in Patients With Refractory Metastatic Soft-Tissue Sarcoma. *Clin Cancer Res* (2018) 24(21):5233–8. doi: 10.1158/1078-0432.ccr-17-3766
9. Zhou AP, Bai Y, Song Y, Luo H, Ren XB, Wang X, et al. Anlotinib Versus Sunitinib as First-Line Treatment for Metastatic Renal Cell Carcinoma: A Randomized Phase II Clinical Trial. *Oncol Aug* (2019) 24(8):e702–8. doi: 10.1634/theoncologist.2018-0839
10. Cheng Y, Wang Q, Li K, Shi J, Liu Y, Wu L, et al. Overall Survival (OS) Update in ALTER 1202: Anlotinib as Third-Line or Further-Line Treatment in Relapsed Small-Cell Lung Cancer (SCLC). *Ann Oncol* (2019) 10/01:30. doi: 10.1093/annonc/mdz264.002
11. Roviello G, Sobhani N, Generali D. Bevacizumab in Small Cell Lung Cancer. *Ann Trans Med* (2017) 5(17):361. doi: 10.21037/atm.2017.06.44
12. Kalemkerian GP, Schneider BJ. Advances in Small Cell Lung Cancer. *Hematology/oncol Clinics North America* (2017) 31(1):143–56. doi: 10.1016/j.hoc.2016.08.005
13. Ready NE, Pang HH, Gu L, Otterson GA, Thomas SP, Miller AA, et al. Chemotherapy With or Without Maintenance Sunitinib for Untreated Extensive-Stage Small-Cell Lung Cancer: A Randomized, Double-Blind, Placebo-Controlled Phase II Study-CALGB 30504 (Alliance). *J Clin Oncol* (2015) 33(15):1660–5. doi: 10.1200/jco.2014.57.3105
14. Han JY, Kim HT, Lim KY, Yoon SJ, Lee DH, Lee JS. Randomized Phase II Study of Maintenance Irinotecan Therapy Versus Observation Following Induction Chemotherapy With Irinotecan and Cisplatin in Extensive Disease Small Cell Lung Cancer. *J Thorac Oncol* (2008) 3(9):1039–45. doi: 10.1097/JTO.0b013e3181834f8e
15. Hanna NH, Sandier AB, Loehrer PJ C.OMMAS.R.X.X.X., Ansari R, Jung SH, Lane K, et al. Maintenance Daily Oral Etoposide Versus No Further Therapy Following Induction Chemotherapy With Etoposide Plus Ifosfamide Plus Cisplatin in Extensive Small-Cell Lung Cancer: A Hoosier Oncology Group Randomized Study. *Ann Oncol* (2002) 13(1):95–102. doi: 10.1093/annonc/mdf014
16. Schiller JH, Adak S, Cella D, DeVore RF3rd, Johnson DH. Topotecan Versus Observation After Cisplatin Plus Etoposide in Extensive-Stage Small-Cell Lung Cancer: E7593–a Phase III Trial of the Eastern Cooperative Oncology Group. *J Clin Oncol* (2001) 19(8):2114–22. doi: 10.1200/jco.2001.19.8.2114
17. O'Brien ME, Ciuleanu TE, Tsekov H, Shparyk Y, Cuceviá B, Juhasz G, et al. Phase III Trial Comparing Supportive Care Alone With Supportive Care With Oral Topotecan in Patients With Relapsed Small-Cell Lung Cancer. *J Clin Oncol* (2006) 24(34):5441–7. doi: 10.1200/jco.2006.06.5821
18. Inoue A, Sugawara S, Yamazaki K, Maemondo M, Suzuki T, Gomi K, et al. Randomized Phase II Trial Comparing Amrubicin With Topotecan in Patients With Previously Treated Small-Cell Lung Cancer: North Japan Lung Cancer Study Group Trial 0402. *J Clin Oncol* (2008) 26(33):5401–6. doi: 10.1200/jco.2008.18.1974
19. Baize N, Monnet I, Greillier L, Geier M, Lena H, Janicot H, et al. Carboplatin Plus Etoposide Versus Topotecan as Second-Line Treatment for Patients With Sensitive Relapsed Small-Cell Lung Cancer: An Open-Label, Multicentre, Randomised, Phase 3 Trial. *Lancet Oncol* (2020) 21(9):1224–33. doi: 10.1016/s1470-2045(20)30461-7
20. Spigel DR, Vicente D, Ciuleanu TE, Gettinger S, Peters S, Horn L, et al. Second-Line Nivolumab in Relapsed Small-Cell Lung Cancer: CheckMate 331 (☆). *Ann Oncol* (2021) 32(5):631–41. doi: 10.1016/j.annonc.2021.01.071
21. Ragavan M, Das M. Systemic Therapy of Extensive Stage Small Cell Lung Cancer in the Era of Immunotherapy. *Curr Treat Options Oncol* (2020) 21(8):64. doi: 10.1007/s11864-020-00762-8
22. Zhang K, Ma X, Gao H, Wang H, Qin H. Efficacy and Safety of Anlotinib in Advanced Non-Small Cell Lung Cancer. *A Real-World Study* (2020) 12:3409–17. doi: 10.2147/cmar.s246000

20

Pembrolizumab Plus Chemotherapy or Anlotinib *vs.* Pembrolizumab Alone in Patients with Previously Treated EGFR-Mutant NSCLC

Ya Chen[‡], Zhengyu Yang[‡], Yanan Wang[‡], Minjuan Hu, Bo Zhang, Yanwei Zhang, Fangfei Qian, Wei Zhang[†] and Baohui Han[*†]*

Department of Pulmonary, Shanghai Chest Hospital, Shanghai Jiao Tong University, Shanghai, China

***Correspondence:**
Baohui Han
18930858216@163.com
Wei Zhang
zhweui2002@hotmail.com*

[†]These authors have contributed equally to this work

[‡]These authors share first authorship

Objectives: More and more encouraging evidence revealed that immunotherapy could improve clinical outcomes in patients with previously treated non-small cell lung cancer (NSCLC) with epidermal growth factor receptor (EGFR) variations. However, immunotherapy is still a controversy for NSCLC patients with EGFR mutation.

Method: In this retrospective analysis, we compared the clinical efficacy of pembrolizumab monotherapy (PM), pembrolizumab combined with chemotherapy (P+C) and pembrolizumab combined with anlotinib (P+A) in NSCLC patients with EGFR mutation who had failed on EGFR-TKI and platinum-based chemotherapy.

Result: Eighty-six patients were included in this study. The overall median progression free survival (PFS) was 3.24 months. Multivariate analysis suggested that $EGFR^{L858R}$ and combined therapy were positive prognostic factors of PFS. The overall median OS was 12.28 months. Multivariate analysis found that high PD-L1 expression (≥50%) and combined therapy seemed to be positive prognostic factors of OS. Among the population, 32 patients received PM, 26 patients received P+C and 28 patients received P+A. Up to Jan 30, 2021, the median progression-free survival was 1.5 months in the PM group, 4.30 months in the P+C group and 3.24 months in the P+A group. The median OS were 7.41, 14.92 and 15.97 months, respectively. The ORR were 3.1%, 23.1% and 21.4%.

Conclusion: The addition of chemotherapy or antiangiogenic therapy to pembrolizumab resulted in significantly longer PFS, OS and ORR than pembrolizumab alone in our study. $EGFR^{L858R}$ might be a positive prognostic factor of PFS and high PD-L1 expression might be a positive prognostic factor of OS.

Keywords: non-small cell lung cancer, pembrolizumab, epidermal growth factor receptor, antiangiogenic agent, chemotherapy

INTRODUCTION

Targeted therapy has revolutionized the treatment landscape for patients with non-small cell lung cancer (NSCLC) with epidermal growth factor receptor (EGFR) mutations. Treatment with EGFR-TKIs, which have been developed to the third generation, provides better disease control and longer survival for patients with EGFR mutations (1). At the same time, screening for PD-L1 expression has become standard practice with the rise of immunotherapy. Of interest, the presence of EGFR mutations has been reported to upregulate the expression of PD-L1 (2–7). However, several studies have revealed that high PD-L1 expression predicted poor response to EGFR-TKIs in patients with EGFR-mutant NSCLC and correlated with primary resistance to EGFR-TKIs (8–10). Nevertheless, EGFR-TKIs have shown overwhelming advantages over standard chemotherapy in patients with EGFR-mutant NSCLC. EGFR-TKIs are recommended as the first-line treatment in this population according to the NCCN guidelines. However, treatment options after the development of TKI resistance need to be further explored. Given the growing emphasis on molecular profiling and detection of PD-L1, more detailed treatment guidance is needed for the critical population of patients with advanced NSCLC with both high PD-L1 and EGFR mutations.

Recently, the use of immune checkpoint inhibitors (ICIs) has greatly altered the standard of care for patients with advanced NSCLC without targetable EGFR or ALK genetic aberrations depending on the patient's PD-L1 expression level. However, immunotherapy is still a controversial for patients with EGFR mutations because several clinical studies, including Checkmate057, Keynote010, POPLAR and OAK, have revealed that immunotherapy failed to improve clinical outcomes in patients with advanced NSCLC with EGFR mutations (11–15). However, the final OS data of the ATLANTIC trial showed that durvalumab improved clinical activity across all cohorts in patients with previously treated advanced NSCLC, including those with EGFR mutations (16). In addition, JAMA oncol reported that the combination of pembrolizumab plus docetaxel improved clinical outcomes in patients with previously treated NSCLC with EGFR variations (17). Furthermore, the ABCP group in the IMPOWER150 trial also prolonged the OS of patients with sensitive EGFR mutations (18). These encouraging results underline the necessity for further investigation into immunotherapy in patients with NSCLC with EGFR mutations. In this study, we collected the clinical records of patients with NSCLC with EGFR mutations who received pembrolizumab at our institution, including pembrolizumab monotherapy (PM), pembrolizumab combined with chemotherapy (P+C) and pembrolizumab combined with anlotinib (P+A). Anlotinib is an antiangiogenic agent that inhibiting VEGFR, FGFR, and PDGFR and has been approved by China National Medical Products Administration (NMPA) (19). In addition, it has been proved to be effective in NSCLC patients with EGFR mutations (20). In this study, we explored the efficacy of PD-1 in previously treated NSCLC patients with EGFR mutation.

MATERIAL AND METHODS

Patients

The medical records of patients with advanced NSCLC with EGFR mutations received pembrolizumab treatment at the Shanghai Chest Hospital between Dec 1, 2017 and Oct 30, 2020 were screened. Eighty-six patients met the following inclusion criteria: (1) stage IV NSCLC (2) positive EGFR mutation [exon 19 deletion mutation ($EGFR^{D19}$), exon 21 L858R mutation ($EGFR^{L858R}$), secondary exon 20 T790M mutation and other uncommon sensitive mutation such as G719X, L861R] (3) patients had disease progressed with at least 1 approved EGFR-TKI (patients with 20T790M mutation must had failed on osimertinib) and platinum-based chemotherapy following standard treatment guideline; (4) patients received PM, P+C or P+A (5) Eastern Cooperative Oncology Group performance status (ECOG PS) 0-1. Therapeutic schedule was decided by physician under the principle that patients at high risk of bleeding should not be treated with P+A, patients with severe adverse effects to previous chemotherapy should not chose P+C as priority. This study was approved by the Institutional Review Board of Shanghai Chest Hospital and performed following the declaration of Helsinki.

Treatment and Clinical Response Evaluation

Among the three groups (PM, P+C and P+A), pembrolizumab was administered 200mg intravenously every 3 weeks. Chemotherapy was administrated following the standard NCCN guidelines. Chemotherapy regimens included docetaxel combined with carboplatin (DC) and nab-paclitaxel combined with carboplatin (TC). Antiangiogenic agent was anlotinib (given orally, 8mg once daily on days 1–14 of a 21-day cycle). Disease stage was decided on the 8th edition of the American Joint Committee on Cancer (AJCC) tumor-node-metastasis (TNM) classification. Enhanced chest computed tomography (CT) scan and abdominal ultrasound scan were examined every 4 weeks for therapeutic response evaluation. Enhanced brain magnetic resonance imaging (MRI) was examined every 4-6 months if no lesion at baseline and no symptoms thereafter. The response was evaluated according to the Response Evaluation Criteria in Solid Tumors (RECIST) version 1.1.

Detection of Gene and Programmed Death Ligand 1 (PD-L1) Tumor Proportion Score (TPS)

The tissue sample was biopsied at the time of disease diagnosis and disease progression. EGFR detection was performed by the amplification refractory mutation system (ARMS) or by next generation sequencing (NGS). PD-L1 expression was assessed at the time of disease progression, right before the initiation of immunotherapy. TPS was detected by the PD-L1 IHC 22C3 pharmDx assay and was classified into TPS<0, 1-49% and ≥50%.

Statistical Analysis

The χ2 test was used for comparison of categorical variables. The primary endpoints were PFS (from immunotherapy initiation to disease progression or the last follow-up); OS (from immunotherapy initiation to death or the last follow-up) and ORR (the ratio of complete and partial response). The median PFS and OS was estimated using the Kaplan-Meier method and compared by the log-rank test. Hazard ratios (HR) and 95% confidence intervals were estimated by a stratified Cox proportional-hazards model. To avoid the influence of confounding factors, factors with p values less than 0.1 in univariate analysis were included in multivariate analysis. All statistical analyses were performed using SPSS version 22.0 (IBM Corporation, Armonk, NY, USA).

RESULTS

Clinical Features

Eighty-six patients who met the eligibility criteria were included in this study. Of these, most patients were male (55.8%) and non-smoker (52.3%) and had received third or more lines of therapy (**Table 1**). 17 patients (19.8%) had brain metastasis. The most common EGFR mutation type was $EGFR^{L858R}$ (54.6%), followed by $EGFR^{D19}$ (25.6%), uncommon sensitive mutation (10.5%) and T790M (9.3%). 75 patients were screened for PD-L1 expression levels immediately before immunotherapy, 17 (19.8%) of whom had a TPS of 0%, 32 (37.2%) of whom had a TPS of 1-49% and 26 (30.2%) of whom had a TPS of 50% or greater.

Progression-Free Survival

PD occurred in 64 (74.4%) patients in the overall population, including 26 (81.3%) patients in PM group, 12 (46.2%) patients in P+C group and 26 (92.9%) patients in P+A group. The overall median PFS was 3.24 months (95% CI: 2.46–4.02) (**Figure 1A**). Univariate analysis found that brain metastasis (p = 0.024), PD-L1 expression [p (1-49% vs 0) = 0.027, p (≥50% vs 0) =0.004)] and therapy [p (P+C vs PM) <0.001, p (P+A vs PM) = 0.002)] were associated with PFS (**Table 2**). Multivariate analysis found that patients with $EGFR^{L858R}$ had longer PFS than those with $EGFR^{D19}$ (p=0.024), patients in P+C group (p<0.001) and P+A group (p<0.001) had longer PFS than those in PM group (**Table 2**). These results suggested that EGFR mutation type and treatments were independent prognostic factors of PFS.

Overall Survival

Death occurred in 35 (40.7%) patients in the overall population, including 18 (56.3%) patients in PM group, 6

TABLE 1 | Clinicopathological characteristics of 86 EGFR-mutated patients treated with pembrolizumab.

Characteristics	Number	Percent (%)
Age(median age, Range)	62(39-80)	-
Sex		
Male	48	55.8%
Female	38	44.2%
Smoking history		
Yes	41	47.7%
No	45	52.3%
Recurrence after surgery		
Yes	39	45.3%
No	47	54.7%
Treatment line of PD-1 Inhibitors		
Second line	4	4.7%
Third or after line	82	95.3%
Brain metastasis		
Yes	17	19.8%
No	69	80.2%
PD-L1 TPS		
<1%	17	19.8%
1~49%	32	37.2%
≥50%	26	30.2%
Unknown	11	12.8%
EGFR mutation subtype		
19del	22	25.6%
21L858R	47	54.6%
T790M	8	9.3%
Other	9	10.5%
Treatment		
PM	32	37.2%
P+C	26	30.2%
P+A	28	32.6%

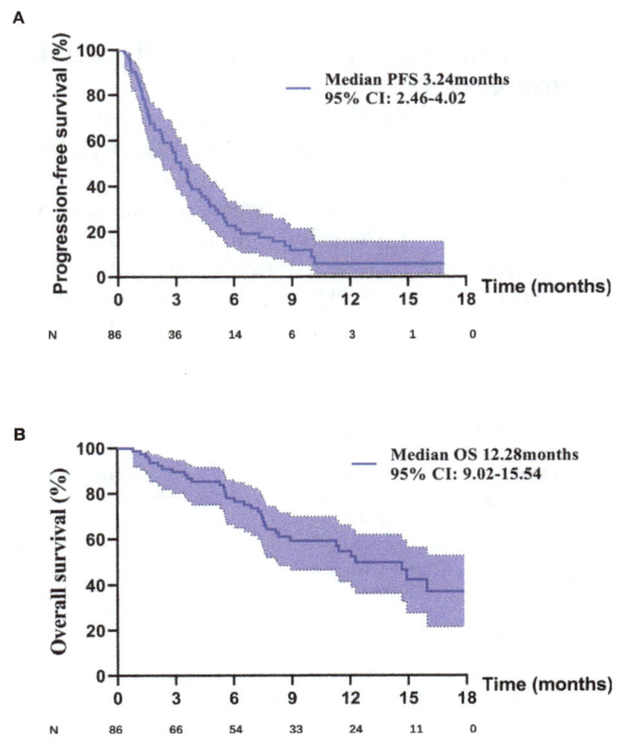

FIGURE 1 | **(A)** The PFS curve of overall patients. **(B)** The OS curve of overall patients.

TABLE 2 | Univariate and multivariable analyses for covariables associated with progression free survival.

Characteristics	Category	Univariate analysis HR (95 %CI)	p	Multivariate analysis HR (95 %CI)	p
Age	≤65 vs >65 years	0.71 (0.43-1.19)	0.194		
Sex	Male vs female	0.88 (0.53-1.46)	0.630		
Smoking history	Yes vs no	1.43 (0.88-2.35)	0.153		
Treatment line	Second line vs posterior line	1.15 (0.36-3.68)	0.814		
Brain	Yes vs No	1.40 (1.05-1.87)	0.024	0.74 (0.39-1.41)	0.361
PD-L1 expression	1-49% vs 0	0.46 (0.23-0.92)	0.027	0.47 (0.22-1.03)	0.058
	≥50% vs 0	0.33 (0.16-0.70)	0.004	0.46 (0.21-1.02)	0.057
	Unknown vs 0	0.71 (0.32-1.61)	0.414	0.60 (0.25-1.42)	0.246
EGFR mutation	21L858R vs 19del	0.60 (0.33-1.09)	0.092	0.41 (0.19-0.90)	0.024
	T790M vs 19del	0.83 (0.33-2.11)	0.691	0.47 (0.17-1.26)	0.133
	Others vs 19del	0.47 (0.19-1.14)	0.095	0.38 (0.14-1.04)	0.059
Therapy	I+C vs IM	0.22 (0.11-0.45)	<0.001	0.16 (0.07-0.37)	<0.001
	I+A vs IM	0.41 (0.23-0.73)	0.002	0.31 (0.16-0.57)	<0.001
	I+C vs I+A	0.53 (0.27-1.06)	0.071	0.55 (0.25-1.19)	0.126

(23.1%) patients in P+C group and 11 (39.3%) patients in P+A group. The overall median OS was 12.28 months (95% CI: 9.02–15.54) (**Figure 1B**). Univariate analysis found that PD-L1 expression [p (≥50% vs 0) =0.007)] and therapy [p (P+C vs PM) =0.021, p (P+A vs PM) =0.020)] were associated with OS (**Table 3**). Multivariate analysis, including brain metastasis, PD-L1 expression and therapy, found that patients with high PD-L1 expression (≥50%) had longer OS than those with negative expression (p=0.039), patients in P+C group (p=0.035) and P+A group (p=0.019) had longer OS than those in PM group (**Table 3**). Hence, high PD-L1 expression and combined therapy seemed to be positive prognostic factors of OS.

Survival Analysis of Patients in Different Therapy Group

We divided the patients into three groups according to the therapy they received (32 patients in PM group, 26 patients in P+C group and 28 patients in P+A group). The baseline characteristics among the three groups were shown in **Table 4**. There were no statistically significant differences in characteristics among the three groups, indicating that no large selection bias existed. The median PFS was 1.5 months (95% CI: 1.19-1.81) in the PM group, 4.30 months (95% CI: 3.21-5.39) in the P+C group and 3.24 (95% CI: 0.96-5.52) months in the P+A group (**Figure 2A**). The median OS of PM, P+A and P+C were 7.41 (95% CI: 4.30-10.52), 14.92 (95% CI: 9.75-20.09) and 15.97 (9.57-22.37) months, respectively (**Figure 2B**). P+C group showed a significant PFS and OS benefit over PM group (p<0.001 and p=0.021). P+A group also revealed a significant PFS and OS benefit over PM group (p=0.002 and p=0.020). The ORR of PM, P+C and P+A group were 3.1%, 23.1% and 21.4% (**Figure 3**). The difference of objective tumor response showed us the superiority of combined therapy over monotherapy [P+C vs PM (p=0.038), P+A vs PM (p=0.041)]. The DCR were 40.6%, 42.3% and 64.3%.

Subgroup Analysis of Patients in P+C and P+A Group

Survival analysis, including PFS, OS and ORR had demonstrated the superiority of combination therapy (P+C and P+A) over monotherapy (PM). However, no significant difference was found between P+C and P+A. We conducted a subgroup analysis of the patients in the P+C and P+A groups to determine the specific characteristics of each treatment. The subgroup analysis of the PFS showed that patients of

TABLE 3 | Univariate and multivariable analyses for covariables associated with overall survival.

Characteristics	Category	Univariate analysis HR (95 %CI)	p	Multivariate analysis HR (95 %CI)	p
Age	≤65 vs >65 years	0.65 (0.32-1.22)	0.168		
Sex	Male vs female	0.67 (0.33-1.35)	0.264		
Smoking history	Yes vs No	1.50 (0.76-2.96)	0.242		
Treatment line	Second line vs posterior line	0.47 (0.14-1.54)	0.211		
Brain	No vs Yes	0.51 (0.24-1.09)	0.082	1.31 (0.88-1.93)	0.180
PD-L1 expression	1-49% vs 0	0.64 (0.30-1.59)	0.339	0.94 (0.35-2.48)	0.895
	≥50% vs 0	0.22 (0.07-0.67)	0.007	0.30 (0.10-0.94)	0.039
	Unknown vs 0	1.74 (0.67-4.55)	0.257	2.27 (0.84-6.15)	0.107
EGFR mutation	21L858R vs 19del	0.79 (0.36-1.72)	0.557		
	T790M vs 19del	0.83 (0.32-4.32)	0.802		
	Others vs 19del	0.58 (0.18-1.86)	0.361		
Therapy	I+C vs IM	0.34 (0.13-0.85)	0.021	0.35 (0.13-0.93)	0.035
	I+A vs IM	0.41 (0.19-0.87)	0.020	0.40 (0.19-0.86)	0.019
	I+C vs I+A	0.82 (0.30-2.23)	0.700	0.88 (0.31-2.46)	0.807

<65years old (HR=0.32, 95%CI: 0.11-0.95), male patients (HR=0.25, 95%CI: 0.09-0.70), patients that relapsed after surgery (HR=0.25, 95%CI: 0.08-0.78) and patients with EGFR^{D19} (HR=0.20, 95%CI: 0.05-0.78) preferred P+C to P+A (**Figure 4A**). However, no difference was found in OS subgroup analysis (**Figure 4B**).

DISCUSSION

To our knowledge, this is the first study to directly compare the efficacy of PD-1 inhibitor monotherapy, PD-1 inhibitor plus chemotherapy and PD-1 inhibitor plus antiangiogenic agents in patients with previously treated advanced NSCLC with EGFR mutations. In this retrospective study, the addition of chemotherapy or anlotinib to pembrolizumab resulted in significantly prolonger PFS, OS and ORR compared with pembrolizumab alone. The median PFS and OS of the whole population in the present study were 3.24 and 12.28 months, respectively. Of interest, the univariate analysis and multivariate analysis found that combined therapies (P+C and P+A) were positive prognostic factors for both the PFS and OS.

The feasibility of immunotherapy for patients with EGFR mutation has long been controversial. A phase II study (NCT02879994) of pembrolizumab in TKI naive patients with EGFR mutations, advanced NSCLC and PD-L1-positive tumors was suspended due to lack of efficacy, which indicating that pembrolizumab was not suitable as a first-line treatment in this population (21). Besides, Checkmate057, Keynote010, POPLAR and OAK trials showed us the poor efficacy of PD-1/PD-L1 monotherapy in patients with EGFR mutations who had progressed after platinum-based doublet chemotherapy and treatment with EGFR-TKIs (12–15). However, the final overall survival update of the ATLANTIC trial demonstrated a promising OS benefit across all cohorts, especially in patients with EGFR mutations (16). The median OS of patients with NSCLC with EGFR mutations (TPS ≥ 25%) was 16.1 months, which was longer than that observed in patients with TPS ≥ 25% EGFR −/ALK− tumors (median OS of 10.9 months) (16). Of note, the median PFS and OS following PM treatment in our cohort were 1.50 and 7.41 months, respectively, which was consistent with the Keynote010 trial and failed to copy the success of ATLANTIC. This might be due to the difference between PD-1 inhibitors and PD-L1 inhibitors (12).

Recently, Christian et al. reported the results of a phase II clinical trial evaluating the effect of ICI (pembrolizumab) plus

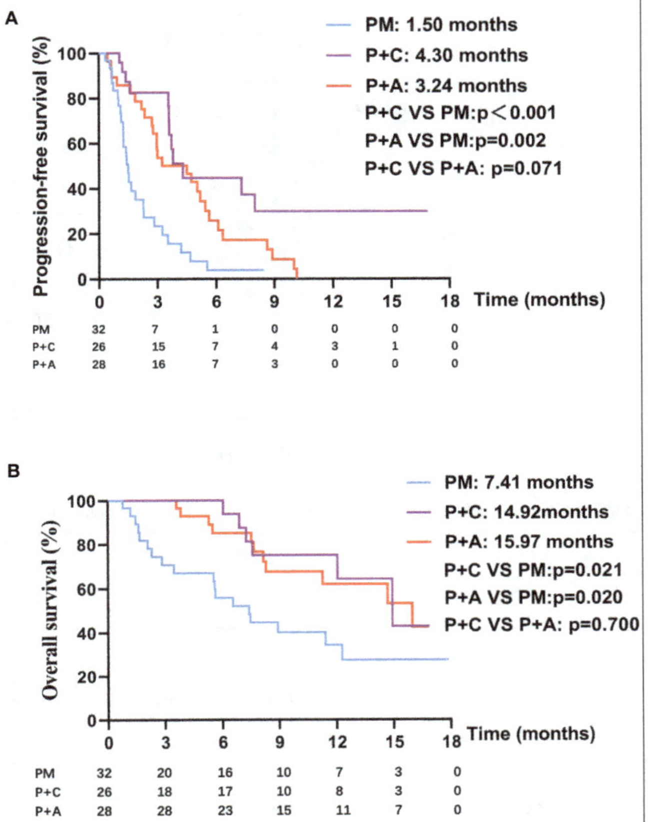

FIGURE 2 | **(A)** The PFS curve of patients in PM, P+C and P+A groups. **(B)** The OS curve of patients in PM, P+C and P+A groups.

TABLE 4 | Clinicopathological characteristics of all patients with different treatments.

Characteristics	Monotherapy (N=17) (%)	With chemotherapy (N=15) (%)	With anlotinib (N=14) (%)	p value
Age				
Median, range	61(39-80)	66(54-78)	59 (41-78)	0.081
Sex				0.763
Male	19 (59.4)	13 (50.0)	16 (57.1)	
Female	13 (40.6)	13 (50.0)	12 (42.9)	
Smoking history				0.471
Yes	18 (56.2)	11 (42.3)	12 (42.9)	
No	14 (43.8)	15 (57.7)	16 (57.1)	
Recurrence after surgery				0.800
Yes	16 (50.0)	11 (42.3)	12 (42.9)	
No	16 (50.0)	15 (57.7)	16 (57.1)	
Treatment line of PD-1 Inhibitors				0.862
Second line	2 (6.3)	1 (3.8)	1 (3.6)	
Third/after line	30 (93.7)	25 (96.2)	27 (96.4)	
Brain metastasis				0.700
Yes	6 (18.8)	5 (19.2)	6 (21.4)	
No	26 (81.2)	21 (80.8)	22 (78.6)	
PD-L1 TPS				0.131
<1%	8 (25.0)	1 (3.8)	8 (28.6)	
1~49%	13 (40.6)	13 (50.0)	6 (21.4)	
≥50%	9 (28.1)	8 (30.8)	9 (32.1)	
Unknown	2 (6.3)	4 (15.4)	5 (17.9)	
EGFR mutation subtype				0.152
19del	5 (1.6)	6 (23.1)	11 (39.3)	
21L858R	21 (65.6)	17 (65.4)	9 (32.1)	
T790M	3 (9.4)	1 (3.8)	4 (14.3)	
Others	3 (9.4)	2 (7.7)	4 (14.3)	

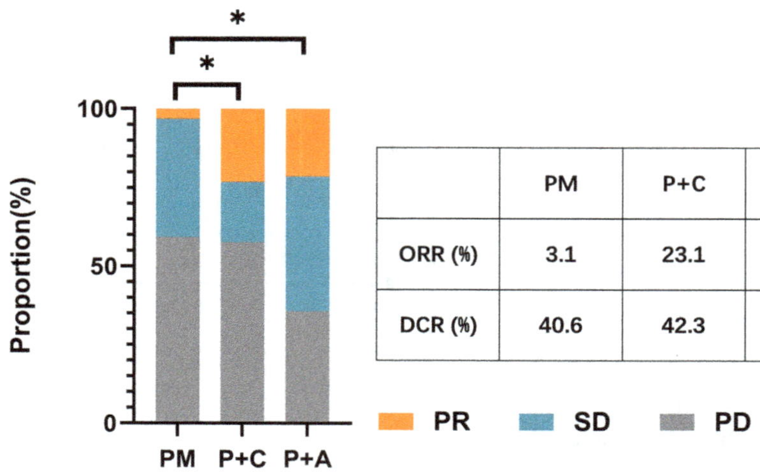

	PM	P+C	P+A	p
ORR (%)	3.1	23.1	21.4	0.031*
DCR (%)	40.6	42.3	64.3	0.576

FIGURE 3 | The ORR and DCR of patients in PM, P+C and P+A groups. * represents a statistically significant difference.

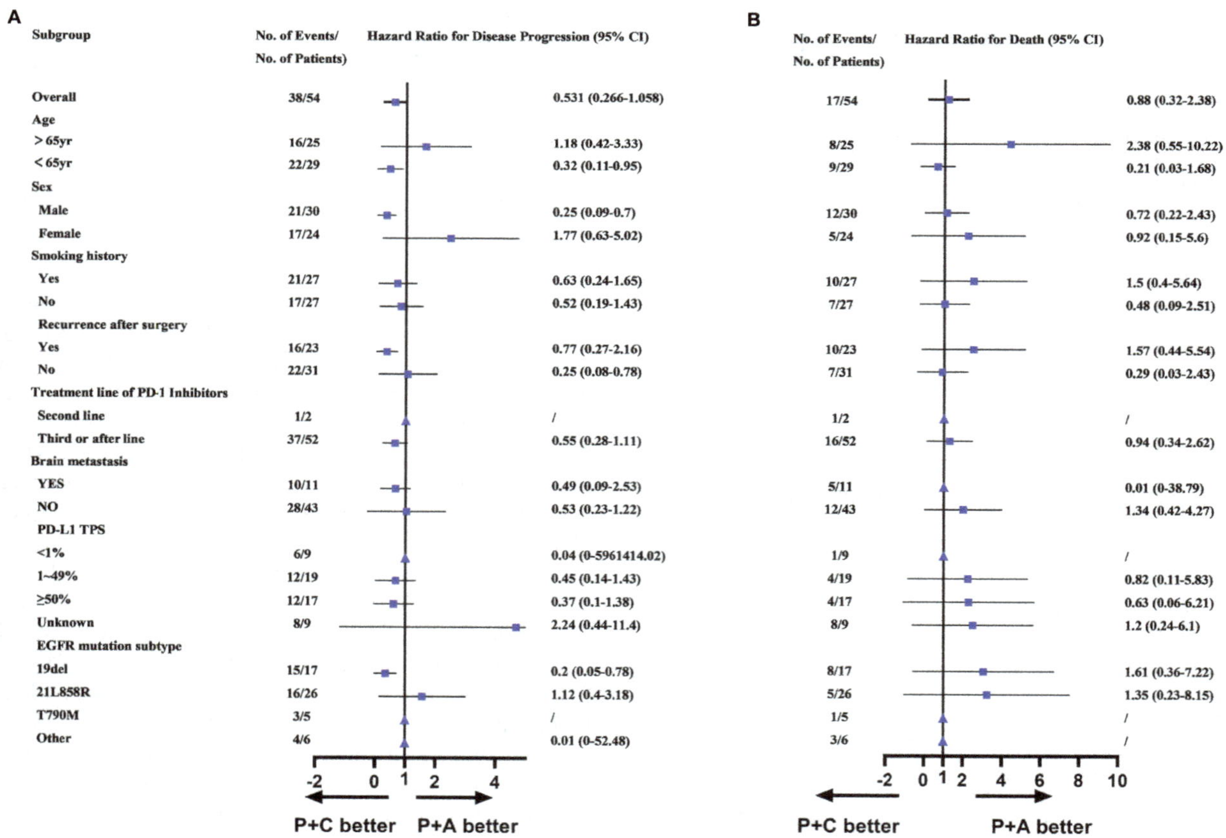

FIGURE 4 | **(A)** Subgroups analysis of PFS in P+C and P+A groups. **(B)** Subgroups analysis of OS in P+C and P+A groups. (▲Represented HR cannot be calculated due to the sample.

chemotherapy (docetaxel) vs chemotherapy (docetaxel) alone in previously treated patients with advanced NSCLC, including patients with sensitizing EGFR mutations who had experienced disease progression after platinum-based chemotherapy. For patients with EGFR variations, the PFS (6.8 vs 3.5 months) and ORR (58.3% vs 23.1%) were statistically significantly different in favor of the combination arm, which highlighted the efficacy of the combination of immunotherapy and chemotherapy. Similarly, another phase II study of immunotherapy (toripalimab) plus chemotherapy in patients with EGFR-mutant advanced NSCLC patients found that the combined treatment yielded encouraging PFS (7.0 months) and ORR (50%) (22). In our cohort, the median PFS and ORR of P+C treatment were 4.30 months and 23.1%, respectively. Our cohort's PFS rate and ORR were lower than those reported in the aforementioned, which probably because our patients were more heavily treated. Nevertheless, our study verified the benefit of the combination treatment.

The IMPOWER150 trial revealed encouraging PFS and OS following immunotherapy, albeit in a combination therapy pattern, in patients with NSCLC with EGFR mutations (18, 23). The OS was greater in the ABCP arm (29.4 months) than in the BCP arm (18.1 months) but the difference was not statistically significant (HR, 0.60; 95% CI, 0.31-1.14), which might be due to the study's small sample size, which might due to the small sample (24). In contrast, the IMPOWER130 trial revealed no significant PFS or OS benefit for patients with EGFR and ALK alterations. This difference in results highlighted the necessity of antiangiogenic agents and supported the hypothesis that antiangiogenic agents could enhance immune efficacy, which might be due to the remarkable improvement of antigen-specific T-cell migration, in patients with NSCLC with EGFR mutations in response to antiangiogenic treatment (25). Similarly, the combination of ICIs and antiangiogenic agents in our cohort also yielded greater PFS (HR, 0.41; 95% CI, 0.23-0.73) and OS (HR, 0.41; 95% CI, 0.19-0.87) than ICIs alone. Meanwhile, Zhai et al. found that anlotinib combined with PD-1 inhibitors showed promising efficacy as a third- or further-line treatment for NSCLC (26). The combination treatment achieved a median OS of 17.3 months, which was similar to the OS of 15.97 months in the P+A group in our cohort. This encouraging result suggested that the combination of immunotherapy and antiangiogenic agents might overcome the barriers associated with immunotherapy for patients with EGFR- mutant NSCLC patients.

Our study demonstrated the superiority of combination therapy (pembrolizumab plus anlotinib or pembrolizumab plus chemotherapy) intuitively. However, was found in the survival analysis between the group that received P+A and the group that received P+C. Future research studies with a larger sample size are needed to define the subgroups of patients to determine precise treatment strategies.

Hastings, K. et al. found that different EGFR mutation subtypes responded to ICIs differently (27). $EGFR^{L858R}$ resulted in longer PFS and OS than $EGFR^{D19}$, which might be due to the higher tumor mutation burden (TMB) in the $EGFR^{L858R}$ group. Consistent with the previous findings, our multivariate analysis in our study also found that $EGFR^{L858R}$ was associated with a longer PFS than $EGFR^{D19}$ (HR:0.41, p=0.024). However, no OS benefit of $EGFR^{L858R}$ was found, which might be due to the small sample size.

There is no doubt that the expression level of PD-L1 is correlated with the efficacy of pembrolizumab in patients with NSCLC without EGFR mutations (28). Meanwhile, several studies have found that patients with EGFR mutations and PD-L1+ were more likely to respond to ICI monotherapy or ICI plus chemotherapy than those who were PD-L1 negative (22, 29, 30). However, some studies did not address the problem that chemotherapy and EGFR-TKIs might affect the expression of PD-L1. Hence, we utilized the tumor samples that were re-biopsied immediately before immunotherapy to detect PD-L1 expression to reduce bias (31, 32). We assessed the relationship between the efficacy of ICIs and PD-L1 expression and revealed that patients with PD-L1≥50% had longer OS than the OS of the PD-L1 negative group (HR:0.30, p=0.039).

Our study is limited by its retrospective nature. First, the data was collected from one center and the sample size was relatively small. Also, selection bias existed inevitable due to unavoidable missing data. However, the baseline clinical characteristics of patients in the PM, P+C and P+A group were balanced well, indicating that no large selection bias existed. Additionally, the heterogeneity of PD-L1 expression within tumors was inevitably existed though all detection were performed under guideline.

In summary, our analysis revealed that pembrolizumab plus chemotherapy or antiangiogenic agents could significantly prolong the PFS, OS and ORR compared with those observed following treatment with pembrolizumab alone in previously treated patients with advanced NSCLC with EGFR mutations. Our findings highlight the efficacy of the combination strategy of immunotherapy in this specific population. We also found that immunotherapy might be a more promising therapeutic agent for patients with $EGFR^{L858R}$ and patients with PD-L1≥50%. Based on the current findings, we hold the opinion that relevant clinical trials are urgently needed. The efficacy and safety of immunotherapy plus chemotherapy or antiangiogenic therapy in patients with EGFR-mutant NSCLC, especially those with high PD-L1 expression, should be further explored in clinical trials that provide strong evidence-based medicine data.

AUTHOR CONTRIBUTIONS

YC, ZY, and YW have substantial contributions to the conception or design of the work, the collection and analysis of data, and the writing and editing of the article. The rest authors have given substantial contributions to the work by providing editing and writing assistance. All authors contributed to the article and approved the submitted version.

ACKNOWLEDGMENTS

The authors thank all the patients and their families for their contributions to this study.

REFERENCES

1. Remon J, Ahn MJ, Girard N, Johnson M, Kim DW, Lopes G, et al. Advanced-Stage Non-Small Cell Lung Cancer: Advances in Thoracic Oncology 2018. *J Thorac Oncol* (2019) 14(7):1134–55. doi: 10.1016/j.jtho.2019.03.022
2. Chen N, Fang W, Zhan J, Hong S, Tang Y, Kang S, et al. Upregulation of PD-L1 by EGFR Activation Mediates the Immune Escape in EGFR-Driven NSCLC: Implication for Optional Immune Targeted Therapy for NSCLC Patients with EGFR Mutation. *J Thorac Oncol* (2015) 10(6):910–23. doi: 10.1097/JTO.0000000000000500
3. Liu J, Liu Y. Molecular diagnostic characteristics based on the next generation sequencing in lung cancer and its relationship with the expression of PD-L1. *Pathol Res Pract* (2020) 216(2):152797. doi: 10.1016/j.prp.2019.152797
4. Soo RA, Lim SM, Syn NL, Teng R, Soong R, Mok TSK, et al. Immune checkpoint inhibitors in epidermal growth factor receptor mutant non-small cell lung cancer: Current controversies and future directions. *Lung Cancer* (2018) 115:12–20. doi: 10.1016/j.lungcan.2017.11.009
5. Tung JN, Lin PL, Wang YC, Wu DW, Chen CY, Lee H. PD-L1 confers resistance to EGFR mutation-independent tyrosine kinase inhibitors in non-small cell lung cancer via upregulation of YAP1 expression. *Oncotarget* (2018) 9(4):4637–46. doi: 10.18632/oncotarget.23161
6. Yoneshima Y, Ijichi K, Anai S, Ota K, Otsubo K, Iwama E, et al. PD-L1 expression in lung adenocarcinoma harboring EGFR mutations or ALK rearrangements. *Lung Cancer* (2018) 118:36–40. doi: 10.1016/j.lungcan.2018.01.024
7. Dietel M, Savelov N, Salanova R, Micke P, Bigras G, Hida T, et al. Real-world prevalence of programmed death ligand 1 expression in locally advanced or metastatic non-small-cell lung cancer: The global, multicenter EXPRESS study. *Lung Cancer* (2019) 134:174–9. doi: 10.1016/j.lungcan.2019.06.012
8. Hsu KH, Huang YH, Tseng JS, Chen KC, Ku WH, Su KY, et al. High PD-L1 expression correlates with primary resistance to EGFR-TKIs in treatment naive advanced EGFR-mutant lung adenocarcinoma patients. *Lung Cancer* (2019) 127:37–43. doi: 10.1016/j.lungcan.2018.11.021
9. Su S, Dong ZY, Xie Z, Yan LX, Li YF, Su J, et al. Strong Programmed Death Ligand 1 Expression Predicts Poor Response and De Novo Resistance to EGFR Tyrosine Kinase Inhibitors Among NSCLC Patients With EGFR Mutation. *J Thorac Oncol* (2018) 13(11):1668–75. doi: 10.1016/j.jtho.2018.07.016
10. Dong ZY, Zhang JT, Liu SY, Su J, Zhang C, Xie Z, et al. EGFR mutation correlates with uninflamed phenotype and weak immunogenicity, causing impaired response to PD-1 blockade in non-small cell lung cancer. *Oncoimmunology* (2017) 6(11):e1356145. doi: 10.1080/2162402x.2017.1356145
11. Matsumoto Y, Koh Y. Tumor immune microenvironment of EGFR-mutant non-small-cell lung cancer and its impact on therapeutic efficacy. *Immunotherapy* (2020) 12(7):431–7. doi: 10.2217/imt-2019-0213
12. Herbst RS, Baas P, Kim DW, Felip E, Perez-Gracia JL, Han JY, et al. Pembrolizumab versus docetaxel for previously treated, PD-L1-positive, advanced non-small-cell lung cancer (KEYNOTE-010): a randomised controlled trial. *Lancet* (2016) 387(10027):1540–50. doi: 10.1016/S0140-6736(15)01281-7
13. Borghaei H, Paz-Ares L, Horn L, Spigel DR, Steins M, Ready NE, et al. Nivolumab versus Docetaxel in Advanced Nonsquamous Non-Small-Cell Lung Cancer. *N Engl J Med* (2015) 373(17):1627–39. doi: 10.1056/NEJMoa1507643
14. Rittmeyer A, Barlesi F, Waterkamp D, Park K, Ciardiello F, von Pawel J, et al. Atezolizumab versus docetaxel in patients with previously treated non-small-cell lung cancer (OAK): a phase 3, open-label, multicentre randomised controlled trial. *Lancet* (2017) 389(10066):255–65. doi: 10.1016/S0140-6736(16)32517-X
15. Fehrenbacher L, Spira A, Ballinger M, Kowanetz M, Vansteenkiste J, Mazieres J, et al. Atezolizumab versus docetaxel for patients with previously treated non-small-cell lung cancer (POPLAR): a multicentre, open-label, phase 2 randomised controlled trial. *Lancet* (2016) 387(10030):1837–46. doi: 10.1016/S0140-6736(16)00587-0
16. Garassino MC, Cho BC, Kim JH, Mazières J, Vansteenkiste J, Lena H, et al. Final overall survival and safety update for durvalumab in third- or later-line advanced NSCLC: The phase II ATLANTIC study. *Lung Cancer* (2020) 147:137–42. doi: 10.1016/j.lungcan.2020.06.032
17. Arrieta O, Barron F, Ramirez-Tirado LA, Zatarain-Barron ZL, Cardona AF, Diaz-Garcia D, et al. Efficacy and Safety of Pembrolizumab Plus Docetaxel vs Docetaxel Alone in Patients With Previously Treated Advanced Non-Small Cell Lung Cancer: The PROLUNG Phase 2 Randomized Clinical Trial. *JAMA Oncol* (2020) 6(6):856–64. doi: 10.1001/jamaoncol.2020.0409
18. Reck M, Mok TSK, Nishio M, Jotte RM, Cappuzzo F, Orlandi F, et al. Atezolizumab plus bevacizumab and chemotherapy in non-small-cell lung cancer (IMpower150): key subgroup analyses of patients with EGFR mutations or baseline liver metastases in a randomised, open-label phase 3 trial. *Lancet Respir Med* (2019) 7(5):387–401. doi: 10.1016/s2213-2600(19)30084-0
19. Zhou M, Chen X, Zhang H, Xia L, Tong X, Zou L, et al. China National Medical Products Administration approval summary: anlotinib for the treatment of advanced non-small cell lung cancer after two lines of chemotherapy. *Cancer Commun (London England)* (2019) 39(1):36. doi: 10.1186/s40880-019-0383-7
20. Han B, Li K, Wang Q, Zhang L, Shi J, Wang Z, et al. Effect of Anlotinib as a Third-Line or Further Treatment on Overall Survival of Patients With Advanced Non-Small Cell Lung Cancer: The ALTER 0303 Phase 3 Randomized Clinical Trial. *JAMA Oncol* (2018) 4(11):1569–75. doi: 10.1001/jamaoncol.2018.3039
21. Lisberg A, Cummings A, Goldman JW, Bornazyan K, Reese N, Wang T, et al. A Phase II Study of Pembrolizumab in EGFR-Mutant, PD-L1+, Tyrosine Kinase Inhibitor Naive Patients With Advanced NSCLC. *J Thorac Oncol* (2018) 13(8):1138–45. doi: 10.1016/j.jtho.2018.03.035
22. Zhou C. A multi-center phase II study of toripalimab with chemotherapy in patients with EGFR mutant advanced NSCLC patients resistant to EGFR TKIs: Efficacy and biomarker analysis. *J Clin Oncol* (2020) 38(suppl; abstr e21618). doi: 10.1200/JCO.2020.38.15_suppl.e21618
23. Socinski MA, Jotte RM, Cappuzzo F, Orlandi F, Stroyakovskiy D, Nogami N, et al. Atezolizumab for First-Line Treatment of Metastatic Nonsquamous NSCLC. *N Engl J Med* (2018) 378(24):2288–301. doi: 10.1056/NEJMoa1716948
24. Socinski MA, Mok TS, Nishio M, Jotte RM, Cappuzzo F, Orlandi F, et al. Abstract CT216: IMpower150 final analysis: Efficacy of atezolizumab (atezo) + bevacizumab (bev) and chemotherapy in first-line (1L) metastatic nonsquamous (nsq) non-small cell lung cancer (NSCLC) across key subgroups. *Cancer Res* (2020) 80(16 Supplement):CT216–CT. doi: 10.1158/1538-7445.Am2020-ct216
25. Wallin JJ, Bendell JC, Funke R, Sznol M, Korski K, Jones S, et al. Atezolizumab in combination with bevacizumab enhances antigen-specific T-cell migration in metastatic renal cell carcinoma. *Nat Commun* (2016) 7:12624. doi: 10.1038/ncomms12624
26. Zhai C, Zhang X, Ren L, You L, Pan Q, Pan H, et al. The Efficacy and Safety of Anlotinib Combined With PD-1 Antibody for Third-Line or Further-Line Treatment of Patients With Advanced Non-Small-Cell Lung Cancer. *Front Oncol* (2021) 10:619010. doi: 10.3389/fonc.2020.619010
27. Hastings K, Yu HA, Wei W, Sanchez-Vega F, DeVeaux M, Choi J, et al. EGFR mutation subtypes and response to immune checkpoint blockade treatment in non-small-cell lung cancer. *Ann Oncol* (2019) 30(8):1311–20. doi: 10.1093/annonc/mdz141
28. Aguilar EJ, Ricciuti B, Gainor JF, Kehl KL, Kravets S, Dahlberg S, et al. Outcomes to first-line pembrolizumab in patients with non-small-cell lung cancer and very high PD-L1 expression. *Ann Oncol* (2019) 30(10):1653–9. doi: 10.1093/annonc/mdz288

29. Liu SY, Dong ZY, Wu SP, Xie Z, Yan LX, Li YF, et al. Clinical relevance of PD-L1 expression and CD8+ T cells infiltration in patients with EGFR-mutated and ALK-rearranged lung cancer. *Lung Cancer* (2018) 125:86–92. doi: 10.1016/j.lungcan.2018.09.010
30. Haratani K, Hayashi H, Tanaka T, Kaneda H, Togashi Y, Sakai K, et al. Tumor immune microenvironment and nivolumab efficacy in EGFR mutation-positive non-small-cell lung cancer based on T790M status after disease progression during EGFR-TKI treatment. *Ann Oncol* (2017) 28(7):1532–9. doi: 10.1093/annonc/mdx183
31. Lacour M, Hiltbrunner S, Lee SY, Soltermann A, Rushing EJ, Soldini D, et al. Adjuvant Chemotherapy Increases Programmed Death-Ligand 1 (PD-L1) Expression in Non-small Cell Lung Cancer Recurrence. *Clin Lung Cancer* (2019) 20(5):391–6. doi: 10.1016/j.cllc.2019.05.013
32. Kim TJ, Hong SA, Kim O, Kim SJ, Yang JH, Joung EK, et al. Changes in PD-L1 expression according to tumor infiltrating lymphocytes of acquired EGFR-TKI resistant EGFR-mutant non-small-cell lung cancer. *Oncotarget* (2017) 8 (64):107630–9. doi: 10.18632/oncotarget.22582

21

Efficacy and Safety of Anti-PD-1 Plus Anlotinib in Patients with Advanced Non–Small-Cell Lung Cancer after Previous Systemic Treatment Failure

Peiliang Wang [1,2], *Xiaozhuang Fang* [1,3], *Tianwen Yin* [1,2], *Hairong Tian* [1,2], *Jinming Yu* [1,2] *and Feifei Teng* [1,2]*

[1] Department of Radiation Oncology, Shandong Cancer Hospital and Institute, Cheeloo College of Medicine, Shandong University, Jinan, China, [2] Department of Radiation Oncology, Shandong Cancer Hospital and Institute, Shandong First Medical University and Shandong Academy of Medical Sciences, Jinan, China, [3] Department of Hepatobiliary Surgery, Shandong Cancer Hospital and Institute, Cheeloo College of Medicine, Shandong University, Jinan, China

***Correspondence:**
Feifei Teng
tengfeifei16@126.com

Background: Pre-clinical and clinical evidences support that simultaneous blockade of programmed death-1 (PD-1) and vascular endothelial growth factor receptor (VEGFR) can enhance antigen-specific T-cell migration, and show tolerable toxicity with favorable antitumor activity in patients. In this study, we aimed to assess the safety and efficacy of anlotinib, a novel multitarget tyrosine kinase inhibitor for VEGFR, platelet-derived growth receptor (PDGFR), and the stem cell-factor receptor (c-Kit), combined with anti-PD-1 treatment in patients with advanced NSCLC.

Methods: Sixty-seven patients with previously treated advanced NSCLC receiving anti-PD-1 agents concomitant with anlotinib were retrospectively enrolled in an IRB approved study. Anti-PD-1 agents including pembrolizumab, nivolumab, camrelizumab, toripalimab, sintilimab, and tislelizumab were administered every two or three weeks until disease progression or unacceptable toxicity was reached. Anlotinib was administered orally once daily on days 1–14 of a 21-day cycle. The safety and tolerability of the combination treatment were assessed by the incidence of adverse events. The efficacy of the treatment was assessed by the tumor response and survival.

Results: With a median follow-up period of 8.7 months, treatment-related adverse events occurred in 85% (57/67) of patients and grade 3–4 adverse events were observed in 27 patients (40%). No unexpected adverse events or significantly increased toxicities were observed. Complete response was not observed, 19 patients had partial response (28.4%), 39 had stable disease (58.2%) and 9 had progressive disease (13.4%). The overall response (ORR) and disease control rates (DCR) were 28.4% and 86.6%, respectively. The median progression-free survival (PFS) was 6.9 months (95% CI, 5.5-8.3 months) and overall survival (OS) was 14.5 months (95% CI, 10.9-18.1 months). The benefit of anti-PD-1 plus anlotinib was also observed in patients with EGFR mutation positive, liver metastases and brain metastases.

Conclusion: Anti-PD-1 treatment concomitant with anlotinib has tolerable toxicity and favorable antitumor activity in patients with previously treated advanced NSCLC. Our results add to the growing evidence that supports the benefits of combining immunotherapy with antiangiogenic drugs. This combination could be further evaluated with or without chemotherapy, since no additional toxicity was observed in the combination treatment.

Keywords: anlotinib, anti-PD-1, non–small cell lung cancer, combination therapy, immune checkpoint inhibitors

INTRODUCTION

Tumors can evade immune-mediated killing through the interaction between PD-L1 mainly expressed by themselves and PD-1, the inhibitory receptor primarily located on tumor infiltrating T cells, which leads to T cell exhaustion. Immune checkpoint inhibitors (ICIs) targeting the PD-L1–PD-1 axis have shown superior survival outcomes compared with cytotoxic chemotherapies in patients with advanced non–small cell lung cancer (NSCLC) (1–3). Several ICIs targeting PD-1 have been approved by the U.S. Food and Drug Administration (FDA) for the clinical treatment of advanced NSCLC, including durvalumab as consolidation treatment in stage III NSCLC patients (4), pembrolizumab(PD-L1≥1) as a single agent or combined with chemotherapy for first-line treatment of patients with metastatic NSCLC (5, 6), nivolumab, pembrolizumab or atezolizumab as second-line treatment in advanced NSCLC (1, 7, 8). Despite anti-PD-1 or anti-PD-L1 clinical trials producing unprecedented positive clinical outcomes, responses are achieved only in about 20% of unselected patients (8, 9), highlighting the need to identify novel combination treatments that broaden the benefit of anti-PD-1/PD-L1 therapies.

Abnormal tumor vasculature might be one of the mechanisms of resistance to immunotherapy. It can exert immunosuppressive effects including the inhibition the maturation of dendritic cells (DCs), the prevention of T cells infiltration into tumors, and the induction of regulating cells (Tregs) and Myeloid-Derived Suppressor Cells (MDSCs) (10, 11). Substantial data has accumulated showing that antiangiogenic therapies targeting the vascular endothelial growth factor (VEGF) or VEGF receptor-2 (VEGFR-2) can modulate the tumor immunosuppressive microenvironment and might help to reverse resistance to immunotherapy (12–14). A translational study, in Colon-26 adenocarcinoma model, shows that simultaneous blockade of PD-1 and VEGFR enhance ICI-induced effects such as reinforcement of antigen presentation and increase of T cells infiltration (15). In a phase Ia/b trial that assessed the preliminary antitumor activity of ramucirumab (anti-VEGFR2 antibody) combined with pembrolizumab in NSCLC patients, 30% of the patients achieved an objective response, with a median PFS of 9.7 months and a median OS of 26.2 months (16). In a phase III study, a benefit was seen in patients with chemotherapy-naive NSCLC when treated with atezolizumab plus bevacizumab with chemotherapy versus bevacizumab with chemotherapy (OS: HR, 0.78 [95% CI 0.62–0.96]; ORR, 64% vs. 48%, respectively) (17), suggesting the clinical benefit of combining anti-angiogenetics with checkpoint blockades.

Anlotinib (AL3818) hydrochloride is a novel small-molecule inhibitor targeting multiple receptor tyrosine kinases involved in tumor angiogenesis, proliferative signaling and tumor microenvironment (18, 19). Anlotinib mainly inhibits VEGF/VEGFR signaling by selectively targeting VEGFR-2,-3 and the fibroblast growth factor receptors (FGFR-1,-2,-3,-4), and also suppresses the activity of the platelet-derived growth factor receptors α/β (PDGFRα/β), c-FMS c-Kit, Aurora-B, and discoidin domain receptor 1 (DDR1) (20). In phase 3 of the ALTER randomized clinical trial, anlotinib has shown antitumor activity as ≥ 3 lines of treatment in patients with advanced NSCLC, with a prolonged median overall survival (OS) versus placebo (9.6 months for anlotinib vs 6.3 months for placebo; P =0.002) (21). Anlotinib also shows encouraging efficacy and a manageable toxicity in a broad range of malignancies, including soft tissue sarcoma (Clinical Trials.gov: NCT01878448), medullary thyroid cancer (Clinical Trials.gov: NCT01874873), and renal cell cancer (Clinical Trials.gov: NCT02072044). According to the results, anlotinib received its first approval as a third-line treatment for advanced NSCLC and its second approval as a second-line treatment for advanced soft-tissue sarcoma in the People's Republic of China. At present, although preclinical trials have shown that the combined antiangiogenic and anti-PD-1 therapy has a positive application prospect, the safety and efficacy of anlotinib combined with anti-PD-1 are still unknown.

This study is intended to evaluate the antitumor activity and safety of anti-PD-1 plus anlotinib in advanced NSCLC. We also explored the clinical efficacy of the combination treatments in key subgroups of patients, including patients with EGFR mutations and patients with baseline liver metastases.

METHODS

Patient Selection and Procedures

We retrospectively enrolled patients with histologically confirmed advanced NSCLC who experienced disease progression after ≥1 systemic treatment. An Eastern Cooperative Oncology Group (ECOG) performance status of 0–2 and measurable disease based on Response Evaluation Criteria in Solid Tumors (RECIST) version 1.1 were also required.

Patients received one of the following anti-PD-1 agents until disease progression, clinical deterioration, or unacceptable toxicity: sintilimab (Innovent Biologics, China), toripalimab (Shangha Merck & Co.), camrelizumab (Jiangsu Hengrui Medicine, China), nivolumab (Bristol-Myers Squibb, USA), pembrolizumab (Merck & Co., USA), or tislelizumab (BeiGene, China). Anlotinib (Chia Tai Tianqing Pharmaceutical, China) was administered orally, once daily (8 mg, 10 mg or 12 mg) on days 1–14 of a 21-day cycle.

The authors are accountable for all aspects of the work in ensuring that questions related to the accuracy or integrity of any part of the work are appropriately investigated and resolved. The study was conducted in accordance with the Declaration of Helsinki (as revised in 2013). The study was approved by the Research Ethics Board of Shandong Cancer Hospital, and individual consent for this retrospective analysis was waived.

Outcomes

Safety and tolerability was evaluated throughout the study using the National Cancer Institute Common Terminology Criteria for Adverse Events, version 4.0. Measurable disease was assessed and documented before initiating treatment and at least one imaging follow-up had been scheduled for each patient. Radiological assessments of target and non-target lesions were performed every six weeks during the treatment phase until confirmation of disease progression was made. Tumor response was evaluated using RECIST 1.1. Objective tumor responses included complete response (CR), partial response (PR), stable disease (SD), and progressive disease (PD). Progression-free survival (PFS) denoted the time between the first anti-PD-1 dosing day and the documented progression or mortality from any cause. Overall survival (OS) denoted the time between the first anti-PD-1 dosing day and mortality or the last follow-up.

Statistical Analyses

Survival analyses were performed using the Kaplan-Meier method and the comparison of survival times was performed using the log-rank test. Univariate and multivariate analyses were conducted using the Cox proportional hazards model to analyze factors associated with treatment response and survival. Covariates with p values <0.1 on univariate analyses were incorporated in the multivariate model, which was constructed using the enter method. All other statistical analyses were performed using SPSS 24.0 (IBM, Armonk, NY, USA), and a p-value of <0.05 was considered statistically significant.

RESULTS

Patients and Treatment

A total of 67 consecutive patients were enrolled between August, 2018 and September, 2020. Baseline demographic and clinical characteristics are listed in **Table 1**. The median age was 60 years (range: 33 to 77 years), and 47 of the patients (70%) were males. More than three quarters of the patients (56 patients, 84%) were diagnosed as having stage IV and more than half of the patients (38 patients, 57%) had >3 metastatic sites. 41 patients (61%) were diagnosed with adenocarcinoma. Among the 39 patients whose dates of EGFR testing were available, nine (23%) patients were positive for EGFR mutation. Unfortunately, the PD-L1 status was only assessed in nine patients, since the biopsy samples were not

TABLE 1 | Baseline Characteristics of Study Population.

Characteristic	Patients (N=67)
Age, median (range, year)	60 (33-77)
Sex, n (%)	
Male	47 (70%)
Female	20 (30%)
ECOG performance status, n (%)	
0	19 (28%)
1-2	48(72%)
Smoking status, n (%)	
≥10 pack-years	32 (48%)
<10 pack-years	35 (52%)
Histology, n (%)	
Squamous	26 (39%)
Adenosquamous	41 (61%)
Surgery treatment, n (%)	
Yes	24 (36%)
No	43 (64%)
Stage	
III	11 (16%)
IV	56 (84%)
Anlotinib dose, n (%)	
8mg	7 (10%)
10mg	32 (48%)
12mg	28 (42%)
EGFR mutation, n (%)	
EGFR(+)	9 (13%)
EGFR(-)	30 (45%)
Unknown	28 (42%)
PD-L1 status, n (%)	
Positive(TPS≥1%)	4 (6%)
Negative(TPS<1%)	5 (7%)
Not reported	58 (87%)
Liver metastases, n (%)	
Absent	49 (73%)
Present	18 (27%)
Brain metastases, n (%)	
Absent	51 (76%)
Present	16 (24%)
Metastatic sites, n (%)	
≤3	29 (43%)
>3	38 (57%)
Previous systemic therapy, n (%)	
1	21 (31%)
≥2	46 (69%)
Anti-PD-1drugs	
sintilimab	28 (42%)
toripalimab	13 (19%)
camrelizumab	12 (18%)
nivolumab	7 (10%)
tislelizuma	4 (6%)
pembrolizumab	3 (4%)

ECOG, Eastern Cooperative Oncology Group; EGFR, epidermal growth factor receptor; TPS, tumor proportion score.

sufficient in most patients. Presence of liver metastases at baseline was reported in 18 (27%) patients and 16 (24%) patients had brain metastases. Of the 67 patients, 21 (31%) received previous first-line systemic therapy, whereas 46 (69%) received previous second- or further-line systemic therapy. Sintilimab (28 patients), toripalimab (13 patients), and camrelizumab (12 patients) were the three main anti-PD-1 drugs, accounting for 79% of the total population.

Safety

The overall incidence of adverse events was 85% (57 of 56), and most of these observed adverse events were grade 1–2 (**Table 2**). Grade 3–4 treatment-related adverse events occurred in 27 patients (40%). No fatal adverse events were observed. 8 patients (12%) underwent anlotinib dose modification due to adverse events. These grade 3–4 adverse events were hypertension (12 patients, 18%), transaminitis (6 patients, 9%), diarrhea (4 patients, 6%), hypothyroidism (4 patient, 6%), hand-foot syndrome (3 patients, 4%), mouth ulceration (3 patients, 4%), headache/dizziness (1 patients, 1%), rash (1 patients, 1%), neutropenia (1 patients, 1%), and thrombocytopenia (1 patients, 1%). The combination of anti-PD-1 and anlotinib was safe, with no new toxicity signals compared with monotherapy (**Table 2**).

Efficacy

The median follow-up period was 8.7 months (range: 1.5 to 23.6 months). As shown in the waterfall plot (**Figure 1**), 19 patients obtained PR, 39 patients exhibited SD, 9 patients developed PD, and none of the patients achieved CR, yielding an overall response rate (ORR) of 28.4% and disease control rate (DCR) of 86.6%. The maximum percent change in target lesion size from the baseline was -70% (**Figure 1**). The median PFS was 6.9 months (95% CI 5.5–8.3 months), and median OS was 14.5 months (95% CI, 10.9–18.1 months) (**Figures 2A, B**). In the full analysis set, death occurred in 21 (31%) patients by the cutoff date; 46 (69%) patients were alive and 26 (39%) patients were being treated at the time of analysis.

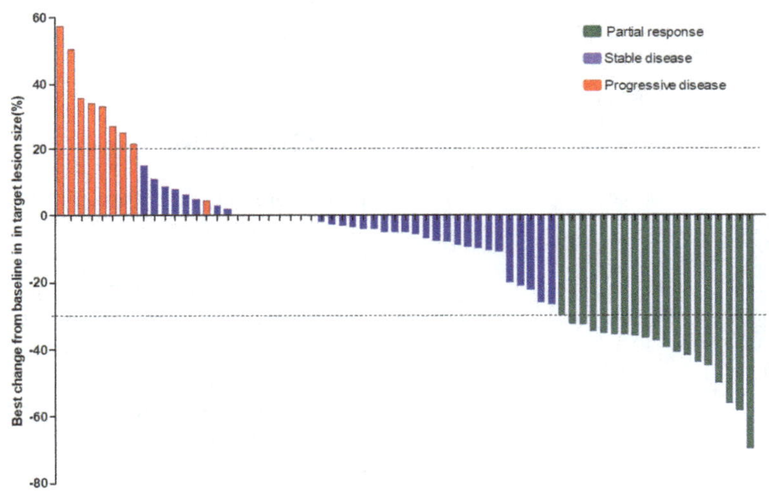

FIGURE 1 | Waterfall plot illustrating maximum change in target lesion size (N = 56).

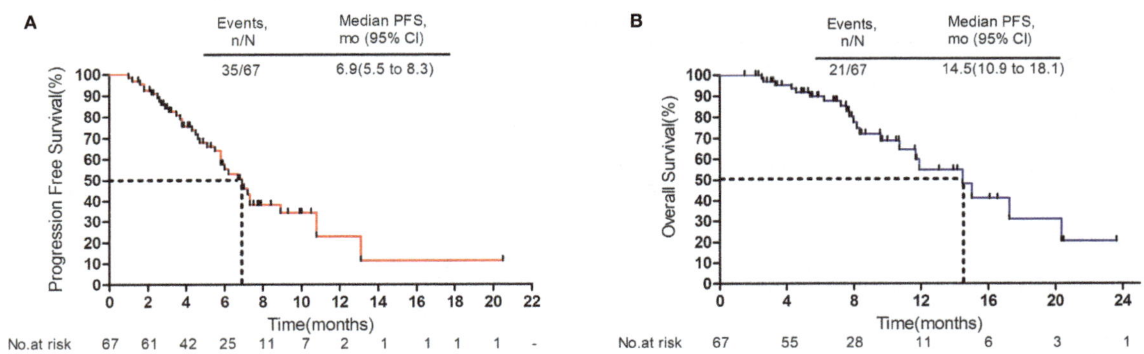

FIGURE 2 | Survival outcomes. **(A)** Progression-free survival. **(B)** Overall survival. Mo, months; CI, confidence interval.

Based on the key subgroup analyses of patients with EGFR mutations, baseline liver metastases or brain metastases, the median PFS was 7.2 months, 6.9 months, and 5.8 months respectively; the median OS was 9.6 months, 11.9 months, and 8.3 months respectively (**Figure 3**).

We also performed exploratory analyses to determine whether any clinical or pathologic features were associated with PFS and OS. In univariate cox analysis, histology and metastatic sites were associated with PFS (p=0.049, p=0.018 respectively) (**Table 3**); Metastatic sites (p=0.006) and metastases brain (p=0.024) were significantly associated with OS (**Table 4**). The number of previous systemic therapies, anlotinib dose, ECOG performance status, and TN stage and liver metastases status were not found to be associated with any predictive effects. In multivariate analysis, only the number of metastatic sites was found to independently predict PFS and OS (**Tables 3, 4**). Patients with < 3 metastatic sites showed better survival to the combination treatment (PFS: HR, 2.267; 95% CI, 1.084–4.742; p=0.030; OS: HR, 3.474; 95% CI, 1.193–10.113; p=0.022).

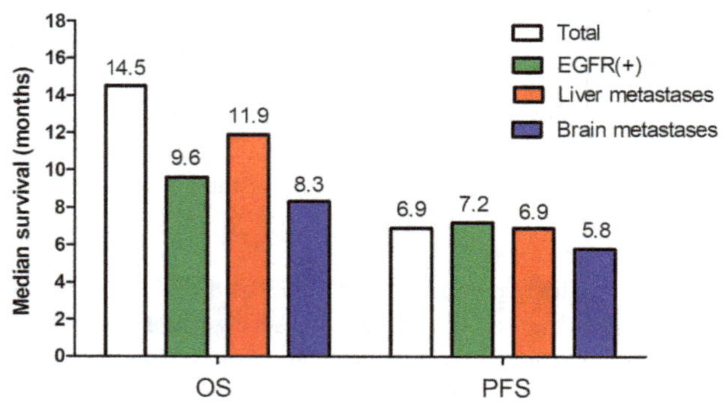

FIGURE 3 | Survival outcomes for key subgroups (EGFR positive, liver metastases, brain metastases).

TABLE 2 | Treatment-Related Adverse Events with at Least 10% Incidence in Study Population.

	No. (%) of Patients (n = 67)		
	All grades	**Grades 1-2**	**Grades 3-4**
Any adverse event	57(85)	49(73)	27 (40)
Hypertension	40(60)	28 (42)	12 (18)
Fatigue	37 (55)	37(55)	0
Transaminitis	36 (54)	30 (45)	6 (9)
Diarrhoea	20 (30)	16 (24)	4 (6)
Headache/Dizziness	18 (27)	17 (25)	1(1)
Rash	14 (21)	13(19)	1 (1)
Neutropenia	14 (21)	13 (19)	1 (1)
Nausea	13 (19)	13 (19)	0
Cough	12 (18)	12 (18)	0
Hand-foot syndrome	11 (16)	8 (12)	3 (4)
Proteinuria	10 (15)	10 (15)	0
Pruritus	9 (13)	9 (13)	0
Dyspnea	9 (13)	9 (13)	0
Hypothyroidism	9 (13)	5 (7)	4 (6)
Thrombocytopenia	8 (12)	7(10)	1 (1)
Mouth ulceration	7 (10)	4 (6)	3 (4)

DISCUSSION

In the present study, anti-PD-1 treatment concomitant with anlotinib has tolerable toxicity and favorable antitumor activity in patients with previously treated advanced NSCLC. As a potential effective treatment regimen, some clinical trials are underway to assess the efficacy of the combination of checkpoint inhibitors with anti-angiogenetics. Our results provided more evidence for the following clinical trials.

Immune checkpoint inhibitors as second or third-line monotherapy has shown limited therapeutic benefit in patients with NSCLC. In the CheckMate 057 (22) and KEYNOTE-001 (8)

TABLE 3 | Univariate and Multivariate Cox Regression Analysis of Factors Associated with PFS.

Characteristics	Univariate analysis			Multivariate analysis		
	HR	**95% CI**	**p value**	**HR**	**95% CI**	**p value**
Age (≤60 vs >60)	1.253	0.643-2.443	0.508			NI
Gender (Male vs Female)	1.224	0.571-2.627	0.603			NI
Smoking (<10 pack-years vs ≥10 pack-years)	0.772	0.397-1.499	0.444			NI
ECOG performance status (1-2 vs 0)	1.544	0.780-3.097	0.210			NI
Histology (Squamous vs Adenosquamous)	0.745	0.373-1.489	0.405			NI
Surgery treatment (Yes vs No)	0.483	0.234-0.997	**0.049**	0.526	0.254-1.090	0.084
T Stage (T1-2 vs T3-4)	1.244	0.40-2.417	0.520			NI
N stage (N0-1 vs N2-3)	0.451	0.157-1.289	0.137			NI
Previous systemic therapy (1 vs ≥2)	0.969	0.469-2.005	0.933			NI
Anlotinib dose (8mg/10mg vs 12mg)	1.146	0.859-1.530	0.354			NI
Metastatic sites (>3 vs ≤3)	2.431	1.166-5.066	**0.018**	2.267	1.084-4.742	**0.030**
Liver metastases(Absent vs Present)	0.821	0.381-1.769	0.615			NI
Brain metastases(Absent vs Present)	0.702	0.341-1.565	0.387			NI

ECOG, Eastern Cooperative Oncology Group; EGFR, epidermal growth factor receptor; HR, hazard ratio; CI, confidence interval; NI, not included in multivariate model; Boldness indicates p-value less than 0.05.

TABLE 4 | Univariate and Multivariate Cox Regression Analysis of Factors Associated with OS.

Characteristics	Univariate analysis			Multivariate analysis		
	HR	95% CI	p value	HR	95% CI	p value
Age (≤60 vs >60)	0.638	0.260-1.562	0.325			NI
Gender (Male vs Female)	0.740	0.298-1.838	0.516			NI
Smoking (<10 pack-years vs ≥10 pack-years)	1.056	0.434-2.570	0.905			NI
ECOG performance status (1-2 vs 0)	1.691	0.709-4.033	0.236			NI
Histology (Squamous vs Adenosquamous)	1.448	0.599-3.496	0.411			NI
Surgery treatment (Yes vs No)	0.667	0.267-1.666	0.386			NI
T Stage (T1-2 vs T3-4)	0.856	0.343-2.139	0.740			NI
N stage (N0-1 vs N2-3)	0.904	0.325-2.513	0.847			NI
Previous systemic therapy (1 vs ≥2)	1.520	0.548-4.212	0.421			NI
Anlotinib dose (8mg/ 10mg vs 12mg)	0.945	0.683-1.308	0.732			NI
Metastatic sites (>3 vs ≤3)	4.178	1.510-11.558	**0.006**	3.474	1.193-10.113	**0.022**
Liver metastases(Absent vs Present)	0.924	0.331-2.577	0.880			NI
Brain metastases(Absent vs Present)	0.342	0.125-0.871	**0.024**	0.551	0.201-1.513	0.247

ECOG, Eastern Cooperative Oncology Group; EGFR, epidermal growth factor receptor; HR, hazard ratio; CI, confidence interval; NI, not included in multivariate model; Boldness indicates p-value less than 0.05.

studies, the ORRs of anti-PD-1 monotherapy were 19% (median PFS of 2.3 months) and 19.4% (median PFS of 3.7 months), respectively. Our results demonstrated the efficacy of anti-PD-1 plus anlotinib, as shown by the ORR of 28.4% and DCR of 86.6%, with a median PFS of 6.9 months (95% CI, 5.5-8.3 months), which was superior to that of anti-PD-1 monotherapy in the second-line setting. The most common toxic effects for the anti-PD-1 plus anlotinib combination therapy were of grade one or two severity, with few patients discontinuing treatment due to adverse events. Although the proportion of patients having grade 3–4 adverse events was higher than that previously reported for anti-PD-1 monotherapy (40% vs 7-10%) (7, 8, 22), most of these events did not affect treatment or could be resolved.

The use of immune checkpoint inhibitors (anti-PD-1 or anti-PD-L1) as monotherapy has shown poor outcome in patients with EGFR mutations (3, 23). Data from IMpower150 showed that the combination of atezolizumab, bevacizumab, carboplatin, and paclitaxel provided OS and PFS benefits to patients with sensitizing EGFR mutations compared to patients who received the standard-of-care bevacizumab, carboplatin, and paclitaxel regimen (24). In our study, the EGFR-positive group had a mPFS of 7.2 months and a mOS of 9.6 months. Immune checkpoint inhibitor monotherapy has also shown minimal therapeutic benefit in patients with liver metastases—a common metastatic site for NSCLC and a negative prognostic indicator (25–27). According to our results, the patients with liver metastasis had a mPFS of 6.9 months and a mOS of 11.9 months. In addition, there is a paucity of data on anti-PD-1 plus antiangiogenesis therapy among patients with brain metastases. Our results indicated that median PFS was 5.8 months, and median OS was 8.3 months in patients with brain metastases. Whether the clinical benefit can extend across these subgroups with EGFR genetic alterations, baseline liver metastases or brain metastases should be further studied in future randomized trials.

The limitation of immunotherapy in solid tumors is the activation of multiple immunosuppressive components in the tumor microenvironment (28). A low level expression of the PD-L1 in tumors alone cannot explain the lack of responsiveness in the majority of patients, nor can a low number of tumor mutational burden (TMB). The VEGF-VEGFR signaling can contribute to local and systemic immunosuppression through a variety of mechanisms. The excessive activation of VEGF-VEGFR pathways can directly inhibit the trafficking of immune cells to the tumor by inhibiting upregulation of the expression of intercellular adhesion molecule-1(ICAM-1) and vascular cell adhesion molecule-1 (VCAM-1) (11, 29). In addition, VEGF also reprogrammed the immunosuppressive microenvironment through various mechanisms, such as boosting immunosuppressive cytokines (IL-10, TGF β), enhancing expression of inhibitory checkpoints (such as PD1, CTLA4, and LAG-3) in $CD8^+$ T cells, and increasing the presence of MDSCs and Treg (30, 31). Thus, antiangiogenics that normalize the tumor microenvironment could potentially improve immunotherapy effectiveness. This was confirmed in a pre-clinical study, which suggested that the application of anti-VEGF-A antibody (sunitinib) in CT26 tumor-bearing mice increases the infiltration of cytotoxic tumor-infiltrating lymphocytes (TIL) and decreases PD-1 expression in $CD8^+$T cells (32). Moreover, another research provided evidence that anti-PD-L1 therapy, in reverse, can make tumors sensitive to antiangiogenic therapy and improve its efficacy (33).

Our study has some limitations. The retrospective nature and relatively small sample size were two major limitations, which mean selection bias could not be ruled out. Given that this study was a single-arm study, we could not formally establish the role of the combination therapy over anti-PD-1 monotherapy. Additionally, we enrolled a heterogeneous patient population treated using a variety of anti-PD-1 drugs and did not have a study design with sufficient power for subgroup analyses with respect to PD-L1 status. Date on survival in specific subgroup (EGFR, liver metastasis, brain metastasis) was only descriptive due to the small sample size. However, our study's findings may still be deemed as meaningful due to the limited number of similar prospective clinical studies in the literature.

Although the combination of antiangiogenic therapy and immunotherapy has been proved to be a very promising treatment in many solid tumors, some issues must be addressed prior to clinical practice application. It is important to identify the optimal dosing and timing to make the combination therapy more effective. Moreover, the exploration of predictive biomarkers is helpful in screening which cancer types and stages would benefit more from this treatment.

CONCLUSION

Our findings show that the combination of anlotinib and anti-PD-1 drugs has promising efficacy and manageable toxic effects as a second- or further-line treatment for patients with previously treated advanced NSCLC. The results further demonstrate the clinical applicability of dual inhibition of the VEGF-VEGFR2 and PD-1-/PD-L1 pathways. Given these findings, prospective investigation is warranted to explored with or without chemotherapy, particularly for patients with tumors for which immune checkpoint inhibitor monotherapy was not superior to chemotherapy.

AUTHOR CONTRIBUTIONS

Conception and design: PW, FT, and JY. Provision of study materials or patients: PW. Collection and assembly of data: PW, XF, TY, and HT. Data analysis and interpretation: PW and FT. Manuscript writing and final approval of manuscript: all authors. All authors contributed to the article and approved the submitted version.

ACKNOWLEDGMENTS

We appreciate the patients who participated in this study. We also thank our colleges for their devoted support.

REFERENCES

1. Rittmeyer A, Barlesi F, Waterkamp D, Park K, Ciardiello F, von Pawel J, et al. Atezolizumab versus docetaxel in patients with previously treated non-small-cell lung cancer (OAK): a phase 3, open-label, multicentre randomised controlled trial. *Lancet* (2017) 389:255–65. doi: 10.1016/S0140-6736(16)32517-X
2. Reck M, Rodriguez-Abreu D, Robinson AG, Hui R, Csoszi T, Fulop A, et al. Pembrolizumab versus chemotherapy for PD-L1–positive non–small-cell lung cancer. *N Engl J Med* (2016) 375:1823–33. doi: 10.1056/NEJMoa1606774
3. Herbst RS, Baas P, Kim DW, Felip E, Perez-Gracia JL, Han JY, et al. Pembrolizumab versus docetaxel for previously treated, PD-L1-positive, advanced non-small-cell lung cancer (KEYNOTE-010): A randomised controlled trial. *Lancet* (2016) 387:1540–50. doi: 10.1016/S0140-6736(15)01281-7
4. Antonia SJ, Villegas A, Daniel D, Vicente D, Murakami S, Hui R, et al. Durvalumab after Chemoradiotherapy in Stage III Non–Small-Cell Lung Cancer. *N Engl J Med* (2017) 377:1919–29. doi: 10.1056/NEJMoa1709937
5. Mok TSK, Wu Y-L, Kudaba I, Kowalski DM, Cho BC, Turna HZ, et al. Pembrolizumab versus chemotherapy for previously untreated, PD-L1-expressing, locally advanced or metastatic non-small-cell lung cancer (KEYNOTE-042): A randomised, open-label, controlled, phase 3 trial. *Lancet* (2019) 393:1819–30. doi: 10.1016/S0140-6736(18)32409-7
6. Gandhi L, Rodríguez-Abreu D, Gadgeel S, Esteban E, Felip E, De Angelis F, et al. Pembrolizumab plus chemotherapy in metastatic non–small-cell lung cancer. *N Engl J Med* (2018) 378:2078–92. doi: 10.1056/NEJMoa1801005
7. Brahmer J, Reckamp KL, Baas P, Crino L, Eberhardt WE, Poddubskaya E, et al. Nivolumab versus docetaxel in advanced squamous-cell non-small-cell lung cancer. *N Engl J Med* (2015) 373:123–35. doi: 10.1056/NEJMoa1504627
8. Garon EB, Rizvi NA, Hui R, Leighl N, Balmanoukian AS, Eder JP, et al. Pembrolizumab for the treatment of non-small-cell lung cancer. *N Engl J Med* (2015) 372:2018–28. doi: 10.1056/NEJMoa1501824
9. Almutairi AR, Alkhatib N, Martin J, Babiker HM, Garland LL, McBride A, et al. Comparative efficacy and safety of immunotherapies targeting the PD-1/PD-L1 pathway for previously treated advanced non-small cell lung cancer: A Bayesian network meta-analysis. *Crit Rev Oncol Hematol* (2019) 142:16–25. doi: 10.1016/j.critrevonc.2019.07.004
10. Hegde PS, Wallin JJ, Mancao C. Predictive markers of anti-VEGF and emerging role of angiogenesis inhibitors as immunotherapeutics. *Semin Cancer Biol* (2018) 52:117–24. doi: 10.1016/j.semcancer.2017.12.002
11. Hendry SA, Farnsworth RH, Solomon B, Achen MG, Stacker SA, Fox SB. The role of the tumor vasculature in the host immune response: Implications for therapeutic strategies targeting the tumor microenvironment. *Front Immunol* (2016) 7:621. doi: 10.3389/fimmu.2016.00621
12. Kashyap AS, Schmittnaegel M, Rigamonti N, Pais-Ferreira D, Mueller P, Buchi M, et al. Optimized antiangiogenic reprogramming of the tumor microenvironment potentiates CD40 immunotherapy. *Proc Natl Acad Sci USA* (2020) 117:541–51. doi: 10.1073/pnas.1902145116
13. Qiang H, Chang Q, Xu J, Qian J, Zhang Y, Lei Y, et al. New advances in antiangiogenic combination therapeutic strategies for advanced non-small cell lung cancer. *J Cancer Res Clin Oncol* (2020) 146:631–45. doi: 10.1007/s00432-020-03129-6
14. Zhou S, Zhang H. Synergies of targeting angiogenesis and immune checkpoints in cancer: From mechanism to clinical applications. *Anticancer Agents Med Chem* (2020) 20:768–76. doi: 10.2174/1871520620666200207091653
15. Yasuda S, Sho M, Yamato I, Yoshiji H, Wakatsuki K, Nishiwada S, et al. Simultaneous blockade of programmed death 1 and vascular endothelial growth factor receptor 2 (VEGFR2) induces synergistic anti-tumour effect in vivo. *Clin Exp Immunol* (2013) 172:500–6. doi: 10.1111/cei.12069
16. Herbst RS, Arkenau HT, Santana-Davila R, Calvo E, Paz-Ares L, Cassier PA, et al. Ramucirumab plus pembrolizumab in patients with previously treated advanced non-small-cell lung cancer, gastro-oesophageal cancer, or urothelial carcinomas (JVDF): A multicohort, non-randomised, open-label, phase 1a/b trial. *Lancet Oncol* (2019) 20:1109–23. doi: 10.1016/S1470-2045(19)30458-9
17. Socinski MA, Jotte RM, Cappuzzo F, Orlandi F, Stroyakovskiy D, Nogami N, et al. Atezolizumab for first-line treatment of metastatic nonsquamous NSCLC. *N Engl J Med* (2018) 378:2288–301. doi: 10.1056/NEJMoa1716948
18. Khalil DN, Smith EL, Brentjens RJ, Wolchok JD. The future of cancer treatment: Immunomodulation, CARs and combination immunotherapy. *Nat Rev Clin Oncol* (2016) 13:273–90. doi: 10.1038/nrclinonc.2016.25
19. Gao Y, Liu P, Shi R. Anlotinib as a molecular targeted therapy for tumors. *Oncol Lett* (2020) 20:1001–14. doi: 10.3892/ol.2020.11685
20. Sun Y, Niu W, Du F, Du C, Li S, Wang J, et al. Safety, pharmacokinetics, and antitumor properties of anlotinib, an oral multi-target tyrosine kinase inhibitor, in patients with advanced refractory solid tumors. *J Hematol Oncol* (2016) 9:105. doi: 10.1186/s13045-016-0332-8
21. Han B, Li K, Wang Q, Zhang L, Shi J, Wang Z, et al. Effect of anlotinib as a third-line or further treatment on overall survival of patients with advanced

non-small cell lung cancer: The ALTER 0303 phase 3 randomized clinical trial. *JAMA Oncol* (2018) 4:1569–75. doi: 10.1001/jamaoncol.2018.3039

22. Borghaei H, Paz-Ares L, Horn L, Spigel DR, Steins M, Ready NE, et al. Nivolumab versus Docetaxel in Advanced Nonsquamous Non-Small-Cell Lung Cancer. *N Engl J Med* (2015) 373:1627–39. doi: 10.1056/NEJMoa1507643
23. Cavanna L, Citterio C, Orlandi E. Immune checkpoint inhibitors in EGFR-mutation positive TKI-treated patients with advanced non-small-cell lung cancer network meta-analysis. *Oncotarget* (2019) 10:209–15. doi: 10.18632/oncotarget.26541
24. Reck M, Mok TSK, Nishio M, Jotte RM, Cappuzzo F, Orlandi F, et al. Atezolizumab plus bevacizumab and chemotherapy in non-small-cell lung cancer (IMpower150): Key subgroup analyses of patients with EGFR mutations or baseline liver metastases in a randomised, open-label phase 3 trial. *Lancet Respir Med* (2019) 7:387–401. doi: 10.1016/S2213-2600(19)30084-0
25. Riihimaki M, Hemminki A, Fallah M, Thomsen H, Sundquist K, Sundquist J, et al. Metastatic sites and survival in lung cancer. *Lung Cancer* (2014) 86:78–84. doi: 10.1016/j.lungcan.2014.07.020
26. Kitadai R, Okuma Y, Hakozaki T, Hosomi Y. The efficacy of immune checkpoint inhibitors in advanced non-small-cell lung cancer with liver metastases. *J Cancer Res Clin Oncol* (2020) 146:777–85. doi: 10.1007/s00432-019-03104-w
27. Tumeh PC, Hellmann MD, Hamid O, Tsai KK, Loo KL, Gubens MA, et al. Liver metastasis and treatment outcome with Anti-PD-1 monoclonal antibody in patients with melanoma and NSCLC. *Cancer Immunol Res* (2017) 5:417–24. doi: 10.1158/2326-6066.CIR-16-0325
28. Huang Y, Kim BYS, Chan CK, Hahn SM, Weissman IL, Jiang W. Improving immune-vascular crosstalk for cancer immunotherapy. *Nat Rev Immunol* (2018) 18:195–203. doi: 10.1038/nri.2017.145
29. Melder RJ, Koenig GC, Witwer BP, Safabakhsh N, Munn LL, Jain RK. During angiogenesis, vascular endothelial growth factor and basic fibroblast growth factor regulate natural killer cell adhesion to tumor endothelium. *Nat Med* (1996) 2:992–7. doi: 10.1038/nm0996-992
30. Terme M, Pernot S, Marcheteau E, Sandoval F, Benhamouda N, Colussi O, et al. VEGFA-VEGFR pathway blockade inhibits tumor-induced regulatory T-cell proliferation in colorectal cancer. *Cancer Res* (2013) 73:539–49. doi: 10.1158/0008-5472.CAN-12-2325
31. Yang J, Yan J, Liu B. Targeting VEGF/VEGFR to modulate antitumor immunity. *Front Immunol* (2018) 9:978. doi: 10.3389/fimmu.2018.00978
32. Voron T, Colussi O, Marcheteau E, Pernot S, Nizard M, Pointet AL, et al. VEGF-A modulates expression of inhibitory checkpoints on CD8+ T cells in tumors. *J Exp Med* (2015) 212:139–48. doi: 10.1084/jem.20140559
33. Allen E, Jabouille A, Rivera LB, Lodewijckx I, Missiaen R, Steri V, et al. Combined antiangiogenic and anti-PD-L1 therapy stimulates tumor immunity through HEV formation. *Sci Transl Med* (2017) 9:eaak9679. doi: 10.1126/scitranslmed.aak9679

22

A Combination of Cytokine-Induced Killer Cells with PD-1 Blockade and ALK Inhibitor Showed Substantial Intrinsic Variability Across Non-Small Cell Lung Cancer Cell Lines

Yutao Li[1†], Amit Sharma[1,2†], Xiaolong Wu[1], Hans Weiher[3], Dirk Skowasch[4], Markus Essler[5] and Ingo G. H. Schmidt-Wolf[1]*

[1] Department of Integrated Oncology, Center for Integrated Oncology (CIO) Bonn, University Hospital Bonn, Bonn, Germany, [2] Department of Neurosurgery, University Hospital Bonn, Bonn, Germany, [3] Department of Applied Natural Sciences, Bonn-Rhein-Sieg University of Applied Sciences, Rheinbach, Germany, [4] Department of Internal Medicine II, Cardiology, Pneumology and Angiology, University Hospital Bonn, Bonn, Germany, [5] Department of Nuclear Medicine, University Hospital Bonn, Bonn, Germany

***Correspondence:**
Ingo G. H. Schmidt-Wolf
Ingo.Schmidt-Wolf@ukbonn.de

†These authors have contributed equally to this work and share first authorship

Background: Cancer heterogeneity poses a serious challenge concerning the toxicity and adverse effects of therapeutic inhibitors, especially when it comes to combinatorial therapies that involve multiple targeted inhibitors. In particular, in non-small cell lung cancer (NSCLC), a number of studies have reported synergistic effects of drug combinations in the preclinical models, while they were only partially successful in the clinical setup, suggesting those alternative clinical strategies (with genetic background and immune response) should be considered. Herein, we investigated the antitumor effect of cytokine-induced killer (CIK) cells in combination with ALK and PD-1 inhibitors *in vitro* on genetically variable NSCLC cell lines.

Methods: We co-cultured the three genetically different NSCLC cell lines NCI-H2228 (EML4-ALK), A549 (KRAS mutation), and HCC-78 (ROS1 rearrangement) with and without nivolumab (PD-1 inhibitor) and crizotinib (ALK inhibitor). Additionally, we profiled the variability of surface expression multiple immune checkpoints, the concentration of absolute dead cells, intracellular granzyme B on CIK cells using flow cytometry as well as RT-qPCR. ELISA and Western blot were performed to verify the activation of CIK cells.

Results: Our analysis showed that (a) nivolumab significantly weakened PD-1 surface expression on CIK cells without impacting other immune checkpoints or PD-1 mRNA expression, (b) this combination strategy showed an effective response on cell viability, IFN-γ production, and intracellular release of granzyme B in $CD3^+$ $CD56^+$ CIK cells, but solely in NCI-H2228, (c) the intrinsic expression of Fas ligand (FasL) as a T-cell activation marker in CIK cells was upregulated by this additive effect, and (d) nivolumab induced Foxp3 expression in $CD4^+CD25^+$ subpopulation of CIK cells significantly increased. Taken together, we could show that CIK cells in combination with crizotinib and nivolumab can enhance the anti-tumor immune response through FasL activation, leading to increased IFN-γ and granzyme B, but only in NCI-H2228 cells with EML4-ALK rearrangement.

Therefore, we hypothesize that CIK therapy may be a potential alternative in NSCLC patients harboring EML4-ALK rearrangement, in addition, we support the idea that combination therapies offer significant potential when they are optimized on a patient-by-patient basis.

Keywords: cytokine-induced killer cells, immune checkpoint inhibition programmed cell death-1, anaplastic lymphoma kinase, immunotherapy, non-small cell lung cancer

INTRODUCTION

Cancer is a highly dynamic disease where clinical (inter-individual differences), molecular (epigenomics), and yet to be known factors often pose a challenge to find a successful treatment option (1, 2). Although, the traditional therapies (surgery, radiation, and chemotherapy) for cancer are still being used, the maximum therapeutic benefit has been obtained using combination therapies. For instance, Pembrolizumab (anti-PD-1 mAb) in combination with chemotherapy in patients with non-small cell lung cancer (NSCLC) showed better survival compared to those treated only with chemotherapy (3). In a meta-analysis including seven studies (>4000 patients) on pretreated NSCLC, Tartarone et al. showed that among immune checkpoint inhibitors, anti-PD-1 provided greater benefit compared to anti-PD-L1 (4). Similarly, in another independent meta-analysis in which immune checkpoint inhibitors were added to chemotherapy, Petrelli et al. showed that there was a significant overall survival benefit in NSCLC cases with PD-L1 (5). Hence, there is reasonable evidence that modulation of PD-1/PD-L1 associated pathways may have predictive significance for the clinical NSCLC spectrum. Since the combination therapy minimizes the toxic effects on normal cells and induces cytotoxic effects on the cancer cells, it also allows the possibility to further combine more than one inhibitor, especially when considering the mutation/genomic landscape, as shown in a recent clinical trial that combined durvalumab (human IgG1κ monoclonal antibody that blocks PD-L1 binding to PD-1 & CD80) and gefitinib (EGFR tyrosine kinase inhibitor) to treat TKI-naïve patients with EGFR mutation-positive NSCLC (6).

It is also worth mentioning that the effective use of combined cancer therapies remains a challenge, especially when optimization is concerned. This can be evident from a recent clinical trial involving crizotinib (ALK inhibitor) and nivolumab (PD-1 inhibitor) in NSCLC that was discontinued due to the safety concerns (CheckMate 370) (7). However, the clinical trials based on a similar combination strategy such as TKI/ALK inhibitor with ICI are still in progress. Primarily, the concern about short-term gastrointestinal toxicity also emerged in the above-mentioned clinical trial, however, it was resolved with the standard medical care. Notably, the treatment sequence also appeared to be pivotal, as evidenced by the fact that treatment in reverse sequence (osimertinib followed by nivolumab) did not result in higher levels of toxicity compared to treatment with nivolumab followed by osimertinib (8). To mention, the second generation ALK inhibitor ceritinib showed a synergistic effect with PD-1/PD-L1 blockade to provide an improved anti-tumor response along with favorable side effect tolerability *in vivo* NSCLC xenograft model (9) and clinical trial (10). Despite T cells dominated the immune cell composition in NSCLC tumors (11), the function of $CD4^+$ and $CD8^+$ T lymphocytes was dysregulated with decreasing of IFN-γ production (12). In this particular scenario, the inclusion of alternative adjuvant treatments, for instance, cytokine-induced killer (CIK) cells, may help to reshape the therapeutic paradigm in NSCLC patients. CIK cells are heterogeneous *in vitro* expanded T lymphocytes with a natural killer (NK)/T phenotype generated primarily by *ex vivo* incubation of human peripheral blood mononuclear cells (PBMC) or cord blood mononuclear cells. The transfusion of CIK cells after *ex-vivo* expansion in cancer patients has already been tested in more than 80 reported clinical trials (13). Moreover, recent studies provide functional details on the function and optimization of CIK cells to maximize their functional potential (14–16). Of note, there have been autologous and allogeneic clinical trials showing that CIKs immunotherapy has potential benefits in the safety and efficacy of patients with advanced NSCLC (17–21), given that clinical trials of DC-CIK (dendritic cells cytokine-induced killer cells) in combination with chemotherapy for advanced lung cancer have shown very limited success. To improve the efficiency of such therapies, several paradigms have been discussed, including inhibition of inflammatory mediators released by tumor cells in combination with vaccination to reduce recruitment of tumorigenic immune cells to the tumor microenvironment in pre/postoperative advanced lung cancer (22). Certainly, the DCs loaded with tumor antigens along with CIK cells may have a lower risk compared to CAR-T cells alone. To mention, the combination of CIK cells with PD-1 blockade before transfusion might improve the efficiency of CIK therapy for NSCLC patients *in vitro* (23). Alternatively, autologous cytokine-induced killer (CIK) cells enhance the clinical response to PD-1 blocking antibodies in patients with advanced non-small-cell lung cancer (24). Recently, the benefits of combining anti-PD-1 antibody with antiangiogenic drugs anlotinib in NSCLC patients have been reported (25). Although there is some previous evidence of ICIs combinations, there has been no report on the combination of CIK with ALK inhibitors and PD-1 inhibitors neither *in vitro* nor *vivo*.

Considering this, we aim to understand whether pretreated-nivolumab CIK cells before transfusion can enhance the antitumor immune response to NSCLC cell lines at different concentrations of crizotinib *in vitro*. To achieve this, we used three NSCLC cell lines: NCI-H2228 (EML4-ALK), A549 (KRAS mutation), and HCC-78 (ROS1 rearrangement) having different genetic alterations and employing multiple techniques (flow cytometry, intracellular staining for granzyme B, cell viability assays, ELISA, RT-PCR, Western blot).

MATERIAL AND METHODS

Regents and Antibodies

Anti-PD-1 mAb nivolumab (purity 99.50%) and ALK inhibitor crizotinib (purity ≥98% (HPLC) were purchased from Selleckchem Co., Ltd. (Houston, TX). Crizotinib was dissolved in dimethyl sulfoxide (DMSO). DMSO was used as a control for crizotinib and 20 µg/mL IgG4 isotype (Biolegend, San Diego, CA)as a control for nivolumab. Concerning antibodies (Abs): The fluorochrome-conjugated FITC anti-human CD3 antibody (Clone OKT3), brilliant violet 421 anti-human CD8 antibody (RPA-T8), APC anti-human CD4 antibody (Clone OKT4), PE-CD56 (Clone 5.1 H11), APC anti-human PD1 (Clone NAT105), PE anti-human PD-L1(Clone 29E-2A3), APC anti-human CTLA-4 antibody (Clone L3D10), PE anti-human GITR antibody (Clone 621), brilliant violet 421 anti-human CD134 (OX40) antibody (Clone Ber-ACT35), and FITC anti-human/mouse granzyme B antibody (GB11) were purchased from Biolegend (San Diego, CA). For APC-anti-human PD-1 detection, its isotype control is mouse IgG1k, which is not compatible to nivolumab as an IgG4 antibody. Anti-Human Foxp3 Staining Set FITC kit (eBioscience, San Diego, CA) was used to identify Foxp3 $CD4^+CD25^+/CD4^+CD25^-$ cells according to the manufacturer's instructions. For Western blot: Anti-FasL (Biolegend, San Diego, CA) and beta Tubulin Loading Control Monoclonal Antibody (BT7R) (Thermo Fisher Scientific, San Diego, CA) were used.

Cell Culture

CIK cells were generated, as previously described (26, 27). PBMCs required for the experiments were isolated from the blood of healthy donors registered at the blood bank of University Hospital Bonn. Three epithelial lung cancer cell lines: A549 cells (KRAS mutation), HCC-78 (ROS1 rearrangement, SLC34A2-ROS1), and NCI-H2228 (EML4-ALK variant 3) were primarily used in this study. All cell lines were mycoplasma negative and cultured in RPMI medium supplemented with 10% heat-inactivated FBS (Sigma-Aldrich GmbH, Munich, Germany) and 1% penicillin/streptomycin (P/S) (Gibco, Germany) at 37°C (5% CO_2). As mentioned above, to avoid the excessive toxicity of simultaneous treatment of nivolumab and crizotinib, CIK cells were pre-treated with 20 µg/mL anti-PD-1 mAb nivolumab or IgG4 isotype control for 24 h and then co-cultured with the tumor cells along with different concentrations of ALK inhibitor crizotinib.

Cell Viability Assessment by CCK-8 Assay and Cell Death Analysis by Flow Cytometry

CCK-8 cell viability assay was performed, as described by the manufacturer (Dojindo Laboratories, Kumamoto, Japan). NSCLC cells were seeded into 96-well plates ($1x10^4$ cells/well) and treated with various concentrations of crizotinib or DMSO for 24 h in the presence or absence of nivolumab. Similarly, the flow cytometry-based cytotoxicity was performed, as described protocol. Briefly, the target cells were labeled with CFSE (1×10^6 cells in 1 ml PBS with 0.5 uM CFSE, 20 min, 37°C in the dark) and washed twice with warm culture medium. CFSE-labeled 5×10^4 tumor cells were incubated at various concentrations of crizotinib for 24 h with CIK cells pre-incubated with 20 µg/mL nivolumab or IgG 4 isotype (24 h) to perform redirected cytolysis assay at an E/T ratio of 10:1. Following 24 h of culturing, the cells were stained with Hoechst 33258 (Cayman Chemical, Hamburg, Germany) and were quantified using BD FACS Canto II. The absolute number of 3000 beads (Biolegend, San Diego, CA) was acquired by a BD Canto II cytometer. Then the absolute numbers of cells per uL were analyzed by FlowJo V10 software (Tree Star, Ashland, Oregon). The absolute number of cells were calculated according to Precision Count protocol provided by Biolegend Company as follows:

$$Absolute\ Cell\ Count\ (Cells/uL) = (Cell\ Count)/(Precision\ Count\ Beads^{TM})\ x\ Precision\ Count\ Beads^{TM}\ Concentration$$

Intracellular Staining for Granzyme B by Flow Cytometry

A fixable Viability Zombie Aqua™ Dye (Biolegend, San Diego, CA) was used to exclude dead cells from the analysis. Mainly, after staining the surface receptors with PE anti-human CD3 antibody and APC anti-human CD56, the cells were fixed with 100 µL fix solution (eBioscience, San Diego, CA) for 30 min at room temperature (in the dark). Cells were then washed and resuspended in 100 µL 1x permeabilization buffer and stained with FITC anti-human granzyme B antibody for 30 min at room temperature. Subsequently, the cells were washed twice with 2 mL 1x permeabilization buffer, resuspended in DPBS, and recorded with a BD Canto II cytometer.

Enzyme-Linked Immunosorbent Assay (ELISA)

The ELISA assay was performed using the standard protocol. Briefly, 1×10^6 CIK cells incubated with 20 µg/mL nivolumab or IgG4 isotype control for 24 h. After that, CIK cells were co-cultured with 5×10^4 tumor cells in the presence of various concentrations of crizotinib for 24 h. Thereafter, the cell-free supernatant was collected to perform sandwich ELISA assay (IFN Gamma Kit, Invitrogen, Camarillo, CA), according to the manufacturer's instructions.

Reverse Transcription and Quantifying PCR (RT-qPCR)

CIK cells were incubated with 20 ug/mL nivolumab or IgG4 isotype control for 48 h. Afterward, CIK cells were washed twice with cold DPBS. RNA was extracted using RNeasy® Plus Mini Kit (QIAGEN, Hilden, Germany) and cDNA synthesis was performed by SuperScript™ III First-Strand Synthesis Super Mix Kit (Invitrogen, CA), according to the manufacturer's instructions. Quantitative real-time PCR analysis was performed using

QuantStadio 6 Flex Sequence Detection System (384-well, Applied Biosystems, CA) using SYBR® Select Master Mix (Applied Biosystems, CA). For q-PCR, the following primers were used to amplify PD-1 [as described (28)]: forward primer 5#-CAGGG TGACAGAGAAGGG-3#, reverse primer 5#-CCTGGCTCCTAT TGTCCCTC-3#, β-actin: 5#-ACCGCGAGAAGATGACCCA GA3# (forward) and 5#-GGATAGCACAGCCTGGATAGCAA3# (reverse) (obtained by Eurofins Genomics Germany GmbH, Ebersberg, Germany). The relative expression of PD-1 was normalized to β-actin expression by ΔΔCt method. To determine C - reactive protein (CRP) transcription level, the following primers were used to amplify (as described (29)): forward primer 5′- CAG ACAGACATGTCGAGGAAGG-3#, reverse primer 5′- AGGCTT TGAGAGGCTTCGTT-3′, HPRT: 5′-TCAGGCAGTATAATC CAAAGATGGT-3′, (forward) and 5′-AGTCTGGCTTATATC CAACACTTCG-3′ (reverse) (obtained by Eurofins Genomics Germany GmbH, Ebersberg, Germany). The relative expression of c-reaction protein (CRP) was normalized to HPRT expression by the ΔΔCt method.

Western Blot Assay

CIK cells incubated with 20 ug/mL nivolumab and various concentrations of crizotinib for 48 h were washed twice with cold DPBS. Cell pellets were lysed using NuPAGE LDS buffer, lysates were separated on 4-12% Tris-glycine gels and transferred to PVDF membranes. Anti-FasL antibody (Biolegend, San Diego, CA) were used for primary antibody. Beta Tubulin Loading Control Monoclonal Antibody (BT7R) (Thermo Fisher Scientific, Inc. San Diego, CA) was used as a loading control.

LDH Assay for the Assessment Hepatoxicity

The cytotoxicity of a combined nivolumab and crizotinib simultaneously in the absence or presence of CIK cells on hepatocyte-like cell line CCL-13, which exhibits the liver function of primary human hepatocytes, was detected by CyQUANT™ LDH Cytotoxicity Assay Kit (Invitrogen, Inc. San Diego, CA.). Briefly, we co-cultured CIK with $1x10^4$ CCL-13 cell line at an E:T ratio 1:1 in the presence of crizotinib/nivolumab triplicate in 96-well flat plates for 16 h. We calculated the percentage of hepatoxicity with the following formula:

$$\% \text{ hepatoxicity} = \frac{\text{experimental LDH activity} - \text{spontaneous CCL} - 13 \text{ LDH activity} - \text{spontaneous CIK LDH activity}}{\text{Maximum LDH activity} - \text{spontenous CCL} - 13 \text{ LDH activity}}$$

Statistical Analysis

All data were presented as the mean ± SD from at least three independent experiments. FACS data sets were analyzed using FlowJo V10.6 software (FlowJo, LLC, Ashland, Oregon). The statistical analysis was performed using SPSS Statistics 23. The data groups were compared using one-way analysis of variance with Turkey *post hoc* test and Student's t-test. P-values < 0.05 were considered significant differences and are marked: * < 0.05; ** < 0.01; *** < 0.001.

RESULTS

Elevated PD-1/PD-L1 Expression in CIK Subsets After 14 Days of *In Vitro* Expansion

We have previously shown that CIK cells are heterogeneous and are composed of $CD3^+$ $CD8^+$, $CD3^+$ $CD4^+$ and $CD3^+$ $CD56^+$ specifically on Day 14 (30). Therefore, we first determined the phenotypes of PD-1 and PD-L1 CIK cells primarily on Day 0 and Day 14 for these three CIK subsets. The analysis showed that the percentage of $PD\text{-}1^+$ $CD3^+$ $CD4^+$ CIK cells increased significantly after 14 days of expansion compared to Day 0 (**Figures 1A, B**, 20.6 ± 2.0 vs. 4.7 ± 1.0%, P < 0.001). However, no significant difference in the $CD3^+$ $CD56^+$ and $CD3^+$ $CD8^+$ CIK cell subsets was observed (6.2 ± 0.7 vs. 7.7 ± 0.7%, P= 0.177; 10.2 ± 2.1 vs. 7.7 ± 0.8%, P= 0.630, respectively). Similarly, the proportion of $PD\text{-}L1^+$ CIK cells was also increased among the $CD3^+$ $CD56^+$, $CD3^+$ $CD8^+$ and $CD3^+$ $CD4^+$ subsets of CIK cells on Day 14 compared to Day 0 (**Figure 1B**, 39. 5 ± 4.6% vs. 21.4 ± 5.9%, P= 0.025; 35.2 ± 4.5% vs. 12.1 ± 3.3%, P < 0.001; 51.6 ± 8.1% vs. 19.7 ± 4.2%, P= 0.008). To mention, we confirmed that all cell lines expressed PD-L1, but at different levels (**Figure 1C**, NCI-H2228 > HCC-78 > A549, 69.2 ± 8.0% on NCI-H2228, 61.8 ± 4.6% on HCC-78 and 6.0 ± 2.0% on A549).

Nivolumab Harbors the Potential to Block Surface Expression of PD-1 on CIK Cells

Next, we examined the association between CIK cell activation and PD-1 surface expression in the presence of nivolumab and found that PD-1 expression on the surface of $CD3^+$ CIK cells decreased significantly from 6.7 ± 2.7% to 0.4 ± 0.04% after 48 h of treatment with nivolumab compared to the IgG4 isotype control (**Figure 2A**). Also, the assessment of the mean fluorescence intensity (MFI) of surface expression of potential immune-associated markers, including PD-L1, PD-L2, CD28, CTLA-4, GITR, and CD134 on $CD3^+$ CIK cells, showed no alterations (**Figure 2B**). When counting the absolute number of $PD\text{-}1^+$ CIK cells, there was also a notable decrease in both $PD\text{-}1^+$ $CD3^+$ CIK cells and/or $PD\text{-}1^+$ $CD3^+$ $CD56^+$ CIK cells after the nivolumab treatment (**Figure 2C**, 0.01 ± 0.01 vs. 0.57 ± 0.18 cells/μL, P= 0.045; 0.01 ± 0.01 vs. 0.38 ± 0.13 cells/μL, P= 0.036, respectively). Besides, PD-1 mRNA levels were not altered by nivolumab (**Figure 2D**, P= 0.408). These findings suggest that nivolumab blocks PD-1 on the surface of CIK cells. Interestingly, nivolumab caused a significant increase in the levels of $CD4^+$ $CD25^+$ CIK cells expressing Foxp3 (**Figure 2E**, P= 0.044).

Nivolumab Affected the Cell Viability of Crizotinib-Treated NCI-H2228

Considering that nivolumab may reduce the tumor cell viability, we performed the CCK-8 assay and found that the combined treatment of nivolumab with crizotinib significantly impaired the viability of NCI-H2228 cells (**Figure 3A**). Primarily, a significant change was observed when 20 μg/mL nivolumab and 100 nM crizotinib/1000 nM crizotinib were administered in NCI-H2228

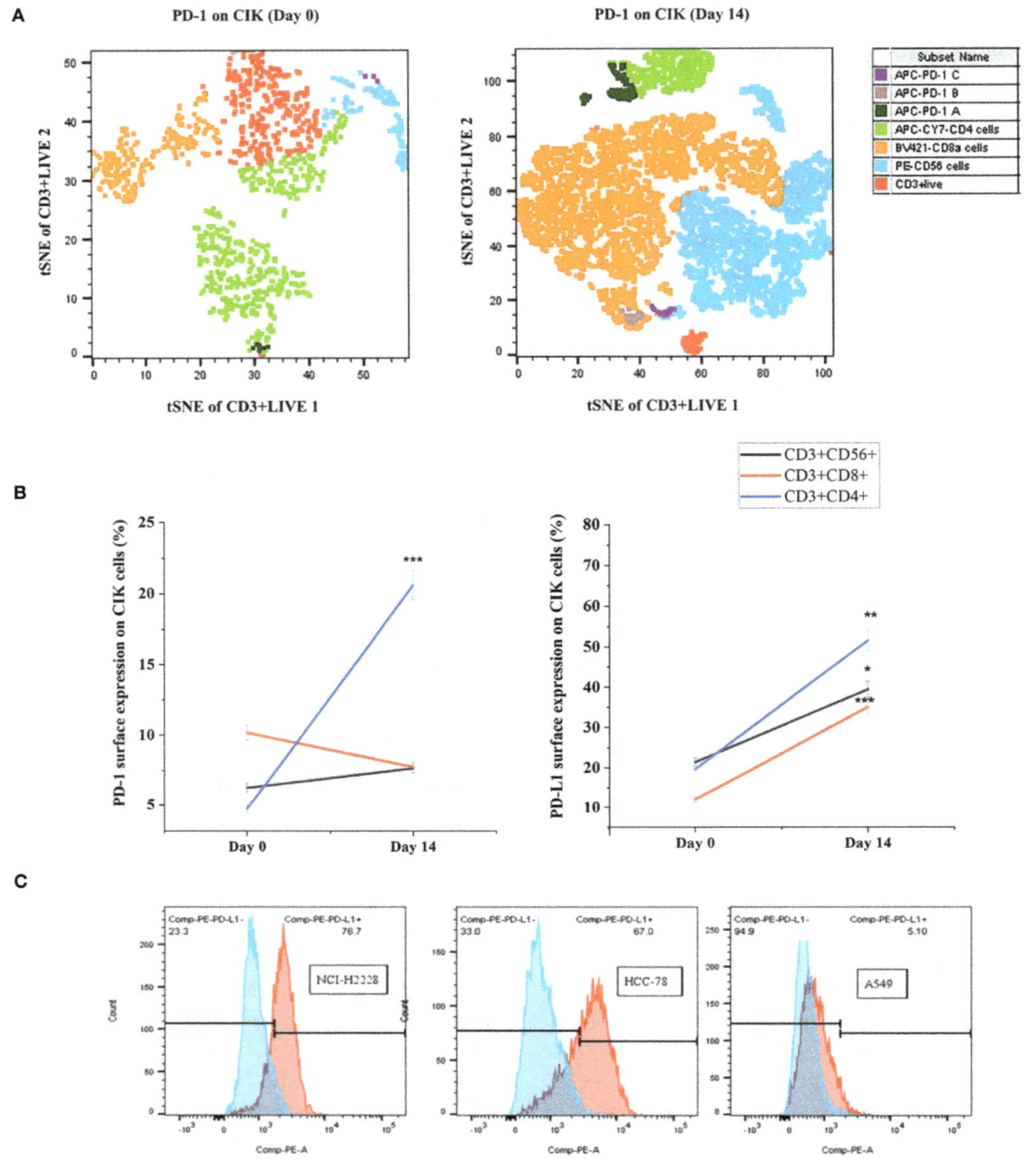

FIGURE 1 | PD-1$^+$/PD-L1$^+$ surface expression on Day 0 and Day 14 of CIK cells. The differential expression of PD-1/PD-L1 phenotypic subsets of CIK cells over *in vitro* culture is shown by flow cytometric analysis. PBMC were isolated from healthy donors and cultured in the presence of IFN- γ on Day 0, anti-human CD3 antibody, IL-1 β and IL-2 on Day 1. After 14 days of expansion with IL-2 induction, CIK cells were investigated by flow cytometric method by staining with FITC-CD3, PE-CD56, APC-Cy7-CD4, Bv421-CD8, and APC-PD-1. Dead CIK cells were gated excluding by 7-AAD. **(A)** The percentage of PD-1 on Day 0 and Day 14 CIK cells represented by tSNE plots using Flowjo V10 software. APC-PD-1 A represented APC-PD-1$^+$ APC-CY7-CD4$^+$ cells; APC-PD-1 B represented APC-PD-1$^+$BV421-CD8a$^+$ cells; APC-PD-1 C represented APC-PD-1$^+$PE-CD56$^+$ cells. **(B)** Summary data of the frequency of PD-1$^+$/PD-L1$^+$ CIK subsets in healthy subjects. **(C)** Variation of PD-L1 surface expression on the 3 NSCLC cell lines, measured by flow cytometry. All data are shown as the mean ± SD. * representative of three independent experiments. *P < 0.05, **P < 0.01, ***P < 0.001 vs. Day 0 CIK cells calculated by Student's t-test. CIK cells derived from three healthy donors.

cells compared to DMSO control (**Figure 3A**, 65.0% ± 3.9% vs. 97.2% ± 3.0%, p < 0.001; 58.3% ± 3.1% vs. 97.2% ± 3.0%, p < 0.001, respectively). However, no such change was observed in the HCC-78 and A549 cell lines as well as CIK cells, suggesting that this effect is cell line (or EML4-ALK variant 3) specific (**Figures 3B–D**).

Nivolumab and Crizotinib Displayed an Additive Effect on the Cytotoxicity

To assess the absolute quantification of dead tumor cells (that may directly reflect the cytotoxic activity of CIK cells), we pre-labelled the NSCLC cells with carboxyfluorescein diacetate succinimidyl ester (CFSE) and co-cultured with nivolumab-

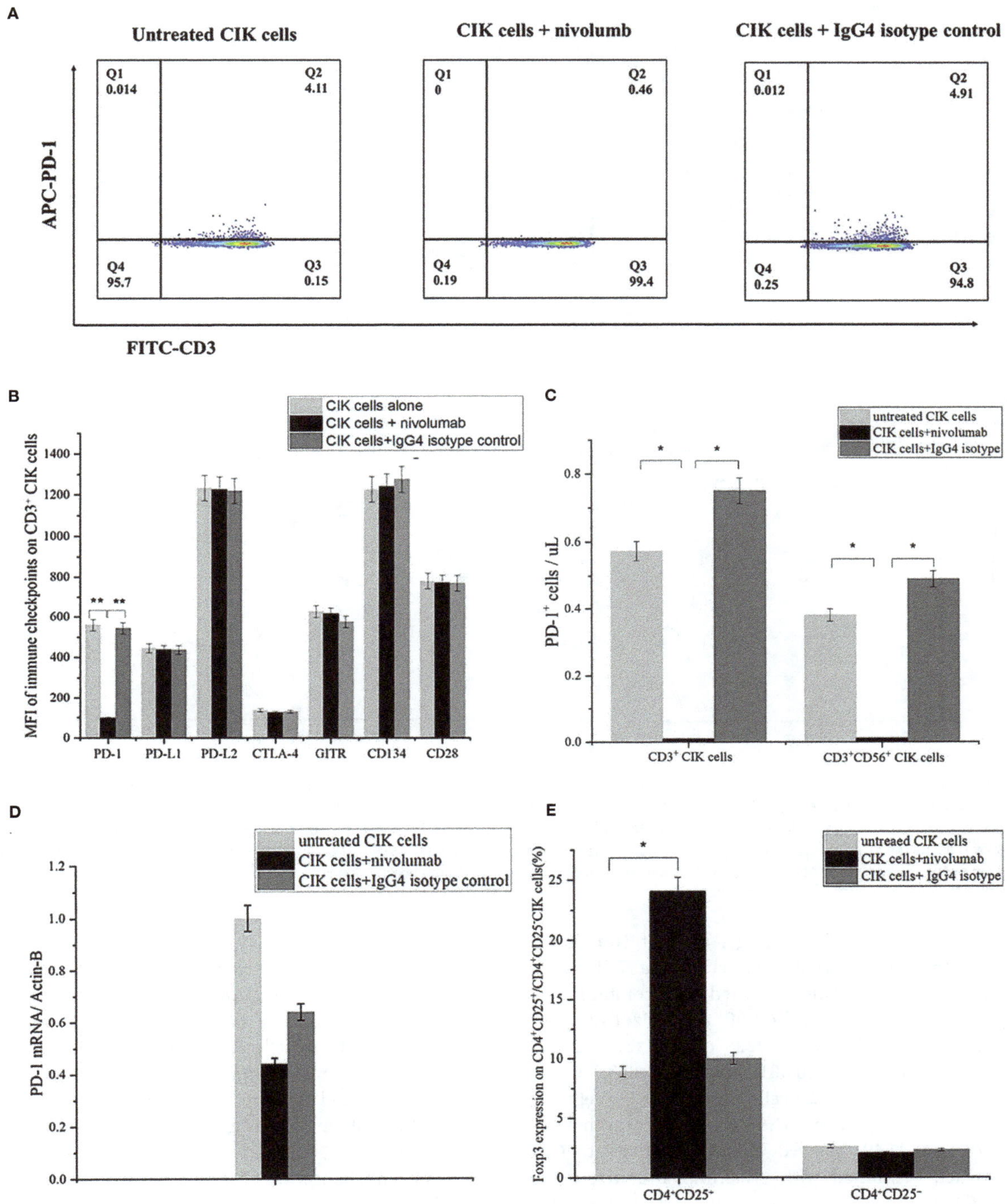

FIGURE 2 | PD-1 expression on CIK cells after treatment with nivolumab for 48 (h) **(A)** PD-1 surface expression on CIK cells in the presence of nivolumab 20 μg/mL for 48 h compared to untreated CIK cells or IgG4 isotype control 20 μg/mL measured by flow cytometry. Dead CIK cells were gated and excluded by 7-AAD. Numbers represent the percentage of the gated population. **(B)** The mean fluorescent intensity (MFI) level of PD-1, PD/L1, PD-L2, CTLA-4, GITR, and CD134 (OX40) on the $CD3^+$ CIK cells was observed after 48 h of treatment with nivolumab by flow cytometry. **(C)** Numbers represent the percentage of the gated population. Quantification of the absolute $PD\text{-}1^+$ CIK cells by count beads. **(D)** Analysis of q-RCR mRNA expression in CIK cells after incubation with nivolumab for 48 (h) PD-1 expression is normalized over β-actin expression. **(E)** Foxp3 expression on $CD4^+$ $CD25^+/CD4^+CD25^-$ CIK cells after 48 h nivolumab treatment. Data from three independent experiments were shown as mean ± SD. Statistical analysis was performed using one-way ANOVA followed by the Tukey–Kramer *post hoc* test. $^*p < 0.05$, $^{**}p < 0.01$ vs. untreated CIK cells or CIK cells treated with IgG4 isotype control. CIK cells derived from three healthy donors.

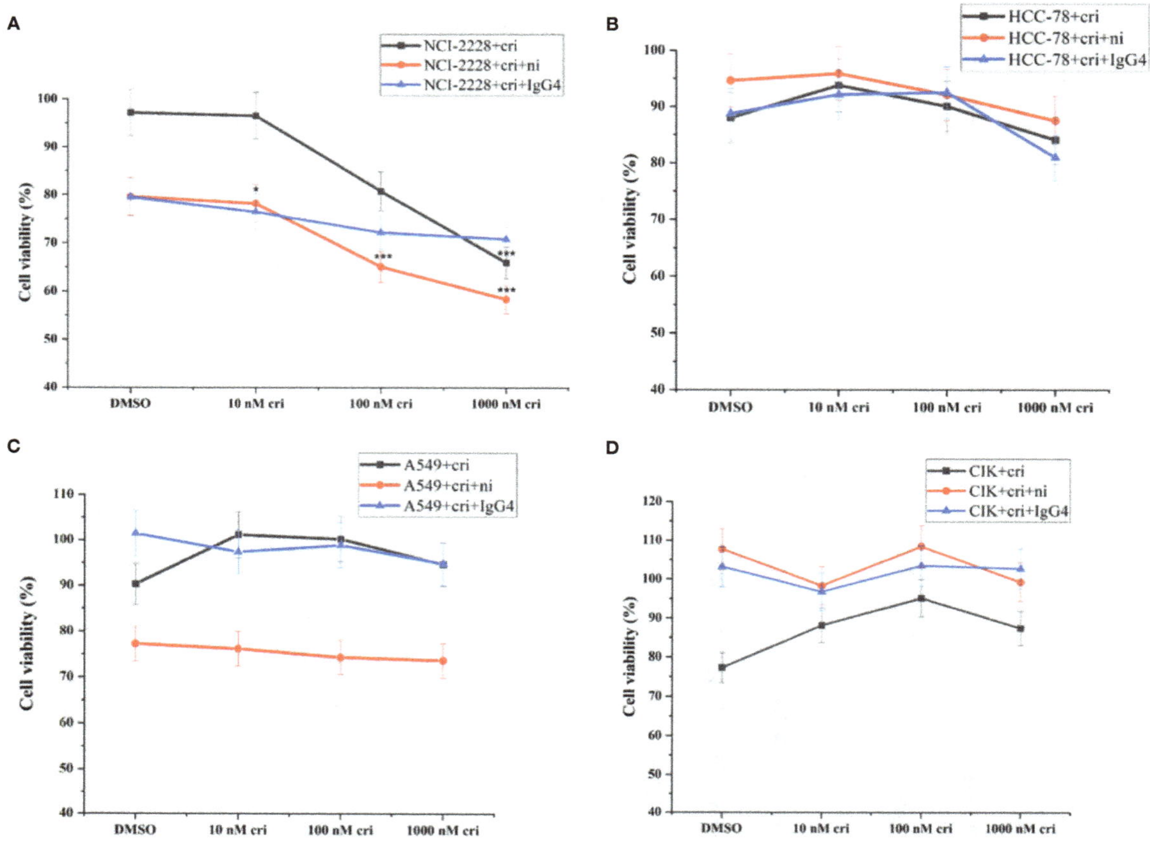

FIGURE 3 | The tumor cell viability after the combination of nivolumab and crizotinib in the absence of CIK cells and CIK cells viability after the combination of nivolumab and crizotinib in the absence of tumor cells. **(A–C)** Tumor cells were pretreated with 20 ug/mL nivolumab for 24 h prior to incubation with crizotinib for 24 h. **(D)** CIK cells were pretreated with 20 ug/mL nivolumab for 24 h prior to incubation with crizotinib for 24 h. Each experiment repeated 3 times and CIK cells derived from four donors. All data are shown as the mean ± SD. *representative of three independent experiments. *P < 0.05, ***P < 0.001 vs. NCI-H2228 treatedwith DMSO control. One-way ANOVA followed by the Tukey–Kramer *post hoc* test was performed. CIK cells derived from three healthy donors.

pretreated CIK cells at an effector-target ratio of 10:1 in the presence of crizotinib. The absolute number of dead NCI-H2228 cells was found to be significantly elevated after combining 10 nM crizotinib/100 nM crizotinb/1000 nM crizotinb with nivolumab compared to the NCI-H2228 control (32.2 ± 3. 9 cells/μL vs. 3.3 ± 0.9 cells/μL, P< 0.001; 30.6 ± 3.8 cells/μL vs. 3.3 ± 0.9 cells/μL, P< 0.001; 24.9 ± 2.7 cells/μL vs. 3.3 ± 0.9 cells/μL, P = 0.004, respectively) (**Figure 4A**). Here again, two other cell lines (HCC-78 and A549) showed weaker sensitivity to CIK cytotoxicity when combined with crizotinib and nivolumab (**Figures 4B, C**). Meanwhile, this combination strategy did not influence the dead cell number in CIK cells (**Figure 4D**).

Cumulative Effect of PD-1 Inhibitor With Crizotinib Influenced Interferon-γ and Intracellular Granzyme B

To investigate the potential variations in immune markers and cytokines primarily associated with the cytotoxicity of CIK cells, we subsequently examined IFN-γ expression (by ELISA) and intracellular expression of granzyme B by flow cytometry (**Figures 5A, B**) and IFN-γ expression by ELISA (**Figure 5C**). CIK cells responded to a combination of PD-1 blockade and crizotinib against NCI-H2228 with a strong secretion of IFN-γ and a significant increase in granzyme B in the $CD3^+$ $CD56^+$ subpopulation of CIK cells. Specifically, in combination with CIK cells, anti-PD-1 and 10 nM crizotinib showed a significant increase compared to either crizotinib or isotype control and/or crizotinib alone (320.3 ± 48.2 vs. 232.8 ± 41.6 pg/mL, P= 0.004; 320.3 ± 48.2 vs. 251.1 ± 40.1 pg/mL, P= 0.022). However, no significant change was observed in the HCC-78 and A549 cell lines (**Supplementary Figure 1**).

Nivolumab Combined Crizotinib Upregulated the Intrinsic FasL Expression in CIK Cells

Considering that cell surface FasL expression is specific to the immune system, we investigated FasL surface expression on the CIK cells. The analysis showed a low level of surface FasL (less than 5%), which was further verified using an additional methodological approach (Western blot) (**Figures 5D, E**).

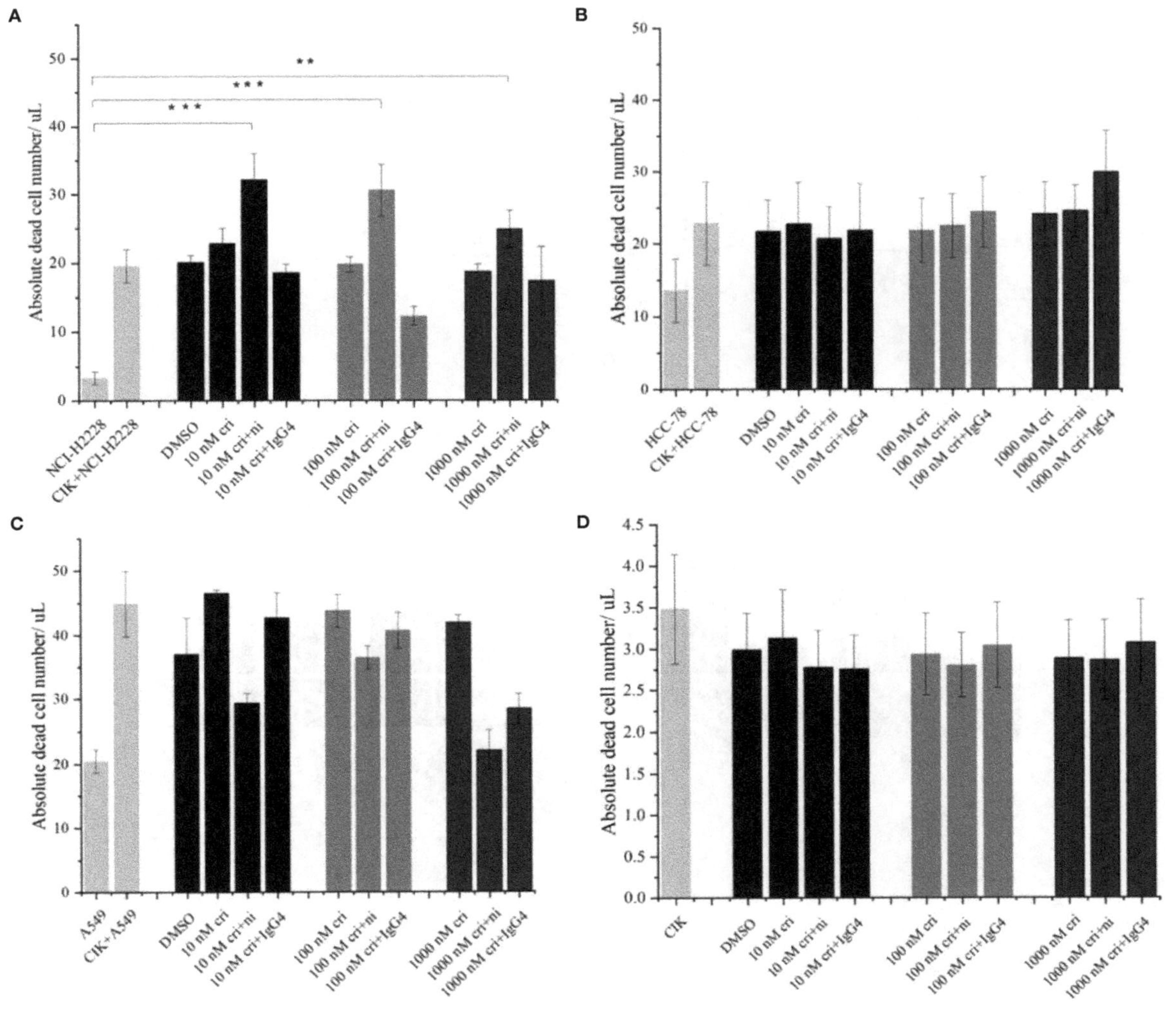

FIGURE 4 | The absolute dead cell concentration after the combination of nivolumab and crizotinib. **(A–C)** The absolute number of dead cells in NSCLC cell lines after the co-culture with 24 h nivolumab-pretreated CIK, and in the presence of crizotinib (for 24 h) were detected by flow cytometry. NSCLC cells were labelled with CFSE and stained with dead cell Dye Hoechst 33258 before data was recorded in the flow cytometer. Dead CFSE$^+$ tumor cells were analyzed by count beads and recorded by absolute cells/µL. **(D)** Similarly, 24 h nivolumab-pretreated CIK incubated with crizotinib (for 24 h) in the absence of tumor cells were stained with dead cell Dye Hoechst 33258 and detected by flow cytometry. Each experiment repeated 3 times and CIK cells derived from three donors. Data from three independent experiments were shown as mean ± SD. Statistical analysis was performed using one-way ANOVA followed by the Tukey–Kramer *post hoc* test. **p < 0.01, ***p < 0.001 vs. untreated NCI-H2228

Importantly, nivolumab combined with 1000 nM crizotinib resulted in significant upregulation of intrinsic FasL expression compared to the untreated CIK control (the band intensity 3.0 ± 0.7 vs. 1.0 ± 0.0, P= 0.028).

CIK Cells Ameliorated the Hepatoxicity in CCL-13 Cell Line Concurrent Incubation With Nivolumab Combined With Crizotinib

To assess the hepatoxicity, LDH release assay was performed. After incubation with CIK cells, cytotoxicity of the simultaneous combination of 1000 nM crizotinib and nivolumab was significantly reduced compared to cytotoxicity without CIK (**Supplementary Figure 2A**, P<0.001). Furthermore, the combination of CIK cells with crizotinib and nivolumab significantly decreased the mRNA expression of C - reactive protein (CRP), which is known to be associated with reactive oxygen species (ROS) (**Supplementary Figure 2B**, P=0.047).

DISCUSSION

Given cancer is quite a complex disease and monotherapies pose a serious challenge regarding patient survival rate, the development of new combination therapies has partially improved patient outcomes. The combined use of therapeutic agents within combination therapy has proven to be

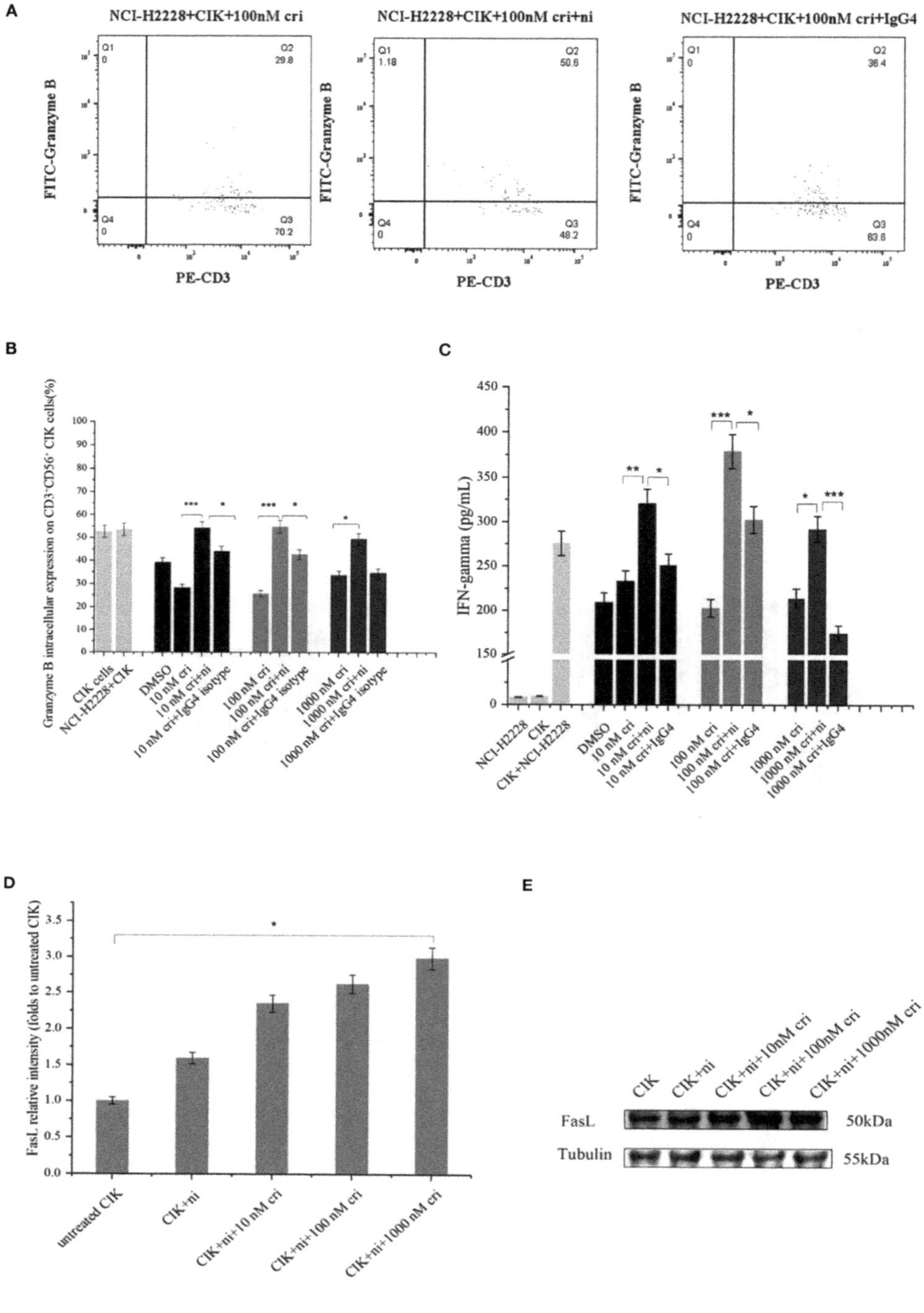

FIGURE 5 | Effects of a combination of blocking PD-1 immune checkpoint and crizotinib on CIK-derived IFN-γ, granzyme B in $CD3^{+}$ $CD56^{+}$ CIK cells. CIK cells were pretreated in the presence or absence of 20 ug/ml nivolumab. At 24 h post mAb treatment in CIK cells, CIK cells were co-cultured with NCI-H2228. **(A)** Intracellular granzyme B expression in $CD3^{+}$ $CD56^{+}$ CIK cells in the presence of PD-1 blockade against NCI-H2228 cells is shown in a dot plot, measured by flow cytometry at different levels of crizotinib. **(B)** Bar plots depict the percentage of intracellular granzyme B expression on CIK cells and **(C)** IFN-γ levels from CIK cells after treatment with a combination of PD-1 blockade and crizotinib on NCI-H2228 target cells. *$p < 0.05$, **$p < 0.01$, ***$p < 0.001$ vs. crizotinib monotherapy or IgG4 isotype control. **(D)** FasL expression was observed by Western blots. CIK cells were treated with nivolumab for 24 h prior to the addition of different concentrations of crizotinib. **(E)** The relative intensities of FasL expression normalized to each Tubulin control without treatment were defined as 1.0. Then, the other relative intensity (folds) was presented. Data were presented as means ± SD of the results from three independent experiments. *$p < 0.05$ vs. CIK control without any treatment. Each experiment repeated 3 times and CIK cells derived from three donors and the data were shown as mean ± SD. Statistical analysis was performed using one-way ANOVA followed by the Tukey–Kramer *post hoc* test.

advantageous (over monotherapy) in several ways, such as enhanced efficacy, reduced side effects, and minimal drug resistance. Of clinical importance, several cancers have been reported to optimize this therapeutic approach, such as renal cell carcinoma, melanoma, Hodgkin's lymphoma, and breast cancer to name a few (31–34). In particular, non-small cell lung cancer (NSCLC) is one of the prominent cancers where a number of studies documenting the clinical outcomes of mono and/or combination therapies have been reported (www.cancer.gov). However, there are serious concerns when the combination of compounds showed a synergistic effect in the preclinical models while failing in the clinical application. As mentioned above, the clinical trial with the combination of crizotinib (ALK inhibitor) and nivolumab (PD-1 inhibitor) was terminated due to safety concerns in NSCLC, while the same combination of compounds showed an improved antitumor response with favorable side-effect tolerability in the *in vivo* model.

In this current study, we investigated whether the inclusion of alternative treatments (for instance, cytokine-induced killer cells) and variable genetic backgrounds (NCI-H2228: EML4-ALK, A549: KRAS mutation, HCC-78: ROS1 rearrangement) within the same cancer type can help to provide an advantageous therapeutic paradigm in NSCLC. In the context of genetic variations, mutations in a few genes (KRAS, EGFR, ALK, ROS1, BRAF, RET, MET, NTRK) have been shown to be clinically relevant and proven to be pivotal to identify patient subgroups with early/advanced-stage patients. Moreover, accumulating data from different ethnic groups has confirmed these previous findings on the NSCLC-associated mutational paradigm and highlighted the potential genetic differences across different racial groups (35–37), given that CIK cells have previously shown positive outcome in NSCLC treatment, and nivolumab has been shown to be highly promising in NSCLC (38). As a proof of concept, we first confirmed that all cell lines expressed PD-L1, but at different levels. Next, we demonstrated that a combination of nivolumab and crizotinib improved the immune function of CIK cells compared to monotherapy with crizotinib, especially in the NSCLC-specific cell line NCI-H2228. We further first verified that PD-1 surface expression on CIK cells decreased dramatically after the treatment with nivolumab and it had no effect on PD-1 mRNA expression in CIK cells. Our findings revealed that PD-1 inhibitors only conjugate on the surface of CIK cells without PD-1 mRNA alternation. Nevertheless, nivolumab was found to bind to T lymphocytes for more than 20 weeks in NSCLC patients, even after stopping treatment, suggesting a sustained therapeutic effect (39). Although one clinical trial reported that treatment of NSCLC patients with anti-PD-1 antibodies nivolumab expanded the levels of effector T cells expressing the costimulatory molecules CD28, CD27, and ICOS (40), we did not observe the similar immuno-logical events (**Figure 2B**). Importantly, our study showed that nivolumab caused an increase in the proportion of Foxp3$^+$ CD4$^+$ CD25$^+$ CIK cells (**Figure 2E**), which is consistent with the previous reports (41). This suggests compensatory expression of immune molecules after PD-1 blockade. Second, we observed that the blocking of the PD-1/PD-L1 pathway by nivolumab increased the cytotoxicity of CIK cells targeted to NCI-H2228 rather than HCC-78 and A549 cells. Additionally, the evidence obtained from multiple markers in our study, such as increased production of IFN-γ from CIK cells, activation of FASL in CIK cells, and increased intracellular expression of granzyme B on CD3$^+$ CD56$^+$ NKT CIK cells, suggest that the combination of nivolumab and crizotinib accelerates the release of immune-related effector molecules. Previously, CIK cells were reported to express a high percentage of granzyme B, a serine protease that together with another protein perforin mediates apoptosis in target cells (42). Similarly, an addition of anti-PD-1 inhibitor has been shown to enhance the granzyme B expression in DC-CIK cells (43). Considering this, we assessed and found an increased level of intracellular granzyme B in PD-1 activated CIK cells after being combined with an ALK inhibitor. FasL, expressed on activated T cells and natural killer (NK) cells, poses another way to kill cancer cells by recruiting Fas-associated protein with DD (FADD) and activating caspase pathways. Notably, Verneris et al. found that CIK cells are resistant to apoptosis by expressing anti-apoptotic genes and can synthesize FasL to induce Fas-dependent apoptosis of sensitive tumor cells (44). In our current study, we are reporting for the first time that a combination of dose-dependent crizotinib and nivolumab can also promote FASL expression in CIK cells, overall suggesting that CIK cells use a different apoptosis pathway to eliminate NSCLC cells *in vitro*. Thus, our findings about the elevated granzyme B levels (along with activation of FASL) in a similar experimental setup suggest a yet unknown mechanism that may be of interest for future NSCLC immunotherapy.

Since our analysis showed predominance in NCI-H2228 compared to HCC-78 and A549 cells, we can assume three possibilities: (1) heterogeneity across cancer cell lines may lead to major discrepancies in the experimental data, as previously discussed by Sharma et al. (45), (2) origin of cell lines, A549 is a lung adenocarcinoma cell line with a mesenchymal signature and is known to be more resistant to the drugs targeting PI3K-AKT pathway (46), and (3) the presence of intrinsic PD-1 protein expression in NSCLC cells that may inhibit tumor cell proliferation and might exert resistance to PD-1/PD-L1 blockades (47). Nevertheless, our study supports the idea that combination therapies have enormous potential if they are optimized on a patient-by-patient basis. Like other cancers, the clonal heterogeneity and the existence of cancer stem cells (CSCs) in lung cancer also continue to be subjects of discussion (48). In an interesting study, six small cell lung cancer (SCLC) cell lines were used to investigate whether CD133 or CD87 could be a potential marker for CSCs (49). The authors showed that both CD133 and CD87 are expressed in the SBC-7 cell line as inadequate markers of CSCs and might be beneficial for predicting chemotherapy resistance. Recently, a study confirmed the identification of CSCs and showed that PD-L1$^+$ CSCs are strongly associated with altered T cell phenotypes and, in particular, the frequency of regulatory molecule-expressing T cells in metastatic lymph nodes of NSCLC patients (50). Of note, our current study mainly concerns enhancing the cytotoxicity and did not emphasize CSCs; however, we cannot exclude the contribution of lung cancer associated CSCs. Certainly, future studies utilizing CIK/ALK/PD inhibitors axis in context with the tumor microenvironment of NSCLCs will be of interest. Here, it is also important to mention CheckMate 370, which was discontinued due to severe hepatotoxicity in 2018. In this context, we also performed analysis to determine whether CIK cells can alleviate the hepatoxicity after incubation with ALK inhibitor and PD-1 inhibitor simultaneously. To achieve this, we used the hepatocyte-like cell line CCL-13, which exhibits the liver function of primary human hepatocytes, and found that: (1) after incubation with CIK cells, the cytotoxicity of the simultaneous combination of crizotinib and nivolumab was significantly reduced as detected by LDH assay. (2) The combination of CIK cells with crizotinib and nivolumab significantly decreased the mRNA expression of C-reactive protein (CRP), which is known to associate with reactive oxygen species (ROS). Therefore, it is reasonable to conclude that CIK cells may have mitigated with hepatotoxicity. In broader terms, the limitations of our study are also worth mentioning, such as (A) we did not investigate the combination of DC-CIK and ALK inhibitor with PD-1 inhibitor, which may exert more potent cytotoxic effects than CIK cells as shown in previous studies (43). (B) The data from a few additional cell lines (e.g., with KRAS, EGFR, and p53 mutation status) would be valuable in this analysis. (C) Our findings require *in vivo* validation. Despite these facts, our data as preclinical model provide an insight about the antitumor immune response by CIK cells in combination with crizotinib and nivolumab.

Based on our results and the existing literature, a few perspectives can be considered for NSCLC, for example, (a) given that response to therapies and improved survival varies significantly in NSCLC subtype, a clear emphasis on precision medicine/therapy should be considered. (b) With the development of second- and third-generation ALK inhibitors, their synergistic effects in preclinical studies, mainly on experimental models associated with NSCLC mutations, may improve their efficacy and resistance problem. (c) As recently proposed, the combinatorial aspect of CIK cell therapy combined with other contemporary anti-cancer therapies in a complementary (rather than competitive) manner may be the key to combat cancer (51), also applies in NSCLC. (d) Identifying a subpopulation of NSCLC patients (with ALK rearrangement) who may benefit from the combination of an ALK inhibitor and PD-1 inhibitor must be stratified according to known risk factors (52) and potential biomarkers (e.g., C-reactive protein levels) (53). In a broader prospective, though different cancers are represented with their unique mutational/epigenomic profiles, they still share few common/overlapping signaling pathways (54) and, therefore, it is important to stratify the uniqueness of each cancer type already in the preclinical models.

CONCLUSIONS

CIK cells in combination with crizotinib and nivolumab can enhance the antitumor immune response through FasL activation, leading to increased IFN-γ and granzyme B, but only in NCI-H2228 cells with EML4-ALK rearrangement. Hence, our study suggests that genetic background plays a significant role, and the combination therapies should be optimized by considering underlying factors (genetic background and immune response) on a patient-by-patient basis.

AUTHOR CONTRIBUTIONS

Conceptualization, YL and IS-W; methodology, YL and XW; validation, YL, XW, AS; formal analysis, YL; data curation, YL, AS, and IS-W; writing—original draft preparation, YL, AS, and IS-W; writing—review and editing, all co-authors; supervision, IS-W, HW, DS, and ME; project administration, IS-W. All authors contributed to the article and approved the submitted version.

REFERENCES

1. Sharma A, Liu H, Herwig-Carl MC, Chand Dakal T, Schmidt-Wolf IGH. Epigenetic Regulatory Enzymes: Mutation Prevalence and Coexistence in Cancers. *Cancer Invest* (2021) 39(3):257–73. doi: 10.1080/07357907.2021.1872593
2. Sharma A, Jamil MA, Nuesgen N, Dauksa A, Gulbinas A, Schulz WA, et al. Detailed Methylation Map of LINE-1 5'-Promoter Region Reveals Hypomethylated CpG Hotspots Associated With Tumor Tissue Specificity. *Mol Genet Genomic Med* (2019) 7(5):e601. doi: 10.1002/mgg3.601
3. Paz-Ares L, Luft A, Vicente D, Tafreshi A, Gümüş M, Mazières J, et al. Pembrolizumab Plus Chemotherapy for Squamous Non-Small-Cell Lung Cancer. *N Engl J Med* (2018) 379(21):2040–51. doi: 10.1056/NEJMoa1810865
4. Tartarone A, Roviello G, Lerose R, Roudi R, Aieta M, Zoppoli P. Anti-PD-1 Versus Anti-PD-L1 Therapy in Patients With Pretreated Advanced Non-Small-Cell Lung Cancer: A Meta-Analysis. *Future Oncol* (2019) 15(20):2423–33. doi: 10.2217/fon-2018-0868
5. Petrelli F, Ferrara R, Signorelli D, Ghidini A, Proto C, Roudi R, et al. Immune Checkpoint Inhibitors and Chemotherapy in First-Line NSCLC: A Meta-Analysis. *Immunotherapy* (2021) 13(7):621 31. doi: 10.2217/imt-2020-0224
6. Creelan BC, Yeh TC, Kim SW, Nogami N, Kim DW, Chow LQM, et al. A Phase 1 Study of Gefitinib Combined With Durvalumab in EGFR TKI-Naive Patients With EGFR Mutation-Positive Locally Advanced/Metastatic Non-Small-Cell Lung Cancer. *Br J Cancer* (2021) 124(2):383–90. doi: 10.1038/s41416-020-01099
7. Spigel DR, Reynolds C, Waterhouse D, Garon EB, Chandler J, Babu S, et al. Phase 1/2 Study of the Safety and Tolerability of Nivolumab Plus Crizotinib for the First-Line Treatment of Anaplastic Lymphoma Kinase Translocation - Positive Advanced Non-Small Cell Lung Cancer (CheckMate 370). *Clin Trial J Thorac Oncol* (2018) 13(5):682–8. doi: 10.1016/j.jtho.2018.02.022
8. Yamaguchi O, Kaira K, Kawasaki T, Mouri A, Hashimoto K, Shiono A, et al. Severe Hepatotoxicity Due to Osimertinib After Nivolumab Therapy in Patients With Non-Small Cell Lung Cancer Harboring EGFR Mutation. *Thorac Cancer* (2020) 11(4):1045–51. doi: 10.1111/1759-7714.13363
9. Du P, Hu T, An Z, Li P, Liu L. *In Vitro* and *In Vivo* Synergistic Efficacy of Ceritinib Combined With Programmed Cell Death Ligand-1 Inhibitor in Anaplastic Lymphoma Kinase-Rearranged non-Small Cell Lung Cancer. *Cancer Sci* (2020) 111(6):1887–98. doi: 10.1111/cas.14397
10. Felip E, de Braud FG, Maur M, Loong HH, Shaw AT, Vansteenkiste JF, et al. Ceritinib Plus Nivolumab in Patients With Advanced ALK-Rearranged Non-Small Cell Lung Cancer: Results of an Open-Label, Multi-Center, Phase 1b Study. *J Thorac Oncol* (2020) 15(3):392–403. doi: 10.1016/j.jtho.2019.10.006

11. Stankovic B, Bjørhovde HAK, Skarshaug R, Aamodt H, Frafjord A, Müller E, et al. Immune Cell Composition in Human Non-Small Cell Lung Cancer. *Front Immunol* (2019) 9:3101. doi: 10.3389/fimmu.2018.03101
12. Sheng SY, Gu Y, Lu CG, Zou JY, Hong H, Wang YF. The Distribution and Function of Human Memory T Cell Subsets in Lung Cancer. *Immunol Res* (2017) 65:639–50. doi: 10.1007/s12026-016-8882-y
13. Zhang Y, Schmidt-Wolf IGH. Ten-Year Update of the International Registry on Cytokine-Induced Killer Cells in Cancer Immunotherapy. *J Cell Physiol* (2020) 235(12):9291–303. doi: 10.1002/jcp.29827
14. Li Y, Sharma A, Bloemendal M, Schmidt-Wolf R, Kornek M, Schmidt-Wolf IGH. PD-1 Blockade Enhances Cytokine-Induced Killer Cell-Mediated Cytotoxicity in B-Cell non-Hodgkin Lymphoma Cell Lines. *Oncol Lett* (2021) 22(2):613. doi: 10.3892/ol.2021.12874
15. Wu X, Sharma A, Oldenburg J, Weiher H, Essler M, Skowasch D. And Schmidt-Wolf I.G.H. NKG2D Engagement Alone Is Sufficient to Activate Cytokine-Induced Killer Cells While 2b4 Only Provides Limited Coactivation. *Front Immunol* (2021) 12:731767. doi: 10.3389/fimmu.2021.731767
16. Zhang Y, Sharma A, Weiher H, Schmid M, Kristiansen G. And Schmidt-Wolf I.G.H. Clinical Studies on Cytokine-Induced Killer Cells: Lessons From Lymphoma Trials. *Cancers* (2021) 13(23):6007. doi: 10.3390/cancers13236007
17. Li DP, Li W, Feng J, Chen K, Tao M. Adjuvant Chemotherapy With Sequential Cytokine-Induced Killer (CIK) Cells in Stage IB Non-Small Cell Lung Cancer. *Oncol Res* (2015) 22(2):67–74. doi: 10.3727/096504014X14024160459168
18. Luo H, Gong L, Zhu B, Huang Y, Tang C, Yu S, et al. Therapeutic Outcomes of Autologous CIK Cells as a Maintenance Therapy in the Treatment of Lung Cancer Patients: A Retrospective Study. *BioMed Pharmacother* (2016) 84:987–93. doi: 10.1016/j.biopha.2016.10.022
19. Wu C, Jiang J, Shi L, Xu N. Prospective Study of Chemotherapy in Combination With Cytokine-Induced Killer Cells in Patients Suffering From Advanced Non-Small Cell Lung Cancer. *Random Controlled Trial Anticancer Res* (2008) 28(6B):3997–4002.
20. Li R, Wang C, Liu L, Du C, Cao S, Yu J, et al. Autologous Cytokine-Induced Killer Cell Immunotherapy in Lung Cancer: A Phase II Clinical Study. *Clin Trial Cancer Immunol Immunother* (2012) 61(11):2125–33. doi: 10.1007/s00262-012-1260-2
21. Gu Y, Lv H, Zhao J, Li Q, Mu G, Li J, et al. Influence of the Number and Interval of Treatment Cycles on Cytokine-Induced Killer Cells and Their Adjuvant Therapeutic Effects in Advanced Non-Small-Cell Lung Cancer (NSCLC). *Int Immunopharmacol* (2017) 50:263–9. doi: 10.1016/j.intimp.2017.07.006
22. Mohsenzadegan M, Peng RW, Roudi R. Dendritic Cell/Cytokine-Induced Killer Cell-Based Immunotherapy in Lung Cancer: What We Know and Future Landscape. *J Cell Physiol* (.(2020) 235(1):74–86. doi: 10.1002/jcp.28977
23. Chen J, Chen Y, Feng F, Chen C, Zeng H, Wen S, et al. Programmed Cell Death Protein-1/Programmed Death-Ligand 1 Blockade Enhances the Antitumor Efficacy of Adoptive Cell Therapy Against Non-Small Cell Lung Cancer. *J Thorac Dis* (2018) 10(12):6711–21. doi: 10.21037/jtd.2018.10.111
24. Han Y, Mu D, Liu T, Zhang H, Zhang J, Li S, et al. Autologous Cytokine-Induced Killer (CIK) Cells Enhance the Clinical Response to PD-1 Blocking Antibodies in Patients With Advanced Non-Small Cell Lung Cancer: A Preliminary Study. *Thorac Cancer* (2021) 12(2):145–52. doi: 10.1111/1759-7714.13731
25. Wang P, Fang X, Yin T, Tian H, Yu J, Teng F. Efficacy and Safety of Anti-PD-1 Plus Anlotinib in Patients With Advanced Non-Small-Cell Lung Cancer After Previous Systemic Treatment Failure-A Retrospective Study. *Front Oncol* (2021) 11:628124. doi: 10.3389/fonc.2021.628124
26. Schmidt-Wolf IG, Negrin RS, Kiem HP, Blume KG, Weissman IL. Use of a SCID Mouse/Human Lymphoma Model to Evaluate Cytokine-Induced Killer Cells With Potent Antitumor Cell Activity. *J Exp Med* (1991) 174(1):139–49. doi: 10.1084/jem.174.1.139
27. Wu X, Zhang Y, Li Y, Schmidt-Wolf IGH. Increase of Antitumoral Effects of Cytokine-Induced Killer Cells by Anti-Body-Mediated Inhibition of MICA Shedding. *Cancers (Basel)* (2020) 12(7):1818. doi: 10.3390/cancers12071818
28. Mariotti FR, Petrini S, Ingegnere T, Tumino N, Besi F, Scordamaglia F, et al. PD-1 in Human NK Cells: Evidence of Cytoplasmic mRNA and Protein Expression. *Oncoimmunology* (2019) 8(3):1557030. doi: 10.1080/2162402X.2018.1557030
29. Chen Y, Meng L, Shang H, Dou Q, Lu Z, Liu L, et al. β2 Spectrin-Mediated Differentiation Repressed the Properties of Liver Cancer Stem Cells Through β-Catenin. *Cell Death Dis* (2018) 9(4):424. doi: 10.1038/s41419-018-0456-6
30. Dehno MN, Li Y, Weiher H, Schmidt-Wolf IGH. Increase in Efficacy of Checkpoint Inhibition by Cytokine-Induced-Killer Cells as a Combination Immunotherapy for Renal Cancer. *Int J Mol Sci* (2020) 21(9):3078. doi: 10.3390/ijms21093078
31. Zhang L, Xie D, Lei Y, Na A, Zhu L. Preclinical Activity of Cobimetinib Alone or in Combination With Chemotherapy and Targeted Therapies in Renal Cell Carcinoma. *Future Oncol* (2021) 17(23):3051–60. doi: 10.2217/fon-2021-0256
32. Sanchez JN, Subramanian C, Chanda M, Shanguan G, Zhang N, Wang T, et al. A Novel C-Terminal Hsp90 Inhibitor KU758 Synergizes Efficacy in Combination With BRAF or MEK Inhibitors and Targets Drug-Resistant Pathways in BRAF-Mutant Melanomas. *Melanoma Res* (2021) 31(3):197–207. doi: 10.1097/CMR.0000000000000734
33. Pezeshki PS, Eskian M, Hamblin MR, Rezaei N. Immune Checkpoint Inhibition in Classical Hodgkin Lymphoma. *Expert Rev Anticancer Ther* (2021) 21(9):1003–16. doi: 10.1080/14737140.2021.1918548
34. Ma H, Li Q, Wang J, Pan J, Su Z, Liu S. Dual Inhibition of Ornithine Decarboxylase and A(1) Adenosine Receptor Efficiently Suppresses Breast Tumor Cells. *Front Oncol* (2021) 11:636373. doi: 10.3389/fonc.2021.636373
35. Wu X, Wang L, Ye Y, Aakre JA, Pu X, Chang GC, et al. Genome-Wide Association Study of Genetic Predictors of Overall Survival for non-Small Cell Lung Cancer in Never Smokers. *Cancer Res* (2013) 73(13):4028–38. doi: 10.1158/0008-5472
36. Arauz RF, Byun JS, Tandon M, Sinha S, Kuhn S, Taylor S, et al. Whole-Exome Profiling of NSCLC Among African Americans. *J Thorac Oncol* (2020) 15 (12):1880–92. doi: 10.1016/j.jtho.2020.08.029
37. Aye PS, McKeage MJ, Tin ST, Khwaounjoo P, Elwood JM. Population-Based Incidence Rates and Increased Risk of EGFR Mutated non-Small Cell Lung Cancer in Māori and Pacifica in New Zealand. *PloS One* (2021) 16(5): e0251357. doi: 10.1371/journal.pone.0251357
38. Sundar R, Cho BC, Brahmer JR, Soo RA. Nivolumab in NSCLC: Latest Evidence and Clinical Potential. *Ther Adv Med Oncol* (2015) 7(2):85–96. doi: 10.1177/1758834014567470
39. Osa A, Uenami T, Koyama S, Fujimoto K, Okuzaki D, Takimoto T, et al. Clinical Implications of Monitoring Nivolumab Immunokinetics in non-Small Cell Lung Cancer Patients. *Observat Stud JCI Insight* (2018) 3(19): e59125. doi: 10.1172/jci.insight.59125
40. Xiong Y, Neskey DM, Horton JD, Paulos CM, Knochelmann HM, Armeson KE, et al. Immunological Effects of Nivolumab Immunotherapy in Patients With Oral Cavity Squamous Cell Carcinoma. *BMC Cancer* (2020) 20(1):229. doi: 10.1186/s12885-020-06726-3
41. He Y, Liu S, Mattei J, Bunn PA Jr, Zhou C, Chan D. The Combination of Anti-KIR Monoclonal Antibodies With an-Ti-PD-1/PD-L1 Monoclonal Antibodies Could be a Critical Breakthrough in Overcoming Tumor Immune Escape in NSCLC. *Drug Design Dev Ther* (2018) 12:981–6. doi: 10.2147/DDDT.S163304
42. Niu C, Jin H, Li M, Xu J, Xu D, Hu J, et al. *In Vitro* Analysis of the Proliferative Capacity and Cytotoxic Effects of Ex Vivo Induced Natural Killer Cells, Cytokine-Induced Killer Cells, and Gamma-Delta T Cells. *BMC Immunol* (2015) 16:61. doi: 10.1186/s12865-015-0124-x
43. Zhang W, Song Z, Xiao J, Liu X, Luo Y, Yang Z, et al. Blocking the PD-1/PD-L1 Axis in Dendritic Cell-Stimulated Cytokine-Induced Killer Cells With Pembrolizumab Enhances Their Therapeutic Effects Against Hepatocellular Carcinoma. *J Cancer.* (2019) 10(11):2578–87. doi: 10.7150/jca.26961
44. Verneris MR, Kornacker M, Mailänder V, Negrin RS. Resistance of Ex Vivo Expanded $CD3^+CD56^+$ T Cells to Fas-Mediated Apoptosis. *Cancer Immunol Immunother* (2000) 49(6):335–45. doi: 10.1007/s002620000111
45. Sharma A, Reutter H, Ellinger J. DNA Methylation and Bladder Cancer: Where Genotype Does Not Predict Phenotype. *Curr Genomics* (2020) 21 (1):34–6. doi: 10.2174/1389202921666200102163422
46. Byers LA, Diao L, Wang J, Saintigny P, Girard L, Peyton M, et al. An Epitheli-Al-Mesenchymal Transition Gene Signature Predicts Resistance to EGFR and PI3K Inhibitors and Identifies Axl as a Therapeutic Target for Overcoming EGFR Inhibitor Resistance. *Clin Cancer Res* (2013) 19(1):279–90. doi: 10.1158/1078-0432.CCR-12-1558

47. Wang X, Yang X, Zhang C, Wang Y, Cheng T, Duan L, et al. Tumor Cell-Intrinsic PD-1 Receptor Is a Tumor Suppressor and Mediates Resistance to PD-1 Blockade Therapy. *Proc Natl Acad Sci USA* (2020) 117(12):6640–50. doi: 10.1073/pnas.1921445117
48. Testa U, Castelli G, Pelosi E. Lung Cancers: Molecular Characterization, Clonal Heterogeneity and Evolution, and Cancer Stem Cells. *Cancers (Basel)* (2018) 10(8):248. doi: 10.3390/cancers10080248
49. Kubo T, Takigawa N, Osawa M, Harada D, Ninomiya T, Ochi N, et al. Subpopulation of Small-Cell Lung Cancer Cells Expressing CD133 and CD87 Show Resistance to Chemotherapy. *Cancer Sci* (2013) 104(1):78–84. doi: 10.1111/cas.12045
50. Raniszewska A, Vroman H, Dumoulin D, Cornelissen R, Aerts JGIV, Domagała-Kulawik J. PD-L1^{+} Lung Cancer Stem Cells Modify the Metastatic Lymph-Node Immunomicroenvironment in Nsclc Patients. *Cancer Immunol Immunother* (2021) 70(2):453–61. doi: 10.1007/s00262-020-02648-y
51. Sharma A, Schmidt-Wolf IGH. 30 Years of CIK Cell Therapy: Recapitulating the Key Breakthroughs and Future Perspective. *J Exp Clin Cancer Res* (2021) 40(1):388. doi: 10.1186/s13046-021-02184-2
52. Hill H, Robinson M, Lu L, Slaughter D, Amin A, Mileham K, et al. Venous Thromboembolism Incidence and Risk Factors in non-Small Cell Lung Cancer Patients Receiving First-Line Systemic Therapy. *Thromb Res* (2021) 208:71–8. doi: 10.1016/j.thromres.2021.10.014
53. Ried JM, Barth DM, Brueckl WM, Zeitler G, Foris V, Mollnar S, et al. C-Reactive Protein (CRP) Levels in Immune Checkpoint Inhibitor Response and Progression in Advanced Non-Small Cell Lung Cancer: A Bi-Center Study. *Cancers (Basel)* (2020) 12(8):2319. doi: 10.3390/cancers12082319
54. Liu H, Li H, Luo K, Sharma A, Sun X. Prognostic Gene Expression Signature Revealed the Involvement of Mutational Pathways in Cancer Genome. *J Cancer* (2020) 11(15):4510–20. doi: 10.7150/jca.40237

23

Immunotherapy in Non-Small Cell Lung Cancer with Actionable Mutations other than *EGFR*

***Karan Seegobin*[1], *Umair Majeed*[1], *Nathaniel Wiest*[2], *Rami Manochakian*[1], *Yanyan Lou*[1] *and Yujie Zhao*[1*]**

[1] Division of Hematology and Oncology, Mayo Clinic, Jacksonville, FL, United States, [2] Department of Medicine, Mayo Clinic, Jacksonville, FL, United States

***Correspondence:**
Yujie Zhao
Zhao.Yujie@mayo.edu

While first line targeted therapies are the current standard of care treatment for non-small cell lung cancer (NSCLC) with actionable mutations, the cancer cells inevitably acquire resistance to these agents over time. Immune check-point inhibitors (ICIs) have improved the outcomes of metastatic NSCLC, however, its efficacy in those with targetable drivers is largely unknown. In this manuscript, we reviewed the published data on ICI therapies in NSCLC with *ALK*, *ROS1*, *BRAF*, *c-MET*, *RET*, *NTRK*, *KRAS*, and *HER2 (ERBB2)* alterations. We found that the objective response rates (ORRs) associated with ICI treatments in lung cancers harboring the *BRAF* (0–54%), *c-MET* (12–49%), and *KRAS* (18.7-66.7%) alterations were comparable to non-mutant NSCLC, whereas the ORRs in *RET* fusion NSCLC (less than10% in all studies but one) and *ALK* fusion NSCLC (0%) were relatively low. The ORRs reported in small numbers of patients and studies of *ROS1* fusion, *NTRK* fusion, and *HER 2* mutant NSCLC were 0–17%, 50% and 7–23%, respectively, making the efficacy of ICIs in these groups of patients less clear. In most studies, no significant correlation between treatment outcome and PD-L1 expression or tumor mutation burden (TMB) was identified, and how to select patients with NSCLC harboring actionable mutations who will likely benefit from ICI treatment remains unknown.

Keywords: targeted mutations, immunotherapy, *c-MET*, *RET*, *BRAF*, *ROS-1*, *ALK*, *NTRK*

INTRODUCTION

NSCLC accounts for 85% of all lung cancers, with lung adenocarcinoma being the major subtype (1). Platinum-based combination chemotherapy is the historical first-line standard of care for patients with advanced NSCLC who have no actionable mutations (2). The introduction of ICIs, such as anti-programmed cell death protein ligand 1 (anti-PD-L1) and anti-programmed cell death protein 1 (anti-PD-1) antibodies, as well as the anti-cytotoxic T-lymphocyte-associated protein 4 (anti-CTLA-4) antibody, have revolutionized the treatment of NSCLC, and is typically offered with or without chemotherapy in the front-line setting for incurable NSCLC that does not have any actionable mutations (2). A number of actionable genetic alterations have been identified in NCSLC, including *ALK*, *ROS1*, *c-MET*, *RET*, *NTRK*, *BRAF* V600E, *KRAS*, and *ERBB2 (HER2)* (3–11). MET, RET, HER2, ALK, NTRK, and ROS-1 are receptor tyrosine kinases; BRAF is a serine/threonine kinase mediating cellular signal from RAS to MEK1/2; KRAS is a RAS protein which functions as a

GDP–GTP-regulated binary on-off switch. While *c-MET, BRAF* and *KRAS* altered NSCLC may develop in both smokers and non-smokers, *ALK, ROS1, RET, NTRK,* and *HER2* alerted NSCLC tend to occur in non-smokers. In patients with actionable driver mutations, namely, *EGFR, ALK, BRAFV600E, RET, c-MET, NTRK* or *ROS1* alterations, the standard of care is to treat with a Food and Drug Administration (FDA) approved targeted agent, which typically can achieve ORRs of 60–80% in treatment naive patients (2, 12). After targeted therapies are exhausted in these patients, systemic therapy with chemotherapy is typically available for them. While incorporating immunotherapy in the regimen is a standard of care option for them, the efficacy of immunotherapy in those with actionable mutations remains poorly defined due to the limited numbers of these patients included in the randomized prospective trials. In addition to the genetic alterations for which targeted therapies have been approved by FDA in the first line setting in NSCLC, *KRAS G12C* has a targeted agent that was approved recently in the beyond first-line setting. Moreover, *HER2* mutations have emerged as new therapeutic targets with promising therapeutic agents in development. The efficacy of ICI in the *KRAS* G12C or *HER2* mutant NSCLC is also of great clinical interest.

In this modern era with a booming number of treatment options for NSCLC and continued improvement in survival, further guidance is needed on what to expect from the use of immunotherapy in those with these genetic abnormalities. The goal of this review is to add valuable information on the use of immunotherapy in NSCLC with actionable alterations in genes including *ALK, ROS1, BRAF, c-MET, RET, NTRK, KRAS,* and *HER2.* Epidermal growth factor receptor (*EGFR*) mutations are not included in this review as they are included in another manuscript by our group which was submitted separately. In this review, we showed that the sensitivity to ICIs can be heterogenous and differs according to the driver alteration considered. *ALK* and *RET* fusions were found to be associated with low responses to ICI while *BRAF, KRAS,* and *c-MET* alterations were associated with responses that were comparable to non-mutant NSCLC, and PD-L1 positive *KRAS* mutant NSCLC may be associated with better outcome when treated with ICI monotherapy as suggested by two retrospective studies. The responses to ICIs are less clear in *HER2, ROS1* or *NTRK* altered NSCLCs due to low patient numbers. While an association between PD-L1 expression level or TMB and the responses to ICI has not been consistently observed across all driver alterations, the overall lack of response to ICI treatment appeared to be more common among NSCLC with driver alterations that are typically associated with non-smokers, raising the question whether the absence of tobacco exposure may predict the lack of benefit from ICI treatment. Moreover, the emerging data in the role of co-mutations in response to ICI had also shed a light in the potential underlining mechanism of resistance to ICI, and particularly in the presence of *KRAS* mutation, co-mutations in *TP53, STK11,* and *KEAP1* have been found to modulate the response to ICIs in several studies (13–15).

ALK

Anaplastic lymphoma kinase (*ALK*), a member of the insulin receptor tyrosine kinase family, has been identified as a fusion partner of nearly 30 different proteins in oncogenic signaling in many different cancer types (3). While there are now over 20 *ALK* fusion partners identified in NSCLC, *EML4* represents the most common fusion partner with 29–33% of gene fusions identified to date (16, 17). The fusion of the 5′ end partner *EML4* to the coding region of the intracellular tyrosine kinase domain of *ALK* leads to aberrant expression of the ALK fusions in the cytoplasm. The domains in the partner proteins also promote dimerization and oligomerization of the fusion proteins, leading to constitutive activation of *ALK* kinase and its downstream signaling pathways including RAS–mitogen-activated protein kinase, phosphoinositide 3-kinase-AKT, and JAK-STAT pathways. This subsequently results in uncontrolled cellular proliferation and promotes survival (3, 18). *ALK* fusions are seen in 3–5% of NSCLC patients and are more common among the following groups: no prior smoking history, adenocarcinoma histology, younger age, female gender, and tumors with wild type *EGFR* and *KRAS* (16, 19–21). Several *ALK* inhibitors have been approved by the FDA for metastatic NSCLC, including crizotinib, brigatinib, alectinib, lorlatinib and ceritinib (22–29). The data on the efficacy of ICIs in the *ALK* fusion positive NSCLC has been scarce. It has been postulated that EML4-ALK oncoprotein can upregulate the PD-L1 expression in lung cancer cells. In one report of 100 patients, fifty patients (50.0%) were PD-L1 negative, 34 patients (34.0%) were PD-L1 low expression (tumor proportion score [TPS] 1–50%), and 16 patients (16.0%) had a strong PD-L1 expression (TPS $\geq$ 50%) (30). Despite the expression of PDL1 in these tumors, the overall response to ICIs in the *ALK* fusion positive population has been disappointing except in one study (**Table 1**).

Although small numbers of patients with *ALK* fusion NSCLC were included in the randomized phase 3 CheckMate 057 and KEYNOTE-010 studies comparing ICI versus docetaxel in

TABLE 1 | Efficacy of ICIs in NSCLS with *ALK* mutations.

Reference	Characteristics	ORR, %	mPFS, months	mOS, months since start of ICI
Mazieres J., et al. (31)	*ALK* (n=23)	0	2.5	17
Gainor JF.,et al. (32)	*ALK* (n=6)	0		
Jahanzeb M., et al. (33)	*ALK* (n=83)		2.34	
Gadgeel SM. et al. (34)	*ALK (n=7)*	28.6%	2.9	2.9

ICIs, immune checkpoint inhibitors; NSCLC, non-small cell lung cancer; ORR, overall response rate; mPFS-median progression-free survival; mOS, median overall survival.

previously treated NSCLC patient population, the outcomes in this specific population were not reported (35, 36).

In a retrospective study using the IMMUNOTARGET registry which included 551 patients receiving ICI monotherapy for advanced NSCLC with at least one oncogenic driver alteration, 23 patients with *ALK* fusion NSCLC were identified (31). The objective response rate to ICI treatment was 0%. The Median PFS was 2.5 (1.5; 3.7) months. The median OS from start of ICI therapy was 17.0 (3.6; NR) months. Among the 10 patients with available PD-L1 status, the median percentage of cells expressing PD-L1 was 7.5% (**Table 1**).

In a retrospective study conducted at the Massachusetts General Hospital, the ORR to ICI treatment among patients with *EGFR* mutations or *ALK* rearrangements was only 1/28 (3.6%) while the ORR among *EGFR WT/ALK*-negative patients was 7/30 (23.3%) (P = 0.053) (32). Since the lone partial response was seen in an *EGFR*-mutant patient, it appeared that none of the six *ALK* fusion NSCLC patients had a response (**Table 1**).

In the randomized Impower130 study, atezolizumab plus chemotherapy (Nab-Paclitaxel and Carboplatin) did not show improved overall survival versus chemotherapy alone in the subset of 44 patients with *EGFR* or *ALK* genomic alterations in the first line setting (37). However, in the Impower150 study, the addition of Atezolizumab to Bevacizumab, Carboplatin, and Paclitaxel improved the median PFS for patients with *EGFR* or *ALK* genomic alteration whose diseases had progressed on TKI or who were unable to tolerate TKI (median, 8.3 months vs. 6.8 months; stratified hazard ratio, 0.61; 95% CI, 0.52 to 0.72). Of note, 34 patients with *ALK* fusion and 80 patients with *EGFR* mutant nonsquamous metastatic lung cancer were included in this study, and information on the benefit of atezolizumab in *ALK* fusion NSCLC was not reported separately (38). In another report of 83 patients with *ALK* mutation treated with ICI, a mPFS of 2.34 months was reported (33).

A recent prospective multicenter trial presented at the World Conference on Lung Cancer evaluated pembrolizumab and chemotherapy in the setting of recurrent *EGFR/ALK*-positive NSCLC. The study enrolled a total of 33 patients, including 26 *EGFR* mutant NSCLC and seven *ALK* fusion positive NSCLC patients. Most of the patients had one prior targeted therapy. No more than one prior line of platinum-based chemotherapy for advanced NSCLC was allowed. In those with ALK-positive tumors, the ORR was seen in 2/7 (28.6%), and the mPFS and mOS were both 2.9 months, suggesting lack of benefit of ICI in this group of patients (34).

BRAF

BRAF is a serine/threonine kinase mediating cellular signal from RAS to MEK1/2, and BRAF activation can result in phosphorylation and activation of extracellular signal-regulated kinase (ERK)1/2, leading to cell survival and proliferation (4). *BRAF* mutations are found in 1.5–3.5% of NSCLC with V600E accounting for approximately half of those mutations (39). Besides adenocarcinoma, *BRAF* mutations have been reported in sarcomatoid carcinomas, large-cell neuroendocrine carcinomas, and squamous cell lung cancer (40, 41). *BRAF* mutations can occur in both smokers and non-smokers (42). Selective kinase inhibitors have been recommended for the first-line and second-line treatments of *BRAF* V600E mutant advanced NSCLC with a reported ORR as high as 64% in this group of patients (39). The outcomes associated with ICIs in this population have been studies in multiple retrospective analyses (**Table 2**). Although the data vary significantly among different studies, responses to ICI have been seen in most of the studies.

In a retrospective study including seven participating Israeli cancer centers reported by Dudnik et al., PD-L1 expression level,

TABLE 2 | Efficacy of ICIs in NSCLS with *BRAF* mutations.

Reference	Characteristics		ORR, %	mPFS, months	mOS, months since start of ICI
Dudnik E., et al. (43)	Total (n=22)		28		
	mutation type	V600E (n=12)	25	3.7	Not reached (median follow-up of 5.5 months)
		nonV600E (n=10)	33	4.1	Not reached (median follow-up of 5.5 months)
	PD-L1 expression	PD-1L ≥50%	36	5.3	
		PDL-1 0-49%	14	2.2	
Rihawi K., et al. (44)	*BRAF*, 2nd line immunotherapy (n=11)		9		10.3
Tan I., et al. (45)	*BRAF*, 1st line immunotherapy (n=3)			0.17, 1.4, and 4.4 for each patient respectively	0.17, 6.8, and 7.5 for each patient respectively
	BRAF, 2nd line immunotherapy (n=8)			2.5	
	BRAF, 1st line chemoimmunotherapy (n=2)			1.5 and 2.1 for each patient respectively	6.6 and 5.6 for each patient respectively
Mazieres J., et al. (31)	*BRAF* (n=43)		24.3	3.1 (1st-3rd line ICI) 2.7 (>3rd line)	20.3
Dudnik E., et al. (46)	*BRAF* V600E (n=5)		25	1.5	NR (not reached)
	BRAF non-*V600E* (n=5)		20	2.6	NR (not reached)
Guisier F., et al. (47)	*BRAF* V600E (n=26)		26.1%	5.3	22.5
	BRAF non-V600E (n=18)		35.3%	4.9	12
Mu Y., et al. (48)	*BRAF*(n=9)		25%	3.0	

ICIs, immune checkpoint inhibitors; NSCLC, non-small cell lung cancer; ORR, overall response rate; mPFS-median progression-free survival; mOS, median overall survival.

tumor mutational burden (TMB), and microsatellite instability status were assessed in both *BRAF* V600E and non-V600E *BRAF* mutation positive NSCLC, and the outcome with ICI treatment was reported (43). High (≥50%) PD-L1 expression was found to be more common in the *non-BRAF* V600E mutant group than the V600E *BRAF* mutant group (50% vs 42%, $p = 0.05$). No MSI-H was found in both groups, and the median TMB was 5 (1–42) muts/Mb and 11 (7–14) muts/Mb in the *BRAF* V600E and the non-V600E *BRAF* mutant groups, respectively. ICI therapy was associated with ORRs of 25 and 33% in the *BRAF* V600E and the non-V600E *BRAF* mutant positive groups, respectively (p = 1.0) (**Table 2**). Among the six patients with high PD-L1 and *BRAF* V600E mutant NSCLC, two patients had major tumor shrinkage while two other patients had hyperprogression (43).

Among the 1,588 advanced non-squamous NSCLC patients enrolled in the Italian Expanded Access Program of second line nivolumab, 210 patients were assessed for *BRAF* mutations, and 11 patients (5%) were found to be positive. Median OS was comparable among different groups, and was found to be 11.0 months (range: 9.8 to 12.2 months), 11.2 months (range: 9.2 to 13.2 months) and 10.3 months (range: 2.1 to 18.5 months) in the population with unknown *BRAF* status, *BRAF* wild-type subgroup, and *BRAF* mutated subgroup, respectively (44) (**Table 2**).

A retrospective study was conducted to evaluate the clinical response to immunotherapy and chemotherapy among 31 patients with *BRAF* mutant metastatic NSCLC treated at the Duke University Hospital (45). PD-L1 expression information was only available for 11 patients. PD-L1 expression levels ranged from 0 to 90%, with six patients with PD-L1 expression levels greater than 50%. TMB was only available on five patients, ranging from 3 to 18 mutations/Mb. The median PFS in patients who received first-line chemotherapy was 6.4 months (95% CI, 2.3 to 13.0) while the PFS of each of the three patients who received first-line immunotherapy was 0.17, 1.4, and 4.4 months. The median OS in patients who received first-line chemotherapy was 18.4 months (95% CI, 7.4 to 28.6), and the OS of each of the three patients who received first-line immunotherapy was 0.17, 6.8, and 7.5 months (**Table 2**).

In the retrospective study using the IMMUNOTARGET registry, among the 43 patients with *BRAF* mutations, PFS was significantly higher in smokers than never smokers (4.1 versus 1.9 months, $P = 0.03$), however shorter in the V600E subgroup (1.8 months) compared with other *BRAF* mutations (4.1 months, $P = 0.20$) (31) (**Table 2**). The ORR was 24.3%. Among the nine patients with available PD-L1 status, the median percentage of cells expressing PD-L1 was 50%.

In the IMAD2 (GFPC 01-2018), a retrospective study that included 21 centers in France reported by Guisier et al., 44 ICI-treated *BRAF* mutant (*BRAF* V600E, n = 26; *BRAF* non-V600E, n = 18) NSCLC patients were identified (47). Most of the patients received ICI in the beyond-first line setting. Response rates for *BRAF*-V600E- and *BRAF*-non-V600E- mutant NSCLC were 26 and 35%, respectively. The median DORs to ICI were NR (95% CI 12.6–NR) and 13.1 months (95% CI 7.6–NR) in the *BRAF*-V600E- and *BRAF*-non-V600E groups. The PFS in the *BRAF*-V600E- and *BRAF*-non-V600E groups were 5.3 months (95% CI 2.1–NR) and 4.9 months (95% CI 2.3–NR), and the OS in the *BRAF*-V600E- and *BRAF*-non-V600E groups were 22.5 months (95% CI 8.3–NR) and 12 months (95% CI 6.8–NR). The 12-month OS in the *BRAF*-V600E- and *BRAF*-non-V600E- groups were 53.4 and 44%, respectively (**Table 2**).

In a cohort of 10 patients with tumors harboring *BRAF* mutations (*BRAF* V600E, n–5; *BRAF* non-V600E, n–5) who received ICI treatment, ORR of 25% (1/4) and 20% (1/5) were seen in patients with *BRAF* V600E mutation and *BRAF* non-V600E mutation, respectively (46). Median PFS comprised 1.5 months (95% CI, 1.2–8.3) in patients with *BRAF* V600E mutation and 2.6 months (95% CI, 2.0–4.2) in patients with *BRAF* non-V600E mutation. Median OS was not reached in patients with *BRAF V600E* mutation (95% CI, 1.2–NR) or *BRAF* non-V600E mutation (95% CI, 2.3–NR) (46) (**Table 2**). Among patients with known PD-L1 TPS, TPS high (≥50%) was seen in 25 and 60% of the *BRAF* V600E- and non-*BRAF* V600E-mutant NSCLC cases, respectively. TMB high (≥10 mut/Mb) was seen in 3 and 1% of the *BRAF* V600E- and non-*BRAF* V600E-mutant NSCLC cases, respectively. No MSI-H/I was seen.

In another report of nine patients with *BRAF* (*BRAF* V600E, n–6; *BRAF* non-V600E, n–3) who received ICI with chemotherapy or antiangiogenic treatment, the ORR was 25% and mPFS was three months (95%CI 2.9, 3.1) (48).

MET

MET is a proto-oncogene receptor tyrosine kinase that mediates cell proliferation, survival, and metastasis (5). Recurrent somatic splice site alterations at *MET exon 14 (METex14)* can result in exon skipping, decreased MET degradation, and MET activation. *METex14* is involved in cancer through promoting angiogenesis, cell migration, and invasion (49, 50). *METex14* occurs in 3–4% of lung cancers and 8–30% of sarcomatoid lung cancers (51, 52). The occurrence of *METex14* appears to be independent of smoking status (53). FDA has granted accelerated approval to capmatinib and tepotinib for adult patients with metastatic NSCLC whose tumors have a mutation that leads to *METex14* alterations (54, 55).

In a retrospective study that included 147 patients with *METex14* lung cancers, PD-L1 expression of ≥50% was identified in 41% of 111 evaluable tumor samples. The median TMB of *METex14* lung cancers was lower than that of unselected non-small-cell lung cancers (NSCLCs). In 24 response-evaluable patients, the ORR was 17% (95% CI 6 to 36%) and the median PFS was 1.9 months (95% CI 1.7–2.7). Responses were not associated with PD-L1 expression ≥50% or high TMB (12) (**Table 3**).

Among the 551 patients in the IMMUNOTARGET registry, 13 patients with *MET* amplification and 23 patients with *METex14* were identified (31). Median OS from ICI initiation of this 36-paitent cohort was 18.4 months (7.0; NR) (31). Progressive disease (PD) was found to be the best response to ICI among 50% of patients, and median PFS was found to be 3.4

TABLE 3 | Efficacy of ICIs in NSCLS with *c-MET* mutations.

Reference	Characteristics	ORR, %	mPFS, months	mOS, months since start of ICI
Sabari JK. et al. (12)	*cMET exon 14* skipping mutation (n=147)	17	1.9	18.2
Mazieres J., et al. (31)	*cMET exon 14* skipping mutation and *cMET* amplification (n=36)	49	3.4	18.4
Guisier F., et al. (47)	*cMET* mutant (n=30)	36	4.9	13.4
Dudnik- E., et al. (46)	*cMET exon 14* skipping mutation (n=148)	12	4	NR (not reached)
	cMET amplification (n=54)	25	4.9	NR (not reached)
Mayenga M., et al. (56)	*cMET exon 14* skipping mutations, 2nd line immunotherapy (n=13)	46.2		

ICIs, immune checkpoint inhibitors; NSCLC, non-small cell lung cancer; ORR, overall response rate; mPFS, median progression-free survival; mOS, median overall survival.

months (1.7; 6.2). Long-term responders were seen in 23.4% of patients (**Table 3**). Among the 15 patients with available PD-L1 status, the median percentage of cells expressing PD-L1 was 30%.

In the French retrospective study IMAD2 (GFPC 01-2018), 30 cases of ICI-treated *MET* mutant NSCLC were identified (47). Most patient received ICI in the beyond-first line setting. The response rate for *MET*-altered NSCLC was 36%. The median duration of response (mDOR) was 10.4 months (95% CI 4.6–NR). The mPFS was 4.9 months ((95% CI 2.0–11.4), and the mOS was 13.4 months (95% CI 9.4–NR) (**Table 3**).

In a retrospective study that included eight cases of NSCLC with *METex14* and four cases of NSCLC with *MET* amplification treated with ICI, median PFS with ICI was 4.0 months (95% CI, 2.4–NR) in patients with *METex14* and 4.9 months (95% CI, 2.4–NR) in patients with *MET* amplification (46). ORR comprised 12% (1/8) and 25% (1/4) in patients with *METex14* and *MET* amplification respectively. Median OS with ICI was not reached in patients with *METex14* (95% CI, 4.1–NR) or in patients with *MET* amplification (95% CI, 3.5–NR) (**Table 3**). Among patients with known PD-L1 TPS, TPS high (≥50%) was seen in 67% of the cases. TMB high (≥10 mut/Mb) or MSI-H/I was not seen.

In a case series, among 13 patients with *METex14* NSCLCs treated with ICI, 46.2% (6/13) patients responded to immunotherapy. Six patients had prolonged duration of responses ranging from 18 months (still ongoing) to 49 months (56).

RET

RET is a proto-oncogene receptor tyrosine kinase that binds with the ligand-co-receptor complex of glial cell line-derived neurotrophic factor (GDNF) family ligands (GFLs) and subsequently activates signaling pathways such as RAS/mitogen activated protein kinase (MAPK), RAS/ERK, phosphatidylinositol 3-kinase (PI3K)/AKT, and c-Jun N-terminal kinase (JNK). Aberrant activation of the RET receptor have been associated with multiple endocrine neoplasia 2 (*MEN2*), sporadic medullary thyroid cancer, papillary thyroid carcinoma (PTC), and non-small cell lung cancer (NSCLC) (6, 7). *RET* rearrangements have been identified in 1–3% of NSCLC and were found to have significantly higher frequencies in younger (<60 years of age), female, non-smokers, and adenocarcinoma histology (57–60). *RET* fusion positive NSCLC is usually associated with low PD-L 1 expression (61). Two potent selective RET inhibitors, selpercatinib and pralsetinib, have been approved by the FDA for *RET* fusion-positive NSCLC (62, 63). The activity of ICI in *RET* altered NSCLC has been evaluated in multiple studies, and the benefit of ICI was found to be low in most of the studies (**Table 4**).

In the French retrospective study IMAD2 (GFPC 01-2018), nine patients with *RET* translocation NSCLC received ICI, all in the beyond-first line setting. The response rate for *RET*-altered NSCLC was 38%. The mDOR response to ICI was 12.1 months (95% CI 8.4–NR). The median PFS was 7.6 months (2.3–NR), and the median OS was not reached (95% CI 26.8–NR) (47) (**Table 4**).

In a single center retrospective study conducted in Korea, the median progression-free survival for ICI among 13 patients with *RET* fusion-positive NSCLC treated with ICI was 2.1 (95% CI: 1.6–2.6) months, and the ORR was 7.7% (64). The median PFS and OS were 2.1 (95% CI: 1.6–2.6) and 12.4 (95% CI: 2.9–21.8) months, respectively. Among patients with PD-L1 expression 25% and above, 2/5 patients demonstrated stable disease, while the best response in the other three patients was disease progression (**Table 4**). In contrast, the ORR and DCR among 46 patients treated with pemetrexed-based regimens in this study was 63.0 and 91.3%, respectively, and the median PFS was 9.0 (95% CI: 6.9–11.2) months.

Among the 16 patients with *RET* fusion-positive NSCLC in the IMMUNOTARGET registry, the median OS from the start of

TABLE 4 | Efficacy of ICIs in NSCLS with *RET* mutations.

Reference	Characteristics	ORR, %	mPFS, months	mOS, months since start of ICI
Guisier F., et al. (47)	*RET* fusion (n=9)	37.5	7.6	NR (not reached)
Lee J., et al. (64)	*RET* fusion (n=13)	7.7	2.1	12.4
Mazieres J., et al. (31)	*RET* fusion (n=16)	6	2.1	21.3
Offin M., et al. (61)	*RET* fusion (n=16)	0	3.4	
Dudnik E., et al. (46)	*RET* fusion (n=4)	0	3	14.9
	RET mutation (n=1)	0	6.9	15.3

ICIs, immune checkpoint inhibitors; NSCLC, non-small cell lung cancer; ORR, overall response rate; mPFS, median progression-free survival; mOS, median overall survival.

ICI therapy was 21.3 (3.8; 28.0), and the median PFS was only 2.1 (1.3; 4.7) (31). The rate of any partial or complete response was very low and was 6.3% (1/16) (**Table 4**). Among the six patients with available PD-L1 status, the median percentage of cells expressing PD-L1 was 26%.

In a retrospective study conducted at the Memorial Sloan Kettering Cancer Center, 13 patients with *RET*-rearranged NSCLC treated with ICI were assessed for clinical and/or radiologic response (30). No response to immunotherapy was observed. The median PFS was 3.4 months (95% CI, 2.1 to 5.6 months). No difference in OS between patients with advanced *RET*-rearranged lung cancers who received immunotherapy (n = 16) and those who did not receive immunotherapy (n = 46), (hazard ratio, 1.4 [95% CI, 0.7 to 2.9]; log-rank P = .35) (**Table 4**). Only one patient was found to have PD-L1 expression ≥50%, and the disease of this patient did not respond to ICI. No patient had TMB >10 mut/Mb.

In the single institution retrospective study published by Dudnik et al., four patients with *RET* fusion NSCLC and one patient with *RET* mutant NSCLC were treated with ICI (46). No objective response was observed. Median PFS was 3.0 months (95% CI, 1.9–3.1) in patients with *RET* fusion and 6.9 months in patient with *RET* mutation. Median OS since start of ICP were 14.9 months (95% CI, 7.2–19.7) in patients with *RET* fusion and 15.3 months in patient with *RET* mutation (**Table 4**). Among patients with known PD-L1 TPS, TPS high (≥50%) was seen in 13 and 0% of the *RET* fusion and the *RET* mutant NSCLC cases, respectively. TMB high or MSI-H/I was not seen.

ROS1

ROS proto-oncogene 1 (*ROS1*) belongs to the subfamily of tyrosine kinase insulin receptors (65). *ROS1* fusion can lead to constitutive activation of kinase activity, resulting in increased cell proliferation, survival, and migration due to the upregulation of JAK/STAT, PI3K/AKT, and MAPK/ERK signaling pathways (8). *ROS1* rearrangements account for 1–2% of NSCLC patients (66, 67). This alteration more frequently occurs in adenocarcinoma and in younger patients with no or light smoking history (68, 69).

Seven patients with *ROS1* fusion NSCLC treated with ICI were identified in the IMMUNOTARGET registry (31). The objective response rate to ICI treatment was 17% (**Table 5**).

In the single institution retrospective study published by Dudnik et al., only one patient with *ROS1* fusion NSCLC treated with ICI was identified, and the reported PFS and OS were both 0.1 month (46) (**Table 5**). Among the five patients with available PD-L1 status, the median percentage of cells expressing PD-L1 was 90%.

In the Japanese retrospective study, 15 *ROS1* altered NSCLC cases were identified. High expression of PD-L1 (>50% of tumor cells by 22C3) were observed in 53% cases, however, no response to immunotherapy was observed (70).

NTRK

The *NTRK* genes (*NTRK1*, *NTRK2* and *NTRK3*) encode tropomyosin receptor kinases (*TRKA*, *TRKB* and *TRKC*) (9). The *TRK* fusion protein leads to constitutive activation of various downstream signal transduction pathways including the PI3k/Akt and RAS/RAF/MAPK pathways, and subsequently causes proliferation of cancer cells (9). Rearrangements including *NTRK1*, *NTRK2*, and *NTRK3* occur in approximately 2–3% of NSCLC patients (10). Selective *TRK* inhibitors, Entrectinib and Larotrectinib, have been approved for patients with *NTRK* fusion-positive solid tumors, including NSCLC (71, 72).

In the single institution retrospective study published by Dudnik et al., two patients with *NTRK* fusion NSCLC were treated with ICI. The objective response rate was 50% (1/2). Median PFS was as not reached (95% CI, 3.2–NR). Median OS since start of ICP not reached (95% CI, NR–NR) (46) (**Table 6**). One patient had PD-L1 TPS ≥50%. No patient had TMB ≥10 muts/Mb.

KRAS G12C

KRAS is one of the RAS proteins (KRAS4A, KRAS4B, NRAS, and HRAS) which function as GDP–GTP-regulated binary on-off switches and regulate cell survival, cell cycle progression, cell polarity, movement, and nuclear transport by transducing signals from transmembrane receptors to cytoplasmic signaling pathways such as the MAPK pathway (10, 11). It is the most common proto-oncogene identified in NSCLC. *KRAS* mutations occur in 15–25% of lung adenocarcinomas and are more prevalent in smokers than nonsmokers (73, 74). Majority of the *KRAS* mutations in NSCLC occur on exon 2 or 3 (G12, G13, and Q61), with the most frequent being the G12C followed by G12V and G12D (75, 76). Sotorasib has been approved by the FDA for patients with *KRAS* G12C mutant locally advanced or metastatic NSCLC in the beyond the first line setting (72). It is associated with an objective response rate of 37.1% in this group of patients (77). The efficacy of ICIs in

TABLE 5 | Efficacy of ICIs in NSCLS with *ROS-1* mutations.

Reference	Characteristics	ORR, %	mPFS, months	mOS, months since start of ICI
Mazieres J., et al. (31)	*ROS1* (n=7)	17		
Dudnik E., et al. (46)	*ROS 1* (n=1)		0.1	0.1

ICIs, immune checkpoint inhibitors; NSCLC, non-small cell lung cancer; ORR, overall response rate; mPFS, median progression-free survival; mOS, median overall survival.

TABLE 6 | Efficacy of ICIs in NSCLS with *NTRK* mutations.

Reference	Characteristics	ORR, %	mPFS, months	mOS, months since start of ICI
Dudnik E., et al. (46)	*NTRK* (n=2)	50%	Not reached	Not reached

ICIs, immune checkpoint inhibitors; NSCLC, non-small cell lung cancer; ORR, overall response rate; mPFS, median progression-free survival; mOS, median overall survival.

KRAS mutant NSCLC has been studied in several retrospective studies, and most of the data support the benefit on ICIs in *KRAS* mutant NSCLC (**Table 7**).

In a retrospective analysis in patients enrolled in the KEYNOTE-042 evaluating pembrolizumab monotherapy vs platinum-based chemotherapy as the first-line therapy among patients with PD-L1-positive (TPS ≥1%) advanced non-squamous histology NSCLC, 301 patients were evaluable by whole-exome sequencing (WES). *KRAS* mutations were found in 69 (23%) patients, among which, 29 (10%) patients were found to have *KRAS* G12C (78). PD-L1 TPS and TMB were found to be higher in patients with *KRAS* mutations than without *KRAS* mutations, although the differences were not significant. The OS associated with pembrolizumab was better than chemotherapy in both the *KRAS* mutant group and *KRAS* G12C subgroup, with the HRs being 0.42 (0.22–0.81) and 0.28 (0.09–0.86), respectively. Conversely, there was no significant OS difference seen between pembrolizumab and chemotherapy in the *KRAS* wild-type patients, and HR was 0.86 (0.63–1.18). A superior PFS was also observed when pembrolizumab was compared with chemotherapy in the *KRAS* mutant patients. The data supported the benefit of single agent pembrolizumab in the PD-1 TPS >1% *KRAS* mutant (including *KRAS* G12C) NSCLC patients, underlining the important role of ICI in the treatment of this group of patients.

The efficacy of ICIs in the first line setting in PD-L1 TPS ≥50% advanced NSCLC was also investigated in a retrospective analysis using the Flatiron Health database (79). Among the1,127 patients with PD-L1 expression of 50% or greater who were treated with either ICI monotherapy or chemoimmunotherapy, 573 (50.8%) had *KRAS* alterations and 554 (49.2%) had wild type *KRAS*. Among the patients treated with ICI monotherapy, a better mOS was seen in the *KRAS* mutant group when compared with the wild-type group (mOS, 21.1 vs 13.6 months; P = .03). Interestingly, this OS advantage was not observed among patients treated with chemoimmunotherapy, and the mOS was 20.0 vs 19.3 months; P = .93 in the *KRAS* mutant and wild type patients. Furthermore, no mOS difference was seen between ICI monotherapy and chemoimmunotherapy in the *KRAS* mutant NSCLC patients (mOS, 21.1 vs 20.0 months; P = .78), suggesting that the use of ICI monotherapy in the PD-L1 TPS ≥50% is an acceptable option in the *KRAS* mutant advanced NSCLC.

The efficacy of chemoimmunotherapy in *KRAS* mutant NSCLC was also analyzed retrospectively in the participants of another randomized trial, the KEYNOTE-189 study of pembrolizumab plus pemetrexed and platinum chemotherapy vs placebo plus chemotherapy as first-line therapy for metastatic non-squamous NSCLC (80). Among the 289 patients who had evaluable WES data, 89 (31%) patients were found to have *KRAS* mutations including *KRAS* G12C, which was found in 37 (13%) patients. As observed in the KEYNOTE-042 study, the higher PD-L1 TPS and TMB tended to be seen with KRAS mutant patients. Although unlike the observation in the KEYNOTE-042, the OS benefit associated with the addition of ICI was only detected in the *KRAS* wild-type patients. PFS improvement associated with the additional of ICI was seen in both the *KRAS* mutant and wild type group but not in the *KRAS* G12C subgroup, which could be related to the small sample number.

In addition to ICI monotherapy and chemoimmunotherapy, the combination of VEGF receptor targeted agent and chemoimmunotherapy represents another first-line treatment option for advanced NSCLC based on the IMpower150 study (84). A *post hoc* analysis evaluated the efficacy outcomes in

TABLE 7 | Efficacy of ICIs in NSCLS with *KRAS* mutations.

Reference	Characteristics	ORR, %	mPFS, months	mOS, months since start of ICI
Mazieres J., et al. (31)	*KRAS* (n=271)	26%	3.2 (1st-3rd line ICI) 3.1 (>3rd line) G12C: 5.5 G12A: 4.4 G12D: 3.2 G12V: 1.9 G12S: 2.1	13.5
Herbst RS., et al. (78)	Any *KRAS* (n=69), first line immunotherapy	56.7%	12	28
	KRAS G12C	66.7%	15	NR
Sun L., et al. (79)	Any *KRAS* (n=573), first line monotherapy or chemoimmunotherapy			21.1 (ICI monotherapy) 20 (chemoimmunotherapy)
Gadgeel SM. et al. (80)	Any *KRAS* (n=89), first line chemoimmunotherapy	40.7%	9	21
	KRAS G12C	50%	11	18
West H., et al. (81)	*KRAS (n=80)* (first line chemoimmunotherapy with VEGFR targeted therapy)		8.11	19.81
	With *mutant STK* and/or *mutant KEPA1 (n=34)*		6.03	11.1
	With wild-type *STK* and wild-type *KEPA1 (n=46)*		15.21	26.18
Passiglia F., et al. (82)	*KRAS*, (n=206)	20%	4	11.2
Jeanson A., et al. (83)	*KRAS* (n=162)	18.7%	3.09	14.29

ICIs, immune checkpoint inhibitors; NSCLC, non-small cell lung cancer; ORR, overall response rate; mPFS, median progression free survival; mOS, median overall survival, HR, hazard ratio, CI, confidence interval.

patients with *KRAS*, *STK11(LKB1)*, and *KEAP1* mutations (81). Among 920 patients included, *KRAS* mutations were found in 80 patients (24.5%), with 39 patients found to have co-occurring mutations in *STK11* and/or *KEAP1*. The addition of ICI improved mOS and PFS in the *KRAS* mutant patients regardless of STK11 and KEAP1 status (**Table 7**), supporting the use of this regimen in *KRAS* mutant NSCLC.

The correlation between STK11/LKB1 genomic alterations and the efficacy of ICI treatment in KRAS mutant NSCLC was also evaluated using the Stand Up To Cancer (SU2C) dataset (13). Unlike the *post hoc* analysis of the IMpower150 study, this study showed that the concurrent *STK11/LKB1* mutation in *KRAS* mutant NSCLC was associated with an inferior ORR to PD-1 blockade when compared with *KRAS* mutation without *STK11/LKB1* mutation and *KRAS* mutation with *P53* mutations groups (7.4, 28.6 and 35.7% (P <0.001)). The details of the ICI therapy in this dataset were not available, and it is unclear whether this group of patients also received angiogenesis targeted agent treatment.

In a systemic review and metanalysis aiming to investigate the predictive clinicopathological characteristics for the relative efficacy of ICIs vs docetaxel in the second-line setting in NSCLCs, the authors analyzed data from five randomized clinical trials involving 3,025 patients (85). ICIs were associated with prolonged overall survival (HR, 0.69; 95% CI, 0.63–0.75; *P* < .001). The survival benefit was also seen among the 148 *KRAS* mutant patients (HR, 0.65; 95% CI, 0.44–0.97; *P* = .03) but not in the 371 *KRAS* wild-type patients (HR, 0.86; 95% CI, 0.67–1.11; P = .24; interaction, P = .24) (85).

The efficacy of ICI in *KRAS* mutant non-squamous NSCLC in the beyond first-line setting was also investigated in patients who received nivolumab in an Italian expanded access program (EAP) study (82). Among the 530 patients evaluated, 206 (39%) had *KRAS* mutations. No significant differences in OS, PFS or ORR were seen between *KRAS* mutant and *KRAS* wild-type patients in this study, supporting that nivolumab should be considered for patients regardless of *KRAS* mutation status. Interestingly, any significantly higher grade and grade 3–4 treatment related adverse events were seen in the *KRAS* mutant group than the wild-type group, although the underlining mechanism for the finding is unknown.

KRAS mutant NSCLC was also evaluated in the IMMUNOTARGET study. Two hundred and seventy-one patients treated with ICIs were found to have *KRAS* mutations. An encouraging ORR of 26% was found, and the mPFS and mOS were 3.2 and 13.5months, respectively (31).

In a single instituation retrospective study conducted in France, a total of 162 *KRAS*-mutant advanced NSCLC were identified among the 282 subjects analyzed. No significant difference was seen in ORR, mPFS or mOS between the *KRAS* mutant and the *KRAS* wild-type groups. The ORR, mPFS, and mOS associated with ICI of *KRAS* mutant NSCLC were 18.7%, 3.09 months and 14.29 months. No significant difference in treamtent outcomes was seen among the KRAS mutation subtypes including G12A, G12C, G12D, G12V, and G13C (83).

HER 2

Human epidermal growth factor 2 (HER2 erbB-2/neu) is one of the four receptor tyrosine kinase members of the human epidermal growth factor receptor family. Upon forming homo- or hetero-dimers with other family members, HER2 becomes activated and signal through the PI3K-AKT and MEK-ERK downstream pathways to activate proliferation (86). In NSCLC, activating *HER2* mutations occur in 2–4% of cases, most commonly in adenocarcinoma histology and never smokers (87). Patients with *HER2* mutant NSCLC have worse OS if treated without HER2 targeted therapy (88). Although there has not been any HER 2 targeted agent approved by NSCLC by the FDA, several agents have showed promising activity. Ado-trastuzumab emtansine, a HER2-targeted antibody-drug conjugate was found to be associated with an ORR of 44% in NSCLC with *HER2* exon 20 insertions and point mutations (89), and another HER2-targeted antibody-drug conjugate, trastuzumab deruxtecan, also showed an encouraging ORR of 55% in patients with metastatic HER2-overexpressing or *HER2*-mutant NSCLC whose disease had relapsed during standard treatment or was refractory to standard treatment (90). Both agents are included as novel therapeutic options for *HER2* mutant NSCLC in the current NCCN guidelines (2). Poziotinib, a tyrosine kinase inhibitor targeting *EGFR/HER2* exon 20 insertion mutation, was found to have an ORR of 27% in HER2 exon 20 mutant NSCLC, gaining fast track designation by FDA (91, 92).

The efficacy of immunotherapy in patients whose cancer harbors *HER2* mutation is largely unknown. The ORR associated with ICI among the 29 patients with exon 20 activating mutations in the IMMUNOTARGET study was only 7%. PFS was 2.5 months, and the 12-month PFS was 13.6 months. The OS was 20.3 months (31). The ORR among the 23 patients with exon 20 insertions included in the IMAD2 study by the French Lung Cancer Group was 27.3%. PFS was similar to the findings in the IMMUNOTARGET study and was 2.2 months, and the 12-month PFS was 22.9%. The mOS was an encouraging 20.4 months (47) (**Table 8**).

TABLE 8 | Efficacy of ICIs in NSCLS with *HER2* mutations.

Reference	Characteristics	ORR, %	mPFS, months	mOS, months since start of ICI
Mazieres J., et al. (31)	*HER2* (n=29)	7%	2.9 (1st-3rd line ICI) 2.0 (>3rd line)	20.3
Guisier F., et al. (47)	*HER2* (n=23), number of lines prior to ICI =one median	27.3%	2.2	20.4

ICIs, immune checkpoint inhibitors; NSCLC, non-small cell lung cancer; ORR, overall response rate; mPFS, median progression-free survival; mOS, median overall survival.

DISCUSSION

To delineate the benefit of ICI treatment in NSCLC harboring actional mutations other than *EGFR* alterations, we reviewed the current available data in this area. We found that the ORR, median PFS, and OS with ICPi varied significantly across genetic alteration subgroups. While the ORR observed in the *BRAF, c-MET*, and *KRAS* altered NSCLC appeared to be similar to what had been observed in the non-selected NSCLC groups, the ORRs in the *ALK* and *RET* altered NSCLC groups were much lower (2).

Unlike *ALK* and *RET* fusions, *BRAF, MET*, and *KRAS* mutations can be seen in both smokers and non-smokers. The higher prevalence of smoking history in these patients could be a potential reason of the higher response rates since smoking has been found to be associated with the benefit derived from ICI treatment in some of the literatures (93, 94), although not confirmed by other studies (95). Other known predictive biomarkers for ICI treatment include PD-L1 expression level, microsatellite instability-high (MSI-H) or mismatch repair deficient (dMMR), and TMB (96–98). A higher percentage of PD-L1 TPS high (67%) was reported in *BRAF* non V600E mutant and *MET* mutant NSCLC in some of the reports (46), and a relatively higher response was seen in patients with PD-L1 TPS high *BRAF* mutant NSCLC (43), albeit the sample numbers was too small to draw any firm conclusion.

The current NCCN guidelines support the use of targeted therapy in the first line setting for advanced NSCLC with actionable genomic alterations involving *EGFR, ALK, ROS1, BRAF, NTRK1/2/3, METex14* skipping, and *RET*. After disease progression, chemoimmunotherapy is recommended for this population based on the guidelines (2). Although most of the chemoimmunotherapy trials excluded the *EGFR* and *ALK* altered NSCLC patients, these groups of patients were evaluated in the IMpower150 study if they have had progression with or unacceptable side effects from treatment with at least one approved tyrosine kinase inhibitor. The data showed improved PFS associated with the additional of atezolizumab to the bevacizumab, carboplatin, and paclitaxel combination in *EGFR* and *ALK* altered NSCLC (9.7 months vs. 6.1 months), providing direct evidence supporting the use of the regimen in this population (38). In our review, while not robust, we see that ICI's do have activity in patients with NSCLC harbouring actionable mutations, and that a response can be seen after progression on targeted therapy, supporting offering chemoimmunotherapy in the post-targeted therapy setting. For *KRAS* G12C NSCLC, ICI monotherapy or chemoimmunotherapy is the current standard of care first line treatment. The data included in this review did confirm the benefits of ICI in the *KRAS* mutant NSCLC, supporting the current treatment approach. The benefit of ICI monotherapy in PD-L1 positive *KRAS* mutant NSLCL was suggested in retrospective studies, warranting further investigation on the selection of ICI monotherapy vs chemoimmunotherapy in this population (78, 79). Furthermore, data from prospective studies will be helpful to identify the best treatment sequence among targeted therapy, ICI, and chemotherapy.

Even in the subgroups where the benefits of ICIs were observed, the ORRs tended to be low. Therefore, developing predictive biomarkers for ICI therapy would be of great importance.

Co-occurring genomic alterations have been reported to be related to responses to immunotherapy through altering the microenvironment. For example, *LKB1/STK11* genomic alterations, a frequent co-occurring mutation in of *KRAS* mutant NSCLC, have been found to be associates with "immune-inert" state (99). This was supported by several studies including a retrospective study conducted in 103 NSCLC patients receiving ICIs. In this study, among the patient with *KRAS* mutations, the presence of concurrent *STK11* mutation or *STK11/TP53* mutations were associated with worse survival with ICI therapy. This association was not observed with chemotherapy, supporting the predictive roles of these co-mutations for ICI therapy in *KRAS* mutant NSCLC (15). The data from a retrospective analysis suggested that co-occurring *LKB1/STK11* mutations in *KRAS* mutant NSCLC may predict lower ORR, while data from another group showed no PFS or OS differences with or without concurrent mutant *LKB1/STK11* and/or mutant *KEPA1* in patients receiving combined chemoimmunotherapy and angiogenesis targeted agent (13, 81), raising the question whether angiogenesis targeted agent may help to overcome the challenge of the immune-inert state. Other co-occurring genomic alterations such as *P53, KEAP1, ATM, PTEN, CDKN2A* are common among *KRAS*-mutant NSCLC, and may play a role in determining response to ICI (100). Furthermore, a recent study showed that co-occurring mutations such as NOTCH and HR pathways were also found to be associated with increased efficacy of immunotherapy in advanced NSCLC (101). Therefore, identifying co-occurring mutations that are responsible for ICI response or resistance could potentially help to identify the candidate for ICI treatments and warrants further investigation in this group of patients.

How to overcome the resistance to ICI therapy is another great challenge. The mechanism of resistance is complex and is a combination of tumor-intrinsic and extrinsic factors. Many factors such as immune contexture and tumor microenvironment, expression of PD-L1 and LAG3, TMB, genetic and epigenetic alterations, antigen-presenting molecules (MHC, HLA) and microbiota may all contribute to the resistance to immunotherapy (102). The tumors with higher initial mutational burdens have been found to be associated with higher sensitivity to ICIs in some studies, although this association may be negated by other factors such as intratumoral heterogeneity and mutations (103). *RET* fusion positive NSCLC was found to have poor response to ICIs, and the alterations appears to be associated with lower TMB. In the analysis by Offin M. et al., the median TMB of *RET* altered NSCLC was significantly lower than that of the *RET* wild-type NSCLCs (1.75 versus 5.27 mutations/Mb, P <.0001) (61). The best outcome in patients in this study was stable disease which only lasted 5.6 months. In the report by Dudnik E. et al, the TBM was low in all 13 patients except one patient who had intermediate TMB, and the ORR in this report was also 0% (46). Nevertheless, an ORR of 37.5% was found among the nine evaluable patients reported by Guisier F. et al. Unfortunately, the TMB information was not available in this study, and it was unclear if the treatments were ICI monotherapy or chemoimmunotherapy. A prospective study to allow uniform treatment and collection of information on biomarkers such as TMB, PD-L1, MSI/MMR, tumor-infiltrating lymphocytes, whole-exome sequencing analysis on tumor samples and intestinal microbiome composition may be helpful to identify the resistance mechanisms.

ALK fusion positive NSCLC showed poor response to ICI in retrospective studies. However, this group of patients did benefit from ICI in the IMpower 150 trial, raising the question if the inhibition of angiogenesis could sensitize cancer cells to ICI therapy. Tumor angiogenesis can lead to immunosuppression through various mechanisms including maintaining an acidic/hypoxic and immunosuppressive environment, development of dysfunctional blood vessels which limits T cell trafficking, and suppression of dendritic cell maturation. Moreover, the angiogenic factors such as VEGF are also immunosuppressive (104). Therefore, further investigation is warranted in co-inhibition of angiogenic factors in NSCLC harboring actionable driver mutations undergoing ICI treatment.

With regard to the combination of ICIs and targeted therapies, a number of studies had evaluated the combiantion of *ALK* TKIs and different ICIs in NSCLC, including the combination of nivolumab with ceritinib or crizotinib and the combiantion of alectinib plus atezolizumab (105–107). However, significant toxicities were observed without survival benefit. In addition, there has been some concerning safety signals where ICI treatment is followed with targeted therapy (108). Reports showed risk of hepatotoxicity in a series of patients with *ALK*, *ROS1*, or *MET* exon 14 alterations who received ICI before crizotinib. Among the eleven patients treated with crizotinib following ICI, five patients (45.5%) developed grade 3 or 4 hepatotoxicity, whereas only 8% of those patients who received crizotinib alone experienced hepatotoxicity. The increased hepatotoxicity in sequentially treated patients led to permanent discontinuation of crizotinib in four of the five patients (108), highlighting the importance of establishing the presence of actionable mutations prior to initiating ICI therapy in patients with advanced NSCLC. The frequency and severity of toxicities associates with sequential use of ICI followed by targeted therapy may vary among different therapeutic agents. In the CodeBreaK100 phase II study evaluating Sotorasib in the beyond first-line setting, even though 91.3% patients had received ICI treatment prior to Sotorasib, the tolerability remained acceptable. Ongoing clinical trials DESTINY-Lung03 (NCT04686305) and the HUDSON trial (NCT03334617) are investigating the combination of T-DXd with immunotherapy, chemotherapy, novel anticancer agents and will hence shed more light on the approach in *HER2* mutant subgroup NSCLC patients.

Our review certainly has limitations. We were unable to comment on the response of *HER2*, *ROS1* and *NTRK* altered NSCLC to ICI as there were few reports in the literature, and the patient numbers in these reports were often very small. The challenges are obviously associated with the low incidences of these alterations. A recent report from Negrao et al. showed that *RET*, *ROS1* and *ALK* alterations were associated with low sensitivity to ICIs. However, there were only three *ROS1* fusion NSCLC patients included in the study, and the outcome of all three alterations were reported collectively (15). Furthermore, we were also unable to compare the responses to ICIs among different alterations which can be better investigated in prospective studies. Moreover, many studies included in this reivew did not have the biomarker information on all the evaluable patients. The ICI treatments and the number of lines of treament received previously by the patients also varied significantly. Additionally, it was not always clear whether the ICI treament was given as a monotherapy or in combination with cytotoxic chemotherapy. Randomized prospective studies would undoubtly provide more definitive information on this topic.

In conclusion, we see low responses to ICI in *ALK and RET* altered NSCLCs whereas *BRAF, KRAS and c-MET alterations* were associated with benefit from ICIs, and PD-L1 positive *KRAS* mutant NSCLCs may be more responsive to ICI monotherapy. Furthermore, the response to ICIs in *KRAS* mutant NSCLCs may vary depending on co-existing mutations, and responses to ICIs in *HER2*, *ROS1* and *NTRK* altered NSCLCs are less clear and varies significantly across a small number of studies. Ultimately, immunotherapy in the second line after progression on targeted agents can be considered as a treatment option at the discretion of treating physicians, following a mutual discussion with patients about the pros and cons of this approach.

AUTHOR CONTRIBUTIONS

All authors contributed equally to the writing, development, editing, and information gathering of the manuscript.

REFERENCES

1. Siegel R, Naishadham D, Jemal A. Cancer Statistics, 2013. *CA Cancer J Clin* (2013) 63(1):11–30. doi: 10.3322/caac.21166
2. *NCCN Clinical Practice Guidelines in Oncology (NCCN Guidelines®): Non-Small Cell Lung Cancer. Version 5.2021*. Available at: https://www.nccn.org/professionals/physician_gls/pdf/nscl.pdf.
3. Hallberg B, Palmer RH. The Role of the ALK Receptor in Cancer Biology. *Ann Oncol* (2016) 27(Suppl 3):iii4–15. doi: 10.1093/annonc/mdw301
4. Marchetti A, Felicioni L, Malatesta S, Grazia Sciarrotta M, Guetti L, Chella A, et al. Clinical Features and Outcome of Patients With Non-Small-Cell Lung Cancer Harboring BRAF Mutations. *J Clin Oncol* (2011) 29(26):3574–9. doi: 10.1200/JCO.2011.35.9638
5. Maulik G, Shrikhande A, Kijima T, Ma PC, Morrison PT, Salgia R. Role of the Hepatocyte Growth Factor Receptor, C-Met, in Oncogenesis and Potential for Therapeutic Inhibition. *Cytokine Growth Factor Rev* (2002) 13(1):41–59. doi: 10.1016/S1359-6101(01)00029-6
6. Li AY, McCusker MG, Russo A, Scilla KA, Gittens A, Arensmeyer K, et al. RET Fusions in Solid Tumors. *Cancer Treat Rev* (2019) 81:101911. doi: 10.1016/j.ctrv.2019.101911
7. Santoro M, Moccia M, Federico G, Carlomagno F. RET Gene Fusions in Malignancies of the Thyroid and Other Tissues. *Genes (Basel)* (2020) 11 (4):424. doi: 10.3390/genes11040424
8. Roskoski R Jr. ROS1 Protein-Tyrosine Kinase Inhibitors in the Treatment of ROS1 Fusion Protein-Driven non-Small Cell Lung Cancers. *Pharmacol Res* (2017) 121:202–12. doi: 10.1016/j.phrs.2017.04.022

9. Miao Q, Ma K, Chen D, Wu X, Jiang S. Targeting Tropomyosin Receptor Kinase for Cancer Therapy. *Eur J Med Chem* (2019) 175:129–48. doi: 10.1016/j.ejmech.2019.04.053
10. Stokoe D, Macdonald SG, Cadwallader K, Symons M, Hancock JF. Activation of Raf as a Result of Recruitment to the Plasma Membrane. *Science* (1994) 264(5164):1463–7. doi: 10.1126/science.7811320
11. Wennerberg K, Rossman KL, Der CJ. The Ras Superfamily at a Glance. *J Cell Sci* (2005) 118(Pt 5):843–6. doi: 10.1242/jcs.01660
12. Sabari JK, Leonardi GC, Shu CA, Umeton R, Montecalvo J, Ni A, et al. PD-L1 Expression, Tumor Mutational Burden, and Response to Immunotherapy in Patients With MET Exon 14 Altered Lung Cancers. *Ann Oncol* (2018) 29 (10):2085–91. doi: 10.1093/annonc/mdy334
13. Skoulidis F, Goldberg ME, Greenawalt DM, Hellmann MD, Awad MM, Gainor JF, et al. STK11/LKB1 Mutations and PD-1 Inhibitor Resistance in KRAS-Mutant Lung Adenocarcinoma. *Cancer Discov* (2018) 8(7):822–35. doi: 10.1158/2159-8290.CD-18-0099
14. Pavan A, Boscolo Bragadin A, Calvetti L, Ferro A, Zulato E, Attili I, et al. Role of Next Generation Sequencing-Based Liquid Biopsy in Advanced Non-Small Cell Lung Cancer Patients Treated With Immune Checkpoint Inhibitors: Impact of STK11, KRAS and TP53 Mutations and Co-Mutations on Outcome. *Trans Lung Cancer Res* (2020) 10(1):202–20. doi: 10.21037/tlcr-20-674
15. Negrao MV, Skoulidis F, Montesion M, Schulze K, Bara I, Shen V, et al. Oncogene-Specific Differences in Tumor Mutational Burden, PD-L1 Expression, and Outcomes From Immunotherapy in Non-Small Cell Lung Cancer. *J ImmunoTherapy Cancer* (2021) 9(8):e002891. doi: 10.1136/jitc-2021-002891
16. Wong DW, Leung EL, So KK, Tam IY, Sihoe AD, Cheng LC, et al. The EML4-ALK Fusion Gene is Involved in Various Histologic Types of Lung Cancers From Nonsmokers With Wild-Type EGFR and KRAS. *Cancer* (2009) 115(8):1723–33. doi: 10.1002/cncr.24181
17. Koivunen JP, Mermel C, Zejnullahu K, Murphy C, Lifshits E, Holmes AJ, et al. EML4-ALK Fusion Gene and Efficacy of an ALK Kinase Inhibitor in Lung Cancer. *Clin Cancer Res* (2008) 14(13):4275–83. doi: 10.1158/1078-0432.CCR-08-0168
18. Sasaki T, Rodig SJ, Chirieac LR, Janne PA. The Biology and Treatment of EML4-ALK Non-Small Cell Lung Cancer. *Eur J Cancer* (2010) 46(10):1773–80. doi: 10.1016/j.ejca.2010.04.002
19. Shaw AT, Yeap BY, Mino-Kenudson M, Digumarthy SR, Costa DB, Heist RS, et al. Clinical Features and Outcome of Patients With Non-Small-Cell Lung Cancer Who Harbor EML4-ALK. *J Clin Oncol* (2009) 27(26):4247–53. doi: 10.1200/JCO.2009.22.6993
20. Soda M, Choi YL, Enomoto M, Takada S, Yamashita Y, Ishikawa S, et al. Identification of the Transforming EML4-ALK Fusion Gene in Non-Small-Cell Lung Cancer. *Nature* (2007) 448(7153):561–6. doi: 10.1038/nature05945
21. Chia PL, Mitchell P, Dobrovic A, John T. Prevalence and Natural History of ALK Positive Non-Small-Cell Lung Cancer and the Clinical Impact of Targeted Therapy With ALK Inhibitors. *Clin Epidemiol* (2014) 6:423–32. doi: 10.2147/CLEP.S69718
22. Cruz BD, Barbosa MM, Torres LL, Azevedo PS, Silva VEA, Godman B, et al. Crizotinib Versus Conventional Chemotherapy in First-Line Treatment for ALK-Positive Non-Small Cell Lung Cancer: A Systematic Review and Meta-Analysis. *Oncol Ther* (2021) 9:505–24. doi: 10.1007/s40487-021-00155-3
23. Chen J, O'Gorman MT, James LP, Klamerus KJ, Mugundu G, Pithavala YK. Pharmacokinetics of Lorlatinib After Single and Multiple Dosing in Patients With Anaplastic Lymphoma Kinase (ALK)-Positive Non-Small Cell Lung Cancer: Results From a Global Phase I/II Study. *Clin Pharmacokinet* (2021) 60:1313–24. doi: 10.1007/s40262-021-01015-z
24. Camidge DR, Kim HR, Ahn MJ, Yang JCH, Han JY, Hochmair MJ, et al. Brigatinib Versus Crizotinib in Advanced ALK Inhibitor-Naive ALK-Positive Non-Small Cell Lung Cancer: Second Interim Analysis of the Phase III ALTA-1l Trial. *J Clin Oncol* (2020) 38(31):3592–603. doi: 10.1200/JCO.20.00505
25. Wu YL, Lu S, Lu Y, Zhou J, Shi YK, Sriuranpong V, et al. Results of PROFILE 1029, a Phase III Comparison of First-Line Crizotinib Versus Chemotherapy in East Asian Patients With ALK-Positive Advanced Non-Small Cell Lung Cancer. *J Thorac Oncol* (2018) 13(10):1539–48. doi: 10.1016/j.jtho.2018.06.012
26. Solomon BJ, Besse B, Bauer TM, Felip E, Soo RA, Camidge DR, et al. Lorlatinib in Patients With ALK-Positive Non-Small-Cell Lung Cancer: Results From a Global Phase 2 Study. *Lancet Oncol* (2018) 19(12):1654–67. doi: 10.1016/S1470-2045(18)30649-1
27. Camidge DR, Kim HR, Ahn MJ, Yang JC, Han JY, Lee JS, et al. Brigatinib Versus Crizotinib in ALK-Positive Non-Small-Cell Lung Cancer. *N Engl J Med* (2018) 379(21):2027–39. doi: 10.1056/NEJMoa1810171
28. Peters S, Camidge DR, Shaw AT, Gadgeel S, Ahn JS, Kim DW, et al. Alectinib Versus Crizotinib in Untreated ALK-Positive Non-Small-Cell Lung Cancer. *N Engl J Med* (2017) 377(9):829–38. doi: 10.1056/NEJMoa1704795
29. Soria JC, Tan DSW, Chiari R, Wu YL, Paz-Ares L, Wolf J, et al. First-Line Ceritinib Versus Platinum-Based Chemotherapy in Advanced ALK-Rearranged Non-Small-Cell Lung Cancer (ASCEND-4): A Randomised, Open-Label, Phase 3 Study. *Lancet* (2017) 389(10072):917–29. doi: 10.1016/S0140-6736(17)30123-X
30. Chang G-C, Yang T-Y, Chen K-C, Hsu K-H, Huang Y-H, Su K-Y, et al. ALK Variants, PD-L1 Expression, and Their Association With Outcomes in ALK-Positive NSCLC Patients. *Sci Rep* (2020) 10(1):21063. doi: 10.1038/s41598-020-78152-1
31. Mazieres J, Drilon A, Lusque A, Mhanna L, Cortot AB, Mezquita L, et al. Immune Checkpoint Inhibitors for Patients With Advanced Lung Cancer and Oncogenic Driver Alterations: Results From the IMMUNOTARGET Registry. *Ann Oncol* (2019) 30(8):1321–8. doi: 10.1093/annonc/mdz167
32. Gainor JF, Shaw AT, Sequist LV, Fu X, Azzoli CG, Piotrowska Z, et al. EGFR Mutations and ALK Rearrangements Are Associated With Low Response Rates to PD-1 Pathway Blockade in Non-Small Cell Lung Cancer: A Retrospective Analysis. *Clin Cancer Res* (2016) 22(18):4585–93. doi: 10.1158/1078-0432.CCR-15-3101
33. Jahanzeb M, Lin HM, Pan X, Yin Y, Baumann P, Langer CJ. Immunotherapy Treatment Patterns and Outcomes Among ALK-Positive Patients With Non-Small-Cell Lung Cancer. *Clin Lung Cancer* (2021) 22(1):49–57. doi: 10.1016/j.cllc.2020.08.003
34. Gadgeel S, Dziubek K, Nagasaka M, Braun T, Hassan K, Cheng H, et al. Pembrolizumab in Combination With Platinum-Based Chemotherapy in Recurrent EGFR/ALK-Positive Non-Small Cell Lung Cancer (NSCLC), in: Abstracts | IASLC 2021 World Conference on Lung Cancer | Worldwide Virtual Event. 2021(WCLC 2021). *Journal of Thoracic Oncology*. Amsterdam: Elsevier (2021). Available at: Dziubek.
35. Borghaei H, Paz-Ares L, Horn L, Spigel DR, Steins M, Ready NE, et al. Nivolumab Versus Docetaxel in Advanced Nonsquamous Non–Small-Cell Lung Cancer. *N Engl J Med* (2015) 373(17):1627–39. doi: 10.1056/NEJMoa1507643
36. Herbst RS, Baas P, Kim D-W, Felip E, Pérez-Gracia JL, Han J-Y, et al. Pembrolizumab Versus Docetaxel for Previously Treated, PD-L1-Positive, Advanced Non-Small-Cell Lung Cancer (KEYNOTE-010): A Randomised Controlled Trial. *Lancet* (2016) 387(10027):1540–50. doi: 10.1016/S0140-6736(15)01281-7
37. West H, McCleod M, Hussein M, Morabito A, Rittmeyer A, Conter HJ, et al. Atezolizumab in Combination With Carboplatin Plus Nab-Paclitaxel Chemotherapy Compared With Chemotherapy Alone as First-Line Treatment for Metastatic Non-Squamous Non-Small-Cell Lung Cancer (IMpower130): A Multicentre, Randomised, Open-Label, Phase 3 Trial. *Lancet Oncol* (2019) 20(7):924–37. doi: 10.1016/S1470-2045(19)30167-6
38. Socinski MA, Jotte RM, Cappuzzo F, Orlandi F, Stroyakovskiy D, Nogami N, et al. Atezolizumab for First-Line Treatment of Metastatic Nonsquamous NSCLC. *N Engl J Med* (2018) 378(24):2288–301. doi: 10.1056/NEJMoa1716948
39. Dong J, Li B, Lin D, Zhou Q, Huang D. Advances in Targeted Therapy and Immunotherapy for Non-Small Cell Lung Cancer Based on Accurate Molecular Typing. *Front Pharmacol* (2019) 10:230–. doi: 10.3389/fphar.2019.00230
40. Leonetti A, Facchinetti F, Rossi G, Minari R, Conti A, Friboulet L, et al. BRAF in Non-Small Cell Lung Cancer (NSCLC): Pickaxing Another Brick in the Wall. *Cancer Treat Rev* (2018) 66:82–94. doi: 10.1016/j.ctrv.2018.04.006
41. Cancer Genome Atlas Research N. Comprehensive Genomic Characterization of Squamous Cell Lung Cancers. *Nature* (2012) 489 (7417):519–25. doi: 10.1038/nature11404
42. Cui G, Liu D, Li W, Fu X, Liang Y, Li Y, et al. A Meta-Analysis of the Association Between BRAF Mutation and Nonsmall Cell Lung Cancer. *Med (Baltimore)* (2017) 96(14):e6552. doi: 10.1097/MD.0000000000006552

43. Dudnik E, Peled N, Nechushtan H, Wollner M, Onn A, Agbarya A, et al. BRAF Mutant Lung Cancer: Programmed Death Ligand 1 Expression, Tumor Mutational Burden, Microsatellite Instability Status, and Response to Immune Check-Point Inhibitors. *J Thorac Oncol* (2018) 13(8):1128–37. doi: 10.1016/j.jtho.2018.04.024
44. Rihawi K, Giannarelli D, Galetta D, Delmonte A, Giavarra M, Turci D, et al. BRAF Mutant NSCLC and Immune Checkpoint Inhibitors: Results From a Real-World Experience. *J Thorac Oncol* (2019) 14(3):e57–9. doi: 10.1016/j.jtho.2018.11.036
45. Tan I, Stinchcombe TE, Ready NE, Crawford J, Datto MB, Nagy RJ, et al. Therapeutic Outcomes in Non-Small Cell Lung Cancer With BRAF Mutations: A Single Institution, Retrospective Cohort Study. *Transl Lung Cancer Res* (2019) 8(3):258–67. doi: 10.21037/tlcr.2019.04.03
46. Dudnik E, Bshara E, Grubstein A, Fridel L, Shochat T, Roisman LC, et al. Rare Targetable Drivers (RTDs) in Non-Small Cell Lung Cancer (NSCLC): Outcomes With Immune Check-Point Inhibitors (ICPi). *Lung Cancer* (2018) 124:117–24. doi: 10.1016/j.lungcan.2018.07.044
47. Guisier F, Dubos-Arvis C, Vinas F, Doubre H, Ricordel C, Ropert S, et al. Efficacy and Safety of Anti-PD-1 Immunotherapy in Patients With Advanced NSCLC With BRAF, HER2, or MET Mutations or RET Translocation: GFPC 01-2018. *J Thorac Oncol* (2020) 15(4):628–36. doi: 10.1016/j.jtho.2019.12.129
48. Mu Y, Yang K, Hao X, Wang Y, Wang L, Liu Y, et al. Clinical Characteristics and Treatment Outcomes of 65 Patients With BRAF-Mutated Non-Small Cell Lung Cancer. *Front Oncol* (2020) 10:603–. doi: 10.3389/fonc.2020.00603
49. Ding S, Merkulova-Rainon T, Han ZC, Tobelem G. HGF Receptor Up-Regulation Contributes to the Angiogenic Phenotype of Human Endothelial Cells and Promotes Angiogenesis In Vitro. *Blood* (2003) 101(12):4816–22. doi: 10.1182/blood-2002-06-1731
50. Bauer TW, Somcio RJ, Fan F, Liu W, Johnson M, Lesslie DP, et al. Regulatory Role of C-Met in Insulin-Like Growth Factor-I Receptor-Mediated Migration and Invasion of Human Pancreatic Carcinoma Cells. *Mol Cancer Ther* (2006) 5(7):1676–82. doi: 10.1158/1535-7163.MCT-05-0175
51. Frampton GM, Ali SM, Rosenzweig M, Chmielecki J, Lu X, Bauer TM, et al. Activation of MET *via* Diverse Exon 14 Splicing Alterations Occurs in Multiple Tumor Types and Confers Clinical Sensitivity to MET Inhibitors. *Cancer Discov* (2015) 5(8):850–9. doi: 10.1158/2159-8290.CD-15-0285
52. Awad MM, Oxnard GR, Jackman DM, Savukoski DO, Hall D, Shivdasani P, et al. MET Exon 14 Mutations in Non-Small-Cell Lung Cancer Are Associated With Advanced Age and Stage-Dependent MET Genomic Amplification and C-Met Overexpression. *J Clin Oncol* (2016) 34(7):721–30. doi: 10.1200/JCO.2015.63.4600
53. Van Der Steen N, Giovannetti E, Pauwels P, Peters GJ, Hong DS, Cappuzzo F, et al. cMET Exon 14 Skipping: From the Structure to the Clinic. *J Thorac Oncol* (2016) 11(9):1423–32. doi: 10.1016/j.jtho.2016.05.005
54. Wolf J, Seto T, Han JY, Reguart N, Garon EB, Groen HJM, et al. Capmatinib in MET Exon 14-Mutated or MET-Amplified Non-Small-Cell Lung Cancer. *N Engl J Med* (2020) 383(10):944–57. doi: 10.1056/NEJMoa2002787
55. Paik PK, Felip E, Veillon R, Sakai H, Cortot AB, Garassino MC, et al. Tepotinib in Non-Small-Cell Lung Cancer With MET Exon 14 Skipping Mutations. *N Engl J Med* (2020) 383(10):931–43. doi: 10.1056/NEJMoa2004407
56. Mayenga M, Assie JB, Monnet I, Massiani MA, Tabeze L, Friard S, et al. Durable Responses to Immunotherapy of Non-Small Cell Lung Cancers Harboring MET Exon-14-Skipping Mutation: A Series of 6 Cases. *Lung Cancer* (2020) 150:21–5. doi: 10.1016/j.lungcan.2020.09.008
57. Kohno T, Ichikawa H, Totoki Y, Yasuda K, Hiramoto M, Nammo T, et al. KIF5B-RET Fusions in Lung Adenocarcinoma. *Nat Med* (2012) 18(3):375–7. doi: 10.1038/nm.2644
58. Li F, Feng Y, Fang R, Fang Z, Xia J, Han X, et al. Identification of RET Gene Fusion by Exon Array Analyses in "Pan-Negative" Lung Cancer From Never Smokers. *Cell Res* (2012) 22(5):928–31. doi: 10.1038/cr.2012.27
59. Kato S, Subbiah V, Marchlik E, Elkin SK, Carter JL, Kurzrock R. RET Aberrations in Diverse Cancers: Next-Generation Sequencing of 4,871 Patients. *Clin Cancer Res* (2017) 23(8):1988–97. doi: 10.1158/1078-0432.CCR-16-1679
60. Lin C, Wang S, Xie W, Chang J, Gan Y. The RET Fusion Gene and Its Correlation With Demographic and Clinicopathological Features of Non-Small Cell Lung Cancer: A Meta-Analysis. *Cancer Biol Ther* (2015) 16 (7):1019–28. doi: 10.1080/15384047.2015.1046649
61. Offin M, Guo R, Wu SL, Sabari J, Land JD, Ni A, et al. Immunophenotype and Response to Immunotherapy of RET-Rearranged Lung Cancers. *JCO Precis Oncol* (2019) 3:1–8. doi: 10.1200/PO.18.00386
62. Drilon A, Oxnard GR, Tan DSW, Loong HHF, Johnson M, Gainor J, et al. Efficacy of Selpercatinib in RET Fusion-Positive Non-Small-Cell Lung Cancer. *N Engl J Med* (2020) 383(9):813–24. doi: 10.1056/NEJMoa2005653
63. Gainor JF, Curigliano G, Kim DW, Lee DH, Besse B, Baik CS, et al. Pralsetinib for RET Fusion-Positive Non-Small-Cell Lung Cancer (ARROW): A Multi-Cohort, Open-Label, Phase 1/2 Study. *Lancet Oncol* (2021) 22(7):959–69. doi: 10.1016/S1470-2045(21)00247-3
64. Lee J, Ku BM, Shim JH, La Choi Y, Sun JM, Lee SH, et al. Characteristics and Outcomes of RET-Rearranged Korean Non-Small Cell Lung Cancer Patients in Real-World Practice. *Jpn J Clin Oncol* (2020) 50(5):594–601. doi: 10.1093/jjco/hyaa019
65. Birchmeier C, Sharma S, Wigler M. Expression and Rearrangement of the ROS1 Gene in Human Glioblastoma Cells. *Proc Natl Acad Sci U S A* (1987) 84(24):9270–4. doi: 10.1073/pnas.84.24.9270
66. Davies KD, Le AT, Theodoro MF, Skokan MC, Aisner DL, Berge EM, et al. Identifying and Targeting ROS1 Gene Fusions in Non-Small Cell Lung Cancer. *Clin Cancer Res* (2012) 18(17):4570–9. doi: 10.1158/1078-0432.CCR-12-0550
67. Facchinetti F, Rossi G, Bria E, Soria JC, Besse B, Minari R, et al. Oncogene Addiction in non-Small Cell Lung Cancer: Focus on ROS1 Inhibition. *Cancer Treat Rev* (2017) 55:83–95. doi: 10.1016/j.ctrv.2017.02.010
68. Lin JJ, Shaw AT. Recent Advances in Targeting ROS1 in Lung Cancer. *J Thorac Oncol* (2017) 12(11):1611–25. doi: 10.1016/j.jtho.2017.08.002
69. Bergethon K, Shaw AT, Ou SH, Katayama R, Lovly CM, McDonald NT, et al. ROS1 Rearrangements Define a Unique Molecular Class of Lung Cancers. *J Clin Oncol* (2012) 30(8):863–70. doi: 10.1200/JCO.2011.35.6345
70. Yoh K, Matsumoto S, Kunimasa K, Kodani M, Nishi K, Nakagawa T, et al. The Efficacy of Immune Checkpoint Inhibitors and PD-L1 Status in Patients With Advanced Non-Small Cell Lung Cancer Harboring Oncogenic Driver Alterations: Immuno-Oncology Biomarker Study in LC-SCRUM-Japan. *J Clin Oncol* (2019) 37(15_suppl):9046–. doi: 10.1200/JCO.2019.37.15_suppl.9046
71. Al-Salama ZT, Keam SJ. Entrectinib: First Global Approval. *Drugs* (2019) 79 (13):1477–83. doi: 10.1007/s40265-019-01177-y
72. Available at: https://www.fda.gov/drugs/resources-information-approved-drugs/fda-grants-accelerated-approval-sotorasib-kras-g12c-mutated-nsclc.
73. Wood K, Hensing T, Malik R, Salgia R. Prognostic and Predictive Value in KRAS in Non-Small-Cell Lung Cancer: A Review. *JAMA Oncol* (2016) 2 (6):805–12. doi: 10.1001/jamaoncol.2016.0405
74. Liu C, Zheng S, Jin R, Wang X, Wang F, Zang R, et al. The Superior Efficacy of Anti-PD-1/PD-L1 Immunotherapy in KRAS-Mutant Non-Small Cell Lung Cancer That Correlates With an Inflammatory Phenotype and Increased Immunogenicity. *Cancer Lett* (2020) 470:95–105. doi: 10.1016/j.canlet.2019.10.027
75. Dogan S, Shen R, Ang DC, Johnson ML, D'Angelo SP, Paik PK, et al. Molecular Epidemiology of EGFR and KRAS Mutations in 3,026 Lung Adenocarcinomas: Higher Susceptibility of Women to Smoking-Related KRAS-Mutant Cancers. *Clin Cancer Res* (2012) 18(22):6169–77. doi: 10.1158/1078-0432.CCR-11-3265
76. El Osta B, Behera M, Kim S, Berry LD, Sica G, Pillai RN, et al. Characteristics and Outcomes of Patients With Metastatic KRAS-Mutant Lung Adenocarcinomas: The Lung Cancer Mutation Consortium Experience. *J Thorac Oncol* (2019) 14(5):876–89. doi: 10.1016/j.jtho.2019.01.020
77. Skoulidis F, Li BT, Dy GK, Price TJ, Falchook GS, Wolf J, et al. Sotorasib for Lung Cancers With KRAS P.G12C Mutation. *N Engl J Med* (2021) 384 (25):2371–81. doi: 10.1056/NEJMoa2103695
78. Herbst RS. LBA4 Association of KRAS Mutational Status With Response to Pembrolizumab Monotherapy Given as First-Line Therapy for PD-L1-Positive Advanced Non-Squamous NSCLC in Keynote-042. *Ann Oncol* (2019) 30(Supplement 11):xi63–xi4. doi: 10.1093/annonc/mdz453.001
79. Sun L, Hsu M, Cohen RB, Langer CJ, Mamtani R, Aggarwal C. Association Between KRAS Variant Status and Outcomes With First-Line Immune Checkpoint Inhibitor-Based Therapy in Patients With Advanced Non-

Small-Cell Lung Cancer. *JAMA Oncol* (2021) 7(6):937–9. doi: 10.1001/jamaoncol.2021.0546

80. Gadgeel S, Rodriguez-Abreu D, Felip E, Esteban E, Speranza G, Reck M, et al. KRAS Mutational Status and Efficacy in KEYNOTE-189: Pembrolizumab (Pembro) Plus Chemotherapy (Chemo) vs Placebo Plus Chemo as First-Line Therapy for Metastatic Non-Squamous NSCLC. *Ann Oncol* (2019) 30:xi64–xi5. doi: 10.1093/annonc/mdz453.002
81. West H, Cappuzzo F, Reck M, Mok T, Jotte RM, Nishio M, et al. IMpower150: A *Post Hoc* Analysis of Efficacy Outcomes in Patients With KRAS, STK11 and KEAP1 Mutations. *Ann Oncol* (2020) 31(10):817–8. doi: 10.1016/j.annonc.2020.08.1579
82. Passiglia F, Cappuzzo F, Alabiso O, Bettini AC, Bidoli P, Chiari R, et al. Efficacy of Nivolumab in Pre-Treated Non-Small-Cell Lung Cancer Patients Harbouring KRAS Mutations. *Br J Cancer* (2019) 120(1):57–62. doi: 10.1038/s41416-018-0234-3
83. Jeanson A, Tomasini P, Souquet-Bressand M, Brandone N, Boucekine M, Grangeon M, et al. Efficacy of Immune Checkpoint Inhibitors in KRAS-Mutant Non-Small Cell Lung Cancer (NSCLC). *J Thorac Oncol* (2019) 14 (6):1095–101. doi: 10.1016/j.jtho.2019.01.011
84. Remon J, Castro-Henriques M, Esteller L, Vives J. Combination of Atezolizumab, Bevacizumab, and Chemotherapy (IMpower 150) in a Patient With NSCLC Having Leptomeningeal Metastases. *JTO Clin Res Rep* (2021) 2(1):100096. doi: 10.1016/j.jtocrr.2020.100096
85. Lee CK, Man J, Lord S, Cooper W, Links M, Gebski V, et al. Clinical and Molecular Characteristics Associated With Survival Among Patients Treated With Checkpoint Inhibitors for Advanced Non–Small Cell Lung Carcinoma: A Systematic Review and Meta-Analysis. *JAMA Oncol* (2018) 4(2):210–6. doi: 10.1001/jamaoncol.2017.4427
86. Lenferink AE, Pinkas-Kramarski R, van de Poll ML, van Vugt MJ, Klapper LN, Tzahar E, et al. Differential Endocytic Routing of Homo- and Hetero-Dimeric ErbB Tyrosine Kinases Confers Signaling Superiority to Receptor Heterodimers. *EMBO J* (1998) 17(12):3385–97. doi: 10.1093/emboj/17.12.3385
87. Ekman S. HER2: Defining a Neu Target in Non-Small-Cell Lung Cancer. *Ann Oncol* (2019) 30(3):353–5. doi: 10.1093/annonc/mdz043
88. Pillai RN, Behera M, Berry LD, Rossi MR, Kris MG, Johnson BE, et al. HER2 Mutations in Lung Adenocarcinomas: A Report From the Lung Cancer Mutation Consortium. *Cancer* (2017) 123(21):4099–105. doi: 10.1002/cncr.30869
89. Li BT, Shen R, Buonocore D, Olah ZT, Ni A, Ginsberg MS, et al. Ado-Trastuzumab Emtansine for Patients With HER2-Mutant Lung Cancers: Results From a Phase II Basket Trial. *J Clin Oncol* (2018) 36(24):2532–7. doi: 10.1200/JCO.2018.77.9777
90. Li BT, Smit EF, Goto Y, Nakagawa K, Udagawa H, Mazières J, et al. Trastuzumab Deruxtecan in HER2-Mutant Non–Small-Cell Lung Cancer. *N Engl J Med* (2021). doi: 10.1056/NEJMoa2112431
91. Elamin YY, Robichaux JP, Carter BW, Altan M, Gibbons DL, Fossella FV, et al. Poziotinib for Patients With HER2 Exon 20 Mutant Non–Small-Cell Lung Cancer: Results From a Phase II Trial. *J Clin Oncol* (2021) 2021: JCO.21.01113. doi: 10.1200/JCO.21.01113
92. Heymach J, Negrao M, Robichaux J, Carter B, Patel A, Altan M, et al. OA02.06 A Phase II Trial of Poziotinib in EGFR and HER2 Exon 20 Mutant Non-Small Cell Lung Cancer (NSCLC). *J Thorac Oncol* (2018) 13(10):S323–S4. doi: 10.1016/j.jtho.2018.08.243
93. Mo J, Hu X, Gu L, Chen B, Khadaroo PA, Shen Z, et al. Smokers or Non-Smokers: Who Benefits More From Immune Checkpoint Inhibitors in Treatment of Malignancies? An Up-to-Date Meta-Analysis. *World J Surg Oncol* (2020) 18(1):15. doi: 10.1186/s12957-020-1792-4
94. Wang X, Ricciuti B, Alessi JV, Nguyen T, Awad MM, Lin X, et al. Smoking History as a Potential Predictor of Immune Checkpoint Inhibitor Efficacy in Metastatic Non-Small Cell Lung Cancer. *J Natl Cancer Inst* (2021). doi: 10.1093/jnci/djab116
95. Chen DL, Li QY, Tan QY. Smoking History and the Efficacy of Immune Checkpoint Inhibitors in Patients With Advanced Non-Small Cell Lung Cancer: A Systematic Review and Meta-Analysis. *J Thorac Dis* (2021) 13 (1):220–31. doi: 10.21037/jtd-20-1953
96. Marabelle A, Le DT, Ascierto PA, Di Giacomo AM, De Jesus-Acosta A, Delord JP, et al. Efficacy of Pembrolizumab in Patients With Noncolorectal High Microsatellite Instability/Mismatch Repair-Deficient Cancer: Results From the Phase II KEYNOTE-158 Study. *J Clin Oncol* (2020) 38(1):1–10. doi: 10.1200/JCO.19.02105
97. Yu Y, Zeng D, Ou Q, Liu S, Li A, Chen Y, et al. Association of Survival and Immune-Related Biomarkers With Immunotherapy in Patients With Non-Small Cell Lung Cancer: A Meta-Analysis and Individual Patient-Level Analysis. *JAMA Netw Open* (2019) 2(7):e196879. doi: 10.1001/jamanetworkopen.2019.6879
98. Kim JY, Kronbichler A, Eisenhut M, Hong SH, van der Vliet HJ, Kang J, et al. Tumor Mutational Burden and Efficacy of Immune Checkpoint Inhibitors: A Systematic Review and Meta-Analysis. *Cancers (Basel)* (2019) 11(11):1798. doi: 10.3390/cancers11111798
99. Skoulidis F, Byers LA, Diao L, Papadimitrakopoulou VA, Tong P, Izzo J, et al. Co-Occurring Genomic Alterations Define Major Subsets of KRAS-Mutant Lung Adenocarcinoma With Distinct Biology, Immune Profiles, and Therapeutic Vulnerabilities. *Cancer Discov* (2015) 5(8):860–77. doi: 10.1158/2159-8290.CD-14-1236
100. Davis AP, Cooper WA, Boyer M, Lee JH, Pavlakis N, Kao SC. Efficacy of Immunotherapy in KRAS-Mutant Non-Small-Cell Lung Cancer With Comutations. *Immunotherapy* (2021) 13(11):941–52. doi: 10.2217/imt-2021-0090
101. Mazzotta M, Filetti M, Occhipinti M, Marinelli D, Scalera S, Terrenato I, et al. Efficacy of Immunotherapy in Lung Cancer With Co-Occurring Mutations in NOTCH and Homologous Repair Genes. *J Immunother Cancer* (2020) 8(2):1–6. doi: 10.1136/jitc-2020-000946
102. Perez-Ruiz E, Melero I, Kopecka J, Sarmento-Ribeiro AB, Garcia-Aranda M, De Las Rivas J. Cancer Immunotherapy Resistance Based on Immune Checkpoints Inhibitors: Targets, Biomarkers, and Remedies. *Drug Resist Update* (2020) 53:100718. doi: 10.1016/j.drup.2020.100718
103. Park YJ, Kuen DS, Chung Y. Future Prospects of Immune Checkpoint Blockade in Cancer: From Response Prediction to Overcoming Resistance. *Exp Mol Med* (2018) 50(8):1–13. doi: 10.1038/s12276-018-0130-1
104. Kashyap AS, Schmittnaegel M, Rigamonti N, Pais-Ferreira D, Mueller P, Buchi M, et al. Optimized Antiangiogenic Reprogramming of the Tumor Microenvironment Potentiates CD40 Immunotherapy. *Proc Natl Acad Sci U S A* (2020) 117(1):541–51. doi: 10.1073/pnas.1902145116
105. Felip E, de Braud FG, Maur M, Loong HH, Shaw AT, Vansteenkiste JF, et al. Ceritinib Plus Nivolumab in Patients With Advanced ALK-Rearranged Non-Small Cell Lung Cancer: Results of an Open-Label, Multicenter, Phase 1b Study. *J Thorac Oncol* (2020) 15(3):392–403. doi: 10.1016/j.jtho.2019.10.006
106. Spigel DR, Reynolds C, Waterhouse D, Garon EB, Chandler J, Babu S, et al. Phase 1/2 Study of the Safety and Tolerability of Nivolumab Plus Crizotinib for the First-Line Treatment of Anaplastic Lymphoma Kinase Translocation - Positive Advanced Non-Small Cell Lung Cancer (CheckMate 370). *J Thorac Oncol* (2018) 13(5):682–8. doi: 10.1016/j.jtho.2018.02.022
107. Kim D-W, Gadgeel SM, Gettinger SN, Riely GJ, Oxnard GR, Mekhail T, et al. Safety and Clinical Activity Results From a Phase Ib Study of Alectinib Plus Atezolizumab in ALK+ Advanced NSCLC (aNSCLC). *J Clin Oncol* (2018) 36 (15_suppl):9009–. doi: 10.1200/JCO.2018.36.15_suppl.9009
108. McCoach CE. A Cautionary Analysis of Immunotherapy Prior to Targeted Therapy. *J Thorac Oncol* (2019) 14(1):8–10. doi: 10.1016/j.jtho.2018.10.009

24

Considerations for the Surgical Management of Thoracic Cancers during the COVID-19 Pandemic: Rational Strategies for Thoracic Surgeons

*Jiahao Zhang†, Yichao Han†, Yajie Zhang†, Dong Dong, Yuqin Cao, Xiang Chen and Hecheng Li**

Department of Thoracic Surgery, Ruijin Hospital, Shanghai Jiao Tong University School of Medicine, Shanghai, China

***Correspondence:**
Hecheng Li
lihecheng2000@hotmail.com

†These authors have contributed equally to this work

Objective: The novel Coronavirus Disease 2019 (COVID-19) has resulted in a global health crisis since first case was identified in December 2019. As the pandemic continues to strain global public health systems, elective surgeries for thoracic cancer, such as early-stage lung cancer and esophageal cancer (EC), have been postponed due to a shortage of medical resources and the risk of nosocomial transmission. This review is aimed to discuss the influence of COVID-19 on thoracic surgical practice, prevention of nosocomial transmission during the pandemic, and propose modifications to the standard practices in the surgical management of different thoracic cancer.

Methods: A literature search of PubMed, Medline, and Google Scholar was performed for articles focusing on COVID-19, early-stage lung cancer, and EC prior to 1 July 2021. The evidence from articles was combined with our data and experience.

Results: We review the challenges in the management of different thoracic cancer from the perspectives of thoracic surgeons and propose rational strategies for the diagnosis and treatment of early-stage lung cancer and EC during the COVID-19 pandemic.

Conclusions: During the COVID-19 pandemic, the optimization of hospital systems and medical resources is to fight against COVID-19. Indolent early lung cancers, such as pure ground-glass nodules/opacities (GGOs), can be postponed with a lower risk of progression, while selective surgeries of more biologically aggressive tumors should be prioritized. As for EC, we recommend immediate or prioritized surgeries for patients with stage Ib or more advanced stage and patients after neoadjuvant therapy. Routine COVID-19 screening should be performed preoperatively before thoracic surgeries. Prevention of nosocomial transmission by providing appropriate personal protective equipment (PPE), such as N-95 respirator masks with eye protection to healthcare workers, is necessary.

Keywords: COVID-19, early-stage lung cancer, esophageal cancer, ground glass opacities, recommendation, prevention of nosocomial transmission in hospitals, thoracic surgeons, surgical treatment

INTRODUCTION

Coronavirus Disease-2019 (COVID-19) is caused by infection of the novel coronavirus severe acute respiratory syndrome coronavirus 2 (SARS-CoV-2) virus, which has widely spread worldwide and resulted in over 1.8 hundred million infection cases and 3,930,000 deaths worldwide (1). The SARS-CoV-2 virus was first identified in the city of Wuhan, China in 2019. SARS-CoV-2 is a highly contagious pathogen transmitted from human to human through exposure to respiratory fluids carrying an infectious virus, and the average reproductive ratio (R_0) for SARS-CoV-2 has been found between 1.4 and 2.5 transmissions by one initial infection (2). The incubation period of SARS-CoV-2 is found most likely to be ≤14 days (median, 5 days) and the average mortality rate of COVID-19 is 3.6% (3) whereas mortality for critical cases reaches up to 60.5% (4). Patients with symptoms can develop fever, cough, fatigue, expectoration, and anhelation as the most common clinical manifestations after being infected by SARS-CoV-2. The elderly or those with previous and current existing chronic medical conditions may suffer from relatively severe viral pneumonia, and then some of these patients may progress to SARS and eventually death (5). Moreover, there are patients who are not yet experiencing onset of symptoms (presymptomatic) and patients without typical symptoms (asymptomatic) of COVID-19 disease (6), which increases the risk of human to human transmission in population.

As the COVID-19 pandemic constantly strains the health systems in almost every nation, interfering with the organization of normal healthcare delivery in severe epidemic areas, it has temporarily postponed a large proportion of elective surgeries for early-stage lung cancers and other thoracic cancers worldwide. The delay of lung cancer resections brings the risk of disease progression. Further, social distancing policies have affected timely evaluation for the initial diagnosis and follow-ups of suspected non-small cell lung cancer (NSCLC) and esophageal cancer (EC) in outpatient clinics. Therefore, based on the case load of COVID-19 in a certain area, the surgical treatment of thoracic cancers needs to overcome these difficulties with appropriate modifications to the standard practices by surgeons and healthcare workers, and certain measures are supposed to be adapted for minimalizing the risk of transmission. This review aims to share and discuss the latest clinical evidence and provide a framework and proposal for modifications to the current practices of managing early-stage NSCLC and EC that contributes to the promptly surgical treatment and safety of patients, and protection for healthcare providers during the ongoing pandemic, from a thoracic surgeon's perspective.

PREVENTING NOSOCOMIAL TRANSMISSION IN THORACIC SURGERY: PREOPERATIVE SCREENING AND PERSONAL PROTECTION

Previous reports have shown that the infection of SARS-CoV-2 in the perioperative period is associated with a relatively poor prognosis for patients who underwent thoracic surgical procedures, and healthcare workers are vulnerable to transmission from infected patients prior to appropriate personal protective equipment (PPE) utilization (7, 8). Thus, preventing and breaking the chains of nosocomial transmission during the pandemic should be the priority of concerns in the thoracic surgery department.

The transmission of the SARS-CoV-2 virus from infected individuals to other people is mainly by inhaling aerosolized droplets containing the virus and direct contact with infected patients. There is no evidence of airborne transmission through aerosols of SARS-CoV-2 up to the present. The smallest aerosolized droplets containing SARS-CoV-2 have been found to be as small as 5 μm, and those droplets can be produced during nearly all procedures concerning the bronchus and upper areo-digestive tract, such as bronchoscopy, endotracheal intubation, endobronchial ultrasound (EBUS), upper endoscopy, or surgeries, involving the bronchus and lung that include radical resection of lung cancer (such as lobectomy, pneumonectomy, segmentectomy, and wedge resections) (2). Surgical damage to the bronchial, upper areo-digestive tract mucosa, or lung parenchyma might lead to aerosolization of the droplets containing the SARS-CoV-2 virus and increase the risk of transmission in the operating room. Similarly, Mckeown and Ivor-Lewis esophagectomy also involves a thoracic phase surgery, which increases the risk of infection.

According to WHO and Central Disease Control, appropriate personal protection equipment is recommended for all medical staff during thoracic surgeries (9). Notably, standard precautions may not work as the optimal protection in the operating room (OR) during procedures with high risks of aerosol-generating as the aerosolized viral particles may not be effectively filtered by a standard droplet mask for their 5 μm diameter. For the optimal personal protection of thoracic surgeons, anesthetists, and other hospital staff inside the operating room, the application of N-95 respirator masks for all aerosol/droplet-generating procedures regardless of the local COVID-19 pandemic status is always recommended (2), and eye-protective goggles for preventing direct liquid splashing should be considered for surgeons and scrub nurses.

Apart from that, current reports suggest a range of 30–60% (10) proportion of patients with asymptomatic COVID-19. Given that the number might be greater than previously expected (2), the risk of COVID-19 transmission from patients without symptoms or with only mild symptoms to other uninfected patients or health hospital staff is unknown, which further

Abbreviations: COVID-19, Coronavirus disease 2019; SARS-CoV-2, Severe acute respiratory syndrome coronavirus; GGOs, Ground-glass opacities; NSCLC, Non-small cell lung cancer; RT-PCR, Real-time polymerase chain reaction; CT, Computed tomography; LDCT, Low-dose CT; VDT, Volume doubling time; NCCN, the National Comprehensive Cancer Network; ACS, the American College of Surgeons; CDC, Centers for Disease Control; OR, Operating room; PPE, Personal protective equipment; HR, Hazard ratio; OR, Odds ratio; RR, Relative risk; nCRT, Neoadjuvant chemoradiation therapy; EC, Esophageal cancer; SCC, Squamous cell carcinoma; AC, Adenocarcinoma; DFS, Disease-free survival; OS, Overall survival; pCR, Pathologic complete response; ER, Endoscopic resection; dCRT, Definitive chemoradiotherapy; TMT, Trimodality therapy; PET-CT, Positron emission tomography-Computed tomography.

increases the difficulty to distinguish nosocomial infection from community infection (2). The potential existence of asymptomatic "super spreader" patients also increases the possibility of nosocomial transmission in the ward and operating theater (8). In order to identify these asymptomatic patients in advance, a routine preoperative screening of SARS-CoV-2 by sampling from nasal or nasopharyngeal swabs and testing the virus RNA by real-time reverse transcription polymerase chain reaction (RT-PCR) is indispensable for alleviating the risk for intraoperative and perioperative nosocomial transmission by asymptomatic patients. Although the accuracy and reliability of the test are influenced by a number of factors that include sampling technique, sampling timing, quality of the testing kits, and the evolution of the disease, routine screening of SARS-CoV-2 by RT-PCR for all patients who are admitted or transferred to the thoracic surgery department is recommended for its convenience and relative reliability, especially for patients who are undergoing procedures with a high risk of transmission, such as bronchoscopy or lung cancer surgery. Considering the false negativity of the RT-PCR test, repeat testing should be considered for negative patients with symptoms or patients with contact history.

Teaching Points

Application of N-95 respirator masks and eye-protective goggles for all aerosol/droplet-generating procedures in the operating room and a routine preoperative screening of SARS-CoV-2 by RT-PCR regardless of the local COVID-19 pandemic status are recommended for alleviating perioperative nosocomial transmission.

TABLE 1 | Radiological differences between Coronavirus Disease-19 (COVID-19) and early-stage lung cancer with GGO features.

	COVID-19	**Early-stage lung cancer**
Spatial location		
Number	Multiple	Solitary
Laterality	Bilateral	Unilateral
Location	Peripheral	Peripheral
Involved lobes	2–4	1
Involved Segments	10–12	1
Component	Pure GGO and mixed GGO	Pure GGO and mixed GGO
Form	Patchy	Oval
Radiographic features	Interlobular septal thickening	Lobulation
	Air bronchogram	Spiculation
	Crazy-paving pattern	Notches
	Reticular pattern	Vascular convergence
	Halo sign	Pleural indentation
Temporal progression		
Progression rate	Rapid	Slow
Disease period	2-6 weeks	VDT of pure GGO: 813 days VDT of mixed GGO: 457 days
Changes on CT	GGOs grow and resolve	GGOs grow
	Lung involvement increases	Increasing or new solid component
	Consolidation	

GGO, ground-glass opacity; VDT, volume doubling time.

DIAGNOSING AND SURGICAL MANAGEMENT OF EARLY-STAGE NSCLC DURING THE COVID-19 PANDEMIC

Comparing and Differentiating COVID-19 From Early-Stage Lung Cancer

During the COVID-19 pandemic, making an accurate diagnosis in asymptomatic patients is more challenging. Computed tomography (CT) scans of patients with COVID-19 without symptoms have sometimes identified related lung lesions (2, 11, 12), and patients with COVID-19 sometimes have presented similarly with early-stage lung cancer on CT scans. It has been reported that most COVID-19 cases are initially featured as patchy or oval ground-glass opacities (GGOs), yet others are featured by consolidative nodules on the chest CT scans, while the progression of virus pneumonia is usually accompanied by the enlargement and consolidation of the GGOs (13, 14). Taking a thorough history, a careful review of imaging, and appropriate testing are required to make an accurate diagnosis. Hereby, we discuss the radiographic similarities and distinctions between early-stage lung cancer and COVID-19 with GGO features that include aspects of spatial location, lesion components, specific radiographic features, and dynamic changes (**Table 1**).

Solitary GGO predominates in early-stage lung cancer, and morbidity of multiple GGOs has been increasing gradually (15). Multiple GGOs can be either unilateral or bilateral, with no obvious preference (16, 17). In contrast, GGO lesions for COVID-19 are usually multiple and located bilaterally (14). Pulmonary involvement is generally more diffuse in patients with COVID-19 and affects more lobes and segments than early lung cancer patients.

Ground-glass opacities are radiologically categorized into pure GGOs, which have no solid component, and part-solid, or mixed GGOs, which contain both a GGO and a solid component (18). Pure GGOs and mixed GGOs are both common on CT scans in COVID-19. In a multicenter retrospective study, 86% of 101 COVID-19 patients were presented with pure GGOs on CT while 64% showed mixed GGOs (19), data from our institution also showed that 100 and 63.6% of 11 patients with COVID-19 had pure GGOs and mixed GGO, respectively (20). On the contrast, although the proportion of pure or mixed GGO in early lung cancer is unclear, a large volume study has shown that 73 cases in 82 pure GGOs and 79 cases in 102 mixed GGOs are confirmed for lung cancers (21, 22). Thus, GGOs in early-stage lung cancer and COVID-19 do not have a predilection toward pure or mixed GGOs. Besides, the patchy form was much more frequent than the oval form in patients with COVID-19 (23), while early lung cancer was more frequently presented as the round or oval form (24).

In addition, studies of patients with COVID-19 discovered that ill-defined margins and air bronchograms are the most common imaging features observed except for GGO, along with thickening of interlobular septal and crazy-paving pattern (11). Reticular patterns, halo signs, air bronchograms, and fibrous stripes can also be seen (23, 25).

The clinical course on CT scans in the two disease entities over time is also significantly different. As an acute disease, COVID-19 has a rapid progression over a period of 2 and 3–6 weeks for mild and severe cases, respectively. Four stages of pneumonia progression on chest CT scan were proposed as the early stage (0–4 days after initial diagnosis) featured by GGOs, progressive stage (5–8 days) featured by increasing total CT score, peak stage (10–13 days) featured by consolidation, and absorption stage (≥14 days) at last (26). During the progressive stage, GGOs grew larger and lung involvement was increased, with the onset of a crazy-paving pattern and consolidation, with the whole process of progression usually within weeks (26). On the contrast, early-stage lung cancers with GGO features are regarded as indolent tumors. These indolent or slow-growing GGOs are often defined by volume doubling time (VDT), i.e., the time required for an enlarging tumor to double its volume. A screening program for early lung cancer in Japan, where 78% were adenocarcinomas, reported mean VDTs of 813 and 457 days for pure GGOs and mixed GGOs, respectively (27), which is distinctly longer than COVID-19 progression. Therefore, although the initial imaging profiles may be similar, the dynamic development of CT findings in early-stage lung cancer is much slower than COVID-19, which can also resolve over time in contrast to malignancy, which emphasizes the follow-up CT imaging for differentiation.

Taken together, the imaging characteristics of COVID-19 are similar but partially different from early-stage lung cancer presenting as GGOs, which can be recognized by thorough and meticulous examination of CT scan on the first diagnosis in clinics. However, to achieve a reliable diagnosis of early lung cancer and to differentiate it from COVID-19, imaging profiles of suspected patients should be sufficiently understood and comprehensively analyzed combined with clinical manifestations, epidemiological history especially contact history with infectious sources, laboratory tests, pathogen screening, CT re-examination, and pathological analysis acquired from surgical treatment (28).

Indication and Triage of Surgical Intervention for Early-Stage Lung Cancers During the COVID-19 Pandemic

The decision on treating suspected early-stage lung cancers, generally by pulmonary resection, depends on the risk evaluation through chest CT imaging. However, the risk of disease progression needs to be balanced with the risk of COVID-19 infection during this COVID-19 pandemic. Prompt surgical treatment for lung cancer has also been challenged by restricted operating room capacity. The optimal treatment decisions for thoracic surgeons during the pandemic can be made by proposing a triage system for NSCLC cases, arranging surgical resection at the appropriate time without significantly increasing the risk of cancer progression.

The American College of Surgeons (ACS) had released a well-considered guideline in late March 2020 for triaging cancer surgery during the pandemic. This guideline outlined the general principles of selection and prioritization for thoracic surgery cases in three outbreak phases of COVID-19 (29). According to ACS and Thoracic Surgery Outcomes Research Network, three phases are proposed according to the COVID-19 trajectory within the hospital and limitations in hospital resources: semi-urgent setting, urgent setting, and fully urgent setting. Elective surgeries, such as resection of lung GGOs, should be restricted to the semi-urgent situation when the volume of patients with COVID-19 is limited and hospital resources are not in scarcity. An analysis of database (30) has found that surgical delay for more than 8 weeks was an independent risk factor related to the progression of operable NSCLC (30). Therefore, the period of delay in early NSCLC patients waiting to have surgery should be less than 2 months to avoid increasing the risk of disease progression (2). Accordingly, surgery for early-stage lung cancer should become one of the top priorities in surgical cases scheduling, especially when oncological results and survival are influenced by progression caused by overlong delay. If necessary, consider those patients as second priority surgical cases if the delay is estimated to be no more than 2 or 3 months (2). According to the ACS Guidelines on Triaging Thoracic Patients, resection should be restricted to the semi-urgent phase and limited to predominantly solid (>50%) or presumed lung cancers >2 cm or nodal positive disease (29).

As for the specific indication for surgical intervention, the National Comprehensive Cancer Network (NCCN) Guidelines have recommended 6 mm as the cutoff values for the evaluation of incidental nodules (31). Intervention should be considered if the nodules develop a solid or invasive component, although the relatively lower risk of progression of an indolent, slow-growing nodule should be balanced with the risks and resource constraints that the local hospital system is facing due to COVID-19 (31).

Non-small cell lung cancer consists of a broad spectrum of different cancer types with growth patterns and grades of malignancy based on their location, image characteristics, pathology type, invasiveness, and tumor differentiation. Interestingly, the tumor's standardized uptake value (SUVmax) from positron emission tomography-Computed tomography (PET-CT) may be related to a higher rate of advanced tumor features, such as mediastinal lymph node metastasis, pleural and pericardial invasion found at operation, and a higher possibility of postoperative pathologic upstaging, but not statistically significantly (12.0 vs. 9.4, $p = 0.08$) (32). Therefore, SUVmax may also be regarded as a factor for deciding the priority of early-stage lung cancer surgeries. Apart from that, a comprehensive triaging system should also be created with consideration of tumor staging, histology, and imaging features, which might indicate invasiveness, to prioritize the more malignant, aggressively behaving tumors for surgical intervention, and postpone the surgery for relatively indolent lesions.

Teaching Points

To accurately differentiate early lung cancer from COVID-19, sufficient understanding and comprehensive analysis of imaging profiles of suspected patients should be combined with clinical manifestations, epidemiological history, laboratory tests, pathogen screening, CT re-examination, and pathological analysis is recommended. A comprehensive triaging system considering tumor staging, histology, and imaging features indicating invasiveness along with SUVmax from PET-CT should be created to prioritize the more malignant, aggressively behaving tumors.

Timing and Consideration of Surgical Management for EC During the COVID-19 Pandemic

Esophageal cancer is an aggressive thoracic malignancy, and the majority of EC patients typically requires neoadjuvant therapy before surgical treatment, except in the earliest stage patients. A typical esophagectomy usually consists of two (Ivor-Lewis) or three (Mckeown) phases, both include a transthoracic phase, except transhiatal esophagectomy (THE). Transthoracic esophagectomy involves dissociation and dissection of the thoracic esophagus, mediastinal lymph node dissection, and esophageal-tubular stomach anastomosis, which facilitates the generation of aerosolized droplets and increases the risk of postoperative pulmonary complications and SARS-CoV-2 infection. Besides, esophagectomies are highly complicated and demanding procedures with a median operation time of 6 h for transthoracic esophagectomy surgeries (33), surgeons thus limited operating room capacity and medical supplies that include qualified PPE also contribute to the delay of a timely esophagectomy for patients. These factors have deeply impacted the timely scheduling of EC surgeries during the COVID-19 pandemic.

In the guidelines published by ACS for the triage of cancer surgery, immediate surgery have been recommended for patients with stage Ib or more advanced stage EC, and EC patients who have finished preoperative neoadjuvant therapy, while considering endoscopic resection (ER) as a minimally invasive treatment through natural orifice for amenable early-stage Ia/b EC patients has also been suggested (34). However, ER treatment should be decided by completely assessing the possibility of paraoesophageal lymph node metastasis, which rarely occurs in carcinoma *in situ* or early-stage EC within the lamina propria. The indication for ER is the same for early esophageal adenocarcinoma and squamous cell carcinoma patients (35).

Esophagectomy plus lymphadenectomy is recommended to be the standard treatment for resectable stage I (cT1bN0) esophageal squamous cell carcinoma (SCC) patients (35). For patients with EC in this stage, minimal evidence exists by now has investigated the influence of surgical delay on the patients' oncological outcomes, but it does suggest that prolonged waiting time before esophagectomy for over 50 days might be related to a decreased survival, thus surgical resection should not be delayed as much as possible (36). Raman (37) found that for patients with T1N0M0 esophageal AC who underwent esophagectomy without preoperative therapy, a delay of less than 50 days led to improved survival (hazard ratio [HR] = 0.991). On the other hand, time to surgery longer than 100 days was related to worse survival (HR = 1.003) and an increased positive margin rate during surgery (odds ratio [OR] = 1.01) (37). One study by Visser (38) also found that overall survival (OS) was worse with each additional week of surgical delay for patients acquiring primary surgeries, but the waiting time (<8 weeks or ≥ 8 weeks) had no statistically significant impact on disease-free survival (DFS) (HR = 1.03, p = 0.443) or OS (HR = 1.06, p = 0.108), and it did not significantly influence DFS (p = 0.884) or OS (p = 0.374) for patients treated with neoadjuvant therapy followed by surgery or primary surgery in total (38).

Apart from primary surgeries, most of the currently existing evidence has investigated the impact of time to surgery after finishing neoadjuvant therapy. The results from the studies that focus on surgery delays after neoadjuvant therapy are mixed. Ranney et al. (39) found that for patients with stages II and III esophageal AC who accepted neoadjuvant chemoradiotherapy (nCRT) and subsequent esophagectomy surgery, long-interval (the time between nCRT and surgery over 56 days) patients had a higher rate of pathologic downstaging (OR = 1.38, p = 0.04), but there was no significant difference in resection margin positivity when compared with short-interval (no more than 56 days) patients (OR = 0.91, p = 0.69). They also found worse OS in the long-interval subgroup (HR = 1.44, $p < 0.001$). Besides, there was a difference in the 30-day postoperative mortality rate but the difference was statistically insignificant (OR = 1.56, p = 0.12) (39). In addition, a meta-analysis evaluating the association between short- and long-term outcomes of EC treatment and the length of the interval between neoadjuvant chemoradiation therapy and surgery indicates that an interval longer than 7–8 weeks has improved the pathologic complete response (pCR) rate [relative risk (RR) = 1.13, p = 0.001] but decreased 2- and 5-year OS (RR = 0.94, p = 0.002; RR = 0.88, p = 0.0009, respectively) (40). A longer interval was also associated with higher 30-day surgical-related perioperative mortality (RR = 1.51, p = 0.0006) (40). Therefore, the optimal interval to surgery following neoadjuvant therapy is possibly approximately 6–8 weeks (36). The interval can be slightly prolonged according to the severity of the epidemic and medical surge capacity in different regions, but we should exert efforts to avoid surgical delay for more than 8 weeks.

Another important note to be considered for patients with EC during the COVID-19 pandemic is that a few studies have revealed a possible equivalence of definitive chemoradiotherapy (dCRT) to trimodality therapy (TMT) that includes nCRT and esophagectomy in OS of loco-regionally advanced, resectable patients with EC (41). In meta-analyses that include 26,917 resectable, curatively treated patients with EC from 33 studies, when analyzing by equal patient groups, there was no significant difference between dCRT and TMT - 3- and 5-year OS with an RR of 0.83 for 2-year OS, 0.81 for 3-year OS, and 0.63 for 5-year OS, respectively (41). In the situation of severe medical resources shortage, especially OR capacity scarcity due to the COVID-19 pandemic, the possibility of dCRT as an alternative for nCRT followed by esophagectomy should be considered.

Teaching Points

Timely scheduling of EC surgeries during COVID-19 is important for improving survival. Immediate surgery should be considered for patients with stage Ib or more advanced stage EC and EC patients who have finished preoperative neoadjuvant therapy. The optimal interval to surgery following neoadjuvant therapy is possibly approximately 6–8 weeks, which can be slightly prolonged but surgical delay for more than 8 weeks should be avoided as much as possible.

CONCLUSION

During the COVID-19 pandemic, the overall priority is patient safety and optimization of hospital systems to fight against COVID-19. Radiological evaluation of lung GGOs should receive adequate attention for suspected early-stage lung cancer patients, and surgeries for lung tumors behaving indolently, such as pure GGO tumors, can likely be postponed, while selective cases that include resection of more biologically aggressive tumors should be prioritized. As for EC treatment during the pandemic, immediate or prioritized surgery for stage Ib or greater operable EC and for patients after neoadjuvant therapy is recommended, and the delay of surgery should not exceed 8 weeks. ER can be considered for amenable early-stage Ia/b EC without risk of lymph node metastasis. dCRT might be considered as an alternative for nCRT followed by esophagectomy for resectable loco-regionally advanced patients with EC in certain circumstances. Preoperative COVID-19 screening is recommended to be routinely and repetitively performed before undergoing any thoracic surgeries. Surgeons should use proper PPE that includes N-95 respirators with eye protection during surgery or direct contact with suspected infected patients.

AUTHOR CONTRIBUTIONS

All authors listed have made a substantial, direct, and intellectual contribution to the work and approved it for publication.

REFERENCES

1. World Health Organization Coronavirus disease. COVID-19 Situation Report. (2019). Available online at: https://www.who.int/. (accessed March 1, 2022).
2. Merritt R E, Kneuertz P J. Considerations for the surgical management of early stage lung cancer during the COVID-19 pandemic. *Clin Lung Cancer.* (2021) 22:156–60. doi: 10.1016/j.cllc.2020.06.024
3. Baud D, Qi X, Nielsen-Saines K, Musso D, Pomar L, Favre G. Real estimates of mortality following COVID-19 infection. *Lancet Infect Dis.* (2020) 20:773. doi: 10.1016/S1473-3099(20)30195-X
4. Yang X, Yu Y, Xu J, Shu H, Xia J, Liu H, et al. Clinical course and outcomes of critically ill patients with SARS-CoV-2 pneumonia in Wuhan, China: a single-centered, retrospective, observational study. *Lancet Respir Med.* (2020) 8:475–81. doi: 10.1016/S2213-2600(20)30079-5
5. Jin YH, Cai L, Cheng ZS, Cheng H, Deng T, Fan Y P, et al. A rapid advice guideline for the diagnosis and treatment of 2019 novel coronavirus (2019-nCoV) infected pneumonia (standard version). *Mil Med Res.* (2020) 7:4. doi: 10.1186/s40779-020-0233-6
6. Majumder J, Minko T. Recent developments on therapeutic and diagnostic approaches for COVID-19. *AAPS J.* (2021) 23:14. doi: 10.1208/s12248-020-00532-2
7. Liu Y, Ning Z, Chen Y, Guo M, Liu Y, Gali NK, et al. Aerodynamic analysis of SARS-CoV-2 in two Wuhan hospitals. *Nature.* (2020) 582:557–60. doi: 10.1038/s41586-020-2271-3
8. Li YK, Peng S, Li LQ, Wang Q, Ping W, Zhang N, et al. Clinical and transmission characteristics of Covid-19 - a retrospective study of 25 cases from a single thoracic surgery department. *Curr Med Sci.* (2020) 40:295–300. doi: 10.1007/s11596-020-2176-2
9. United States Centers for Disease Control and Prevention Interim infection and control reccomendations for patients with suspected or confirmed coronavirus disease (COVID-19) in healthcare settings. Available online at: https://www.cdc.gov/coronavirus/2019-ncov/infection-control/control-reccomendations.html [EB/OL] (accessed March 1, 2022).
10. Qian G, Yang N, Ma A, Wang L, Li G, Chen X, et al. COVID-19 transmission within a family cluster by presymptomatic carriers in China. *Clin Infect Dis.* (2020) 71:861–2. doi: 10.1093/cid/ciaa316
11. Shi H, Han X, Jiang N, Cao Y, Alwalid O, Gu J, et al. Radiological findings from 81 patients with COVID-19 pneumonia in Wuhan, China: a descriptive study. *Lancet Infect Dis.* (2020) 20:425–34. doi: 10.1016/S1473-3099(20)30086-4
12. Ng MY, Lee E, Yang J, Yang F, Li X, Wang H, et al. Imaging profile of the COVID-19 infection: radiologic findings and literature review. *Radiol Cardiothorac Imaging.* (2020) 2:e200034. doi: 10.1148/ryct.2020200034
13. Pan Y, Guan H, Zhou S, Wang Y, Li Q, Zhu T, et al. Initial CT findings and temporal changes in patients with the novel coronavirus pneumonia (2019-nCoV): a study of 63 patients in Wuhan, China. *Eur Radiol.* (2020) 30:3306–9. doi: 10.1007/s00330-020-06731-x
14. Chung M, Bernheim A, Mei X, Zhang N, Huang M, Zeng X, et al. CT imaging features of 2019 novel coronavirus (2019-nCoV). *Radiology.* (2020) 295:202–7. doi: 10.1148/radiol.2020200230
15. Hiramatsu M, Inagaki T, Inagaki T, Matsui Y, Satoh Y, Okumura S, et al. Pulmonary ground-glass opacity (GGO) lesions-large size and a history of lung cancer are risk factors for growth. *J Thorac Oncol.* (2008) 3:1245–50. doi: 10.1097/JTO.0b013e318189f526
16. Kim HK, Choi YS, Kim J, Shim YM, Lee KS, Kim K. Management of multiple pure ground-glass opacity lesions in patients with bronchioloalveolar carcinoma. *J Thorac Oncol.* (2010) 5:206–10. doi: 10.1097/JTO.0b013e3181c422be
17. Liu M, He WX, Song N, Yang Y, Zhang P, Jiang GN. Discrepancy of epidermal growth factor receptor mutation in lung adenocarcinoma presenting as multiple ground-glass opacities. *Eur J Cardiothorac Surg.* (2016) 50:909–13. doi: 10.1093/ejcts/ezw113
18. MacMahon H, Naidich DP, Goo JM, Lee KS, Leung A, Mayo JR, et al. Guidelines for management of incidental pulmonary nodules detected on CT images: from the fleischner society 2017. *Radiology.* (2017) 284:228–43. doi: 10.1148/radiol.2017161659
19. Zhao W, Zhong Z, Xie X, Yu Q, Liu J. Relation between chest CT findings and clinical conditions of coronavirus disease (COVID-19) pneumonia: a multicenter study. *AJR Am J Roentgenol.* (2020) 214:1072–7. doi: 10.2214/AJR.20.22976
20. Cheng Z, Lu Y, Cao Q, Qin L, Pan Z, Yan F, et al. Clinical features and chest CT manifestations of coronavirus disease 2019 (COVID-19) in a single-center study in Shanghai, China. *AJR Am J Roentgenol.* (2020) 215:121–6. doi: 10.2214/AJR.20.22959
21. Yankelevitz DF, Yip R, Smith JP, Liang M, Liu Y, Xu DM, et al. CT screening for lung cancer: nonsolid nodules in baseline and annual repeat rounds. *Radiology.* (2015) 277:555–64. doi: 10.1148/radiol.2015142554
22. Henschke CI, Yip R, Smith JP, Wolf AS, Flores RM, Liang M, et al. CT screening for lung cancer: part-solid nodules in baseline and annual repeat rounds. *AJR Am J Roentgenol.* (2016) 207:1176–84. doi: 10.2214/AJR.16.16043

23. Yang W, Cao Q, Qin L, Wang X, Cheng Z, Pan A, et al. Clinical characteristics and imaging manifestations of the 2019 novel coronavirus disease (COVID-19): a multi-center study in Wenzhou city, Zhejiang, China. *J Infect.* (2020) 80:388–93. doi: 10.1016/j.jinf.2020.02.016
24. Yu H, Liu S, Zhang C, Li S, Ren J, Zhang J, et al. Computed tomography and pathology evaluation of lung ground-glass opacity. *Exp Ther Med.* (2018) 16:5305–9. doi: 10.3892/etm.2018.6886
25. Zhou Z, Guo D, Li C, Fang Z, Chen L, Yang R, et al. Coronavirus disease 2019: initial chest CT findings. *Eur Radiol.* (2020) 30:4398–406. doi: 10.1007/s00330-020-06816-7
26. Pan F, Ye T, Sun P, Gui S, Liang B, Li L, et al. Time course of lung changes at chest CT during recovery from coronavirus disease 2019 (COVID-19). *Radiology.* (2020) 295:715–21. doi: 10.1148/radiol.2020200370
27. Hasegawa M, Sone S, Takashima S, Li F, Yang ZG, Maruyama Y, et al. Growth rate of small lung cancers detected on mass CT screening. *Br J Radiol.* (2000) 73:1252–9. doi: 10.1259/bjr.73.876.11205667
28. Zhang YJ, Yang WJ, Liu D, Cao YQ, Zheng YY, Han YC, et al. COVID-19 and early-stage lung cancer both featuring ground-glass opacities: a propensity score-matched study. *Transl Lung Cancer Res.* (2020) 9:1516–27. doi: 10.21037/tlcr-20-892
29. American College of Surgeons ACS guidelines for triage and management of elective cancer surgery cases during the acute and recovery phases of coronavirus disease 2019 (COVID-19). Available online at: https://www.facs.org/media/files/covid19/acs_triage_and_management_elective_cancer_surgery_during_acute_and_recovery_phases.ashx [EB/OL] (accessed March 1, 2022).
30. Fujimoto H, Asai K, Watanabe T, Kanazawa H, Hirata K. Association of six-minute walk distance (6MWD) with resting pulmonary function in patients with chronic obstructive pulmonary disease (COPD). *Osaka City Med J.* (2011) 57:21–9.
31. National Comprehensive Cancer Network. Non-Small Cell Lung Cancer (Version 5.2021). Available online at: https://www.nccn.org/professionals/physician_gls/pdf/nscl.pdf (accessed June 15, 2021).
32. Verma S, Chan J, Chew C, Schultz C, PET-SUV. Max and upstaging of lung cancer. *Heart Lung Circ.* (2019) 28:436–42. doi: 10.1016/j.hlc.2017.12.011
33. Hulscher JB, van Sandick JW, de Boer AG, Wijnhoven BP, Tijssen JG, Fockens P, et al. Extended transthoracic resection compared with limited transhiatal resection for adenocarcinoma of the esophagus. *N Engl J Med.* (2002) 347:1662–9. doi: 10.1056/NEJMoa022343
34. Antonoff M, Backhus L, Boffa DJ, Broderick SR, Brown LM, Carrott P, et al. COVID-19 guidance for triage of operations for thoracic malignancies: a consensus statement from thoracic surgery outcomes research network. *Ann Thorac Surg.* (2020) 110:692–6. doi: 10.1016/j.athoracsur.2020.03.005
35. Fligor SC, Tsikis ST, Wang S, Ore AS, Allar BG, Whitlock AE, et al. Recent progress in multidisciplinary treatment for patients with esophageal cancer. *Surg Today.* (2020) 50:12–20. doi: 10.1007/s00595-019-01878-7
36. Raman V, Jawitz OK, Voigt SL, Yang CJ, Wang H, Harpole DH, et al. Time to surgery in thoracic cancers and prioritization during COVID-19: a systematic review. *J Thorac Dis.* (2020) 12:6640–54. doi: 10.21037/jtd-20-2400
37. Visser E, Leeftink AG, van Rossum PS, Siesling S, van Hillegersberg R, Ruurda JP. Effect of time to surgery on outcomes in stage I esophageal adenocarcinoma. *J Thorac Cardiovasc Surg.* (2020) 159:1626–35. doi: 10.1016/j.jtcvs.2019.09.123
38. Visser E, Leeftink A G, van Rossum P S, Siesling S, van Hillegersberg R, Ruurda J P. Waiting time from diagnosis to treatment has no impact on survival in patients with esophageal cancer. *Ann Surg Oncol.* (2016) 23:2679–89. doi: 10.1245/s10434-016-5191-6
39. Ranney DN, Mulvihill MS, Yerokun BA, Fitch Z, Sun Z, Yang CF, et al. Surgical resection after neoadjuvant chemoradiation for oesophageal adenocarcinoma: what is the optimal timing? *Eur J Cardiothorac Surg.* (2017) 52:543–51. doi: 10.1093/ejcts/ezx132
40. Qin Q, Xu H, Liu J, Zhang C, Xu L, Di X, et al. Does timing of esophagectomy following neoadjuvant chemoradiation affect outcomes? A meta-analysis. *Int J Surg.* (2018) 59:11–8. doi: 10.1016/j.ijsu.2018.09.013
41. Voeten DM, den Bakker CM, Heineman DJ, Ket J, Daams F, van der Peet DL. Definitive chemoradiotherapy versus trimodality therapy for resectable oesophageal carcinoma: meta-analyses and systematic review of literature. *World J Surg.* (2019) 43:1271–85. doi: 10.1007/s00268-018-04901-z

25

Homozygous Co-Deletion of Type I Interferons and *CDKN2A* Genes in Thoracic Cancers: Potential Consequences for Therapy

Marion Grard[1,2†], *Camille Chatelain*[1,2†], *Tiphaine Delaunay*[1,2], *Elvire Pons-Tostivint*[1,2,3], *Jaafar Bennouna*[1,2,3] and *Jean-François Fonteneau*[1,2*]

[1] *Université de Nantes, Inserm, CRCINA, Nantes, France,* [2] *Labex IGO, Immunology Graft Oncology, Nantes, France,* [3] *CHU de Nantes, oncologie thoracique et digestive, Université de Nantes, Nantes, France*

Correspondence:
Jean-François Fonteneau
jean-francois.fonteneau@inserm.fr

†*These authors have contributed equally to this work and share first authorship*

Homozygous deletion (HD) of the tumor suppressor gene *CDKN2A* is the most frequent genetic alteration in malignant pleural mesothelioma and is also frequent in non-small cell lung cancers. This HD is often accompanied by the HD of the type I interferons (IFN I) genes that are located closed to the *CDKN2A* gene on the p21.3 region of chromosome 9. IFN I genes encode sixteen cytokines (IFN-α, IFN-β...) that are implicated in cellular antiviral and antitumor defense and in the induction of the immune response. In this review, we discuss the potential influence of IFN I genes HD on thoracic cancers therapy and speak in favor of better taking these HD into account in patients monitoring.

Keywords: lung cancer, mesothelioma, type I interferon, CDKN2A (p16), homozygous deletion, immunotherapy, STING

FREQUENT HOMOZYGOUS CO-DELETION OF THE *CDKN2A* TUMOR SUPPRESSOR GENE AND THE IFN I GENES IN THORACIC CANCERS

Non-small cell lung cancer (NSCLC) is the most common cause of cancer death worldwide often due to long-term tobacco smoking. Malignant pleural mesothelioma (MPM) is a rare cancer that is mainly due to asbestos exposure. As other cancers, some genomic alterations are found in NSCLC and MPM tumor cells, especially in locus containing tumor suppressor genes. These alterations are in part responsible for the disease.

In MPM cells, the most frequent genomic alteration is the homologous deletion (HD) in the p21.3 region of chromosome 9 (1–6). These HDs are variable in length but they mainly overlap at the level of the cyclin-dependent kinase inhibitor 2A (*CDKN2A*) tumor suppressor gene located in this region (**Figures 1A, B**). Fluorescence *in situ* hybridization (FISH) studies reported that *CDKN2A* gene HDs are found in 60 to 80% of patients (3–6). Copy number alteration study from The Cancer Genome Atlas (TCGA) reported a lower frequency of 44% of patients with *CDKN2A* gene HD in MPM (**Figure 1B**) (7). However, TCGA study is performed on tumor biopsies that often contain non-malignant cells. These non-malignant cells may mask *CDKN2A* gene HD that are only present in tumor cells. Thus, some patients with *CDKN2A* gene HD were probably not detected in the TCGA study.

In NSCLC, *CDKN2A* gene HDs were also identified in the 1990s (8–10). They were then found more frequently in a subset of patient with intact retinoblastoma (rb) pathway (11). FISH studies on 85 and 19 NSCLC patients reported *CDKN2A* gene HD in 21 and 29% of patients respectively (12, 13), and FISH study on 31 squamous cell carcinoma (SqCC) patients reported them in 16% (14). TCGA study on 1144 NSCLC patients (660 lung adenocarcinoma and 484 lung SqCC) reported *CDKN2A* gene HD in 21% of patients (**Figure 1C**) (15).

The *CDKN2A* gene encodes several proteins, notably $p16^{INK4a}$ and $p14^{arf}$ that are implicated in the regulation of the cell cycle. $p16^{INK4a}$ binds to cyclin-dependent kinase 4 and 6 (CDK4/6) and inhibits its capacity with cyclin D1 to phosphorylate rb protein and the translocation of the transcription factor E2F from the cytoplasm to the nucleus (16). In absence of $p16^{INK4a}$, E2F translocates to the nucleus and allows the transition from G1 phase to S phase of the cell cycle. $p14^{arf}$ also acts as a tumor suppressor *via* the p53 pathway and its absence favors the entry in the cell cycle.

Close to *CDKN2A* gene, *CDKN2B* and *MTAP* are two other genes that are often co-deleted with *CDKN2A* in MPM (**Figure 1B**) and NSCLC (**Figure 1C**). *CDKN2B* encode the $p15^{Ink4b}$ protein that interacts with CDK4/6 and inhibits its activation by cyclin D and thus acts as a tumor suppressor (17). *MTAP* encodes the S-methyl-5'-thioadenosine phosphorylase (MTAP) implicated in the polyamine metabolism (18).

Further downstream from *CDKN2A* and *MTAP* in the p21.3 region of human chromosome 9, a cluster of 16 genes encodes the type I interferons (IFN I): IFN-β, IFN-ε, IFN-ω and 13 IFN-α (**Figure 1A**) (19). *IFNB1* is the furthest gene from *CDKN2A*. In the 1990s, IFN I genes HDs were identified in a fraction of NSCLC and MPM patients with *CDKN2A* gene HD (1, 2, 8, 20). We recently reported that in 78 short-term–cultured MPM cell lines, 57 (73%) and 18 (23%) cell lines harbors *CDKN2A* and *IFNBI* genes HD respectively, whereas in TCGA study performed on 82 patients, these percentage where smaller, probably due to non-malignant cells contamination (44 and 9%) (**Figure 1B**) (21). Thus, about 10 to 20% of mesothelioma patients present HD of all the IFN I genes. In NSCLC, the TCGA study on 1,144 patients reported 21 and 7% of patients with *CDKN2A* and *IFNBI* gene HDs respectively (**Figure 1C**). Interestingly, NSCLC patients with IFN I and *CDKN2A* gene

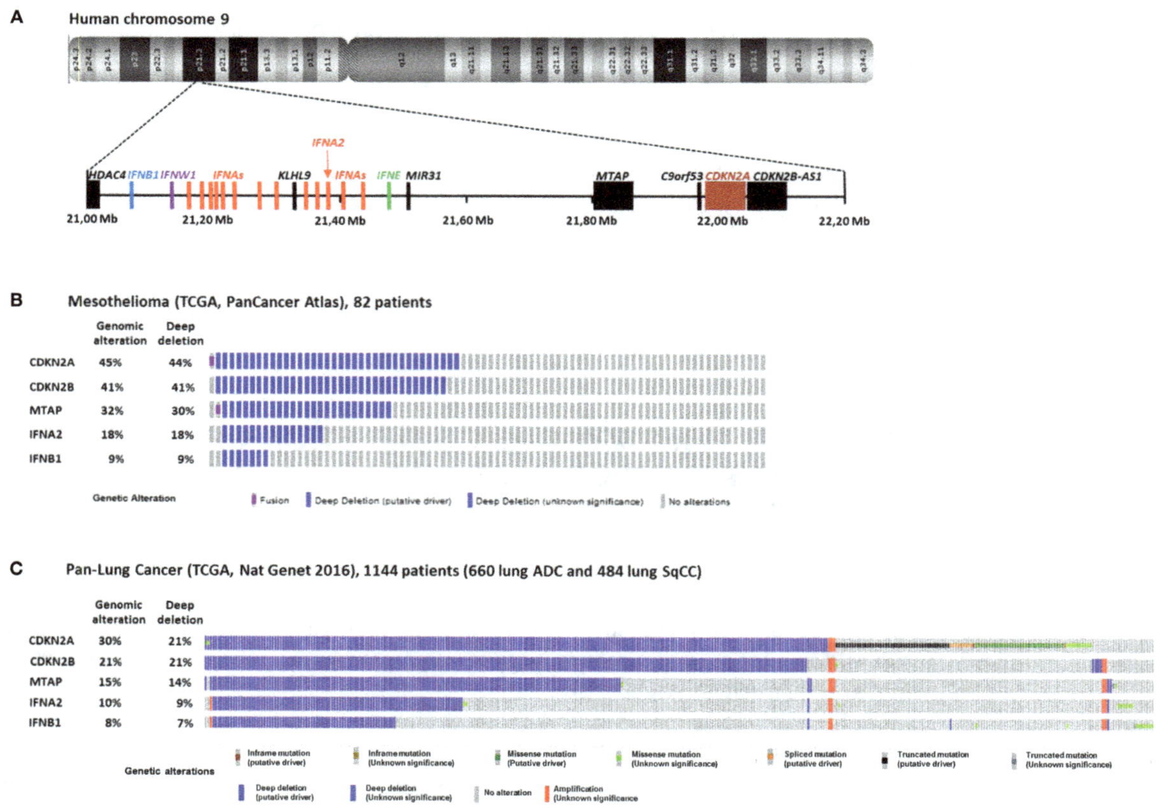

FIGURE 1 | Homozygous Deletions in the p21.3 region of chromosome 9 in MPM and NSCLC. **(A)** Schematic representation of genes present in the p21.3 region of chromosome 9 between positions 21,000,000 and 22,200,000 drawn from UCSC Genome Browser (https://genome.ucsc.edu/). **(B)** Oncoprint representation of *CDKN2A, CDKN2B, MTAP, IFNA2* and *IFNB1* genomic alterations found in tumor samples of 82 MPM patients. Oncoprint was performed with cbioportals website (http://www.cbioportal.org/) using TCGA Pancancer atlas data. **(C)** Oncoprint representation of *CDKN2A, CDKN2B, MTAP, IFNA2* and *IFNB1* genomic alterations found in tumor samples of 1144 NSCLC patients. Oncoprint was performed with cbioportals website (http://www.cbioportal.org/) using TCGA Pan lung cancer data. Only the patients with at least one genomic alteration in the five genes are shown. ADC, adenocarcinoma; SqCC, squamous cell carcinoma.

HDs have a significantly worst disease free survival than patients with only *CDKN2A* gene HD (22), suggesting a tumor suppressor role for IFN I genes in this cancer.

THE TYPE I INTERFERON RESPONSE IN THORACIC CANCERS

Type I interferon (IFN I) response is key in antiviral immune response (**Figure 2**). The IFN I response allows infected and immune cells to report *via* IFN-α and -β secretion the presence of the virus to neighboring cells and to the immune system *via* the IFN-α/-β receptor (IFNAR) which is expressed by virtually all somatic cells (23). The presence of viral genome or intermediaries of its replication is detected by cytoplasmic pattern recognition receptors (PRR) and lead to the production of IFN I *via* two main pathways: the stimulator of interferon genes protein (STING) pathway for DNA viruses and the mitochondrial antiviral-signaling protein (MAVS) pathway for RNA viruses (23, 24). IFN I are also produced by immune cells notably *via* Toll like receptor (TLR) activation, especially plasmacytoid dendritic cells (pDC) (25). IFN-β is expressed by all nucleated cells in response to infection, whereas the IFN-α are mainly produced by immune cells. Among IFN-α, IFN-α2 was the first cytokines to be approved in clinics for cancer treatment in 1986 and is the most studied (26).

Cells exposed to IFN I express hundreds of IFN-stimulated genes (ISGs). Many ISGs encode proteins that induce a state of anti-viral resistance. These antiviral proteins act by blocking the different stages of the viral cycle, from the entry of the virus, through the inhibition of its replication, to the release of its progeny by the infected cell (23, 27). The IFN I also play a crucial role in the induction and the regulation of the antiviral adaptive immune response, notably by favoring antigen cross-priming by dendritic cells (28, 29). However, during chronic infection, prolonged IFN I response can have deleterious effects by inducing immune dysfunctions (30).

IFN I response is often induced during cancer development and treatments. Several pathways are involved in this induction. Presence of mitochondrial or nuclear DNA in the cytoplasm of tumor cells can induce the secretion of IFN I *via* the STING pathway (31–39). Expression of endogenous retrovirus (ERV) under the form of dsRNA due to epigenetic deregulation in tumor cells can also trigger the expression of IFN I *via* the MAVS pathway (35, 40–44). Non-malignant cells from the tumor microenvironment, such as phagocytic cells notably dendritic cells (DC), can also produce IFN I *via* activation of the STING pathway after engulfment of dead tumor cells. This occurs due to

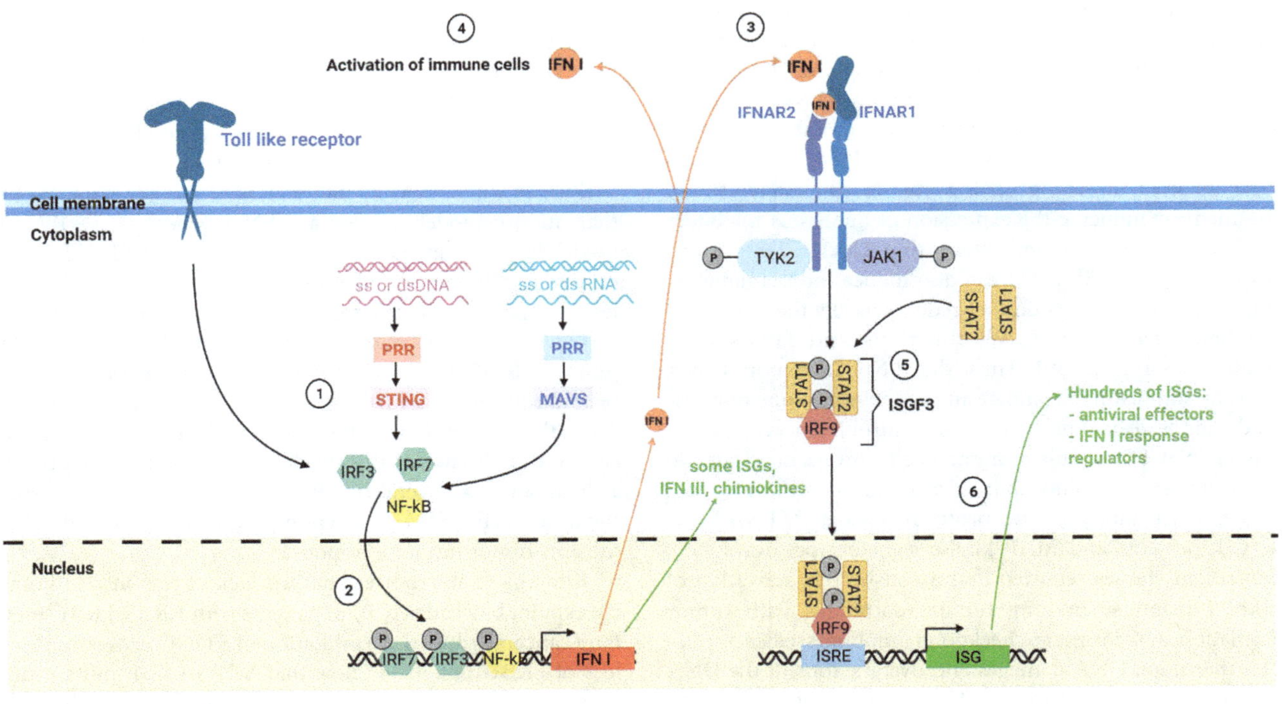

FIGURE 2 | The IFN I response. (1) The IFN I response is triggered by different stimuli such as ssDNA, dsDNA, ssRNA and dsRNA *via* the toll like receptors, the MAVS and the STING pathway. (2) Activation of these pathways induces the nuclear translocation of transcription factors such as IRF3, IRF7 and NF-kB that trigger IFN I production and expression of some interferon stimulated genes (ISGs). (3) Secreted IFN I trigger IFNAR signaling on neighboring cells, notably immune cells. (4) IFN I and other soluble factors of the IFN I response activate the immune response. (5) Activation of IFNAR signaling by IFN I leads to the formation of the interferon stimulated gene factor 3 complex. (6) This complex translocates to the nucleus and activates numerous ISGs with antiviral, immunomodulatory and regulatory functions. PRR, pattern recognition receptors.

accumulation of DNA from engulfed dead tumor cells in DC cytoplasm (39, 45–47). A recent analysis of 31 cancer types in TCGA database by Liu et al. shows that, lung adenocarcinoma, MPM and SqCC are the 3rd, 6th and 8th respectively in the intensity of an IFN I signature based on the expression of 38 ISGs (35). Globally, IFN I signature correlates with the degree of immune cells infiltration, but some tumors with an interferon signature and with no immune cells infiltration were also found.

IFN I signaling is able to modulate the expressions of hundreds of genes (27). This signaling pathway also induces expression of noncoding RNAs including long noncoding RNAs, miRNA and ERV RNA (27, 41, 48). Due to its potential toxicity and inflammatory effects, IFN I production and signaling are tightly regulated by numerous positive and negative regulators, many of which are ISGs (49). Thus, induction of IFN I response in tumors has multiple complex effects that are rather unfavorable to tumor development. The IFN I can restrict tumor growth by reducing proliferation of tumor cells, inducing their apoptosis, limiting their migratory capacity and inhibiting angiogenesis (50, 51). Furthermore, they increase antigen presentation by HLA molecules, stimulate the innate and adaptive antitumor immune response and inhibit CD4+ regulatory T cells (30, 50, 52–56). IFN I were shown to play an important role in tumor immuno-editing in mouse models of chemically-induced and transposable tumors (57). They signal tumor cells to the immune system. They are necessary for the priming of anti-tumor T cell response as the abrogation of IFN I signaling in CD8+ dendritic cells blocks their capacity to cross-present antigens in mouse (54, 55). They also participate in the activation of anti-tumor NK cell response (56). Induction of anti-tumor NK and T cell responses lead to the secretions of the type II interferon-gamma (IFN-γ) that will further shapes the immunogenicity and the immunosuppressive microenvironment of the tumor with the IFN I (58). Indeed, IFN I are also involved in setting up the immunosuppressive tumor environment by inducing the expression of numerous inhibitory molecules such as PD1 and PDL1 that block CD8+ T cell cytotoxicity (30, 50, 58). IFN I can also induce Indoleamine 2,3-dioxygenase (IDO) expression that reduces locally the amount of tryptophan needed for T cell functions and favors their differentiation in Treg (59). Thus, the IFN I in tumors play a dual role by stimulating the innate and adaptive immune response and inducing feedback mechanisms to control its magnitude.

IFN I in NSCLC modulates numerous pathways implicated in proliferation, survival and apoptosis of tumor cells including JAK/STAT, Src kinases, Vav proto-oncogene, PTEN/PI3-K/AKT, Crk proteins and MAP kinase signaling pathways (51). Several recent studies reported that a constitutive activation of the IFN I response in lung tumors correlates with tumor inflammation and immune checkpoint inhibitors efficacy (60–62). Furthermore, DNA damages and dysfunctions of the DNA damage response are inducers of the IFN I response and have been linked to immune checkpoint efficiency (37, 63). The renewed interest in IFN I response also comes from the observation that they are necessary for the radiotherapy abscopal response (64–67), and that they participate in the induction of the antitumor immune response by chemotherapy (68). This is also due to the identification of new potential immune checkpoint such as ADAR and Trex1 which are ISG that functions as negative regulators of the IFN I response by inactivating the nucleic acids that stimulate this response (35, 40, 65, 66). By blocking ADAR or Trex function, IFN I response is amplified which promotes the antitumor immune response. Thus, there is still a great interest to adapt treatments or find new therapeutic strategies to activate the IFN I response locally especially in cold tumors with no or low immune cells infiltrate.

POTENTIAL CONSEQUENCES OF IFN I GENES HD FOR THORACIC CANCERS THERAPY

Given the central role of IFN I response in tumor immune surveillance, the frequent loss of all copies of IFN I genes that accompanied *CDKN2A* gene HD in tumor cells likely plays a role in tumor immune escape. In NSCLC, like in other cancers, patients with only *CDKN2A* gene HD have a longer survival compared to patients with IFN I and *CDKN2A* genes HD (22). Thus, IFN I genes act as tumor suppressors genes in malignant cells. Beside this study of Ye et al., nothing is known on the prognostic value and immunotherapy biomarker potential of IFN I genes HD in NSCLC, MPM and other cancers. These deletions were described as early as the mid-1990s and yet they have not been well documented. It may be because they were discovered in studies focusing on the *CDKN2A* tumor suppressor gene HD. Furthermore, reports that IFN I treatment in NSCLC and MPM has limited clinical benefit at that time, may have decrease the interest of studying IFN I gene HD. Finally, most studies on the role of IFN I on antitumor immune response were performed with IFNARko mouse models that are easier to obtain than mouse models ko for all IFN I genes. These IFNARko models are instrumental to understand the role of IFN I signaling on tumor cells and the different subtypes of immune cells but are less suitable to study the source of the IFN I production.

Questions arise regarding presence of IFN I genes HD in tumor cells. There are several potential cellular sources of IFN I secretion in tumors, that are basically tumor and immune cells. Thus, the first question is the role of IFN I production by tumor cells and if absence of this production is compensated by other cellular sources. Several recent studies suggest that triggering of the tumor cells IFN I production play a role in the induction of the anti-tumor immune response.

Kitajima et al. reported that the lack of response to immune checkpoint blockade (ICB) of patients with KRAS-LKB1–mutant lung cancers is due to the inhibition of STING expression *via* the loss of LKB1 (62). They show that KRAS-LKB1–mutant tumor cells are not able to sense cytoplasmic dsDNA *via* the STING pathway, and to produce IFN I in response. In consequence, T cells infiltration and PD-L1 expression in KRAS-LKB1-mutant tumors is reduced and ICB therapy is ineffective.

Demaria's team showed that triggering of tumor cell IFN I response is necessary for induction of anti-tumor immune response by radiotherapy (64, 65). They first reported that abscopal response in mouse is abrogated when cancer cells in the irradiated tumor do not express cGAS/STING or overexpress the exonuclease Trex1 (65). Irradiation induces the presence of cytoplasmic DNA that triggers the IFN-β production *via* the STING pathway and lead to the expression of the ISG Trex1. This ISG is an exonuclease that degrades DNA in the cytoplasm and thus decreases IFN I response by tumor cells and triggering of the antitumor immune response. By inactivating Trex1 in tumor cells, the IFN I response induced by irradiation is increased, as well as the antitumor immune response. Thus, tumor cell IFN I response is essential for abscopal effect of radiation in that mouse model. Demaria's team then showed that combination of radiotherapy and anti-CTLA4 blockade in NSCLC patients that have failed anti-CTLA4 alone or in combination with chemotherapy, induced IFN-β in the blood and an antitumor T cell response in responding patients (64).

These studies highlight the important role on the antitumor immune response of triggering the IFN I response *via* the STING pathway in tumor cells. However, IFN I response in tumor cells can also be induced by the sensing of endogenous dsRNA *via* the MAVS pathway and that also plays a role in the stimulation of the antitumor immune response (35, 40–44). Best evidences come from the study of an ISG, the adenosine deaminase acting on RNA (ADAR) that acts on the MAVS pathway like Trex1 does on the STING pathway (35, 40). The ADAR protein, by converting A to I, disrupts the normal A:U pairing which destabilizes the dsRNA into ssRNA. dsRNA edited by ADAR are no longer able to trigger the IFN I response by the dsRNA cytoplasmic sensor Mda5. Thus like Trex1, ADAR inactivates the stimuli at the origin of the IFN I production by tumor cells. In a mouse model, Ishizuka et al. reported that loss of *ADAR1* in tumor cells overcomes the resistance to immune checkpoint inhibitors by increasing the IFN I response *via* the MAVS pathway and, thus, the inflammation of the tumor microenvironment (40). This results was confirmed by Liu et al., that show that both, the MAVS and the STING pathway are needed to maintain the IFN I response in tumor cells that have lost ADAR (35).

Altogether these studies on the STING and the MAVS pathway show that triggering of the IFN I response in tumor cells is central to inflame the microenvironment. However, it does not establish clearly that IFN I production by tumor cells is required. Indeed, in these studies, the MAVS or the STING pathway is inactivated. This inactivation impairs IFN I production and also the expression of lots of other genes. Indeed, when the MAVS or the STING pathway are triggered, activated transcription factors such as IRF3 and NF-kB not only induce IFN I production, but also the expression of many other genes with many being ISG (**Figure 2**). In MPM cell lines that have lost IFN I genes, exposition to attenuated measles virus still resulted in the induction of expression of a small subset of genes (21). Among these genes, some may play a role in the inflammation of the microenvironment, such as the chemokines CCL5, CXCL10 and CXCL11, or the type III interferons. Thus, triggering of the IFN I response in tumor cells that have lost IFN I genes may still conserve a certain capacity to inflame the microenvironment. By studying patients with IFN I genes HD tumors, we would better understand the IFN I contribution of tumor cells versus non-malignant cells in cancer development and therapies. We would also better define the contribution of IFN I versus other cytokines/chemokines induced by the triggering of the MAVS or the STING pathway.

IFN I genes HD may also be interesting for new cancer therapies such as antitumor virotherapy using oncolytic replicative viruses. We studied the replication and oncolytic activity of the attenuated Schwarz strain of measles virus (MV) on 22 human MPM cell lines and four types of healthy cell (fibroblasts, mesothelial, endothelial and lung epithelial cells) (69). We found that the healthy cells and seven MPM cell lines were resistant to MV replication due to a protective functional IFN I response. The 15 others MPM cell lines were permissive to MV replication and lysis due to a defective IFN I response. Among these 15 cell lines, 11 were unable to produce IFN I when exposed to MV. We showed later that eight of these 11 cell lines have lost both copies of the IFN I genes (21). The three others cells line have at least one copy of IFN I genes but are not able to produce IFN I in response to the virus suggesting another type of defects of the IFN I response in these MPM cells lines (69). These 11 MV-sensitive MPM cell lines that are unable to produce IFN I in response to MV become MV-resistant if exposed to exogenous IFN I, suggesting that IFNAR signaling is functional in these cell lines. The four other MV-sensitive MPM cell lines were able to produce IFN I in response to MV, but unable to control viral replication suggesting a defect of the IFN I response in IFNAR signaling. This defective IFNAR signaling has been previously reported in tumor cells of some patients with MPM (70). It has been associated to mark decrease of IFNAR, IRF9 and PKR expression and to tumor sensitivity to an oncolytic vesicular stomatitis virus. These studies illustrate the diversity of defects found in the IFN I response from one patients to another in MPM. Such converging selection of tumor cells with a deficient IFN I response highlights the tumor suppressive role of this response.

Other questions are still pending regarding IFN I genes HD. These HD are diverse in length (**Figure 2**). For some patients, only a part of IFN I genes are lost and *IFNB1* gene that encodes IFN-β is preserved (**Figure 1**). Consequences of these partial losses are also to define. During tumor development, do these HD appear concomitantly to *CDKN2A* HD or do they appear later conferring an additional advantage to the tumor variant that carries them? The best techniques for detecting IFN I genes HD is probably FISH assay that can be performed cost effectively on paraffin-embedded tissue and allow to identify homozygous and hemizygous deletions at the single cell level (71). It can also be performed by polymerase chain reaction-based techniques or whole exome sequencing on tumor biopsies, but large amount of non-malignant cells in the biopsy may hide the deletions.

With the success of cancer immunotherapy and recent advances in understanding the IFN I tumor suppressor role, IFN I genes HD should be studied and taken into account in the monitoring of MPM and NSCLC patients. This would likely lead to new strategies and improvements of immunotherapy.

AUTHOR CONTRIBUTIONS

Literature review: MG, CC, and JFF. All authors contributed to the article and approved the submitted version.

ACKNOWLEDGMENTS

We thank Dr. Didier Jean for his insightful discussion. **Figure 2** was created with BioRender.com.

REFERENCES

1. Cheng JQ, Jhanwar SC, Klein WM, Bell DW, Lee WC, Altomare DA, et al. p16 Alterations and Deletion Mapping of 9p21-p22 in Malignant Mesothelioma. *Cancer Res* (1994) 54(21):5547–51.
2. Xio S, Li D, Vijg J, Sugarbaker DJ, Corson JM, Fletcher JA. Codeletion of p15 and p16 in Primary Malignant Mesothelioma. *Oncogene* (1995) 11(3):511–5.
3. Cheng YY, Yuen ML, Rath EM, Johnson B, Zhuang L, Yu TK, et al. CDKN2A and MTAP Are Useful Biomarkers Detectable by Droplet Digital PCR in Malignant Pleural Mesothelioma: A Potential Alternative Method in Diagnosis Compared to Fluorescence in Situ Hybridisation. *Front Oncol* (2020) 10:579327. doi: 10.3389/fonc.2020.579327
4. Illei PB, Rusch VW, Zakowski MF, Ladanyi M. Homozygous Deletion of CDKN2A and Codeletion of the Methylthioadenosine Phosphorylase Gene in the Majority of Pleural Mesotheliomas. *Clin Cancer Res* (2003) 9(6):2108–13.
5. Hwang HC, Sheffield BS, Rodriguez S, Thompson K, Tse CH, Gown AM, et al. Utility of BAP1 Immunohistochemistry and p16 (Cdkn2a) FISH in the Diagnosis of Malignant Mesothelioma in Effusion Cytology Specimens. *Am J Surg Pathol* (2016) 40(1):120–6. doi: 10.1097/PAS.0000000000000529
6. Marshall K, Jackson S, Jones J, Holme J, Lyons J, Barrett E, et al. Homozygous Deletion of CDKN2A in Malignant Mesothelioma: Diagnostic Utility, Patient Characteristics and Survival in a UK Mesothelioma Centre. *Lung Cancer* (2020) 150:195–200. doi: 10.1016/j.lungcan.2020.10.020
7. Hmeljak J, Sanchez-Vega F, Hoadley KA, Shih J, Stewart C, Heiman D, et al. Integrative Molecular Characterization of Malignant Pleural Mesothelioma. *Cancer Discovery* (2018) 8(12):1548–65. doi: 10.1158/2159-8290.CD-18-0804
8. Dreyling MH, Bohlander SK, Adeyanju MO, Olopade OI. Detection of CDKN2 Deletions in Tumor Cell Lines and Primary Glioma by Interphase Fluorescence in Situ Hybridization. *Cancer Res* (1995) 55(5):984–8.
9. Kamb A, Gruis NA, Weaver-Feldhaus J, Liu Q, Harshman K, Tavtigian SV, et al. A Cell Cycle Regulator Potentially Involved in Genesis of Many Tumor Types. *Science* (1994) 264(5157):436–40. doi: 10.1126/science.8153634
10. Nobori T, Miura K, Wu DJ, Lois A, Takabayashi K, Carson DA. Deletions of the Cyclin-Dependent Kinase-4 Inhibitor Gene in Multiple Human Cancers. *Nature* (1994) 368(6473):753–6. doi: 10.1038/368753a0
11. Shapiro GI, Edwards CD, Kobzik L, Godleski J, Richards W, Sugarbaker DJ, et al. Reciprocal Rb Inactivation and p16INK4 Expression in Primary Lung Cancers and Cell Lines. *Cancer Res* (1995) 55(3):505–9.
12. Okami K, Cairns P, Westra WH, Linn JF, Ahrendt SA, Wu L, et al. Detailed Deletion Mapping at Chromosome 9p21 in Non-Small Cell Lung Cancer by Microsatellite Analysis and Fluorescence in Situ Hybridization. *Int J Cancer* (1997) 74(6):588–92. doi: 10.1002/(sici)1097-0215(19971219)74:6<588::aid-ijc5>3.0.co;2-q
13. Panani AD, Maliaga K, Babanaraki A, Bellenis I. Numerical Abnormalities of Chromosome 9 and p16CDKN2A Gene Deletion Detected by FISH in non-Small Cell Lung Cancer. *Anticancer Res* (2009) 29(11):4483–7.
14. Dessy E, Rossi E, Berenzi A, Tironi A, Benetti A, Grigolato P. Chromosome 9 Instability and Alterations of p16 Gene in Squamous Cell Carcinoma of the Lung and in Adjacent Normal Bronchi: FISH and Immunohistochemical Study. *Histopathology* (2008) 52(4):475–82. doi: 10.1111/j.1365-2559.2008.02969.x
15. Campbell JD, Alexandrov A, Kim J, Wala J, Berger AH, Pedamallu CS, et al. Distinct Patterns of Somatic Genome Alterations in Lung Adenocarcinomas and Squamous Cell Carcinomas. *Nat Genet* (2016) 48(6):607–16. doi: 10.1038/ng.3564
16. Burkhart DL, Sage J. Cellular Mechanisms of Tumour Suppression by the Retinoblastoma Gene. *Nat Rev Cancer* (2008) 8(9):671–82. doi: 10.1038/nrc2399
17. Kim WY, Sharpless NE. The Regulation of INK4/ARF in Cancer and Aging. *Cell* (2006) 127(2):265–75. doi: 10.1016/j.cell.2006.10.003
18. Urso L, Cavallari I, Sharova E, Ciccarese F, Pasello G, Ciminale V. Metabolic Rewiring and Redox Alterations in Malignant Pleural Mesothelioma. *Br J Cancer* (2020) 122(1):52–61. doi: 10.1038/s41416-019-0661-9
19. Diaz MO. The Human Type I Interferon Gene Cluster. *Semin Virol* (1995) 6 (3):143–9. doi: 10.1006/smvy.1995.0019
20. Mead LJ, Gillespie MT, Irving LB, Campbell LJ. Homozygous and Hemizygous Deletions of 9p Centromeric to the Interferon Genes in Lung Cancer. *Cancer Res* (1994) 54(9):2307–9.
21. Delaunay T, Achard C, Boisgerault N, Grard M, Petithomme T, Chatelain C, et al. Frequent Homozygous Deletions of Type I Interferon Genes in Pleural Mesothelioma Confer Sensitivity to Oncolytic Measles Virus. *J Thorac Oncol* (2020) 15(5):827–42. doi: 10.1016/j.jtho.2019.12.128
22. Ye Z, Dong H, Li Y, Ma T, Huang H, Leong HS, et al. Prevalent Homozygous Deletions of Type I Interferon and Defensin Genes in Human Cancers Associate With Immunotherapy Resistance. *Clin Cancer Res* (2018) 24 (14):3299–308. doi: 10.1158/1078-0432.CCR-17-3008
23. Schneider WM, Chevillotte MD, Rice CM. Interferon-Stimulated Genes: A Complex Web of Host Defenses. *Annu Rev Immunol* (2014) 32:513–45. doi: 10.1146/annurev-immunol-032713-120231
24. Iwasaki A. A Virological View of Innate Immune Recognition. *Annu Rev Microbiol* (2012) 66:177–96. doi: 10.1146/annurev-micro-092611-150203
25. Brubaker SW, Bonham KS, Zanoni I, Kagan JC. Innate Immune Pattern Recognition: A Cell Biological Perspective. *Annu Rev Immunol* (2015) 33:257–90. doi: 10.1146/annurev-immunol-032414-112240
26. Paul F, Pellegrini S, Uze G. Ifna2: The Prototypic Human Alpha Interferon. *Gene* (2015) 567(2):132–7. doi: 10.1016/j.gene.2015.04.087
27. Schoggins JW. Interferon-Stimulated Genes: What Do They All do? *Annu Rev Virol* (2019) 6(1):567–84. doi: 10.1146/annurev-virology-092818-015756
28. Crouse J, Kalinke U, Oxenius A. Regulation of Antiviral T Cell Responses by Type I Interferons. *Nat Rev Immunol* (2015) 15(4):231–42. doi: 10.1038/nri3806
29. Schiavoni G, Mattei F, Gabriele L. Type I Interferons as Stimulators of DC-Mediated Cross-Priming: Impact on Anti-Tumor Response. *Front Immunol* (2013) 4:483. doi: 10.3389/fimmu.2013.00483
30. Snell LM, McGaha TL, Brooks DG. Type I Interferon in Chronic Virus Infection and Cancer. *Trends Immunol* (2017) 38(8):542–57. doi: 10.1016/j.it.2017.05.005
31. Mackenzie KJ, Carroll P, Martin CA, Murina O, Fluteau A, Simpson DJ, et al. cGAS Surveillance of Micronuclei Links Genome Instability to Innate Immunity. *Nature* (2017) 548(7668):461–5. doi: 10.1038/nature23449
32. McArthur K, Whitehead LW, Heddleston JM, Li L, Padman BS, Oorschot V, et al. BAK/BAX Macropores Facilitate Mitochondrial Herniation and mtDNA Efflux During Apoptosis. *Science* (2018) 359(6378):eaao6047. doi: 10.1126/science.aao6047
33. Harding SM, Benci JL, Irianto J, Discher DE, Minn AJ, Greenberg RA. Mitotic Progression Following DNA Damage Enables Pattern Recognition Within Micronuclei. *Nature* (2017) 548(7668):466–70. doi: 10.1038/nature23470
34. Marcus A, Mao AJ, Lensink-Vasan M, Wang L, Vance RE, Raulet DH. Tumor-Derived Cgamp Triggers a STING-Mediated Interferon Response in Non-Tumor Cells to Activate the NK Cell Response. *Immunity* (2018) 49 (4):754–63.e4. doi: 10.1016/j.immuni.2018.09.016
35. Liu H, Golji J, Brodeur LK, Chung FS, Chen JT, deBeaumont RS, et al. Tumor-Derived IFN Triggers Chronic Pathway Agonism and Sensitivity to ADAR Loss. *Nat Med* (2019) 25(1):95–102. doi: 10.1038/s41591-018-0302-5
36. Vanpouille-Box C, Demaria S, Formenti SC, Galluzzi L. Cytosolic DNA Sensing in Organismal Tumor Control. *Cancer Cell* (2018) 34(3):361–78. doi: 10.1016/j.ccell.2018.05.013
37. Mouw KW, Goldberg MS, Konstantinopoulos PA, D'Andrea AD. Dna Damage and Repair Biomarkers of Immunotherapy Response. *Cancer Discovery* (2017) 7(7):675–93. doi: 10.1158/2159-8290.CD-17-0226
38. Yamazaki T, Kirchmair A, Sato A, Buque A, Rybstein M, Petroni G, et al. Mitochondrial DNA Drives Abscopal Responses to Radiation That Are

Inhibited by Autophagy. *Nat Immunol* (2020) 21(10):1160–71. doi: 10.1038/s41590-020-0751-0
39. Ahn J, Xia T, Konno H, Konno K, Ruiz P, Barber GN. Inflammation-Driven Carcinogenesis is Mediated Through STING. *Nat Commun* (2014) 5:5166. doi: 10.1038/ncomms6166
40. Ishizuka JJ, Manguso RT, Cheruiyot CK, Bi K, Panda A, Iracheta-Vellve A, et al. Loss of ADAR1 in Tumours Overcomes Resistance to Immune Checkpoint Blockade. *Nature* (2019) 565(7737):43–8. doi: 10.1038/s41586-018-0768-9
41. Canadas I, Thummalapalli R, Kim JW, Kitajima S, Jenkins RW, Christensen CL, et al. Tumor Innate Immunity Primed by Specific Interferon-Stimulated Endogenous Retroviruses. *Nat Med* (2018) 24(8):1143–50. doi: 10.1038/s41591-018-0116-5
42. Panda A, de Cubas AA, Stein M, Riedlinger G, Kra J, Mayer T, et al. Endogenous Retrovirus Expression is Associated With Response to Immune Checkpoint Blockade in Clear Cell Renal Cell Carcinoma. *JCI Insight* (2020) 5 (11):e137569. doi: 10.1172/jci.insight.121522
43. Roulois D, Loo Yau H, Singhania R, Wang Y, Danesh A, Shen SY, et al. Dna-Demethylating Agents Target Colorectal Cancer Cells by Inducing Viral Mimicry by Endogenous Transcripts. *Cell* (2015) 162(5):961–73. doi: 10.1016/j.cell.2015.07.056
44. Sun S, Frontini F, Qi W, Hariharan A, Ronner M, Wipplinger M, et al. Endogenous Retrovirus Expression Activates Type-I Interferon Signaling in an Experimental Mouse Model of Mesothelioma Development. *Cancer Lett* (2021) 507:26–38. doi: 10.1016/j.canlet.2021.03.004
45. Woo SR, Fuertes MB, Corrales L, Spranger S, Furdyna MJ, Leung MY, et al. STING-Dependent Cytosolic DNA Sensing Mediates Innate Immune Recognition of Immunogenic Tumors. *Immunity* (2014) 41(5):830–42. doi: 10.1016/j.immuni.2014.10.017
46. Barber GN. STING: Infection, Inflammation and Cancer. *Nat Rev Immunol* (2015) 15(12):760–70. doi: 10.1038/nri3921
47. Xu MM, Pu Y, Han D, Shi Y, Cao X, Liang H, et al. Dendritic Cells But Not Macrophages Sense Tumor Mitochondrial DNA for Cross-priming Through Signal Regulatory Protein Alpha Signaling. *Immunity* (2017) 47(2):363–73.e5. doi: 10.1016/j.immuni.2017.07.016
48. Suarez B, Prats-Mari L, Unfried JP, Fortes P. LncRNAs in the Type I Interferon Antiviral Response. *Int J Mol Sci* (2020) 21(17):6447. doi: 10.3390/ijms21176447
49. Arimoto KI, Miyauchi S, Stoner SA, Fan JB, Zhang DE. Negative Regulation of Type I IFN Signaling. *J Leukoc Biol* (2018) 103:1099–116. doi: 10.1002/JLB.2MIR0817-342R
50. Zhou L, Zhang Y, Wang Y, Zhang M, Sun W, Dai T, et al. A Dual Role of Type I Interferons in Antitumor Immunity. *Adv Biosyst* (2020) 4(11):e1900237. doi: 10.1002/adbi.201900237
51. Galani V, Kastamoulas M, Varouktsi A, Lampri E, Mitselou A, Arvanitis DL. Ifns-Signaling Effects on Lung Cancer: An Up-to-Date Pathways-Specific Review. *Clin Exp Med* (2017) 17(3):281–9. doi: 10.1007/s10238-016-0432-3
52. Zitvogel L, Galluzzi L, Kepp O, Smyth MJ, Kroemer G. Type I Interferons in Anticancer Immunity. *Nat Rev Immunol* (2015) 15(7):405–14. doi: 10.1038/nri3845
53. Vidal P. Interferon Alpha in Cancer Immunoediting: From Elimination to Escape. *Scand J Immunol* (2020) 91(5):e12863. doi: 10.1111/sji.12863
54. Diamond MS, Kinder M, Matsushita H, Mashayekhi M, Dunn GP, Archambault JM, et al. Type I Interferon is Selectively Required by Dendritic Cells for Immune Rejection of Tumors. *J Exp Med* (2011) 208 (10):1989–2003. doi: 10.1084/jem.20101158
55. Fuertes MB, Kacha AK, Kline J, Woo SR, Kranz DM, Murphy KM, et al. Host Type I IFN Signals are Required for Antitumor CD8+ T Cell Responses Through CD8{alpha}+ Dendritic Cells. *J Exp Med* (2011) 208(10):2005–16. doi: 10.1084/jem.20101159
56. Swann JB, Hayakawa Y, Zerafa N, Sheehan KC, Scott B, Schreiber RD, et al. Type I IFN Contributes to NK Cell Homeostasis, Activation, and Antitumor Function. *J Immunol* (2007) 178(12):7540–9. doi: 10.4049/jimmunol.178.12.7540
57. Dunn GP, Bruce AT, Sheehan KC, Shankaran V, Uppaluri R, Bui JD, et al. A Critical Function for Type I Interferons in Cancer Immunoediting. *Nat Immunol* (2005) 6(7):722–9. doi: 10.1038/ni1213
58. Benci JL, Xu B, Qiu Y, Wu TJ, Dada H, Twyman-Saint Victor C, et al. Tumor Interferon Signaling Regulates a Multigenic Resistance Program to Immune Checkpoint Blockade. *Cell* (2016) 167(6):1540–54.e12. doi: 10.1016/j.cell.2016.11.022
59. Lemos H, Mohamed E, Huang L, Ou R, Pacholczyk G, Arbab AS, et al. Sting Promotes the Growth of Tumors Characterized by Low Antigenicity Via IDO Activation. *Cancer Res* (2016) 76(8):2076–81. doi: 10.1158/0008-5472.CAN-15-1456
60. Della Corte CM, Sen T, Gay CM, Ramkumar K, Diao L, Cardnell RJ, et al. Sting Pathway Expression Identifies Nsclc With an Immune-Responsive Phenotype. *J Thorac Oncol* (2020) 15(5):777–91. doi: 10.1016/j.jtho.2020.01.009
61. Thompson JC, Hwang WT, Davis C, Deshpande C, Jeffries S, Rajpurohit Y, et al. Gene Signatures of Tumor Inflammation and Epithelial-to-Mesenchymal Transition (EMT) Predict Responses to Immune Checkpoint Blockade in Lung Cancer With High Accuracy. *Lung Cancer* (2020) 139:1–8. doi: 10.1016/j.lungcan.2019.10.012
62. Kitajima S, Ivanova E, Guo S, Yoshida R, Campisi M, Sundararaman SK, et al. Suppression of STING Associated With LKB1 Loss in KRAS-Driven Lung Cancer. *Cancer Discovery* (2019) 9(1):34–45. doi: 10.1158/2159-8290.CD-18-0689
63. Ricciuti B, Recondo G, Spurr LF, Li YY, Lamberti G, Venkatraman D, et al. Impact of DNA Damage Response and Repair (Ddr) Gene Mutations on Efficacy of PD-(L)1 Immune Checkpoint Inhibition in Non-Small Cell Lung Cancer. *Clin Cancer Res* (2020) 26(15):4135–42. doi: 10.1158/1078-0432.CCR-19-3529
64. Formenti SC, Rudqvist NP, Golden E, Cooper B, Wennerberg E, Lhuillier C, et al. Radiotherapy Induces Responses of Lung Cancer to CTLA-4 Blockade. *Nat Med* (2018) 24(12):1845–51. doi: 10.1038/s41591-018-0232-2
65. Vanpouille-Box C, Alard A, Aryankalayil MJ, Sarfraz Y, Diamond JM, Schneider RJ, et al. DNA Exonuclease Trex1 Regulates Radiotherapy-Induced Tumour Immunogenicity. *Nat Commun* (2017) 8:15618. doi: 10.1038/ncomms15618
66. Diamond JM, Vanpouille-Box C, Spada S, Rudqvist NP, Chapman JR, Ueberheide BM, et al. Exosomes Shuttle Trex1-Sensitive IFN-Stimulatory dsDNA From Irradiated Cancer Cells to Dcs. *Cancer Immunol Res* (2018) 6 (8):910–20. doi: 10.1158/2326-6066.CIR-17-0581
67. Skoulidis F, Goldberg ME, Greenawalt DM, Hellmann MD, Awad MM, Gainor JF, et al. Stk11/Lkb1 Mutations and PD-1 Inhibitor Resistance in KRAS-Mutant Lung Adenocarcinoma. *Cancer Discov* (2018) 8(7):822–35. doi: 10.1158/2159-8290.CD-18-0099
68. Yum S, Li M, Chen ZJ. Old Dogs, New Trick: Classic Cancer Therapies Activate Cgas. *Cell Res* (2020) 30(8):639–48. doi: 10.1038/s41422-020-0346-1
69. Achard C, Boisgerault N, Delaunay T, Roulois D, Nedellec S, Royer PJ, et al. Sensitivity of Pleural Mesothelioma to Oncolytic Measles Virus Depends on Defects of the Type I Interferon Response. *Oncotarget* (2015) 6(42):44892–904. doi: 10.18632/oncotarget.6285
70. Saloura V, Wang LC, Fridlender ZG, Sun J, Cheng G, Kapoor V, et al. Evaluation of an Attenuated Vesicular Stomatitis Virus Vector Expressing Interferon-Beta for Use in Malignant Pleural Mesothelioma: Heterogeneity in Interferon Responsiveness Defines Potential Efficacy. *Hum Gene Ther* (2010) 21(1):51–64. doi: 10.1089/hum.2009.088
71. Husain AN, Colby TV, Ordonez NG, Allen TC, Attanoos RL, Beasley MB, et al. Guidelines for Pathologic Diagnosis of Malignant Mesothelioma 2017 Update of the Consensus Statement From the International Mesothelioma Interest Group. *Arch Pathol Lab Med* (2018) 142(1):89–108. doi: 10.5858/arpa.2017-0124-RA

26

How to Better Understand the Influence of Host Genetics on Developing an Effective Immune Response to Thoracic Cancers

*Kiarash Behrouzfar[1,2], Kimberley Burton[1,2], Steve E. Mutsaers[2,3], Grant Morahan[4], Richard A. Lake[1] and Scott A. Fisher[1,2]**

[1] National Centre for Asbestos Related Diseases (NCARD), University of Western Australia, Nedlands, WA, Australia, [2] School of Biomedical Sciences, University of Western Australia, Nedlands, WA, Australia, [3] Institute for Respiratory Health, University of Western Australia, Nedlands, WA, Australia, [4] Centre for Diabetes Research, Harry Perkins Institute of Medical Research, Nedlands, WA, Australia

***Correspondence:**
Scott A. Fisher
scott.fisher@uwa.edu.au

Thoracic cancers pose a significant global health burden. Immune checkpoint blockade therapies have improved treatment outcomes, but durable responses remain limited. Understanding how the host immune system interacts with a developing tumor is essential for the rational development of improved treatments for thoracic malignancies. Recent technical advances have improved our understanding of the mutational burden of cancer cells and changes in cancer-specific gene expression, providing a detailed understanding of the complex biology underpinning tumor-host interactions. While there has been much focus on the genetic alterations associated with cancer cells and how they may impact treatment outcomes, how host genetics affects cancer development is also critical and will greatly determine treatment response. Genome-wide association studies (GWAS) have identified genetic variants associated with cancer predisposition. This approach has successfully identified host genetic risk factors associated with common thoracic cancers like lung cancer, but is less effective for rare cancers like malignant mesothelioma. To assess how host genetics impacts rare thoracic cancers, we used the Collaborative Cross (CC); a powerful murine genetic resource designed to maximize genetic diversity and rapidly identify genes associated with any biological trait. We are using the CC in conjunction with our asbestos-induced MexTAg mouse model, to identify host genes associated with mesothelioma development. Once genes that moderate tumor development and progression are known, human homologues can be identified and human datasets interrogated to validate their association with disease outcome. Furthermore, our CC–MexTAg animal model enables in-depth study of the tumor microenvironment, allowing the correlation of immune cell infiltration and gene expression signatures with disease development. This strategy provides a detailed picture of the underlying biological pathways associated with mesothelioma susceptibility and progression; knowledge that is crucial for the rational development of new diagnostic and therapeutic strategies. Here we discuss the influence of host genetics on developing an effective immune response to thoracic cancers. We highlight current knowledge gaps, and with a focus on mesothelioma, describe the development and application of the CC-MexTAg to overcome limitations and illustrate how the knowledge gained from this unique study will inform the rational design of future treatments of mesothelioma.

Keywords: thoracic malignancies, tumor immune microenvironment, mesothelioma, Collaborative Cross, MexTAg, host genetics

INTRODUCTION

Thoracic cancers including lung cancer (LC), malignant mesothelioma and thymic epithelial tumors (TETs) are among the most lethal cancers (1). In addition to conventional treatment options for thoracic cancers such as surgery, chemotherapy and radiotherapy, immune based treatments including immune checkpoint therapies, have improved treatment outcome for some patients (2, 3).

Cancer immunotherapy aims to restore or enhance the host's immune system to recognize and eliminate cancer cells (4). Although immunotherapies have improved treatment outcomes for some thoracic cancers, success is often limited to a subset of patients, while prognosis for the majority of patients remains dismal (5). This dichotomy in response, highlights the need to better understand interactions between thoracic cancer cells and the host immune system that underpin an effective response to cancer immunotherapy.

Advances in high-throughput sequencing technologies and associated computational analysis pipelines allow us to investigate the interplay between tumor cells and the immune microenvironment (6, 7). These technologies enable us to broaden our knowledge of the immunobiology of tumor-host interactions by identifying immune-related genetic alterations associated with cancer development (6, 7). While genetic alterations associated with immune response in thoracic cancers have been exploited to improve treatment outcome (8, 9), the development of strong, durable responses occurs in a limited subset of patients (10); further highlighting the importance of understanding the role of host genetics, in addition to tumor genetics, in thoracic cancer development, for predicting response to immunotherapies (9, 11–13).

In this review, we discuss how host genetics affects the development of an effective immune response to thoracic cancers. We highlight knowledge gaps in our current understanding and acknowledge the limitations related to identifying host genetic factors associated with thoracic cancer susceptibility and development of effective anti-tumor immunity. Finally, we propose our unique murine model; the MexTAg Collaborative Cross (CC–MexTAg), as a strategy to overcome current limitations of conventional genetic studies in mesothelioma, to improve our knowledge about the impact of host genetics on initiating immune responses and the developing tumor microenvironment.

HOST GENETIC FACTORS AND THORACIC CANCER SUSCEPTIBILITY

To date, many rare, high penetrance genetic variants such as *BRCA1, BRCA2, TP53, APC, and PTEN* have been associated with a genetic predisposition to cancer (14–16). However, these genetic alterations only account for a small proportion of heritable cancer genetic risk variants (14, 15). In fact, the combination of genetic variation in common low penetrance alleles and rare moderate-risk alleles has been recognized as the major genetic contributors to heritable cancer genetic predisposition (17–19).

Common low-penetrance genetic variants, including single-nucleotide polymorphisms (SNPs), have been identified by GWAS (20). These genetic studies determine the frequency of SNPs in patients compared to healthy individuals (20). More than 450 genetic variants associated with increased cancer risk for breast, prostate, colorectal and lung cancer have been identified; supporting the polygenic pattern of susceptibility in these cancers (18).

Lung Cancer

Lung cancer is the most prevalent thoracic cancer, and chromosomal positions 15q25, 5p15.33 and 6p21 have been identified as susceptibility loci (21, 22). However, whether 15q25 is truly an independent susceptibility locus for lung cancer remains contentious, as genetic variants of nicotinic acetylcholine receptor (CHRNA) genes, which have been strongly associated with nicotine dependence and smoking behavior (23–26), are also present at this loci. Furthermore, genetic variants in 15q25 are mainly frequent in European populations and not Asian populations (23). Other independent susceptibility loci, 6p21 and 5p15, show significant levels of genetic polymorphisms associated with lung cancer risk in Asian populations, including Japanese and Korean. However, there are different risk variants within 6p21 locus observed between Asian and European populations (27).

A large meta-analysis of GWAS on Chinese and European populations identified 19 susceptibility loci significantly associated with non-small cell lung cancer (NSCLC) risk (28). Using identified genetic factors, this study proposed the polygenic risk score (PRS) strategy as an effective risk indicator of lung cancer, independent from age and smoking pack-year (28). However, the utility of the PRS strategy may be limited, as it was only used to predict lung cancer risk among the Chinese population, not in other cohorts comprised of different ethnicity and effect size for genetic variants (28). Furthermore, most genetic variants were only associated with a small improvement in the prediction of lung cancer risk, and were not any greater than major risk factors such as smoking and age (29–31).

Malignant Mesothelioma

Malignant mesothelioma is a relatively rare thoracic cancer, inextricably linked to asbestos exposure. The relatively low number of samples available for study means that conventional genetic studies are often underpowered (1). Consequently, despite using separate and well-characterized cohorts of control and mesothelioma patients, numerous GWAS studies have failed to identify common genetic risk factors that can be considered broadly associated with mesothelioma (32–34).

Germline mutations in *BAP1* and some DNA repair genes have been considered as predisposing genetic factors associated with mesothelioma development (34–36). However, these genetic risk factors are not specific for mesothelioma alone and can predispose people to other cancers such as uveal melanoma (37).

Thymic Epithelial Tumors

Thymic epithelial tumors (TETs) are rare thoracic cancers arising from epithelial cells of the thymus, and can be categorized as either thymomas or thymic carcinomas (38). Our current knowledge of the etiology and genomic alterations of TETs remains limited, and like mesothelioma, the small number of patients available for study often restricts the power of conventional genetic analyses (39, 40). Although we could not find any published GWAS associated with any form of TETs, Wang et. al., identified mutated *TP53* as the most frequent genetic alteration in TET patients (40). The authors used comparative sequence analysis to show a higher mutation incidence in epigenetic regulatory genes in thymic carcinoma compared to thymoma patients (40). Additionally, a study by Cortes-Ledesma et. al., demonstrated a strong causal relationship between the loss of the highly-specialized DNA repair enzyme tyrosyl-DNA phosphodiesterase 2 (*TDP2*) and increased thymic-derived cancer predisposition in ataxia telangiectasia affected individuals (41).

THE IMPORTANCE OF HOST GENETICS IN CANCER SUSCEPTIBILITY: SHAPING OF THE TUMOR IMMUNE MICROENVIRONMENT

The tumor microenvironment (TME) consists of a variety of immune cells, endothelial cells, fibroblasts and associated tissue cells, and develops in part from the dynamic interactions between the developing tumor and the surrounding host tissue (42). One way to describe how host-tumor interactions play a significant role in shaping the tumor microenvironment, is through the impact on 'field effect' around the tumor (43). In the context of cancer development, the term 'field effect' refers to pre-neoplastic cellular and molecular changes that arise as a consequence of long-term exposure to environmental carcinogens in morphologically healthy tissues, promoting a 'field of susceptibility' to neoplasia initiation and progression (44). For instance, the presence of a high burden and pervasive positive selection of somatic driver mutations has been identified in normal human skin (45). In a cohort of patients undergoing blepharoplasty, positively selected 'driver' mutations were found in 18–32% of normal skin cells taken from 234 biopsies of sun-exposed eyelid epidermis. These data suggest that the frequency of driver mutations in physiologically normal skin cells is surprisingly high, with multiple driver mutations in cancer associated genes found in many 'normal' cells that had not yet acquired malignant potential. These findings raise the question as to what combination of intrinsic (additional mutations) or extrinsic (host genetics/anti-tumor immunity) changes are required for cellular transformation to proceed?

In addition to driver mutations, epigenetic alterations including DNA methylation and histone modifications can play a role in establishing a field effect contributing to cancer development (46, 47). A number of studies have indicated the influence of an epigenetic field effect around the tumor by identifying aberrant DNA methylation profiles in both tumor and normal adjacent tissues (48–52).

THE EFFECT OF KNOWN HOST GENETIC FACTORS ON TUMOR IMMUNE MICROENVIRONMENT OF THORACIC CANCERS

The influence of host genetics on the development of thoracic cancers remains poorly understood. Shen et. al., performed enrichment analysis of GWAS data to identify shared genomic regions and pathways between host genetic variants and somatic mutations in lung cancer (53). They identified an association between the SNP rs36600 at 22q12.2 and somatic mutations within *ARID1A* (53), a member of the SWI/SNF chromatin remodeling complexes associated with many cancers (54). Mutations in *ARID1A* and *ARID1B* are also associated with improved response to NSCLC patients receiving immune checkpoint blockade (ICB) therapy (55). Elevation of the tumor mutational burden, enhanced antigen presentation and cellular immunity, and increased PD-L1 expression, are all correlated with the presence of ARID1A and ARID1B mutations; suggesting that mutated ARID1A and ARID1B could serve as novel biomarkers to predict sensitivity and prognosis to ICB in advanced NSCLC patients (55). Additionally, rare missense variants in genes encoding SWI/SNF chromatin remodeling components and genes encoding the histone methyl transferases, *SETD2* and *SETDB1*, were identified in a cohort of Japanese mesothelioma patients (56).

Furthermore, *TRB*:rs1964986 and *IDO1*:rs10108662 have been identified as the two most significant SNPs associated with the risk of disease recurrence and death respectively in early stage lung cancer (57). When assessing the functionality of T cells between low and high-risk groups relative to healthy controls (57), high-risk subjects exhibited lower cytotoxicity and reduced granulation of T cells, as demonstrated by increased expression of T cell inhibitory checkpoint gene Indoleamine 2, 3-dioxygenase (*IDO1*) and decreased expression of the T cell cytotoxicity genes *IL2*, Perforin 1 (*PRF*) and Granzyme B (*GZMB*). These data support the hypothesis that mutations of host immune genes affect the TME and thus, prognosis of NSCLC *via* suppression of T cell antitumor immunity (57).

Additionally, epigenetic alterations of tissues derived from NSCLC patients revealed the upregulation of *CTLA4*, *PDCD1 via* hypomethylation in tumors *versus* non-tumor tissues (58). Effects of epigenetic alterations in shaping immune tumor microenvironment was also demonstrated by strong correlation between site-specific DNA methylation of CpG markers of cancers and transcription of genes associated with immune infiltration (59).

In contrast to NSCLC, there are limited published studies that investigate the role of host genetic factors in shaping the tumor immune microenvironment of mesothelioma and TETs. Costa et. al., identified lower expression of miR-320 in mesothelioma tumors compared to normal tissues by performing differential miRNA expression analysis on 14 formalin-fixed paraffin-embedded tumors and six normal controls (60). They also identified an association between p53-induced expression of miR-320, miR-200a and miR-34a with reduced expression of *PD-L1* in mesothelioma cell lines (60). These data indicate defective p53-induced miRNA response as a possible contributor to immune evasion in mesothelioma by increasing tumor *PD-L1* expression (60). Reduced expression of major histocompatibility complex (*MHC*) and autoimmune regulator (*AIRE*) genes has been associated with defective T cell maturation in thymoma patients (61, 62) and as such, the reduced expression of *MHC* and *AIRE* were proposed as genetic alterations explaining the association between thymomas and autoimmune disorders (61).

More recently, a number of studies have significantly advanced our understanding of the molecular biology of mesothelioma (63–67). Through the application of next generation sequencing technologies and innovative bioinformatic analyses, these studies have demonstrated the complex heterogeneity within and between tumors; expanding the classic epithelioid, biphasic and sarcomatoid paradigm to at least 4 distinct molecular subtypes, with a molecular gradient along the epithelial-to mesenchymal transition spectrum separating the two extreme epithelioid-like and mesenchymal-like groups (63, 65–67). Additionally, the NSG approach has further advanced our knowledge of the key mutational events associated with mesothelioma, linking a number of unique cancer signaling pathways with mesothelioma (64, 65). However, despite these advances, our understanding of how host genetics impacts mesothelioma onset remains underdeveloped.

In summary, studies investigating the role of immune related genetic factors in NSCLC have identified suggestive genetic variants capable of shaping the tumor immune microenvironment and affecting cellular immunity. However, there are a limited number of studies identifying immune related genetic factors in mesothelioma and TETs, highlighting the dearth in our knowledge of, and ability to identify how host genetic factors shape the immune tumor microenvironment of rare thoracic cancers.

OVERCOMING LIMITATIONS FOR IDENTIFYING HOST GENETIC FACTORS ASSOCIATED WITH THORACIC CANCERS

GWAS have been used to identify susceptibility loci in common cancers such as breast, prostate, colorectal and lung cancer (22, 68), but they have been less effective for rare cancers including mesothelioma (32). In fact, the suitability of GWAS for rare cancers is often restricted by the relatively small number of patients available for studies; thus any identified genetic variants are often limited to the study cohort and not likely to have a significant influence on disease outcome (32, 34, 68–71). Furthermore, the absence of standardized protocols for collecting environmental exposure data in addition to the lack of accurate, consistent and defined phenotypic data to match with genomic information, are additional potential limitations for human genetic studies of thoracic cancers (72–74).

To overcome these limitations, mouse models that can faithfully mimic human cancer development, in a well-controlled and modulated environment are needed for identifying translatable host genetic variants (75). Moreover, such mouse models need to be sufficiently genetically diverse to maximize the chance of genetic polymorphisms associated with cancer development. The ideal mouse model would enable rapid identification of genes associated with cancer homologous to human genetic studies (7).

ADVANCEMENTS IN RECOMBINANT INBRED MOUSE MODELS FOR HOST GENETIC STUDIES OF THORACIC CANCERS

Recombinant inbred (RI) mice are generated by breeding two or more different mouse strains to genetic stability (76). Historically, RI mice have been used to identify genomic regions, referred to as quantitative trait loci (QTLs), that are associated with particular disease phenotypes (77). The main advantage to using RI mouse strains compared to classical simple (F2) cross breeding is their improved reproducibility due to the ability to test a phenotype in any number of individuals with the same defined genetic constitution (77). The use of RI mice allows unknown genes to be integrated into the known genetic map by comparing the inheritance pattern of an unknown gene or trait in a panel of RI strains with that of known markers. Therefore, these models have been widely used as a robust and rapid method of gene mapping of polygenic traits and diseases (77).

USE OF CLASSICAL AND TRADITIONAL RECOMBINANT INBRED MOUSE MODELS

Classical mouse genetic studies identified *Kras2* as a major lung cancer susceptibility locus using the F2 progeny of A/J (susceptible) and C3H/He (resistant) mouse strains in a urethane-induced lung cancer model (78). Similarly, experiments involving the progeny of BALB/c and SWR/J mouse strains identified *Par2* and *Par4* as modifier loci that specifically affected tumor initiation, progression and lung tumor multiplicity (79). Additional, whole-genome linkage disequilibrium analysis on 25 inbred mouse strains identified 63 markers including *Kras* and *Pas1* loci, supporting the association of *Kras* loci with lung cancer susceptibility (80). Traditionally, bi-parental RI mouse strains were used for identifying susceptibility loci of diseases with polygenic pattern of inheritance (78, 81, 82). However, the usefulness of traditional bi-parental RI mouse strains in genetic studies is limited by the inherent low genetic diversity associated with using only two parental genomes, which have large 'identical by descent' (IBD) regions in which both parental strains have the same alleles (83). Such IBD regions are 'blind spots', having little or no variation, thus limiting the potential for gene mapping (84).

THE COLLABORATIVE CROSS (CC)

The Collaborative cross (CC) is a powerful mouse genetic resource, comprising hundreds of independent RI mouse strains developed from eight founder strains selected to maximize genetic diversity (84–86). The CC harnesses 90% of the common allelic diversity of the entire mouse species (84) and has enhanced mapping ability due to the much greater degree of polymorphisms derived from the eight diverse founder strains, rather than the two somewhat similar strains used in conventional RI mapping, as well as the greater number of strains available. Conventional mapping of simple Mendelian traits requires approximately 100 backcrossed mice to obtain 1 cM (approximately 2 megabase pairs; Mbp) resolution. The same resolution can be obtained by testing ~26 BXD RI strains. In contrast, with as few as 70 CC strains, mapping resolution can be less than 40 thousand bp, i.e. approximately to the single gene level (85) and even achieve down-to-the-base resolution (87). Thus, the CC allows mapping of loci with unprecedented accuracy. The CC has been successfully used to study diseases with polygenic inheritance such as melanoma, prostate cancer, diabetes and osteoporosis (86, 88–91). It is also powerful in allowing development of novel disease models (92).

The application of the CC to understanding cancer has been best studied for melanoma and skin cancer. A series of investigations made several important discoveries, such as that every stage of melanoma progression was subject to control by genetic variation (88); that UV–induced and spontaneous cancers were mediated by different genetic mechanisms (93) the specific mutation causing nevus development was identified (94); and the molecular mechanism for giant congenital nevi was defined (95).

USING GENETICALLY ENGINEERED MOUSE MODELS FOR STUDYING THE IMPACT OF HOST GENETICS ON THORACIC CANCER DEVELOPMENT

Numerous genetically engineered mice models have been developed for modelling and studying genetic heterogeneity of human malignancies (96). Recent technical advances in the manipulation and sequencing of mouse genomes has promoted the use of mouse models as an experimentally tractable system for testing hypotheses generated from human genetic studies (96). Such engineered models have also allowed the identification of novel candidate mechanisms linking the impact of host genetics and cancer development (96, 97). As the development and use of genetically engineered mouse models is time-consuming and expensive, the generation of models with high tumor penetrance and short cancer latency are often favored, as they are more viable in terms of research time and cost (75, 98).

Kras2^{LA2} and *Trp53*$^{\mathrm{LSL\text{-}R172H/þ}}$ mice are the most common used models in host genetic studies of lung cancer (96, 99, 100). However, mice with mutations in *Kras2* and *Trp53* are highly predisposed to other cancers (101, 102) and cancer development can be triggered by spontaneous oncogene recombination events; thus these models are not necessarily lung cancer specific and therefore some mechanisms of carcinogenesis may not accurately recapitulate human disease (99, 100).

There are many excellent mouse models for mesothelioma research that mimic the genetic defects found in human disease. Knockout (KO) mouse models with heterozygous mutations in *Bap1*, *CDKN2A*, neurofibromin 2 (*Nf2*), or *p53* have been used to study the effect of genetic alterations on asbestos-induced mesothelioma susceptibility (103–112). These studies demonstrate significantly higher incidence of mesothelioma in the presence, or absence of asbestos in mice with *Bap*$^{(+/-)}$ and *Nf2*$^{(+/-)}$ mutations compared to wild-type (wt) mice (103–112). However, all animal models have their limitations. While some conditional KO models demonstrate increased mesothelioma incidence, they also have moderate to high levels of unrelated (non-mesothelioma) cancers; presumable a consequence of off-target deletion of key tumor suppressor genes (105, 108, 110). However, recently published CRE-mediated conditional KO models only develop disease in CRE-expressing tissues (109, 113). Mesothelioma incidence in *Bap1*$^{(+\backslash-)}$ mice ranged between 36-60% depending on asbestos doses (41, 106). However, while *Bap1*$^{(+\backslash-)}$ mice develop mesothelioma, they also develop other cancers such as uveal and cutaneous melanoma (37). Furthermore, *Bap1*$^{(+\backslash-)}$ mice develop mesothelioma after exposure to doses of asbestos fibers that are unlikely to induce mesothelioma in wt mice (106).

ASBESTOS INDUCED MESOTHELIOMA MexTAg MOUSE MODEL

There is no absolute consensus over which is the best model system for studying mesothelioma; some groups prefer to use conditional knockout models, as they replicate the genetic deletions observed in human disease, while others prefer alternative models that require asbestos induction and have limited unrelated cancer development. We developed the transgenic C57BL/6 MexTAg mouse model expressing SV40 large T antigen directed to mesothelial cells by use of cell-type specific mesothelin promoter as a tool for the pre-clinical evaluation of asbestos-induced mesothelioma (114). Importantly, MexTAg mice develop mesothelioma with similar pathology to humans, but only after asbestos exposure (115). Furthermore, MexTAg mice have high disease incidence (> 85%) and are less likely to develop unrelated tumors compared to wild type mice or some heterozygous or conditional knockout models (103–112). Comparing gene expression profiles of MexTAg mice and wt mesothelioma with their counterpart normal mesothelial cells, exhibits overlapping gene expression profiles, suggesting a similar overall mechanism of mesothelioma development in transgenic MexTAg mice (116). Expression of the TAg transgene does not affect the overall mechanism of mesothelioma development, but rather phenocopies *p16* loss (117) and as a consequence onset of disease is more rapid, significantly increasing the incidence and rate of mesothelioma development compared to wt mice (114).

USING THE CC-MexTAg MOUSE MODEL TO ASSESS THE IMPACT OF HOST GENETICS ON THE DEVELOPING ANTI-TUMOR IMMUNE RESPONSE TO MESOTHELIOMA

To investigate how host genetics might impact asbestos related disease development (ARD), it is important to use a model in which only ARD (and not unrelated tumors) occur and high incidence. We developed the MexTAg Collaborative Cross to investigate how a hosts' genetic background influences the development of mesothelioma in asbestos-exposed individuals. Combining the genetic diversity inherent in the CC with the high incidence of asbestos–induced disease and rare onset of unrelated spontaneous tumors of MexTAg mice, provides an ideal model to define with unprecedented accuracy the genes and associated pathways that affect susceptibility and resistance to disease. In this model, the F1 progeny of CC x MexTAg mice (CC–MexTAg mice) are exposed to asbestos and monitored for up to 18 months, or until asbestos related disease (ARD) developed and progressed to a clearly defined endpoint. ARD phenotypic traits such as overall survival, disease latency and progression for each CC–MexTAg group, can be analyzed using the GeneMiner™ bioinformatic portal (87), where candidate modifier genes are mapped with ARD phenotype as a quantitative trait. Genome wide scans defined chromosomal locations of peak SNPs associated with each of the characterized ARD phenotypes. To date, we have generated and asbestos-exposed over 2500 individual CC–MexTAg mice progeny of 72 unique CC strains. At the time of writing 55 CC–MexTAg groups that have completed the observation period. These preliminary data indicate greater than 3-fold variation in median overall survival. This shows the power of the CC approach, given that the parental MexTAg mice survive 365 days. An additional 20 CC–MexTAg groups remain under study, and we envisage accrual of complete data by late 2021.

Importantly, the development of the CC–MexTAg model has not only enabled data collection on numerous ARD phenotypic traits, but has enabled the generation of a large repository of tumor samples and tumor-derived cell lines, collected from animals that are either relatively resistant or highly sensitive to asbestos-induced cancer. Given recent insights provided by the CheckMate 743 study demonstrating for the first time first-line immune checkpoint blockade (nivolumab plus ipilimumab) provided a significant and clinically meaningful improvement in overall survival *versus* platinum plus pemetrexed chemotherapy for mesothelioma (118), this unique biological resource can be exploited for comprehensive genetic and immunohistological analysis on tumors collected from CC-MexTAg mice (**Figure 1**). The CCMT biobank will complement many of the recent 'multi-omic' informed human mesothelioma datasets, helping to overcome some of the limitations associated with conventional genetic studies aimed at identifying the role of host genetic factors associated with the development and immunological control of rare thoracic cancers like mesothelioma.

We believe this strategy will not only allow identification of host modifier genes associated with ARD development, but when correlated with data on immune microenvironment will help elucidate what is required to generate an effective immune response to asbestos induced cancers. In addition, our strategy provides a rational approach that could be applied to other thoracic cancers by taking advantage of the power of CC to define a protective host genetic background.

SUMMARY AND CONCLUDING REMARKS

Thoracic cancers are a leading cause of death worldwide. While advances have been made in our understanding of how genetic alternations impact cancer development and treatment outcomes for common thoracic malignancies like lung cancer, our knowledge remains limited for less common cancers such as mesothelioma and TETs. Moreover, there is a paucity in our understanding of the complex biological interplay between the tumor and the immune microenvironment. Understanding how the host immune system interacts with a developing tumor is essential for the rational development of new or improved treatment regimens for thoracic malignancies. An often overlooked characteristic of the tumor host interaction, is the influence a hosts' background genetics has on tumor development and how this affects treatment response. While previous conventional genomic studies are often limited to more common cancers, recent technical advances in computation biology, combined with the use of 'system genetics' approaches, now provide

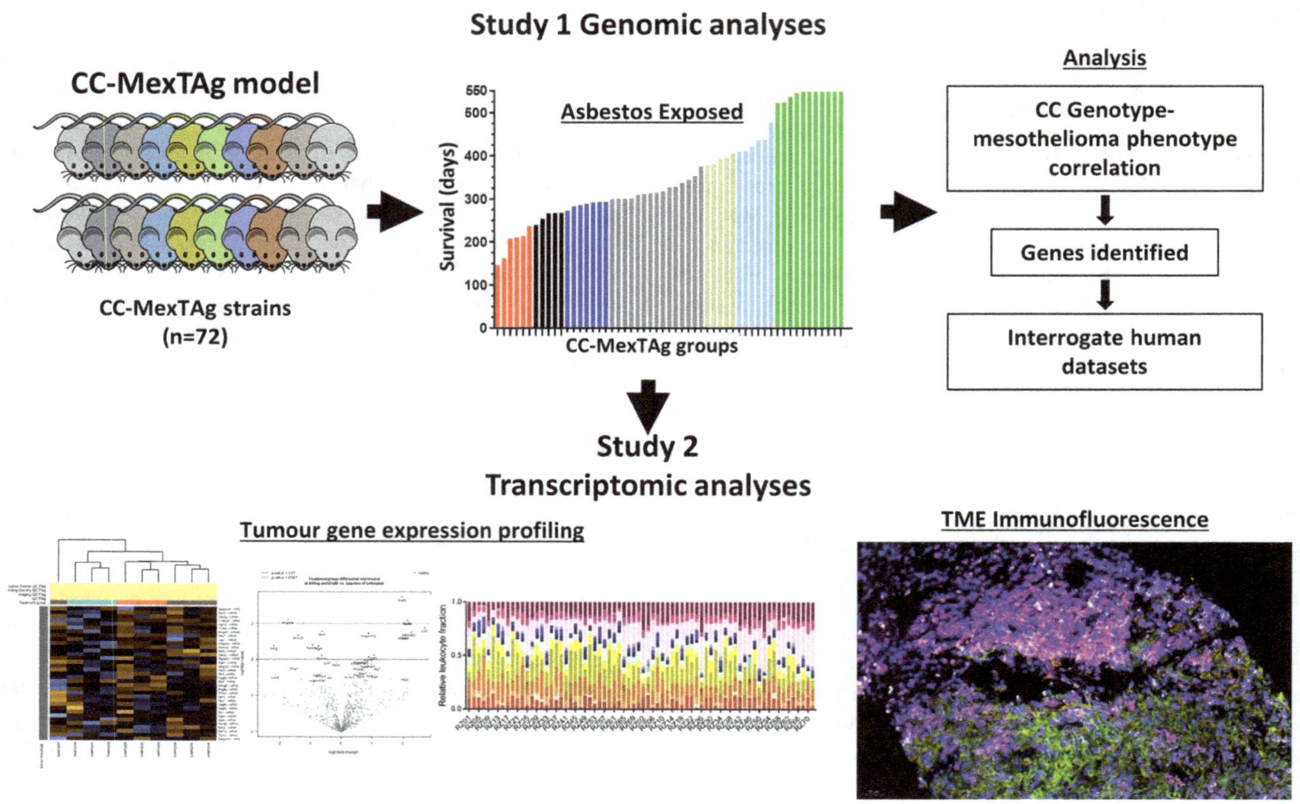

FIGURE 1 | A schematic of the CC-MexTAg experimental design. *The generation of CC-MexTAg mice and their exposure to asbestos (Study 1):* Briefly, candidate modifier genes will be mapped with mesothelioma-free survival, as a quantitative trait using the GeneMiner Bioinformatics pipeline. Genome wide scans will be used to define chromosomal locations of peak single nucleotide polymorphism (SNPs) associated with each of the characterized mesothelioma phenotypes, such as disease progression, latency, overall survival, and mesothelioma incidence. *Gene expression analysis and immunofluorescence analysis of tumors collected from CC-MexTAg mice exposed to asbestos (Study 2):* Comprehensive analyses of gene expression profiles and immune cell infiltrate of the tumor microenvironment will be performed to identify any differences between distinct CC-MexTAg groups. These data will be correlated back to phenotypic data from Study 1, to build a broader understanding of the impact of host genetics on asbestos related disease development.

a framework for investigating more rare thoracic malignancies such as mesothelioma and TETs. To address these issues, we have developed the MexTAg Collaborative cross to identify host genes that affect asbestos-related disease. The CC-MexTAg mouse model embraces a systems genetics approach, linking the power of CC's defined host background genetics, with gene expression analysis and unparalleled detailed spatial assessment of the immunological milieu of asbestos-induced mesothelioma. This unique model allows rapid identification of key host modifier genes and a comprehensive genomic and histopathological analyses of biological pathways associated with asbestos-induced mesothelioma development. These data can then be validated by interrogating the numerous data sets produced from current human genetic studies.

In conclusion, the CC-MexTAg mouse model, particularly in combination with contemporaneous tumor expression data, will provide a detailed picture of the role of modifier genes and their biological pathways associated with immune response in mesothelioma. Such data is essential to help identify potential druggable and translatable targets for the development of better treatment options and developing an effective anti-tumor immune response in malignant mesothelioma patients.

AUTHOR CONTRIBUTIONS

SF, KBe, SM and RK contributed to conception and design of the review. SF, KBu and KBe performed, collected and analyzed CC–MexTAg data. KBe and SF wrote the first draft of the manuscript. RK, SM, KBu, and GM wrote sections of the manuscript. All authors contributed to the article and approved the submitted version.

REFERENCES

1. Siesling S, van der Zwan JM, Izarzugaza I, Jaal J, Treasure T, Foschi R, et al. Rare Thoracic Cancers, Including Peritoneum Mesothelioma. *Eur J Cancer* (2012) 48(7):949–60. doi: 10.1016/j.ejca.2012.02.047
2. Duruisseaux M, Rouquette I, Adam J, Cortot A, Cazes A, Gibault L, et al. Efficacy of PD-1/PD-L1 Immune Checkpoint Inhibitors and PD-L1 Testing in Thoracic Cancers. *Ann Pathol* (2017) 8(1):61–78. doi: 10.1016/j.annpat.2016.12.009
3. Facchinetti F, Marabelle A, Rossi G, Soria J-C, Besse B, Tiseo M. Moving Immune Checkpoint Blockade in Thoracic Tumors Beyond NSCLC. *J Thorac Oncol* (2016) 11(11):1819–36. doi: 10.1016/j.jtho.2016.05.027
4. Gasparri ML, Ruscito I, Taghavi K, Farooqi AA, Papadia A, Focaccetti C, et al. The Immunobiology of Cancer: From Tumor Escape to Cancer Immunoediting Towards Immunotherapy in Gynecologic Oncology. In: Farooqi A, Ismail M. eds. *Molecular Oncology: Underlying Mechanisms and Translational Advancements*. Cham: Springer (2017). p. 193–204. doi: 10.1007/978-3-319-53082-6_9
5. Byers LA, Rudin CM. Small Cell Lung Cancer: Where do We Go From Here? *Cancer* (2015) 121(5):664–72. doi: 10.1002/cncr.29098
6. Kiyotani K, Park J-H, Inoue H, Husain A, Olugbile S, Zewde M, et al. Integrated Analysis of Somatic Mutations and Immune Microenvironment in Malignant Pleural Mesothelioma. *Oncoimmunology* (2017) 6(2): e1278330. doi: 10.1080/2162402X.2016.1278330
7. Li H, Auwerx J. Mouse Systems Genetics as a Prelude to Precision Medicine. *Trends Genet* (2020) 36(4):259–72. doi: 10.1016/j.tig.2020.01.004
8. Izzi V, Masuelli L, Tresoldi I, Foti C, Modesti A, Bei R. Immunity and Malignant Mesothelioma: From Mesothelial Cell Damage to Tumor Development and Immune Response-Based Therapies. *Cancer Lett* (2012) 322(1):18–34. doi: 10.1016/j.canlet.2012.02.034
9. Freudenstein D, Litchfield C, Caramia F, Wright G, Solomon BJ, Ball D, et al. Tp53 Status, Patient Sex, and the Immune Response as Determinants of Lung Cancer Patient Survival. *Cancers* (2020) 12(6):1535. doi: 10.3390/cancers12061535
10. Topalian SL, Hodi FS, Brahmer JR, Gettinger SN, Smith DC, McDermott DF, et al. Safety, Activity, and Immune Correlates of Anti–PD-1 Antibody in Cancer. *N Engl J Med* (2012) 366(26):2443–54. doi: 10.1056/NEJMoa1200690
11. Wang E, Uccellini L, Marincola FM. A Genetic Inference on Cancer Immune Responsiveness. *Oncoimmunology* (2012) 1(4):520–5. doi: 10.4161/onci.19531
12. Sui X, Ma J, Han W, Wang X, Fang Y, Li D, et al. The Anticancer Immune Response of anti-PD-1/PD-L1 and the Genetic Determinants of Response to anti-PD-1/PD-L1 Antibodies in Cancer Patients. *Oncotarget* (2015) 6 (23):19393. doi: 10.18632/oncotarget.5107
13. Lim YW, Chen-Harris H, Mayba O, Lianoglou S, Wuster A, Bhangale T, et al. Germline Genetic Polymorphisms Influence Tumor Gene Expression and Immune Cell Infiltration. *Proc Natl Acad Sci* (2018) 115(50):E11701–10. doi: 10.1073/pnas.1804506115
14. Chubb D, Broderick P, Dobbins SE, Frampton M, Kinnersley B, Penegar S, et al. Rare Disruptive Mutations and Their Contribution to the Heritable Risk of Colorectal Cancer. *Nat Commun* (2016) 7(1):1–7. doi: 10.1038/ncomms11883
15. Yurgelun MB, Kulke MH, Fuchs CS, Allen BA, Uno H, Hornick JL, et al. Cancer Susceptibility Gene Mutations in Individuals With Colorectal Cancer. *J Clin Oncol* (2017) 35(10):1086. doi: 10.1200/JCO.2016.71.0012
16. AlDubayan SH, Giannakis M, Moore ND, Han GC, Reardon B, Hamada T, et al. Inherited DNA-Repair Defects in Colorectal Cancer. *Am J Hum Genet* (2018) 102(3):401–14. doi: 10.1016/j.ajhg.2018.01.018
17. Khera AV, Chaffin M, Aragam KG, Haas ME, Roselli C, Choi SH, et al. Genome-Wide Polygenic Scores for Common Diseases Identify Individuals With Risk Equivalent to Monogenic Mutations. *Nat Genet* (2018) 50 (9):1219–24. doi: 10.1038/s41588-018-0183-z
18. Sud A, Kinnersley B, Houlston RS. Genome-Wide Association Studies of Cancer: Current Insights and Future Perspectives. *Nat Rev Cancer* (2017) 17 (11):692–704. doi: 10.1038/nrc.2017.82
19. Frank SA. Genetic Predisposition to Cancer—Insights From Population Genetics. *Nat Rev Genet* (2004) 5(10):764–72. doi: 10.1038/nrg1450
20. Stadler ZK, Thom P, Robson ME, Weitzel JN, Kauff ND, Hurley KE, et al. Genome-Wide Association Studies of Cancer. *J Clin Oncol* (2010) 28 (27):4255. doi: 10.1200/JCO.2009.25.7816
21. Wang Y, McKay JD, Rafnar T, Wang Z, Timofeeva MN, Broderick P, et al. Rare Variants of Large Effect in BRCA2 and CHEK2 Affect Risk of Lung Cancer. *Nat Genet* (2014) 46(7):736–41. doi: 10.1038/ng.3002
22. Timofeeva MN, Hung RJ, Rafnar T, Christiani DC, Field JK, Bickeböller H, et al. Influence of Common Genetic Variation on Lung Cancer Risk: Meta-Analysis of 14 900 Cases and 29 485 Controls. *Hum Mol Genet* (2012) 21 (22):4980–95. doi: 10.1093/hmg/dds334
23. McKay JD, Hung RJ, Han Y, Zong X, Carreras-Torres R, Christiani DC, et al. Large-Scale Association Analysis Identifies New Lung Cancer Susceptibility Loci and Heterogeneity in Genetic Susceptibility Across Histological Subtypes. *Nat Genet* (2017) 49(7):1126–32. doi: 10.1038/ng.3892
24. Kaur-Knudsen D, Nordestgaard BG, Bojesen SE. CHRNA3 Genotype, Nicotine Dependence, Lung Function and Disease in the General Population. *Eur Respir J* (2012) 40(6):1538–44. doi: 10.1183/09031936.00176811
25. Pérez-Morales R, González-Zamora A, González-Delgado MF, Calleros Rincón EY, Olivas Calderon EH, Martínez-Ramírez OC, et al. Chrna3 rs1051730 and CHRNA5 rs16969968 Polymorphisms Are Associated With Heavy Smoking, Lung Cancer, and Chronic Obstructive Pulmonary Disease in a Mexican Population. *Ann Hum Genet* (2018) 82(6):415–24. doi: 10.1111/ahg.12264
26. Wang Y, Broderick P, Matakidou A, Eisen T, Houlston RS. Role of 5p15. 33 (Tert-CLPTM1L), 6p21. 33 and 15q25. 1 (Chrna5-CHRNA3) Variation and Lung Cancer Risk in Never-Smokers. *Carcinogenesis* (2010) 31(2):234–8. doi: 10.1093/carcin/bgp287
27. Miki D, Kubo M, Takahashi A, Yoon K-A, Kim J, Lee GK, et al. Variation in TP63 Is Associated With Lung Adenocarcinoma Susceptibility in Japanese and Korean Populations. *Nat Genet* (2010) 42(10):893–6. doi: 10.1038/ng.667
28. Dai J, Lv J, Zhu M, Wang Y, Qin N, Ma H, et al. Identification of Risk Loci and a Polygenic Risk Score for Lung Cancer: A Large-Scale Prospective Cohort Study in Chinese Populations. *Lancet Respir Med* (2019) 7(10):881–91. doi: 10.1016/S2213-2600(19)30144-4
29. Bossé Y, Amos CI. A Decade of GWAS Results in Lung Cancer. *Cancer Epidemiol Biomarkers Prev* (2018) 27(4):363–79. doi: 10.1158/1055-9965.EPI-16-0794
30. Sampson JN, Wheeler WA, Yeager M, Panagiotou O, Wang Z, Berndt SI, et al. Analysis of Heritability and Shared Heritability Based on Genome-Wide Association Studies for 13 Cancer Types. *JNCI: J Natl Cancer Inst* (2015) 107(12):djv279. doi: 10.1093/jnci/djv279
31. Lichtenstein P, Holm NV, Verkasalo PK, Iliadou A, Kaprio J, Koskenvuo M, et al. Environmental and Heritable Factors in the Causation of Cancer—Analyses of Cohorts of Twins From Sweden, Denmark, and Finland. *N Engl J Med* (2000) 343(2):78–85. doi: 10.1056/NEJM200007133430201
32. Cadby G, Mukherjee S, Musk AWB, Reid A, Garlepp M, Dick I, et al. A Genome-Wide Association Study for Malignant Mesothelioma Risk. *Lung Cancer* (2013) 82(1):1–8. doi: 10.1016/j.lungcan.2013.04.018
33. Tunesi S, Ferrante D, Mirabelli D, Andorno S, Betti M, Fiorito G, et al. Gene–Asbestos Interaction in Malignant Pleural Mesothelioma Susceptibility. *Carcinogenesis* (2015) 36(10):1129–35. doi: 10.1093/carcin/bgv097
34. Matullo G, Guarrera S, Betti M, Fiorito G, Ferrante D, Voglino F, et al. Genetic Variants Associated With Increased Risk of Malignant Pleural Mesothelioma: A Genome-Wide Association Study. *PLoS One* (2013) 8(4): e61253. doi: 10.1371/journal.pone.0061253
35. Dianzani I, Gibello L, Biava A, Giordano M, Bertolotti M, Betti M, et al. Polymorphisms in DNA Repair Genes as Risk Factors for Asbestos-Related Malignant Mesothelioma in a General Population Study. *Mutat Res/Fundam Mol Mech Mutagen* (2006) 599(1-2):124–34. doi: 10.1016/j.mrfmmm.2006.02.005
36. Testa JR, Cheung M, Pei J, Below JE, Tan Y, Sementino E, et al. Germline BAP1 Mutations Predispose to Malignant Mesothelioma. *Nat Genet* (2011) 43(10):1022–5. doi: 10.1038/ng.912
37. Carbone M, Ferris LK, Baumann F, Napolitano A, Lum CA, Flores EG, et al. BAP1 Cancer Syndrome: Malignant Mesothelioma, Uveal and Cutaneous

Melanoma, and Mbaits. *J Trans Med* (2012) 10(1):179. doi: 10.1186/1479-5876-10-179
38. Travis WD, Brambilla E, Burke AP, Marx A, Nicholson AG. Introduction to the 2015 World Health Organization Classification of Tumors of the Lung, Pleura, Thymus, and Heart. *J Thorac Oncol* (2015) 10(9):1240–2. doi: 10.1097/JTO.0000000000000663
39. Girard N. Thymic Tumors: Relevant Molecular Data in the Clinic. *J Thorac Oncol* (2010) 5(10):S291–S5. doi: 10.1097/JTO.0b013e3181f209b9
40. Wang Y, Thomas A, Lau C, Rajan A, Zhu Y, Killian JK, et al. Mutations of Epigenetic Regulatory Genes Are Common in Thymic Carcinomas. *Sci Rep* (2014) 4:7336. doi: 10.1038/srep07336
41. Álvarez-Quilón A, Terrón-Bautista J, Delgado-Sainz I, Serrano-Benítez A, Romero-Granados R, Martínez-García PM, et al. Endogenous Topoisomerase II-mediated DNA Breaks Drive Thymic Cancer Predisposition Linked to ATM Deficiency. *Nat Commun* (2020) 11(1):1–14. doi: 10.1038/s41467-020-14638-w
42. Whiteside TL. The Tumor Microenvironment and Its Role in Promoting Tumor Growth. *Oncogene* (2008) 27(45):5904–12. doi: 10.1038/onc.2008.271
43. Stearman RS, Dwyer-Nield L, Grady MC, Malkinson AM, Geraci MW. A Macrophage Gene Expression Signature Defines a Field Effect in the Lung Tumor Microenvironment. *Cancer Res* (2008) 68(1):34–43. doi: 10.1158/0008-5472.CAN-07-0988
44. Lochhead P, Chan AT, Nishihara R, Fuchs CS, Beck AH, Giovannucci E, et al. Etiologic Field Effect: Reappraisal of the Field Effect Concept in Cancer Predisposition and Progression. *Modern Pathol* (2015) 28(1):14–29. doi: 10.1038/modpathol.2014.81
45. Martincorena I, Roshan A, Gerstung M, Ellis P, Van Loo P, McLaren S, et al. Tumor Evolution. High Burden and Pervasive Positive Selection of Somatic Mutations in Normal Human Skin. *Science* (2015) 348(6237):880–6. doi: 10.1126/science.aaa6806
46. Klutstein M, Moss J, Kaplan T, Cedar H. Contribution of Epigenetic Mechanisms to Variation in Cancer Risk Among Tissues. *Proc Natl Acad Sci U S A* (2017) 114(9):2230–4. doi: 10.1073/pnas.1616556114
47. Bezu L, Wu Chuang A, Liu P, Kroemer G, Kepp O. Immunological Effects of Epigenetic Modifiers. *Cancers* (2019) 11(12):1911. doi: 10.3390/cancers11121911
48. Yang B, Bhusari S, Kueck J, Weeratunga P, Wagner J, Leverson G, et al. Methylation Profiling Defines an Extensive Field Defect in Histologically Normal Prostate Tissues Associated With Prostate Cancer. *Neoplasia* (2013) 15(4):399–408. doi: 10.1593/neo.13280
49. Yang B, Etheridge T, McCormick J, Schultz A, Khemees TA, Damaschke N, et al. Validation of an Epigenetic Field of Susceptibility to Detect Significant Prostate Cancer From non-Tumor Biopsies. *Clin Epigenet* (2019) 11(1):168. doi: 10.1186/s13148-019-0771-5
50. Pereira AL, Magalhaes L, Moreira FC, Reis-das-Merces L, Vidal AF, Ribeiro-Dos-Santos AM, et al. Epigenetic Field Cancerization in Gastric Cancer: microRNAs as Promising Biomarkers. *J Cancer* (2019) 10(6):1560–9. doi: 10.7150/jca.27457
51. Sugai T, Yoshida M, Eizuka M, Uesugii N, Habano W, Otsuka K, et al. Analysis of the DNA Methylation Level of Cancer-Related Genes in Colorectal Cancer and the Surrounding Normal Mucosa. *Clin Epigenet* (2017) 9:55. doi: 10.1186/s13148-017-0352-4
52. Daniunaite K, Sestokaite A, Kubiliute R, Stuopelyte K, Kettunen E, Husgafvel-Pursiainen K, et al. Frequent DNA Methylation Changes in Cancerous and Noncancerous Lung Tissues From Smokers With non-Small Cell Lung Cancer. *Mutagenesis* (2020) 35(5):373–9. doi: 10.1093/mutage/geaa022
53. Wang Y, Wang C, Zhang J, Zhu M, Zhang X, Li Z, et al. Interaction Analysis Between Germline Susceptibility Loci and Somatic Alterations in Lung Cancer. *Int J Cancer* (2018) 143(4):878–85. doi: 10.1002/ijc.31351
54. Bitler BG, Fatkhutdinov N, Zhang R. Potential Therapeutic Targets in ARID1A-mutated Cancers. *Expert Opin Ther Targets* (2015) 19(11):1419–22. doi: 10.1517/14728222.2015.1062879
55. Sun D, Tian L, Zhu Y, Wo Y, Liu Q, Liu S, et al. Subunits of ARID1 Serve as Novel Biomarkers for the Sensitivity to Immune Checkpoint Inhibitors and Prognosis of Advanced non-Small Cell Lung Cancer. *Mol Med* (2020) 26 (1):1–9. doi: 10.1186/s10020-020-00208-9
56. Yoshikawa Y, Emi M, Nakano T, Gaudino G. Mesothelioma Developing in Carriers of Inherited Genetic Mutations. *Trans Lung Cancer Res* (2020) 9 (Suppl 1):S67. doi: 10.21037/tlcr.2019.11.15
57. Wang Q, Gu J, Wang L, Chang DW, Ye Y, Huang M, et al. Genetic Associations of T Cell Cancer Immune Response-Related Genes With T Cell Phenotypes and Clinical Outcomes of Early-Stage Lung Cancer. *J ImmunoTher Cancer* (2020) 8(2):e000336. doi: 10.1136/jitc-2019-000336
58. Marwitz S, Scheufele S, Perner S, Reck M, Ammerpohl O, Goldmann T. Epigenetic Modifications of the Immune-Checkpoint Genes CTLA4 and PDCD1 in non-Small Cell Lung Cancer Results in Increased Expression. *Clin Epigenet* (2017) 9:51. doi: 10.1186/s13148-017-0354-2
59. Bacolod MD, Barany F, Fisher PB. Can CpG Methylation Serve as Surrogate Markers for Immune Infiltration in Cancer? *Adv Cancer Res* (2019) 143:351–84. doi: 10.1016/bs.acr.2019.03.007
60. Costa C, Indovina P, Mattioli E, Forte IM, Iannuzzi CA, Luzzi L, et al. P53-Regulated miR-320a Targets PDL1 and Is Downregulated in Malignant Mesothelioma. *Cell Death Dis* (2020) 11(9):1–15. doi: 10.1038/s41419-020-02940-w
61. Weksler B, Lu B. Alterations of the Immune System in Thymic Malignancies. *J Thorac Oncol* (2014) 9(9):S137–42. doi: 10.1097/JTO.0000000000000299
62. Lippner EA, Lewis DB, Robinson WH, Katsumoto TR. Paraneoplastic and Therapy-Related Immune Complications in Thymic Malignancies. *Curr Treat Options Oncol* (2019) 20(7):62. doi: 10.1007/s11864-019-0661-2
63. Wadowski B, De Rienzo A, Bueno R. The Molecular Basis of Malignant Pleural Mesothelioma. *Thorac Surg Clin* (2020) 30(4):383–93. doi: 10.1016/j.thorsurg.2020.08.005
64. Hmeljak J, Sanchez-Vega F, Hoadley KA, Shih J, Stewart C, Heiman D, et al. Integrative Molecular Characterization of Malignant Pleural Mesothelioma. *Cancer Discov* (2018) 8(12):1548–65. doi: 10.1158/2159-8290.CD-18-1181
65. Bueno R, Stawiski EW, Goldstein LD, Durinck S, De Rienzo A, Modrusan Z, et al. Comprehensive Genomic Analysis of Malignant Pleural Mesothelioma Identifies Recurrent Mutations, Gene Fusions and Splicing Alterations. *Nat Genet* (2016) 48(4):407–16. doi: 10.1038/ng.3520
66. Blum Y, Meiller C, Quetel L, Elarouci N, Ayadi M, Tashtanbaeva D, et al. Dissecting Heterogeneity in Malignant Pleural Mesothelioma Through Histo-Molecular Gradients for Clinical Applications. *Nat Commun* (2019) 10(1):1333. doi: 10.1038/s41467-019-09307-6
67. Blum Y, Jaurand MC, De Reynies A, Jean D. Unraveling the Cellular Heterogeneity of Malignant Pleural Mesothelioma Through a Deconvolution Approach. *Mol Cell Oncol* (2019) 6(4):1610322. doi: 10.1080/23723556.2019.1610322
68. Liang B, Ding H, Huang L, Luo H, Zhu X. GWAS in Cancer: Progress and Challenges. *Mol Genet Genomics* (2020) 295(3):537–61. doi: 10.1007/s00438-020-01647-z
69. Pharoah PDP, Tsai Y-Y, Ramus SJ, Phelan CM, Goode EL, Lawrenson K, et al. GWAS Meta-Analysis and Replication Identifies Three New Susceptibility Loci for Ovarian Cancer. *Nat Genet* (2013) 45(4):362–70. doi: 10.1038/ng.2564
70. de Maturana EL, Rava M, Anumudu C, Saez O, Alonso D, Malats N. Bladder Cancer Genetic Susceptibility. A Systematic Review. *Bladder Cancer* (2018) 4 (2):215–26. doi: 10.3233/BLC-170159
71. Need AC, Goldstein DB. Next Generation Disparities in Human Genomics: Concerns and Remedies. *Trends Genet* (2009) 25(11):489–94. doi: 10.1016/j.tig.2009.09.012
72. Murphy S, Churchill S, Bry L, Chueh H, Weiss S, Lazarus R, et al. Instrumenting the Health Care Enterprise for Discovery Research in the Genomic Era. *Genome Res* (2009) 19(9):1675–81. doi: 10.1101/gr.094615.109
73. Galvan A, Ioannidis JP, Dragani TA. Beyond Genome-Wide Association Studies: Genetic Heterogeneity and Individual Predisposition to Cancer. *Trends Genet* (2010) 26(3):132–41. doi: 10.1016/j.tig.2009.12.008
74. Song W, Huang H, Zhang C-Z, Bates DW, Wright A. Using Whole Genome Scores to Compare Three Clinical Phenotyping Methods in Complex Diseases. *Sci Rep* (2018) 8(1):1–10. doi: 10.1038/s41598-018-29634-w
75. Olson B, Li Y, Lin Y, Liu ET, Patnaik A. Mouse Models for Cancer Immunotherapy Research. *Cancer Discov* (2018) 8(11):1358–65. doi: 10.1158/2159-8290.CD-18-0044

76. Nisbet NW. Some Aspects of Immunological Tolerance Investigated by Parent to F1 Hybrid Parabiosis in Mice. *Transplantation* (1971) 11(3):318–24. doi: 10.1097/00007890-197103000-00012
77. Flint J, Eskin E. Genome-Wide Association Studies in Mice. *Nat Rev Genet* (2012) 13(11):807–17. doi: 10.1038/nrg3335
78. Festing MFW, Yang A, Malkinson AM. At Least Four Genes and Sex are Associated With Susceptibility to Urethane-Induced Pulmonary Adenomas in Mice. *Genet Res* (1994) 64(2):99–106. doi: 10.1017/S0016672300032705
79. Manenti G, Gariboldi M, Fiorino A, Zanesi N, Pierotti MA, Dragani TA. Genetic Mapping of Lung Cancer Modifier Loci Specifically Affecting Tumor Initiation and Progression. *Cancer Res* (1997) 57(19):4164–6.
80. Wang D, Lemon WJ, You M. Linkage Disequilibrium Mapping of Novel Lung Tumor Susceptibility Quantitative Trait Loci in Mice. *Oncogene* (2002) 21(44):6858–65. doi: 10.1038/sj.onc.1205886
81. Wakana S, Sugaya E, Naramoto F, Yokote N, Maruyama C, Jin W, et al. Gene Mapping of SEZ Group Genes and Determination of Pentylenetetrazol Susceptible Quantitative Trait Loci in the Mouse Chromosome. *Brain Res* (2000) 857(1-2):286–90. doi: 10.1016/S0006-8993(99)02406-3
82. Williams RW, Bennett B, Lu L, Gu J, DeFries JC, Carosone-Link PJ, et al. Genetic Structure of the LXS Panel of Recombinant Inbred Mouse Strains: A Powerful Resource for Complex Trait Analysis. *Mamm Genome* (2004) 15 (8):637–47. doi: 10.1007/s00335-004-2380-6
83. Threadgill DW, Miller DR, Churchill GA, de Villena FP-M. The Collaborative Cross: A Recombinant Inbred Mouse Population for the Systems Genetic Era. *ILAR J* (2011) 52(1):24–31. doi: 10.1093/ilar.52.1.24
84. Roberts A, Pardo-Manuel de Villena F, Wang W, McMillan L, Threadgill DW. The Polymorphism Architecture of Mouse Genetic Resources Elucidated Using Genome-Wide Resequencing Data: Implications for QTL Discovery and Systems Genetics. *Mamm Genome* (2007) 18(6-7):473–81. doi: 10.1007/s00335-007-9045-1
85. Churchill GA, Airey DC, Allayee H, Angel JM, Attie AD, Beatty J, et al. The Collaborative Cross, a Community Resource for the Genetic Analysis of Complex Traits. *Nat Genet* (2004) 36(11):1133–7. doi: 10.1038/ng1104-1133
86. Morahan G, Balmer L, Monley D. Establishment of "The Gene Mine": A Resource for Rapid Identification of Complex Trait Genes. *Mamm Genome* (2008) 19(6):390–3. doi: 10.1007/s00335-008-9134-9
87. Ram R, Mehta M, Balmer L, Gatti DM, Morahan G. Rapid Identification of Major-Effect Genes Using the Collaborative Cross. *Genetics* (2014) 198 (1):75–86. doi: 10.1534/genetics.114.163014
88. Ferguson B, Ram R, Handoko HY, Mukhopadhyay P, Muller HK, Soyer HP, et al. Melanoma Susceptibility as a Complex Trait: Genetic Variation Controls All Stages of Tumor Progression. *Oncogene* (2015) 34(22):2879–86. doi: 10.1038/onc.2014.227
89. Patel SJ, Molinolo AA, Gutkind S, Crawford NP. Germline Genetic Variation Modulates Tumor Progression and Metastasis in a Mouse Model of Neuroendocrine Prostate Carcinoma. *PLoS One* (2013) 8(4): e61848. doi: 10.1371/journal.pone.0061848
90. Yang CH, Mangiafico SP, Waibel M, Loudovaris T, Loh K, Thomas HE, et al. E2f8 and Dlg2 Genes Have Independent Effects on Impaired Insulin Secretion Associated With Hyperglycaemia. *Diabetologia* (2020) 63 (7):1333–48. doi: 10.1007/s00125-020-05137-0
91. Yuan J, Tickner J, Mullin BH, Zhao J, Zeng Z, Morahan G, et al. Advanced Genetic Approaches in Discovery and Characterization of Genes Involved With Osteoporosis in Mouse and Human. *Front Genet* (2019) 10:288. doi: 10.3389/fgene.2019.00288
92. Weerasekera LY, Balmer LA, Ram R, Morahan G. Characterization of Retinal Vascular and Neural Damage in a Novel Model of Diabetic Retinopathy. *Invest Ophthalmol Vis Sci* (2015) 56(6):3721–30. doi: 10.1167/iovs.14-16289
93. Ferguson B, Handoko HY, Mukhopadhyay P, Chitsazan A, Balmer L, Morahan G, et al. Different Genetic Mechanisms Mediate Spontaneous *Versus* UVR-Induced Malignant Melanoma. *Elife* (2019) 8:e42424. doi: 10.7554/eLife.42424
94. Chitsazan A, Ferguson B, Ram R, Mukhopadhyay P, Handoko HY, Gabrielli B, et al. A Mutation in the Cdon Gene Potentiates Congenital Nevus Development Mediated by NRAS(Q61K). *Pigment Cell Melanom Res* (2016) 29(4):459–64. doi: 10.1111/pcmr.12487
95. Chitsazan A, Ferguson B, Villani R, Handoko HY, Mukhopadhyay P, Gabrielli B, et al. Keratinocyte Sonic Hedgehog Upregulation Drives the Development of Giant Congenital Nevi Via Paracrine Endothelin-1 Secretion. *J Invest Dermatol* (2018) 138(4):893–902. doi: 10.1016/j.jid.2017.10.032
96. Walrath JC, Hawes JJ, Van Dyke T, Reilly KM. Genetically Engineered Mouse Models in Cancer Research. *Adv Cancer Res* (2010) 106:113–64. doi: 10.1016/S0065-230X(10)06004-5
97. Gurumurthy CB, Lloyd KCK. Generating Mouse Models for Biomedical Research: Technological Advances. *Dis Models Mech* (2019) 12(1): dmm029462. doi: 10.1242/dmm.029462
98. Kersten K, de Visser KE, van Miltenburg MH, Jonkers J. Genetically Engineered Mouse Models in Oncology Research and Cancer Medicine. *EMBO Mol Med* (2017) 9(2):137–53. doi: 10.15252/emmm.201606857
99. Johnson L, Mercer K, Greenbaum D, Bronson RT, Crowley D, Tuveson DA, et al. Somatic Activation of the K-ras Oncogene Causes Early Onset Lung Cancer in Mice. *Nature* (2001) 410(6832):1111–6. doi: 10.1038/35074129
100. Kasinski AL, Slack FJ. miRNA-34 Prevents Cancer Initiation and Progression in a Therapeutically Resistant K-ras and p53-induced Mouse Model of Lung Adenocarcinoma. *Cancer Res* (2012) 72(21):5576–87. doi: 10.1158/0008-5472.CAN-12-2001
101. Gormally E, Vineis P, Matullo G, Veglia F, Caboux E, Le Roux E, et al. TP53 and KRAS2 Mutations in Plasma DNA of Healthy Subjects and Subsequent Cancer Occurrence: A Prospective Study. *Cancer Res* (2006) 66(13):6871–6. doi: 10.1158/0008-5472.CAN-05-4556
102. Tang FH, Hsieh TH, Hsu CY, Lin HY, Long CY, Cheng KH, et al. KRAS Mutation Coupled With p53 Loss is Sufficient to Induce Ovarian Carcinosarcomas in Mice. *Int J Cancer* (2017) 140(8):1860–9. doi: 10.1002/ijc.30591
103. Testa JR, Berns A. Preclinical Models of Malignant Mesothelioma. *Front Oncol* (2020) 10:101. doi: 10.3389/fonc.2020.00101
104. Kukuyan AM, Sementino E, Kadariya Y, Menges CW, Cheung M, Tan Y, et al. Inactivation of Bap1 Cooperates With Losses of Nf2 and Cdkn2a to Drive the Development of Pleural Malignant Mesothelioma in Conditional Mouse Models. *Cancer Res* (2019) 79(16):4113–23. doi: 10.1158/0008-5472.CAN-18-4093
105. Fleury-Feith J, Lecomte C, Renier A, Matrat M, Kheuang L, Abramowski V, et al. Hemizygosity of Nf2 is Associated With Increased Susceptibility to Asbestos-Induced Peritoneal Tumours. *Oncogene* (2003) 22(24):3799–805. doi: 10.1038/sj.onc.1206593
106. Napolitano A, Pellegrini L, Dey A, Larson D, Tanji M, Flores EG, et al. Minimal Asbestos Exposure in Germline BAP1 Heterozygous Mice Is Associated With Deregulated Inflammatory Response and Increased Risk of Mesothelioma. *Oncogene* (2016) 35(15):1996–2002. doi: 10.1038/onc.2015.243
107. Shamseddin M, Obacz J, Garnett MJ, Rintoul RC, Francies HE, Marciniak SJ. Use of Preclinical Models for Malignant Pleural Mesothelioma. *Thorax* (2021) thoraxjnl-2020-216602. doi: 10.1136/thoraxjnl-2020-216602
108. Kadariya Y, Cheung M, Xu J, Pei J, Sementino E, Menges CW, et al. Bap1 Is a Bona Fide Tumor Suppressor: Genetic Evidence From Mouse Models Carrying Heterozygous Germline Bap1 Mutations. *Cancer Res* (2016) 76 (9):2836–44. doi: 10.1158/0008-5472.CAN-15-3371
109. Badhai J, Pandey GK, Song JY, Krijgsman O, Bhaskaran R, Chandrasekaran G, et al. Combined Deletion of Bap1, Nf2, and Cdkn2ab Causes Rapid Onset of Malignant Mesothelioma in Mice. *J Exp Med* (2020) 217(6):e20191257. doi: 10.1084/jem.20191257
110. Jongsma J, van Montfort E, Vooijs M, Zevenhoven J, Krimpenfort P, van der Valk M, et al. A Conditional Mouse Model for Malignant Mesothelioma. *Cancer Cell* (2008) 13(3):261–71. doi: 10.1016/j.ccr.2008.01.030
111. Robinson C, Solin JN, Lee YCG, Lake RA, Lesterhuis WJ. Mouse Models of Mesothelioma: Strengths, Limitations and Clinical Translation. *Lung Cancer Manage* (2014) 3(5):397–410. doi: 10.2217/lmt.14.27
112. Xu J, Kadariya Y, Cheung M, Pei J, Talarchek J, Sementino E, et al. Germline Mutation of Bap1 Accelerates Development of Asbestos-Induced Malignant Mesothelioma. *Cancer Res* (2014) 74(16):4388–97. doi: 10.1158/0008-5472.CAN-14-1328
113. Farahmand P, Gyuraszova K, Rooney C, Raffo-Iraolagoitia XL, Johnson E, Chernova T, et al. Asbestos Accelerates Disease Onset in a Genetic Model of Malignant Pleural Mesothelioma. *BioRxiv* (2020). doi: 10.1101/2020.06.16.154815

114. Robinson C, Van Bruggen I, Segal A, Dunham M, Sherwood A, Koentgen F, et al. A Novel SV40 Tag Transgenic Model of Asbestos-Induced Mesothelioma: Malignant Transformation is Dose Dependent. *Cancer Res* (2006) 66(22):10786–94. doi: 10.1158/0008-5472.CAN-05-4668

115. Robinson C, Walsh A, Larma I, O'Halloran S, Nowak AK, Lake RA. MexTAg Mice Exposed to Asbestos Develop Cancer That Faithfully Replicates Key Features of the Pathogenesis of Human Mesothelioma. *Eur J Cancer* (2011) 47(1):151–61. doi: 10.1016/j.ejca.2010.08.015

116. Robinson C, Dick IM, Wise MJ, Holloway A, Diyagama D, Robinson BWS, et al. Consistent Gene Expression Profiles in MexTAg Transgenic Mouse and Wild Type Mouse Asbestos-Induced Mesothelioma. *BMC Cancer* (2015) 15 (1):983. doi: 10.1186/s12885-015-1953-y

117. De Luca A, Baldi A, Esposito V, Howard CM, Bagella L, Rizzo P, et al. The Retinoblastoma Gene Family pRb/p105, p107, pRb2/p130 and Simian Virus-40 Large T-Antigen in Human Mesotheliomas. *Nat Med* (1997) 3(8):913–6. doi: 10.1038/nm0897-913

118. Baas P, Scherpereel A, Nowak AK, Fujimoto N, Peters S, Tsao AS, et al. First-Line Nivolumab Plus Ipilimumab in Unresectable Malignant Pleural Mesothelioma (CheckMate 743): A Multicentre, Randomised, Open-Label, Phase 3 Trial. *Lancet* (2021) 397(10272):375–86. doi: 10.1016/S0140-6736(20)32714-8

27

A Panel of Five-lncRNA Signature as a Potential Biomarker for Predicting Survival in Gastric and Thoracic Cancers

Jiayue Shao[1†], Wei Lyu[2†], Jiehao Zhou[3,4], Wenhui Xu[3,4], Dandan Wang[3,4], Shanshan Liang[3,4], Jiayin Zhao[3,4] and Yujing Qin[3,4]*

[1] Department of Medical Oncology, Cancer Hospital, Harbin Medical University, Harbin, China, [2] Department of Pathology, Guangdong Women and Children Hospital, Guangzhou, China, [3] Department of Gastroenterology, Heilongjiang Provincial Hospital, Harbin, China, [4] Department of Gastroenterology, Heilongjiang Provincial Hospital, Harbin Institute of Technology, Harbin, China

***Correspondence:**
Yujing Qin
cream2010@163.com

† These authors have contributed equally to this work

Dysfunctional long non-coding RNAs (lncRNAs) have been found to have carcinogenic and/or tumor inhibitory effects in the development and progression of cancer, suggesting their potential as new independent biomarkers for cancer diagnosis and prognosis. The exploration of the relationship between lncRNAs and the overall survival (OS) of different cancers opens up new prospects for tumor diagnosis and treatment. In this study, we established a five-lncRNA signature and explored its prognostic efficiency in gastric cancer (GC) and several thoracic malignancies, including breast invasive carcinoma (BRCA), esophageal carcinoma, lung adenocarcinoma, lung squamous cell carcinoma (LUSC), and thymoma (THYM). Cox regression analysis and lasso regression were used to evaluate the relationship between lncRNA expression and survival in different cancer datasets from GEO and TCGA. Kaplan-Meier survival curves indicated that risk scores characterized by a five-lncRNA signature were significantly associated with the OS of GC, BRCA, LUSC, and THYM patients. Functional enrichment analysis showed that these five lncRNAs are involved in known biological pathways related to cancer pathology. In conclusion, the five-lncRNA signature can be used as a prognostic marker to promote the diagnosis and treatment of GC and thymic malignancies.

Keywords: long non-coding RNA, gastric cancer, overall survival, thoracic malignancy, prognosis

INTRODUCTION

Long non-coding RNAs (lncRNAs) play an important regulatory role at the transcriptional, post-transcriptional, and epigenetic levels and also participate in multiple aspects of gene regulation and a variety of biological processes (Kopp and Mendell, 2018). As a type of non-coding RNA, lncRNA, which has no protein-coding ability and is more than 200 bp in length, can be transcribed by RNA polymerase II. Abnormal lncRNA expression has also been observed in many complex human diseases, especially cancer. Cancer-related lncRNAs show abnormal expression patterns in a tissue-or cancer-specific manner, indicating their potential as new independent biomarkers for cancer diagnosis and prognosis (Wang et al., 2015; Tate et al., 2019). For example, the lncRNA MALAT1 can regulate multiple biological processes during the development of several cancers.

The diagnostic and prognostic significance of MALAT1 has been demonstrated in gliomas and different cancers of the breast, lung, ovary, pancreas, and prostate (Goyal et al., 2021). The overexpression of the lncRNA GHET1 predicts unfavorable survival and clinical parameters in patients with various cancers (Jiang et al., 2019).

Gastric cancer (GC) is the fourth most common malignant tumor and the third leading cause of cancer-related death (Siegel et al., 2021). Although the treatment of GC has made great progress in recent years, the prognosis remains poor, with a 5 years survival rate of less than 40% (Allemani et al., 2018). In addition, the pathology of several thoracic malignancies, including lung cancer, esophageal cancer, and breast cancer, is found to exhibit dysregulated lncRNA expression in a variety of malignancies. Traditional classification methods are not effective, and molecular biological markers can reveal tumor progression and survival in cancer patients. Thus, identifying specific lncRNAs to predict prognosis is very important for improving patient survival.

To establish a novel risk-stratification lncRNA signature panel in different cancers, we collected lncRNA expression data and clinical information of GC and several thoracic malignancies, such as breast invasive carcinoma (BRCA), esophageal carcinoma (ESCA), lung adenocarcinoma (LUAD), lung squamous cell carcinoma (LUSC), and thymoma (THYM) patients from different independent databases to identify and develop a novel lncRNA-based signature panel as an independent predictor of cancer prognosis. Univariate and multivariate Cox regression analyses were used to explore the prognostic efficiency of lncRNAs. Five potential lncRNA biomarkers significantly related to the survival of GC patients were identified, and a risk score model was established using the coefficients of multivariate Cox regression analysis to predict the survival of patients. Furthermore, this model was applied to several thoracic malignancies in the TCGA database. We found that this five-lncRNA signature could also divide patients into different risk groups in BRCA, LUSC, and THYM. Furthermore, the possible molecular mechanisms related to the occurrence and progression of these prognostic lncRNAs were investigated using functional analysis. In conclusion, the five-lncRNA signature panel offers a potential platform for risk stratification in patients with GC and several thoracic malignancies, which has great implications in the clinical management of patients and contributes to disease diagnosis.

MATERIALS AND METHODS

Data Collection

The gene expression profiles and corresponding clinical information of GC and several thoracic cancers used in this study were obtained from the publicly available Gene Expression Omnibus (Barrett et al., 2013) (GEO)[1] database and The Cancer Genome Atlas (Tomczak et al., 2015) (TCGA)[2] database. GSE62254 (n = 300) and GSE15459 (n = 192) datasets were collected from GEO. The datasets of BRCA (n = 1,089), ESCA (n = 163), LUAD (n = 515), LUSC (n = 497), and THYM (n = 119) were collected from TCGA.

Identification of Potential lncRNA Biomarkers

The GSE62254 series samples were randomly generated in a training set and a test set. Univariate Cox regression analysis was performed on the training set to evaluate the correlation between the expression level of each lncRNA and patient overall survival (OS) (Guo et al., 2019). Lasso regression (Xu et al., 2018; McEligot et al., 2020), which solves the over-fitting problem and can directly reduce some repetitive unnecessary parameters to zero in the parameter reduction process, was used to further screen the results from univariate Cox regression. The results of lasso algorithm screening were used to construct a multivariate Cox risk regression model, where OS was the dependent variable and the other clinical information was the covariate. We retained the lncRNA (p < 0.01) as the final biomarker, which is significantly related to the OS of GC patients. When using the Cox risk regression model, the PH hypothesis test (Zhang et al., 2018) was also used to test whether the data conformed to the Cox regression model. To verify the reliability of the risk score model, we used the test set as well as two other sets of data for validation.

Statistical Analysis

The Kaplan-Meier survival curve (Ranstam and Cook, 2017) was used to prove the difference in OS between the high-risk and low-risk groups, and a bilateral logarithmic rank test was used to evaluate whether the difference was statistically significant (Guyot et al., 2012). Univariate and multivariate Cox regression analyses were performed for each dataset, with OS as the dependent variable and lncRNA risk score as explanatory variables. All analyses were conducted using R (v3.4.1) software.

Functional Enrichment Analysis

Pearson correlation analysis was used to evaluate the co-expression relationship of biomarker lncRNAs related to the OS of GC patients and mRNA. We used the cor.test function in R to calculate the correlation coefficient and significance level between the lncRNA and protein-coding genes. We defined the significant correlation level as a $p < 0.05$ and ranked the positive and negative correlation coefficients. The top 100 protein-coding genes were used for subsequent functional analysis. Functional enrichment of the R package clusterProfiler (Yu et al., 2012) was used to analyze the functional enrichment of mRNAs co-expressed with biomarker lncRNAs to predict the biological function of these biomarkers (Zhou et al., 2019).

Combination of Biomarkers From Gastric Cancer and Prognosis of Thoracic Malignancies

The RNA-seq profiles of thoracic malignancies, including BRCA, ESCA, LUAD, LUSC, and THYM, were downloaded from TCGA.

[1]https://www.ncbi.nlm.nih.gov/geo/

[2]https://portal.gdc.cancer.gov/

Furthermore, we used a univariate Cox risk regression model to explore the association between biomarkers discovered in GC and other thoracic malignancies.

RESULTS

Five lncRNAs Identified to Be Associated With GC Prognosis

To explore the lncRNAs related to the OS of GC patients, microarray profiles from GSE62254, which have appropriate sample abundance and clinical data, were used to construct regression models. The workflow of the analysis pipeline is shown in **Figure 1A**. For the GSE62254 series, we randomly divided samples into a training set ($n = 150$) and a test set ($n = 150$) with the same amount. In the training set, the expression profile of lncRNA was selected for analysis by univariate Cox regression analysis with OS, including survival time and status as the dependent variable. We found 580 lncRNAs ($p < 0.05$ and PH inspection $p > 0.5$) whose expression levels were significantly related to patient survival. Considering the large abundance of the initially screened features, lasso regression was used for a more rigorous screening (**Figure 1B**). We identified 12 significant candidate markers for lncRNA. Furthermore, we used the selected few candidate lncRNAs to establish a multivariate Cox regression model. When considering the interaction between lncRNAs and clinical features, only five lncRNAs (RP11_71E19.5, RP11_722E23.2, RP11_796E2.4, RP11_95O2.1, and AC004528.4) were significantly associated with patient survival (**Figure 1C**). At the same time, the PH hypothesis test results showed that there was no obvious correlation between the Schoenfeld residual and the rank of survival time (**Figures 1D,E**). We used these five biomarker lncRNAs to construct a risk score model independent of other clinical features.

Evaluating the lncRNA Contribution for Risk Prediction Model

For the multivariate Cox risk prediction results, we used the nomogram method to build a more intuitive prediction model of 1 and 3 years survival time probabilities. We found that the characteristic lncRNAs that are more relevant to the patient's survival will increase in scores under the same gene expression fluctuations (**Figure 2A**). To evaluate the contribution of the prediction model, we used a calibration curve to show the predicted survival probability of the prediction model for 1 and 3 years. We found that the fluctuation of the fitting results was not obvious, suggesting that the risk regression model we built was reasonable (**Figure 2B**). A receiver operating characteristic curve was also computed to evaluate the sensitivity and specificity of the predictive model. We found that the AUC value of the prediction model at different time points was approximately 0.8, and it had the best predictive ability (AUC = 0.82) at 19.2 months (**Figure 2C**). Taken together, these results suggest that the risk prediction model built with five biomarker lncRNAs has a good contribution to the prediction of the survival time of GC patients.

Construction of a Risk Score Model for GC

Using the coefficients obtained from the multivariate Cox regression analysis, we constructed a risk scoring model (Wang et al., 2019; Guo et al., 2020) to predict the patient's OS, as shown below: risk score = (−10.14 * expression value of RP11-71E19.5) + (−3.59 * expression value of RP11-722E23.2) + (4.98 * expression value of RP11-796E2.4) + (−9.868541 * expression value of RP11-95O2.1) + (−7.857590 * expression value of AC004528.4). Based on this model, a risk score was calculated for each patient in the training set, and patients were divided into a high-risk group ($n = 75$) and a low-risk group ($n = 75$) using the median risk score as the cut-off point. We found that there was a significant difference in the OS between the high-risk group and the low-risk group, and the p-value of the logarithmic rank test was less than 0.0001 in the Kaplan-Meier curve (**Figure 3A**). Univariate Cox regression analysis also revealed that risk scores constructed from five biomarker lncRNAs were significantly associated with OS ($p < 0.01$). We also evaluated the relationship between the risk score and the distribution of lncRNA expression in the training set. The expression of RP11-796E2.4 in the high-risk score tended to be upregulated, while the expression of the remaining four lncRNAs tended to be downregulated (**Figure 3B**). We also applied a risk score model to calculate the risk score of each sample in the test dataset. Similar to the result predicted by the risk score obtained in the training set, the test data set also found that patients with high-risk scores had significantly worse OS than patients with low-risk scores (**Figures 3C,D**).

Validating Risk Score Models in Multiple Expression Profiles

To further investigate the robustness and practical application of the five-lncRNA risk scoring model, GSE15459 and RNA-seq profiles of GC from TCGA were also used to validate the risk scoring model. We divided the samples from the GSE15459 series into the high-risk group ($n = 96$) and the low-risk group ($n = 96$). There was a significant difference in the OS between the two groups (**Figure 4A**). Univariate Cox regression analysis also showed that the risk score was significantly correlated with OS ($p = 0.0309$, $HR = 1.000187$). We found that the risk score distribution, survival status, and lncRNA expression of all patients were consistent with those observed in the training dataset (**Figure 4B**). In the TCGA dataset, 380 patients in the TCGA data set were divided into a high-risk group ($n = 190$) and a low-risk group ($n = 190$). The results of univariate Cox regression analysis also showed that the risk score was significantly correlated with OS (**Figures 4C,D**). All these results indicate that the risk score model has a better universality.

Cancer-Promoting Function of mRNA Co-expressed With Five lncRNAs

To explore the functional significance of five lncRNA biomarkers in the occurrence and development of gastric carcinoma, bioinformatics analysis was carried out to predict the function of lncRNAs. We extracted these five lncRNA expression profiles

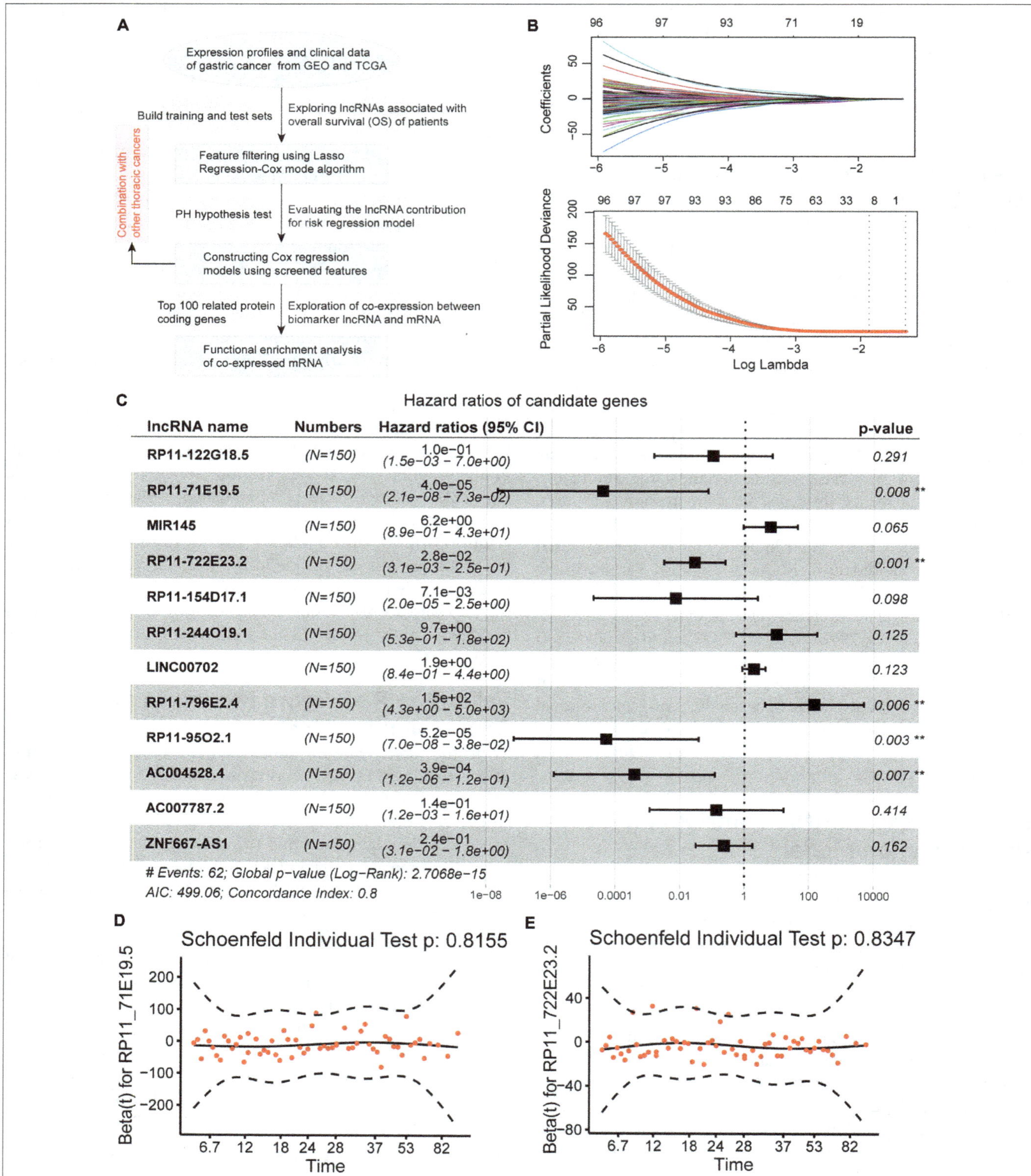

FIGURE 1 | Identification of lncRNAs associating with gastric cancer prognosis. **(A)** The workflow of our analysis pipeline. **(B)** Lasso regression model screened characteristic lncRNAs. Variation curve of regression coefficient and β value. **(C)** Forest plot of multivariate Cox regression results, which include *p*-value and confidence interval of hazard ratios. **(D,E)** The diagram shows the results of the PH hypothesis test. The horizontal axis represents the survival time, and the vertical axis represents the Schoenfeld residual.

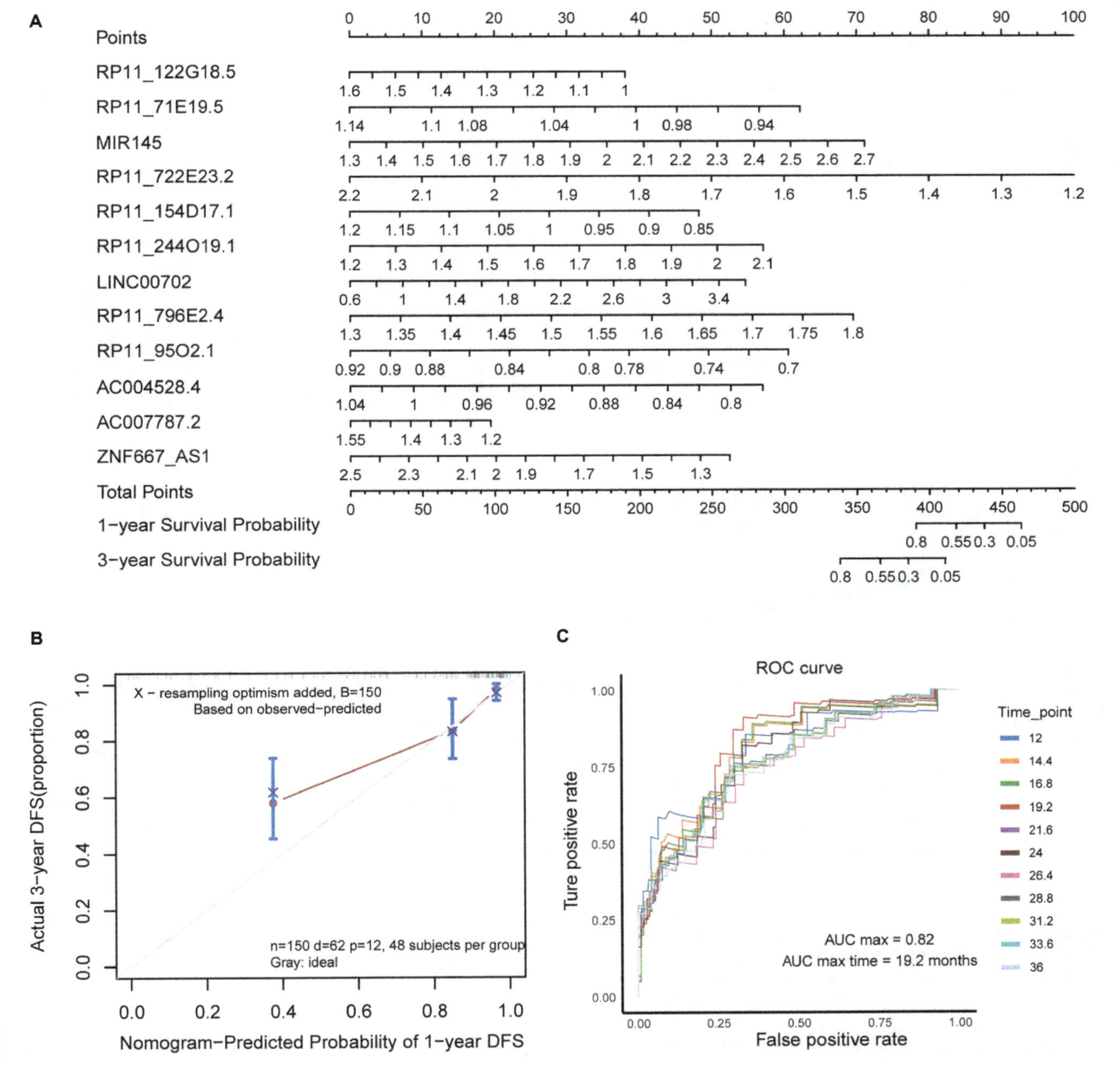

FIGURE 2 | Evaluating the lncRNA contribution for risk prediction model. **(A)** The nomogram shows the prediction model of survival probability. **(B)** Calibration curve of the nomogram. **(C)** The ROC curve reflects the performance of the Cox risk regression model in predicting the probability of survival of patients at different time nodes.

and all mRNA expression profiles from the GSE62254 dataset and calculated the Pearson correlation coefficient between each pair of lncRNAs and mRNAs. We found that the mRNAs related to these five lncRNAs had no significant intersection (**Figure 5A**), indicating that the five lncRNAs have independent roles in carcinogenic mechanisms.

Functional enrichment analysis was performed to reveal the functional mechanism of biomarker lncRNAs. We found many biological pathways (BPs) influenced by mRNAs that correlate with biomarker lncRNA. For lncRNA RP11-722E23.2, the function was mainly enriched in energy metabolism (**Figure 5B**). Variation in lncRNA RP11-796E2.4 and RP11-95O2.1 expression mainly affects immune regulation, which is essential for the recognition and elimination of gastric tumor cells (**Figures 5C,D**; Chen et al., 2007; Amedei et al., 2012). AC004528.4 was mainly involved in the epithelial-mesenchymal transition, which regulates the invasion and metastasis of cancer cells (Lamouille et al., 2014;

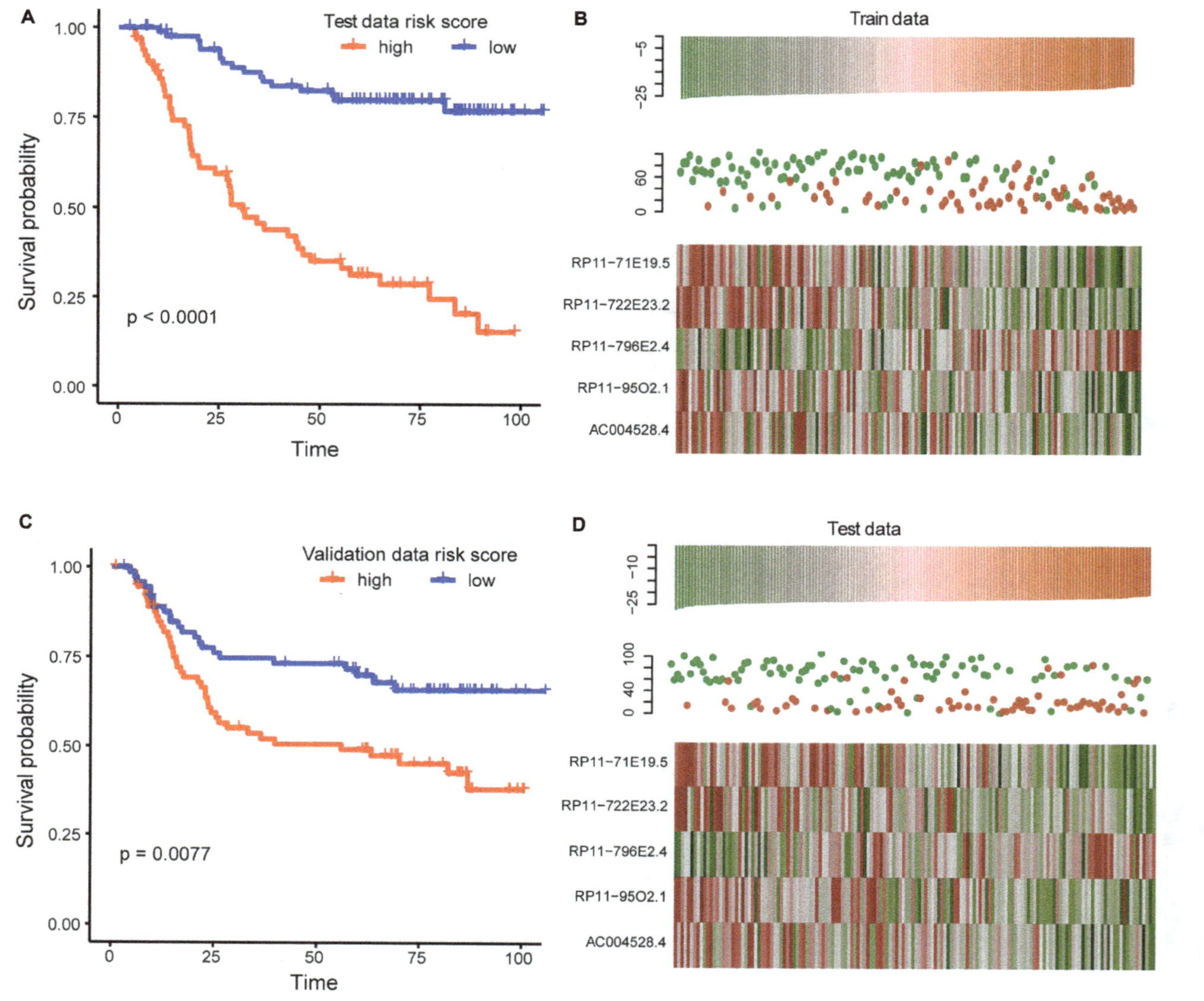

FIGURE 3 | Survival analysis in training and testing dataset. **(A)** Kaplan-Meier curve reflects the difference of overall survival (OS) between high and low-risk score samples for the training set. **(B)** This graph reflects the expression levels of biomarkers for the training set as well as the survival status and risk scores of the patients. **(C)** The same as in **(A)** but for the test set. **(D)** The same as in **(B)** but for the test set.

Dongre and Weinberg, 2019; **Figure 5E**). RP11-71E19.5 mainly regulated the ion channels and contractile activity of gastric muscle cells (**Figure 5F**). These results indicate that lncRNAs can promote the occurrence and development of GC through multiple mechanisms.

Exploring the Prognostic Efficiency of Five lncRNAs in Thoracic Malignancies

Furthermore, we evaluated the prognostic performance of these five-lncRNA signatures in several thoracic cancers, including BRCA, ESCA, LUAD, LUSC, and THYM. The five-lncRNA signature was found to be significantly associated with patient survival in BRCA (HR = 1.952, 95% CI = 1.249–3.051, p = 0.003), LUSC (HR = 2.852, 95% CI = 1.402–5.799, p = 0.003), and THYM (HR = 2.509, 95% CI = 1.335–4.714, p = 0.004) (**Figure 6A**). Patients with different thoracic cancers were ranked and divided into two risk groups based on the median risk score. Kaplan-Meier survival analysis was performed to evaluate the prognostic significance between the two risk groups in each dataset (**Figures 6B–F**). We found that the OS of BRCA patients was significantly different between the high- and low-risk groups (**Figure 6B**). These results were consistent with previous studies that reported that breast cancer with metastasis to the gastric tissue was often mistaken for primary GC (Kim et al., 2018; Birla et al., 2019). However, the survival of patients with other thoracic malignancies did not show sensitivity to these five lncRNAs in GC (**Figures 6C–F**).

Using the median score as a threshold may arbitrarily divide patients with continuous gene expression into different groups

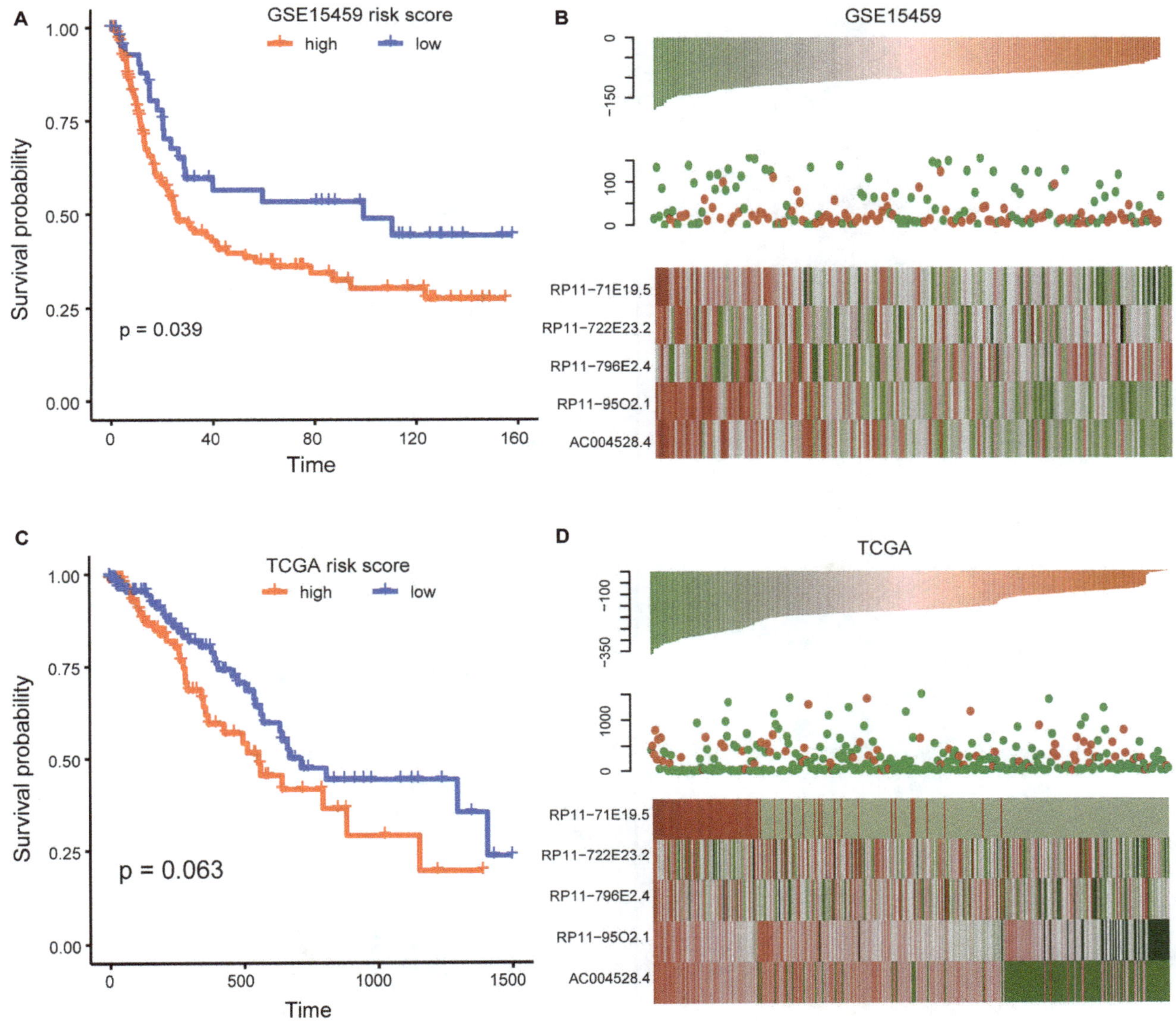

FIGURE 4 | Survival analysis in the GSE15459 and TCGA dataset. **(A)** Kaplan-Meier curve of risk score model based on GSE15459 data. **(B)** Expression pattern of lncRNA and survival status and risk score of patients based onGSE15459 data. **(C)** The same as in **(A)** but for the RNA-seq profile from TCGA. **(D)** The same as in **(B)** but for the RNA-seq profile from TCGA.

and fail to obtain significant survival results. We employed the minimum *p*-value approach for grouping patients and determined the optimal cut-off point for continuous gene expression measurement (Mizuno et al., 2009). Based on this strategy, we re-divided the patients with these thoracic cancers into different groups according to the minimum *p*-value (**Figures 7A–E**). We found that the OS of BRCA (**Figure 7A**), LUSC (**Figure 7D**), and THYM (**Figure 7E**) were significantly different in the high-and low-risk groups, which was consistent with the Cox regression analysis results in **Figure 6A**. Previous studies have also shown that advanced LUSC is often accompanied by gastric metastasis (Li et al., 2018; He et al., 2019). All these results suggest that the similarity in molecular mechanisms between GC and BRCA and LUSC may be caused by a similar localized pathological tissue origin. Taken together, the five-lncRNA signature identified in GC may be a potential prognostic marker for several thoracic malignancies, including BRCA, LUSC, and THYM, which will provide new avenues for the diagnosis and treatment of these cancers.

DISCUSSION

In this study, we identified five lncRNAs related to patient survival in gastric carcinoma and established a risk score model. The reliability of the model was verified using data from other public GCs. Furthermore, these five lncRNAs were also associated with the OS of BRCA, LUSC, and THYM patients. To some

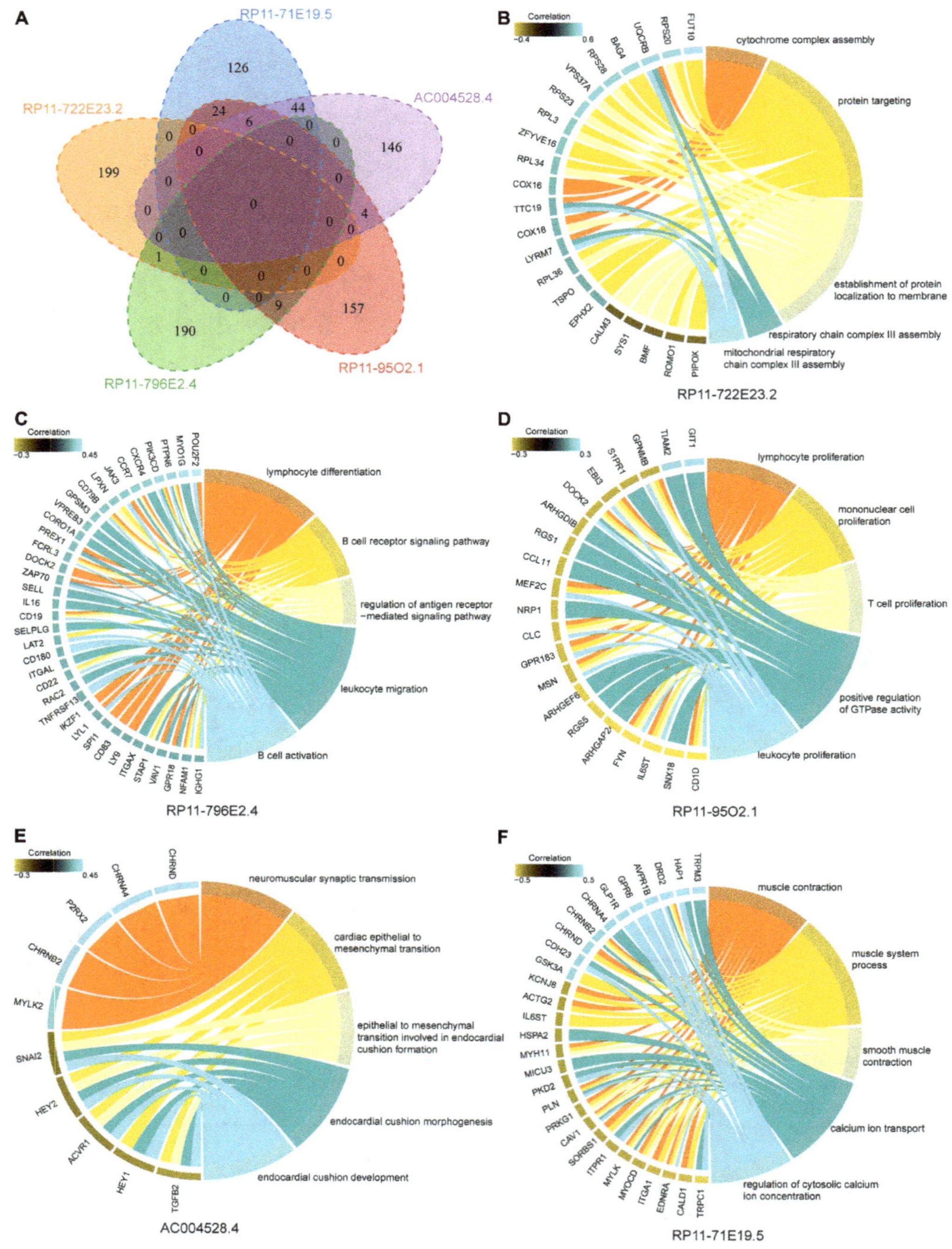

FIGURE 5 | Cancer-promoting function of mRNA co-expressed with five lncRNAs. **(A)** The Venn diagram shows the intersection of mRNAs related to the expression of five biomarker lncRNAs. **(B–F)** The results of functional enrichment of mRNA relating to the expression of lncRNAs. Protein coding genes are on the left side of the circle diagram, and biological pathways (BP) are on the right.

extent, the model has superior performance compared to known traditional clinical parameters. These results demonstrate the potential application of lncRNA as a new independent biomarker for the diagnosis and prognosis of GC.

As one of the common malignant tumors, GC has a high mortality rate (Hartgrink et al., 2009; Smyth et al., 2020). Although treatment has made great progress, the prognosis remains poor. LncRNAs play an important regulatory role at the transcriptional, post-transcriptional, and epigenetic levels and participate in multiple aspects of gene regulation and a variety of biological processes (Batista and Chang, 2013). In recent years, lncRNAs have been found to play an important

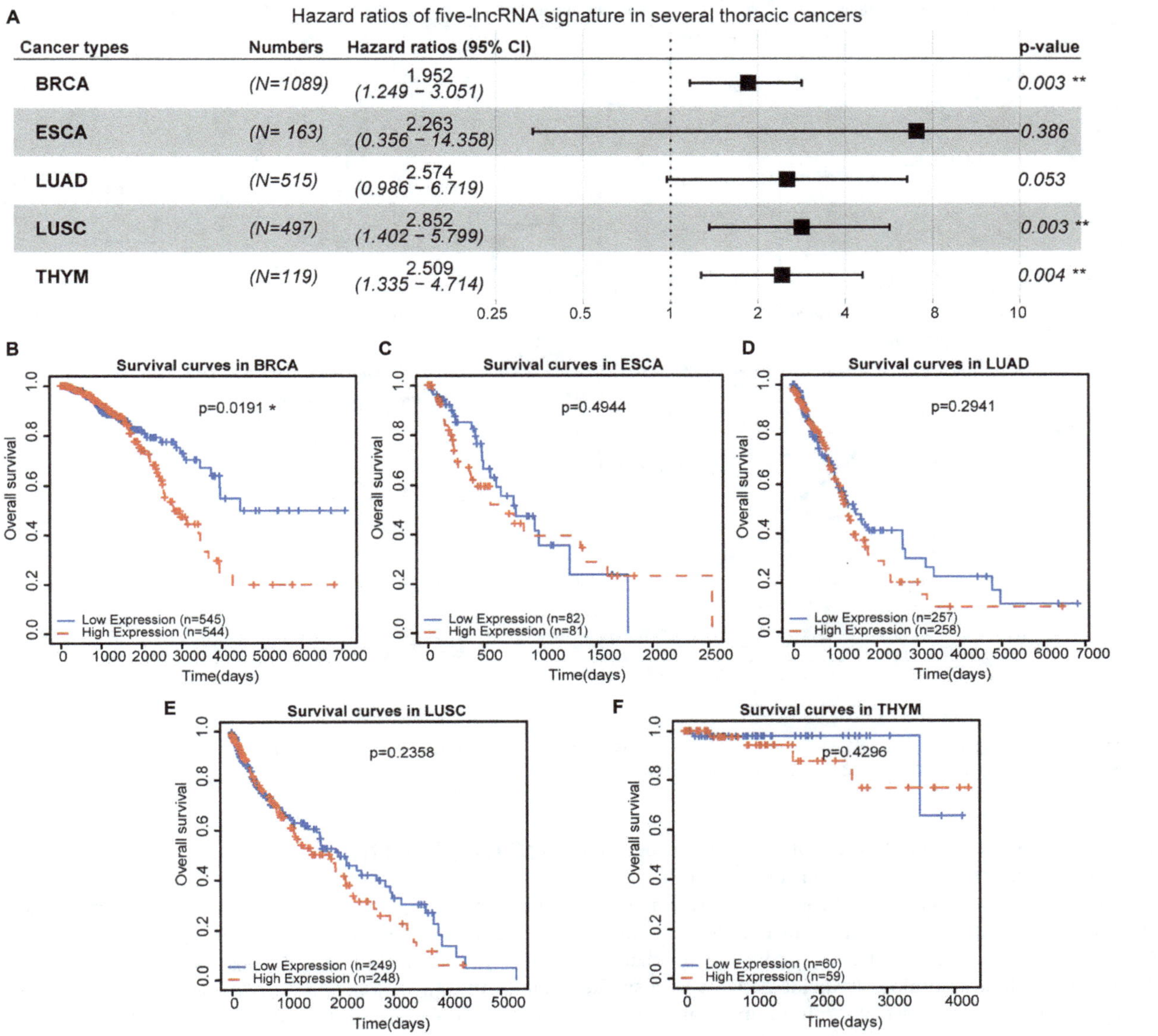

FIGURE 6 | Survival analysis in several thoracic cancers. **(A)** The forest plot demonstrates the risk ratios of five prognosis-related lncRNAs in thoracic cancer. **(B–F)** Kaplan-Meier curves of the five prognostic lncRNAs in thoracic cancers. Patients were divided by the median risk score. $^{**}p < 0.01$.

role in cancer. Therefore, our exploration of biomarkers that affect tumor progression and survival of GC patients is of great significance for the diagnosis and treatment of GC.

We collected several expression profiles and the corresponding clinical information of GC, including GSE62254, GSE15459, and RNA-seq profiles from TCGA. The GSE62254 data were randomly divided into training and test sets. We used the lasso regression-Cox mode algorithm to screen for features related to the patient's OS. Compared with other feature filtering algorithms such as linear regression and ridge regression, the lasso algorithm solves the overfitting problem and can directly reduce some repetitive and unnecessary parameters to zero in the parameter reduction process. Lasso regression performs well in controlling the number of features (Xu et al., 2018; McEligot et al., 2020). Further, multivariate Cox regression analysis identified five lncRNAs that could independently predict the OS of patients. Subsequently, a risk-scoring model was established using the coefficients of multivariate Cox regression analysis. The training data set was divided into high-risk and low-risk groups according to the median risk score, and there was a significant difference in OS between the two groups. We found that the risk score model constructed with five lncRNAs was applicable to multiple GC datasets. We calculated the Pearson correlation coefficient between mRNA and five-lncRNA signature to explore the physiological mechanisms influenced by these biomarkers. Functional analysis suggested that these five lncRNAs play an important role in the initiation and progression of GC through association with known BPs,

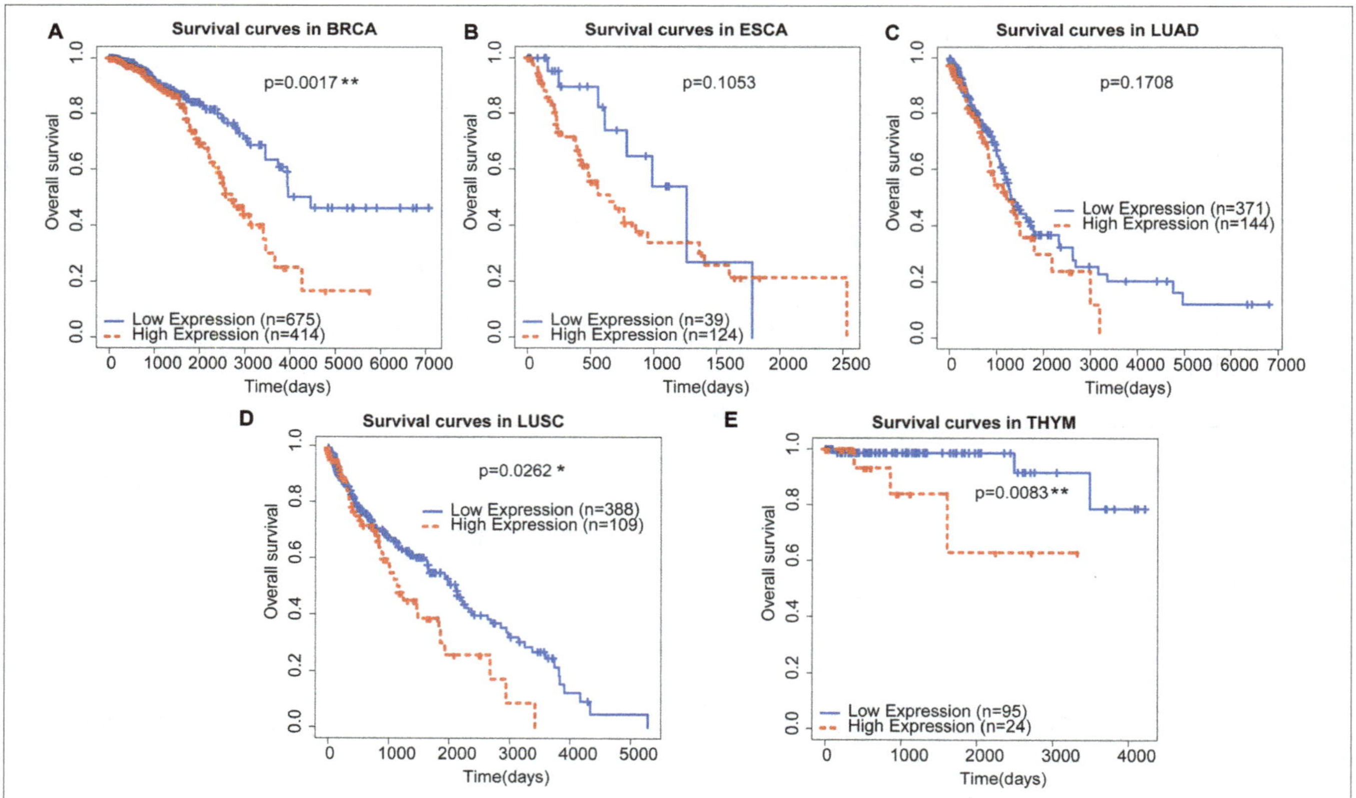

FIGURE 7 | Re-dividing of thoracic cancer patients and survival analysis. **(A–E)** Kaplan-Meier curves of the five prognostic lncRNAs in thoracic cancers. Patients were divided by the optimal cut-off identified from the minimum *p*-value approach.

and further experimental verification of these five prognostic lncRNAs is necessary to understand their function in GC.

Furthermore, we evaluated the prognostic performance of the five-lncRNA signature in several thoracic cancers, including BRCA, ESCA, LUAD, LUSC, and THYM. Since the median can be used as a threshold to arbitrarily divide patients with similar gene expression levels, we used the minimum *p*-value method to obtain the best cut-off point for continuous gene expression (Mizuno et al., 2009). Using this method, we divided the patients with thoracic cancers into different groups according to the minimum *p*-value and found that the five-lncRNA signature could divide patients' OS of BRCA, LUSC, and THYM into different risk groups. To provide a global view of the prognostic efficiency of the five-lncRNA signature in cancers as much as possible, we performed survival analysis in 27 other types of cancers in TCGA. Although the five-lncRNA signature was not a universal marker for all cancers, the results of Cox regression analysis (**Supplementary Figure 1**) and Kaplan-Meier survival curves (**Supplementary Figure 2**) revealed the potential prognostic roles in some other cancers.

CONCLUSION

To summarize, this study offers a risk score model according to research and demonstrate in multiple sets of data. Although we only considered lncRNA expression changes and simple clinical information, the prediction model is reliable after multiple verifications. In addition, the identification of lncRNA biomarkers may bring new insights into the potential molecular basis of cancers.

AUTHOR CONTRIBUTIONS

JS, WL, and YQ conceived and designed the experiments. JZ, WX, and DW analyzed the data. SL and JZ collected the data. JS and WL validated the method and data. JS and YQ wrote this manuscript. All authors read and approved the final manuscript.

REFERENCES

1. Allemani, C., Matsuda, T., di Carlo, V., Harewood, R., Matz, M., Niksic, M., et al. (2018). Global surveillance of trends in cancer survival 2000-14 (CONCORD-3): analysis of individual records for 37 513 025 patients diagnosed with one of 18 cancers from 322 population-based registries in 71 countries. *Lancet* 391, 1023–1075. doi: 10.1016/S0140-6736(17)33326-3

2. Amedei, A., Della Bella, C., Silvestri, E., Prisco, D., and D'Elios, M. M. (2012). T cells in gastric cancer: friends or foes. *Clin. Dev. Immunol.* 2012:690571. doi: 10.1155/2012/690571

3. Barrett, T., Wilhite, S. E., Ledoux, P., Evangelista, C., Kim, I. F., Tomashevsky, M., et al. (2013). NCBI GEO: archive for functional genomics data sets–update. *Nucleic Acids Res.* 41, D991–D995. doi: 10.1093/nar/gks1193
4. Batista, P. J., and Chang, H. Y. (2013). Long noncoding RNAs: cellular address codes in development and disease. *Cell* 152, 1298–1307. doi: 10.1016/j.cell.2013. 02.012
5. Birla, R., Dinu, D., Iosif, C., and Constantinoiu, S. (2019). Gastric metastasis of invasive lobular breast carcinoma, a current diagnostic and treatment challenge - a review. *Chirurgia (Bucur)* 114, 571–578. doi: 10.21614/chirurgia.114.5.571
6. Chen, G., Zhang, F. J., Gong, M., and Yan, M. (2007). Effect of perioperative autologous versus allogeneic blood transfusion on the immune system in gastric cancer patients. *J. Zhejiang Univ. Sci. B* 8, 560–565. doi: 10.1631/jzus.2007. B0560
7. Dongre, A., and Weinberg, R. A. (2019). New insights into the mechanisms of epithelial-mesenchymal transition and implications for cancer. *Nat. Rev. Mol. Cell Biol.* 20, 69–84. doi: 10.1038/s41580-018-0080-4
8. Goyal, B., Yadav, S. R. M., Awasthee, N., Gupta, S., Kunnumakkara, A. B., and Gupta, S. C. (2021). Diagnostic, prognostic, and therapeutic significance of long non-coding RNA MALAT1 in cancer. *Biochim. Biophys. Acta Rev. Cancer* 1875:188502. doi: 10.1016/j.bbcan.2021.188502
9. Guo, Q., He, Y., Sun, L., Kong, C., Cheng, Y., Wang, P., et al. (2019). Identification of potential prognostic TF-associated lncRNAs for predicting survival in ovarian cancer. *J. Cell. Mol. Med.* 23, 1840–1851. doi: 10.1111/jcmm.14084
10. Guo, Q., Wang, J., Gao, Y., Li, X., Hao, Y., Ning, S., et al. (2020). Dynamic TF- lncRNA regulatory networks revealed prognostic signatures in the development of ovarian cancer. *Front. Bioeng. Biotechnol.* 8:460. doi: 10.3389/fbioe.2020. 00460
11. Guyot, P., Ades, A. E., Ouwens, M. J., and Welton, N. J. (2012). Enhanced secondary analysis of survival data: reconstructing the data from published Kaplan-Meier survival curves. *BMC Med. Res. Methodol.* 12:9. doi: 10.1186/1471-2288-12-9
12. Hartgrink, H. H., Jansen, E. P., van Grieken, N. C., and van de Velde, C. J. (2009). Gastric cancer. *Lancet* 374, 477–490. doi:10.1016/S0140-6736(09)60617-6
13. He, Y., Cui, Y., Duan, X., Liu, C., and Cai, X. (2019). Primary lung squamous cell carcinoma with gastric metastasis: a case report. *Thorac. Cancer* 10, 373–377. doi: 10.1111/1759-7714.12940
14. Jiang, Y. F., Zhang, H. Y., Ke, J., Shen, H., Ou, H. B., and Liu, Y. (2019). Overexpression of LncRNA GHET1 predicts an unfavourable survival and clinical parameters of patients in various cancers. *J. Cell. Mol. Med.* 23, 4891–4899. doi: 10.1111/jcmm.14486
15. Kim, D. H., Son, S. M., and Choi, Y. J. (2018). Gastric metastasis from invasive lobular breast cancer, mimicking primary gastric cancer: a case report. *Medicine (Baltimore)* 97:e0258. doi: 10.1097/MD.0000000000010258
16. Kopp, F., and Mendell, J. T. (2018). Functional classification and experimental dissection of long noncoding RNAs. *Cell* 172, 393–407. doi: 10.1016/j.cell.2018. 01.011
17. Lamouille, S., Xu, J., and Derynck, R. (2014). Molecular mechanisms of epithelial-mesenchymal transition. *Nat. Rev. Mol. Cell Biol.* 15, 178–196. doi: 10.1038/ nrm3758
18. Li, X., Li, S., Ma, Z., Zhao, S., Wang, X., and Wen, D. (2018). Multiple gastrointestinal metastases of squamous-cell lung cancer: a case report. *Medicine (Baltimore)* 97:e11027. doi: 10.1097/MD.0000000000011027
19. McEligot, A. J., Poynor, V., Sh arma, R., and Panangadan, A. (2020). Logistic LASSO regression for dietary intakes and breast cancer. *Nutrients* 12:2652. doi: 10.3390/nu12092652
20. Mizuno, H., Kitada, K., Nakai, K., and Sarai, A. (2009). PrognoS can: a new database for meta-analysis of the prognostic value of genes. *BMC Med. Genomics* 2:18. doi: 10.1186/1755-8794-2-18
21. Ranstam, J., and Cook, J. A. (2017). Kaplan-Meier curve. *Br. J. Surg.* 104:442. doi: 10.1002/bjs.10238
22. Siegel, R. L., Miller, K. D., Fuchs, H. E., and Jemal, A. (2021). Cancer statistics, 2021. *CA Cancer J. Clin.* 71, 7–33. doi: 10.3322/caac.21654
23. Smyth, E. C., Nilsson, M., Grabsch, H. I., van Grieken, N. C., and Lordick, F. (2020). Gastric cancer. *Lancet* 396, 635–648. doi: 10.1016/S0140-6736(20)31288-5
24. Tate, J. G., Bamford, S., Jubb, H. C., Sondka, Z., Beare, D. M., Bindal, N., et al. (2019). COSMIC: the catalogue of somatic mutations in cancer. *Nucleic Acids Res.* 47, D941–D947. doi: 10.1093/nar/gky1015
25. Tomczak, K., Czerwinska, P., and Wiznerowicz, M. (2015). The Cancer Genome Atlas (TCGA): an immeasurable source of knowledge. *Contemp. Oncol. (Pozn)* 19, A68–A77. doi: 10.5114/wo.2014.47136
26. Wang, F., Li, X., Zhao, X., and Xue, Y. (2019). Detection of a 5-circRNA signature to improve prognostic prediction in gastric cancer. *J. Investig. Med.* 68, 762–769. doi: 10.1136/jim-2019-001131
27. Wang, P., Ning, S., Zhang, Y., Li, R., Ye, J., Zhao, Z., et al. (2015). Identification of lncRNA-associated competing triplets reveals global patterns and prognostic markers for cancer. *Nucleic Acids Res.* 43, 3478–3489. doi: 10.1093/nar/gkv233
28. Xu, C., Fang, J., Shen, H., Wang, Y. P., and Deng, H. W. (2018). EPS-LASSO: test for high-dimensional regression under extreme phenotype sampling of continuous traits. *Bioinformatics* 34, 1996–2003. doi: 10.1093/bioinformatic s/bty042
29. Yu, G., Wang, L. G., Han, Y., and He, Q. Y. (2012). clusterProfiler: an R package for comparing biological themes among gene clusters. *OMICS* 16, 284–287. doi: 10.1089/omi.2011.0118
30. Zhang, Z., Reinikainen, J., Adeleke, K. A., Pieterse, M. E., and Groothuis-Oudshoorn, C. G. M. (2018). Time-varying covariates and coefficients in Cox regression models. *Ann. Transl. Med.* 6:121. doi: 10.21037/atm.2018. 02.12
31. Zhou, Y., Zhou, B., Pache , L., Chang, M., Khodabakhshi, A. H., Tanaseichuk, O., et al. (2019). Metascape provides a biologist-oriented resource for the analysis of systems-level datasets. *Nat. Commun.* 10:1523. doi: 10.1038/s41467-019- 09234-6

Permissions

All chapters in this book were first published by Frontiers; hereby published with permission under the Creative Commons Attribution License or equivalent. Every chapter published in this book has been scrutinized by our experts. Their significance has been extensively debated. The topics covered herein carry significant findings which will fuel the growth of the discipline. They may even be implemented as practical applications or may be referred to as a beginning point for another development.

The contributors of this book come from diverse backgrounds, making this book a truly international effort. This book will bring forth new frontiers with its revolutionizing research information and detailed analysis of the nascent developments around the world.

We would like to thank all the contributing authors for lending their expertise to make the book truly unique. They have played a crucial role in the development of this book. Without their invaluable contributions this book wouldn't have been possible. They have made vital efforts to compile up to date information on the varied aspects of this subject to make this book a valuable addition to the collection of many professionals and students.

This book was conceptualized with the vision of imparting up-to-date information and advanced data in this field. To ensure the same, a matchless editorial board was set up. Every individual on the board went through rigorous rounds of assessment to prove their worth. After which they invested a large part of their time researching and compiling the most relevant data for our readers.

The editorial board has been involved in producing this book since its inception. They have spent rigorous hours researching and exploring the diverse topics which have resulted in the successful publishing of this book. They have passed on their knowledge of decades through this book. To expedite this challenging task, the publisher supported the team at every step. A small team of assistant editors was also appointed to further simplify the editing procedure and attain best results for the readers.

Apart from the editorial board, the designing team has also invested a significant amount of their time in understanding the subject and creating the most relevant covers. They scrutinized every image to scout for the most suitable representation of the subject and create an appropriate cover for the book.

The publishing team has been an ardent support to the editorial, designing and production team. Their endless efforts to recruit the best for this project, has resulted in the accomplishment of this book. They are a veteran in the field of academics and their pool of knowledge is as vast as their experience in printing. Their expertise and guidance has proved useful at every step. Their uncompromising quality standards have made this book an exceptional effort. Their encouragement from time to time has been an inspiration for everyone.

The publisher and the editorial board hope that this book will prove to be a valuable piece of knowledge for researchers, students, practitioners and scholars across the globe.

List of Contributors

Zuohong Wu, Ke Wang, Deyun Cheng, Weimin Li and Bojiang Chen
Department of Respiratory and Critical Care Medicine, West China Hospital of Sichuan University, Chengdu, China

Xinghong Xian
West China School of Medicine, Sichuan University, Chengdu, China

Ling Peng and De-Guang Mu
Department of Respiratory Disease, Zhejiang Provincial People's Hospital, Hangzhou, China

Wen-Hua Liang
National Clinical Research Center for Respiratory Disease, The First Affiliated Hospital of Guangzhou Medical University, Guangzhou, China

Song Xu
Department of Lung Cancer Surgery, Lung Cancer Institute, Tianjin Medical University General Hospital, Tianjin, China

Shao-Dong Hong
Department of Medical Oncology, Sun Yat-sen University Cancer Center, Guangzhou, China

Justin Stebbing
Division of Cancer, Department of Surgery and Cancer, Imperial College London, London, United Kingdom

Fei Liang
Department of Biostatistics, Zhongshan Hospital, Fudan University, Shanghai, China

Yang Xia
Department of Respiratory and Critical Care Medicine, The Second Affiliated Hospital, School of Medicine, Zhejiang University, Key Laboratory of Respiratory Disease of Zhejiang Province, Hangzhou, China

Mingying Xie
Department of Medical Oncology, The Second Clinical Medical College of Zhejiang Chinese Medical University, Hangzhou, China

Yun Fan
Department of Medical Oncology, The Cancer Hospital of the University of Chinese Academy of Sciences (Zhejiang Cancer Hospital), Hangzhou, China
Institute of Basic Medicine and Cancer (IBMC), Chinese Academy of Sciences, Hangzhou, China
Department of Thoracic Medical Oncology, Zhejiang Cancer Hospital, Hangzhou, China

Guangdie Yang, Jie Wang, Yinan Yao, Jiani Ye and Wenjiang Ma
Department of Respiratory Medicine, The First Affiliated Hospital, College of Medicine, Zhejiang University, Hangzhou, China

Jun Zhao
Department of Respiratory Medicine, The First Affiliated Hospital, College of Medicine, Zhejiang University, Hangzhou, China
Department of Respiratory Medicine, Zhejiang Medical & Health Group Hangzhou Hospital, Hangzhou, China

Zheyan Yu
Department of Respiratory and Critical Care Medicine, Shengzhou People's Hospital, Shaoxing, China

Qiqi Gao
Department of Pathology, The First Affiliated Hospital, College of Medicine, Zhejiang University, Hangzhou, China

Chongya Zhai, Xiaoling Zhang, Lulu Ren, Liangkun You, Qin Pan, Hongming Pan and Weidong Han
Department of Medical Oncology, Sir Run Run Shaw Hospital, College of Medicine, Zhejiang University, Hangzhou, China

Juan Zhou, Jing Zhao, Fei Zhou, Xiangling Chu, Wencheng Zhao, Shengxiang Ren, Caicun Zhou and Chunxia Su
Department of Oncology, Shanghai Pulmonary Hospital & Thoracic Cancer Institute, Tongji University School of Medicine, Shanghai, China

Qingzhu Jia
Department of Oncology, Xinqiao Hospital, Third Military Medical University, Chongqing, China

Qian Chu
Department of Oncology, Tongji Hospital of Tongji Medical College, Huazhong University of Science and Technology, Wuhan, China

Ding Wang
Department of Thoracic Surgery, Cancer Hospital of the University of Chinese Academy of Sciences (Zhejiang Cancer Hospital), Hangzhou, China

Wei Wu
Department of Pathology, Cancer Hospital of the University of Chinese Academy of Sciences (Zhejiang Cancer Hospital), Hangzhou, China

Hongyang Lu
Department of Thoracic Oncology, Cancer Hospital of the University of Chinese Academy of Sciences (Zhejiang Cancer Hospital), Hangzhou, China
Institute of Cancer and Basic Medicine (IBMC), Chinese Academy of Sciences, Hangzhou, China
Zhejiang Key Laboratory of Diagnosis & Treatment Technology on Thoracic Oncology (Lung and Esophagus), Cancer Hospital of the University of Chinese Academy of Sciences (Zhejiang Cancer Hospital), Hangzhou, China

Xiaoling Xu and Yun Fan
Key Laboratory of Head & Neck Cancer Translational Research of Zhejiang Province, Cancer Hospital of the University of Chinese Academy of Sciences (Zhejiang Cancer Hospital), Hangzhou, China
Institute of Cancer and Basic Medicine (IBMC), Chinese Academy of Sciences, Hangzhou, China
Department of Medical Oncology, The Second Clinical Medical College of Zhejiang Chinese Medical University, Hangzhou, China

NaLi
Institute of Cancer and Basic Medicine (IBMC), Chinese Academy of Sciences, Hangzhou, China
Department of Medical Oncology, The Second Clinical Medical College of Zhejiang Chinese Medical University, Hangzhou, China

Wei Chen
Institute of Cancer and Basic Medicine (IBMC), Chinese Academy of Sciences, Hangzhou, China

Sihan Li, Hongwei Zhang and Jun Dang
Department of Radiation Oncology, The First Affiliated Hospital of China Medical University, Shenyang, China

Tingting Liu
Department of Radiation Oncology, Anshan Cancer Hospital, Anshan, China

Jun Chen
Department of Radiation Oncology, Shenyang Chest Hospital, Shenyang, China

Qiao Liu, Xia Luo, Liubao Peng, Lidan Yi, Xiaomin Wan and Chongqing Tan
Department of Pharmacy, The Second Xiangya Hospital of Central South University, Changsha, China

Zhen Zhou
Menzies Institute for Medical Research, University of Tasmania, Hobart, TAS, Australia

Xiaohui Zeng
Department of Nuclear Medicine/PET Image Center, The Second Xiangya Hospital of Central South University, Changsha, China

Li-na He, Xuanye Zhang, Haifeng Li, Wei Du, Wenfeng Fang, Yunpeng Yang, Yan Huang, Shaodong Hong and Li Zhang
State Key Laboratory of Oncology in South China, Guangzhou, China
Collaborative Innovation Center for Cancer Medicine, Guangzhou, China
Department of Medical Oncology, Sun Yat-sen University Cancer Center, Guangzhou, China

Tao Chen
State Key Laboratory of Oncology in South China, Guangzhou, China
Collaborative Innovation Center for Cancer Medicine, Guangzhou, China
Department of Nuclear Medicine, Sun Yat-sen University Cancer Center, Guangzhou, China

Chen Chen
State Key Laboratory of Oncology in South China, Guangzhou, China
Collaborative Innovation Center for Cancer Medicine, Guangzhou, China
Department of Radiation Oncology, Sun Yat-sen University Cancer Center, Guangzhou, China

Yixin Zhou
State Key Laboratory of Oncology in South China, Guangzhou, China
Collaborative Innovation Center for Cancer Medicine, Guangzhou, China
Department of VIP Region, Sun Yat-sen University Cancer Center, Guangzhou, China

Zuan Lin and Hongyun Zhao
State Key Laboratory of Oncology in South China, Guangzhou, China
Collaborative Innovation Center for Cancer Medicine, Guangzhou, China
Department of Clinical Research, Sun Yat-sen University Cancer Center, Guangzhou, China

Shuang Zhao, Panwen Tian and Yalun Li
Department of Respiratory and Critical Care Medicine, West China Hospital, Sichuan University, Chengdu, China

Hao Zeng and Yu-jie Liu
Department of Respiratory and Critical Care Medicine, West China Hospital, West China School of Medicine, Sichuan University, Chengdu, China

Wei-wei Huang and Wei-min Li
Department of Respiratory and Critical Care Medicine, West China Hospital, Sichuan University, Chengdu, China

Qin Huang, Sheng-min Zhao, Ya-lun Li and Pan-wen Tian
Department of Respiratory and Critical Care Medicine, Lung Cancer Treatment Center, West China Hospital, Sichuan University, Chengdu, China

Likui Fang, Wuchen Zhao, Bo Ye and Da Chen
Department of Thoracic Surgery, Affiliated Hangzhou Chest Hospital, Zhejiang University School of Medicine, Hangzhou, China

Wufei Chen, Yanqing Hua, Dingbiao Mao, Hao Wu, Mingyu Tan, Weiling Ma, Xuemei Huang, Jinjuan Lu, Cheng Li and Ming Li
Department of Radiology, Huadong Hospital, Fudan University, Shanghai, China

Xinyi Huang
Department of Oncology, Shandong Provincial Qianfoshan Hospital, Cheeloo College of Medicine, Shandong University, Jinan, China
Department of Oncology, The First Affiliated Hospital of Shandong First Medical University & Shandong Provincial Qianfoshan Hospital, Jinan, China
Shandong Lung Cancer Institute, Jinan, China

Tiantian Tian, Yan Zhang, Pingping Hu and Jiandong Zhang
Department of Oncology, The First Affiliated Hospital of Shandong First Medical University & Shandong Provincial Qianfoshan Hospital, Jinan, China
Shandong Lung Cancer Institute, Jinan, China

Shengjian Zhou
Department of Oncology, Liangshan County People's Hospital, Jining, China

Yuhui Ma, Wanlin Chen and Guangqiang Zhao
First Department of Thoracic Surgery, The Yunnan Cancer Hospital, Kunming, China

Quan Li, Yaxi Du, Xing Liu and Luyao Ma
Department of Key Laboratory of Lung Cancer, Key Laboratory of Lung Cancer Research of Kunming Medical University, Kunming, China

Jingjing Cai and Hongsheng Li
Yunnan Cancer Hospital and The Third Affiliated Hospital of Kunming Medical University, Yunnan Cancer Center, Kunming, China

Yunchao Huang
First Department of Thoracic Surgery, The Yunnan Cancer Hospital, Kunming, China
Yunnan Cancer Hospital and The Third Affiliated Hospital of Kunming Medical University, Yunnan Cancer Center, Kunming, China

Yongchun Zhou
Yunnan Cancer Hospital and The Third Affiliated Hospital of Kunming Medical University, Yunnan Cancer Center, Kunming, China

Ya Chen, Yanan Wang, Zhengyu Yang, Minjuan Hu, Yanwei Zhang, Fangfei Qian, Wei Zhang, Bo Zhang and Baohui Han
Department of Pulmonary, Shanghai Chest Hospital, Shanghai Jiao Tong University, Shanghai, China

Jing Yuan, Feng Cheng, Guodong Xiao, Xiaofeng Wang and Huijie Fan
Department of Oncology, The First Affiliated Hospital of Zhengzhou University, Zhengzhou, China

Peiliang Wang, Tianwen Yin, Hairong Tian, Jinming Yu and Feifei Teng
Department of Radiation Oncology, Shandong Cancer Hospital and Institute, Cheeloo College of Medicine, Shandong University, Jinan, China
Department of Radiation Oncology, Shandong Cancer Hospital and Institute, Shandong First Medical University and Shandong Academy of Medical Sciences, Jinan, China

Xiaozhuang Fang
Department of Radiation Oncology, Shandong Cancer Hospital and Institute, Cheeloo College of Medicine, Shandong University, Jinan, China
Department of Hepatobiliary Surgery, Shandong Cancer Hospital and Institute, Cheeloo College of Medicine, Shandong University, Jinan, China

Yutao Li, Xiaolong Wu and Ingo G. H. Schmidt-Wolf
Department of Integrated Oncology, Center for Integrated Oncology (CIO) Bonn, University Hospital Bonn, Bonn, Germany

Amit Sharma
Department of Integrated Oncology, Center for Integrated Oncology (CIO) Bonn, University Hospital Bonn, Bonn, Germany
Department of Neurosurgery, University Hospital Bonn, Bonn, Germany

Hans Weiher
Department of Applied Natural Sciences, Bonn-Rhein-Sieg University of Applied Sciences, Rheinbach, Germany

Dirk Skowasch
Department of Internal Medicine II, Cardiology, Pneumology and Angiology, University Hospital Bonn, Bonn, Germany

Markus Essler
Department of Nuclear Medicine, University Hospital Bonn, Bonn, Germany

Karan Seegobin, Umair Majeed, Rami Manochakian, Yanyan Lou and Yujie Zhao
Division of Hematology and Oncology, Mayo Clinic, Jacksonville, FL, United States

Nathaniel Wiest
Department of Medicine, Mayo Clinic, Jacksonville, FL, United States

Jiahao Zhang, Yichao Han, Yajie Zhang, Dong Dong, Yuqin Cao, Xiang Chen and Hecheng Li
Department of Thoracic Surgery, Ruijin Hospital, Shanghai Jiao Tong University School of Medicine, Shanghai, China

Marion Grard, Camille Chatelain, Tiphaine Delaunay and Jean-François Fonteneau
Université de Nantes, Inserm, CRCINA, Nantes, France
Labex IGO, Immunology Graft Oncology, Nantes, France

Elvire Pons-Tostivint and Jaafar Bennouna
Université de Nantes, Inserm, CRCINA, Nantes, France
Labex IGO, Immunology Graft Oncology, Nantes, France
CHU de Nantes, oncologie thoracique et digestive, Université de Nantes, Nantes, France

Kiarash Behrouzfar, Kimberley Burton and Scott A. Fisher
National Centre for Asbestos Related Diseases (NCARD), University of Western Australia, Nedlands, WA, Australia
School of Biomedical Sciences, University of Western Australia, Nedlands, WA, Australia

Steve E. Mutsaers
School of Biomedical Sciences, University of Western Australia, Nedlands, WA, Australia
Institute for Respiratory Health, University of Western Australia, Nedlands, WA, Australia

Grant Morahan
Centre for Diabetes Research, Harry Perkins Institute of Medical Research, Nedlands, WA, Australia

Richard A. Lake
National Centre for Asbestos Related Diseases (NCARD), University of Western Australia, Nedlands, WA, Australia

Jiayue Shao
Department of Medical Oncology, Cancer Hospital, Harbin Medical University, Harbin, China

Wei Lyu
Department of Pathology, Guangdong Women and Children Hospital, Guangzhou, China

Jiehao Zhou, Wenhui Xu, Dandan Wang, Shanshan Liang, Jiayin Zhao and Yujing Qin
Department of Gastroenterology, Heilongjiang Provincial Hospital, Harbin, China
Department of Gastroenterology, Heilongjiang Provincial Hospital, Harbin Institute of Technology, Harbin, China

Index

A

Adjuvant Therapy, 145-147

Aging, 127, 130, 132-133

Anaplastic Lymphoma Kinase, 31, 62, 86, 88, 117, 186, 190, 199, 201

Anlotinib, 4, 6-7, 32-35, 37-39, 93-94, 114, 116, 118, 151-153, 155-160, 163, 165-166, 168-174, 177, 187

Anti-angiogenesis, 8, 14, 33, 35, 41, 110, 113, 115-117

Antiangiogenic Agent, 159-160, 165

Apoptosis, 24, 90, 185, 187, 212, 214

Atezolizumab, 8, 10-15, 25, 35, 38, 47, 64, 66-67, 70-71, 84, 90, 114-116, 118, 128, 136, 141-142, 166, 169, 173-175, 191, 197-199, 201

Autoantibody, 40-45, 47

Autoimmune Diseases, 130, 132-133

Autoimmunity, 130, 132

B

Best Supportive Care, 73, 75, 77

Bevacizumab, 8, 10-16, 22, 24, 27, 33, 38, 49-51, 65, 70, 93-94, 96, 114-118, 155-156, 158, 166, 169, 173, 175, 191, 197, 201

Biomarker, 9, 12, 14, 19, 26, 40-41, 44, 46-47, 50, 70, 73, 83, 90-91, 99, 106, 108, 115, 118, 120, 135-136, 139, 141-142, 166, 198, 200, 212, 227-229, 231, 234

Brain Metastases, 61-62, 66, 68-70, 93, 110-111, 114-118, 153-154, 169-170, 172-173

C

Carboplatin, 2, 4, 15-16, 22, 26, 47, 65, 69-71, 93-95, 108, 114, 158, 160, 173, 191, 197, 199

Carcinoembryonic Antigen, 99, 102, 104, 122-123

Cell Surface, 94, 182

Chemoimmunotherapy, 88, 96, 99, 105, 109, 191, 195, 197-198

Chemotherapy, 1-17, 19-22, 26-27, 31, 33, 35, 38-39, 47, 51, 54, 59, 61-62, 65-71, 73, 75, 81, 88, 90, 92-102, 104-108, 111, 114, 116, 118, 120, 136, 141-144, 146-154, 156-160, 163, 165-167, 169, 174-175, 177, 185-189, 191-192, 195, 197-199, 201, 213, 217, 221

Clinical Practice, 41, 57, 69-70, 87, 89, 96, 99, 110, 120, 144, 174, 198

Combination Strategy, 14, 111, 113, 115-116, 165, 176-177, 182

Combination Therapy, 20, 32-34, 38, 40-41, 44-45, 61-63, 65-67, 69, 110-111, 115-116, 152-154, 162, 169, 173-174, 177, 183

Complete Response, 32-33, 35-36, 42, 84, 92, 114, 117, 137, 152, 168, 194, 203, 206

Computed Tomography, 2, 7, 28, 60, 82-83, 91, 100, 119, 126, 144, 160, 203, 205, 208

Cost-effectiveness, 72-73, 77-81

Crizotinib, 28-31, 51, 81, 117, 176-180, 182-186, 190, 198-199

D

Dendritic Cell, 111-112, 117, 127, 130, 133, 169, 187, 198

Deterministic Sensitivity, 72, 76, 78, 80

Disease Control Rate, 19, 33, 35, 42, 113-115, 171

Docetaxel, 2, 4, 19, 21-22, 24-27, 38, 66-67, 69-75, 77-81, 90, 93-94, 108, 116, 118, 133, 141, 149, 160, 165-166, 174-175, 190, 196, 199

F

First-line Treatment, 5, 8-9, 14-15, 20, 24, 31, 40, 47, 65, 67-71, 90, 92-94, 96, 118, 142-146, 152, 158, 160, 166, 169, 174, 186, 199, 201

G

Growth Factor, 19, 22-24, 33, 35, 47, 62, 84, 86, 88, 92-94, 111, 113, 117-120, 126, 149, 156-157, 159-160, 166, 168-169, 172-175, 190, 196, 198, 200, 207

H

Hepatocellular Carcinoma, 83

Human Leukocyte Antigen, 19

Hypoalbuminemia, 29, 31

I

Immune Cell Infiltration, 127-128, 130, 132, 216, 223

Immune Cells, 9, 35, 57, 60, 107, 111-112, 117-118, 128, 130, 132, 173, 211-212, 218

Immune Checkpoint Inhibitor, 1, 8, 40, 62, 70, 110, 174, 188, 200-201

Immunotherapy, 2-3, 5-8, 15-17, 19-20, 24-26, 38, 40-41, 44-45, 47, 49, 51-54, 56, 59-60, 67, 69-71, 73, 75, 83-84, 88, 90, 92-93, 96, 99-100, 102, 104, 107-109, 111, 115-118, 133, 135-136, 142-144, 148, 150, 152, 158-161, 163, 165-166, 189-201, 209, 212-214, 217, 223-224

L

Lesions, 29-30, 33-34, 37, 49, 56, 69-70, 83-89, 110-111, 115, 146, 170, 204-205, 207

Ligand, 2, 6, 8-9, 15-16, 19, 25, 35, 41, 70, 72-75, 77-79, 83, 91, 98-99, 104, 111, 117, 127, 136, 143-144, 160, 166-167, 176, 186-187, 189, 193, 200

Liver Metastases, 106, 118, 151, 153, 155-156, 166, 169-173, 175

Lung Cancer, 1-2, 4, 6-9, 15-17, 19, 21-22, 24-29, 31-33, 36-42, 46-47, 53-55, 59-62, 69-75, 81-83, 88, 90-94, 96-99, 102, 105, 108-110, 113-115, 117-120, 126-130, 133, 135, 141-144, 146, 149-151, 156-160, 166-169, 174-178, 185-191, 193-196, 214-221, 223-225, 228, 237

Lymph Node, 30, 46, 93, 205-207

M

Magnetic Resonance Imaging, 2, 144

Maintenance Therapy, 94, 114, 133, 151-153, 156-157, 187

Meta-analysis, 5, 8-16, 38-39, 47, 61-63, 67, 69-71, 90, 108-109, 133, 142, 147, 149-150, 174-175, 177, 186, 199-201, 206, 208, 217, 224, 237

Monotherapy, 5, 14, 19, 21-22, 24-27, 41-45, 56, 59, 61-63, 65-67, 69-70, 82-83, 87, 90, 109, 113, 116, 142-144, 149, 151, 153, 157, 159-160, 162-163, 165, 171-173, 184-185, 190-191, 195, 197-198, 200

Multivariate Analyses, 46, 88, 151

N

Network Meta-analysis, 8-10, 12, 14-15, 108, 149-150, 174-175

Neutrophils, 111, 113

Next-generation Sequencing, 48-49, 57, 93, 135, 200

Nivolumab, 3-8, 10-15, 19-20, 25-26, 33-35, 37-39, 41, 43, 46-47, 64, 67, 69-75, 77-81, 84, 90, 96-97, 100, 107-109, 114-116, 118, 128, 130, 133, 141-142, 150, 157-158, 166-170, 174-187, 192, 196, 199, 201, 221, 226

Nomogram, 98-101, 104-108, 119, 121-125, 229, 231

O

Objective Response Rate, 31-32, 35-36, 65, 99, 113-115, 149, 152, 191, 194

Overall Response Rate, 19, 84, 92, 193

Overall Survival, 2, 6, 8-9, 14, 19, 31, 33, 36, 38, 41, 47, 57-58, 61-62, 65-68, 73, 75-76, 81, 90, 94, 113-114, 135-136, 138-139, 143-147, 151-152, 155-158, 161-162, 166, 168-171, 174, 177, 187, 190-191, 193-196, 203, 206, 221-222, 227-228, 232

P

Paclitaxel, 2-6, 15-16, 22, 26, 65, 70-71, 108, 114, 144, 160, 173, 191, 197

Partial Remission, 1-4, 24

Partial Response, 29, 33, 35-36, 42, 56, 84, 86, 114, 137, 145-146, 152, 161, 168, 170, 191

Pembrolizumab, 3-7, 9-16, 19-20, 33-39, 41, 43, 47, 56, 64, 66-70, 80-81, 84, 90, 92-97, 99-100, 104-105, 107-109, 113-115, 118, 128, 143-144, 146-147, 149-150, 159-161, 163, 165-166, 168-170, 174, 177, 186-187, 191, 195, 199-201

Prognosis, 5, 7, 9, 17, 19, 23-25, 32, 37, 51, 53-55, 57, 59, 62, 73, 90, 92, 98-99, 101, 104-105, 107-108, 110, 147, 203, 217-219, 224, 227-230, 234-235

Prognostic Factor, 20, 37, 53, 56-57, 59, 89, 91, 98, 104, 159

Prognostic Value, 56, 60, 125, 212, 237

Progression-free Survival, 2, 4, 8, 10, 14, 19, 26, 36, 61, 65-68, 73, 75-78, 82, 87-88, 92, 94, 98-99, 101, 103-107, 113-114, 120, 126, 135-138, 144, 147, 151-152, 155-157, 159, 168, 170-171, 190-191, 193-196

Progressive Disease, 2, 4, 33, 35-36, 84, 86, 168, 170, 192

R

Radiomics, 119-120, 122-126

Radiotherapy, 1-2, 5, 34-35, 83-86, 88, 110, 117, 120, 153, 213, 215, 217

Randomized Trials, 14, 173

S

Second-line Treatment, 19, 21, 33, 72-73, 78, 80, 108, 137, 151-153, 157-158, 169

Sintilimab, 3-5, 7, 10-15, 33-35, 38, 43, 64, 70, 92-95, 100, 114, 118, 168, 170-171

Stable Disease, 2, 4, 33, 35-36, 84, 86, 93, 152, 168, 170, 193, 197

Synergistic Effect, 20, 23, 113, 117, 148, 157, 177, 185

T

Targeted Therapy, 17, 20, 26, 28, 54, 60, 75, 96-97, 120, 160, 166, 174, 191, 195-199

Therapeutic Strategies, 14, 92-93, 99, 117, 126, 174, 212, 216

Third-line Treatment, 169

Transarterial Chemoembolization, 88, 90

Tumor Growth Rate, 82-83, 85, 87-88, 90-91

Tumor Microenvironment, 26, 38, 46, 51, 53-54, 60, 110, 112, 117-118, 173-174, 177, 186, 217-218, 222, 224

Tumor Response, 25, 36, 69, 90, 145, 162, 168, 170, 177, 214

Tumor Vasculature, 38, 111-112, 117, 169, 174

Tumor Volume, 35, 83, 88